THE NATIONAL IMPERATIVE TO IMPROVE
NURSING HOME QUALITY

Honoring Our Commitment to Residents, Families, and Staff

Committee on the Quality of Care in Nursing Homes

Board on Health Care Services

Health and Medicine Division

A Consensus Study Report of

The National Academies of
SCIENCES • ENGINEERING • MEDICINE

THE NATIONAL ACADEMIES PRESS
Washington, D.C.
www.nap.edu

THE NATIONAL ACADEMIES PRESS   500 Fifth Street, NW   Washington, DC 20001

This activity was supported by The John A. Hartford Foundation, The Commonwealth Fund, The Sephardic Foundation on Aging, Jewish Healthcare Foundation, and The Fan Fox & Leslie R. Samuels Foundation. Any opinions, findings, conclusions, or recommendations expressed in this publication do not necessarily reflect the views of any organization or agency that provided support for the project.

International Standard Book Number-13: 978-0-309-68628-0
International Standard Book Number-10: 0-309-68628-8
Digital Object Identifier: https://doi.org/10.17226/26526
Library of Congress Catalog Number: 2022935879

Additional copies of this publication are available from the National Academies Press, 500 Fifth Street, NW, Keck 360, Washington, DC 20001; (800) 624-6242 or (202) 334-3313; http://www.nap.edu.

Copyright 2022 by the National Academy of Sciences. All rights reserved.

Printed in the United States of America.

Suggested citation:
National Academies of Sciences, Engineering, and Medicine. 2022. *The national imperative to improve nursing home quality: Honoring our commitment to residents, families, and staff.* Washington, DC: The National Academies Press. https://doi.org/10.17226/26526.

The National Academies of
SCIENCES · ENGINEERING · MEDICINE

The **National Academy of Sciences** was established in 1863 by an Act of Congress, signed by President Lincoln, as a private, nongovernmental institution to advise the nation on issues related to science and technology. Members are elected by their peers for outstanding contributions to research. Dr. Marcia McNutt is president.

The **National Academy of Engineering** was established in 1964 under the charter of the National Academy of Sciences to bring the practices of engineering to advising the nation. Members are elected by their peers for extraordinary contributions to engineering. Dr. John L. Anderson is president.

The **National Academy of Medicine** (formerly the Institute of Medicine) was established in 1970 under the charter of the National Academy of Sciences to advise the nation on medical and health issues. Members are elected by their peers for distinguished contributions to medicine and health. Dr. Victor J. Dzau is president.

The three Academies work together as the **National Academies of Sciences, Engineering, and Medicine** to provide independent, objective analysis and advice to the nation and conduct other activities to solve complex problems and inform public policy decisions. The National Academies also encourage education and research, recognize outstanding contributions to knowledge, and increase public understanding in matters of science, engineering, and medicine.

Learn more about the National Academies of Sciences, Engineering, and Medicine at **www.nationalacademies.org**.

The National Academies of
SCIENCES • ENGINEERING • MEDICINE

Consensus Study Reports published by the National Academies of Sciences, Engineering, and Medicine document the evidence-based consensus on the study's statement of task by an authoring committee of experts. Reports typically include findings, conclusions, and recommendations based on information gathered by the committee and the committee's deliberations. Each report has been subjected to a rigorous and independent peer-review process and it represents the position of the National Academies on the statement of task.

Proceedings published by the National Academies of Sciences, Engineering, and Medicine chronicle the presentations and discussions at a workshop, symposium, or other event convened by the National Academies. The statements and opinions contained in proceedings are those of the participants and are not endorsed by other participants, the planning committee, or the National Academies.

For information about other products and activities of the National Academies, please visit www.nationalacademies.org/about/whatwedo.

COMMITTEE ON THE QUALITY OF CARE IN NURSING HOMES

BETTY R. FERRELL (*Chair*), Director and Professor, City of Hope National Medical Center, Division of Nursing Research and Education
GREGORY L. ALEXANDER, Professor of Nursing, Columbia University School of Nursing
MARY ERSEK, Senior Scientist, Department of Veteran Affairs; Professor of Palliative Care, University of Pennsylvania Schools of Nursing and Medicine
COLLEEN GALAMBOS, Helen Bader Endowed Chair in Applied Gerontology and Professor, University of Wisconsin–Milwaukee; Adjunct Professor, Medical College of Wisconsin
DAVID C. GRABOWSKI, Professor of Health Care Policy, Harvard Medical School
KATHY GREENLEE, Chief Executive Officer, Greenlee Global LLC
LISA G. KAPLOWITZ, Physician Consultant, COVID Vaccine Unit, Virginia Department of Health
R. TAMARA KONETZKA, Louis Block Professor of Public Health Sciences, University of Chicago
CHRISTINE A. MUELLER, Professor and Senior Executive Associate Dean for Academic Programs, University of Minnesota School of Nursing
MARILYN J. RANTZ, Curators' Professor Emerita, University of Missouri Sinclair School of Nursing
DEBRA SALIBA, Director, Borun Center and Professor of Medicine, University of California, Los Angeles; Physician Scientist, Geriatric Research Education and Clinical Center, Los Angeles Veterans Health Administration; Senior Natural Scientist, RAND
WILLIAM SCANLON, Consultant, West Health
PHILIP D. SLOANE, Goodwin Distinguished Professor of Family Medicine and Geriatrics, School of Medicine and Co-Director, Program on Aging, Disability and Long Term Care, Cecil G Sheps Center for Health Services Research, University of North Carolina at Chapel Hill
DAVID G. STEVENSON, Professor, Department of Health Policy, Vanderbilt University School of Medicine; VA Tennessee Valley Healthcare System, Geriatric Research Education and Clinical Center (GRECC)
JASMINE L. TRAVERS, Assistant Professor, Rory Meyers College of Nursing, New York University
REGINALD TUCKER-SEELEY, Vice President, Health Equity, ZERO-The End of Prostate Cancer; Edward L. Schneider Assistant Professor of Gerontology, Leonard Davis School of Gerontology, University of Southern California

RACHEL M. WERNER, Executive Director, Leonard Davis Institute of Health Economics; Professor of Medicine, University of Pennsylvania; Core Investigator, Crescenz Veterans Affairs Medical Center

Study Staff

LAURENE GRAIG, Study Director
TRACY A. LUSTIG, Study Director
KAITLYN FRIEDMAN, Associate Program Officer *(through December 2021)*
NIKITA VARMAN, Research Associate
RUKSHANA GUPTA, Research Assistant
MICAH WINOGRAD, Financial Officer
ANNE MARIE HOUPPERT, Senior Librarian
SHARYL J. NASS, Director, Board on Health Care Services

Consultants

JOE ALPER, Science Writer
MARISA G. PINEAU, FrameWorks Institute

Reviewers

This Consensus Study Report was reviewed in draft form by individuals chosen for their diverse perspectives and technical expertise. The purpose of this independent review is to provide candid and critical comments that will assist the National Academies of Sciences, Engineering, and Medicine in making each published report as sound as possible and to ensure that it meets the institutional standards for quality, objectivity, evidence, and responsiveness to the study charge. The review comments and draft manuscript remain confidential to protect the integrity of the deliberative process.

We thank the following individuals for their review of this report:

JULIA ADLER-MILSTEIN, University of California, San Francisco
RICHARD D. ALBA, The City University of New York
ALICE BONNER, Institute for Healthcare Improvement
BARBARA BOWERS, University of Wisconsin
KATHY BRADLEY, Our Mother's Voice
STUART M. BUTLER, The Brookings Institution
TOBY S. EDELMAN, Center for Medicare Advocacy
CHARLENE A. HARRINGTON, University of California, San Francisco
BECKY A. KURTZ, Atlanta Regional Commission
NANCY KUSMAUL, University of Maryland Baltimore County
ROBERTA P. LAVIN, University of New Mexico
CARI LEVY, University of Colorado

VINCENT MOR, Brown University
TRICIA NEUMAN, Kaiser Family Foundation
JOSEPH G. OUSLANDER, Florida Atlantic University
KATHLEEN T. UNROE, Indiana University

Although the reviewers listed above provided many constructive comments and suggestions, they were not asked to endorse the conclusions or recommendations of this report nor did they see the final draft before its release. The review of this report was overseen by **CHRISTINE K. CASSEL,** University of California, San Francisco, and **DAVID B. REUBEN,** University of California, Los Angeles. They were responsible for making certain that an independent examination of this report was carried out in accordance with the standards of the National Academies and that all review comments were carefully considered. Responsibility for the final content rests entirely with the authoring committee and the National Academies.

Acknowledgments

The study committee and the Health and Medicine Division (HMD) project staff take this opportunity to recognize and thank the many individuals who shared their time and expertise to support the committee's work and to inform deliberations.

This committee appreciates the sponsors of this study for their generous financial support: The John A. Hartford Foundation, The Commonwealth Fund, Jewish Healthcare Foundation, The Sephardic Foundation on Aging, and The Fan Fox & Leslie R. Samuels Foundation. The contents provided do not necessarily represent the official views of the sponsors.

The committee benefited greatly from discussions with individuals who made presentations during the committee's open sessions and participated in the discussions:

Donald M. Berwick, Institute for Healthcare Improvement
Tom Betlach, Speire Healthcare Strategies
Alice Bonner, Institute for Healthcare Improvement
Wendy Boren, Quality Improvement Program for Missouri
Kathy Bradley, Our Mother's Voice
Scott Brunner, Kansas Department for Aging and Disability Services
Margaret P. Calkins, IDEAS Institute
Eric Carlson, Justice in Aging
Mitzi Daffron, Qsource, Medicare Quality Innovation Network - Quality Improvement Organization for Indiana
John Dicken, U.S. Government Accountability Office
Ruth Ann Dorrill, Office of the Inspector General

Toby S. Edelman, Center for Medicare Advocacy
Barbara Coulter Edwards, BCE Health Policy
Barbara Frank, B&F Consulting, Inc.
John Hagg, Office of the Inspector General
Lacey Hunter, Kansas Department for Aging and Disability Services
Ruth Katz, LeadingAge
Robert G. Kramer, National Investment Center for Seniors Housing and Care, Nexus Insights
Beverley L. Laubert, Ohio Department of Aging
Shari M. Ling, Centers for Medicare & Medicaid Services
Nicky Martin, Quality Improvement Program for Missouri
Richard J. Mollot, The Long-Term Care Community Coalition
Anne Montgomery, Altarum
David A. Nace, AMDA – The Society for Post-Acute and Long-Term Care Medicine, and University of Pittsburgh
Arif Nazir, Signature HealthCARE
Joseph G. Ouslander, Florida Atlantic University
Mary K. Ousley, American Health Care Association
Kezia Scales, PHI
Karen Schoeneman, Karen Schoeneman Consulting
Lori O. Smetanka, The National Consumer Voice for Quality Long-Term Care
Karl Steinberg, AMDA – The Society for Post-Acute and Long-Term Care Medicine, and Mariner Health Central
Amy Stewart, American Association of Post-Acute Care Nursing
Karin J. Wallestad, U.S. Government Accountability Office
Michael Wasserman, California Association of Long-Term Care Medicine
Polly Weaver, Healthcare Management Solutions, LLC
Faith Wiggins, 1199SEIU Funds

The committee is very grateful to these presenters for volunteering to share their knowledge, data, and expert opinions with the committee and the members of the public who attended the committee's open sessions. The committee also appreciates the many nursing home residents, families, and staff who submitted their perspectives and experiences.

Deep appreciation goes to staff at the National Academies of Sciences, Engineering, and Medicine for their efforts and support in the report process, especially to Dana Korsen, Stephanie Miceli, Devona Overton, Marguerite Romatelli, Tina Seliber, Lauren Shern, Leslie Sim, Dorothy Zolandz, and the staff of the National Academies Research Center, including Rebecca Morgan. The committee also gives special thanks to Joe Alper for

ACKNOWLEDGMENTS

his writing and editing contributions, Marissa Pineau for her messaging and framing expertise, and Annalee Gonzales for her graphic design support.

Finally, the committee also recognizes and extends gratitude for all the nursing home residents, families, staff, and organizations that have fought tirelessly to improve nursing home care.

Contents

PREFACE   xvii

ACRONYMS   xxi

ABSTRACT   xxv

SUMMARY   1

1   INTRODUCTION   25
     Study Context, 26
     Study Origin and Statement of Task, 29
     Previous Work of the National Academies, 29
     Study Approach and Scope, 31
     Conceptual Model of Nursing Home Quality, 37
     Organization of the Report, 41
     Conclusion, 42
     References, 42

2   EVOLUTION AND LANDSCAPE OF NURSING
     HOME CARE IN THE UNITED STATES   47
     Brief History of Nursing Homes, 47
     Current Nursing Home Population, 49
     Nursing Home Characteristics, 58
     Factors that Influence the Quality of Care in Nursing Homes, 62
     Critical Impact of COVID-19 on Nursing Homes, 66

Strengthening Connections of Nursing Homes to the
  Community and Broader Health Care System, 72
The Future of Nursing Home Care, 74
References, 76

3   **QUALITY MEASUREMENT AND
  QUALITY IMPROVEMENT**   89
The Purpose of Quality Measurement, 89
Principles and Definitions, 91
Evolution of Quality Measurement in Nursing Homes, 92
Care Compare and the CMS Five-Star Rating System, 94
Resident- and Family-Reported Outcomes:
  Quality of Life, Experience of Care, and Satisfaction, 105
Overview of Quality Improvement, 111
Federal Initiatives for Quality Improvement, 113
State and Local Initiatives for Quality Improvement, 117
Other Approaches to Quality Improvement, 122
Technical Assistance for Quality Improvement, 123
Quality Improvement and Disparities, 125
Coordinated Efforts During the COVID-19 Pandemic, 126
The Future of Quality Improvement in Nursing Homes, 127
Key Findings and Conclusions, 128
References, 130

4   **CARE DELIVERY**   145
Needs-Based Care for Nursing Home Residents, 146
Assessing the Needs of Nursing Home Residents, 148
Providing Care to Address Residents' Needs, 158
Models of Care Delivery, 197
Key Findings and Conclusions, 198
References, 199

5   **THE NURSING HOME WORKFORCE**   221
The Overall Nursing Home Workforce, 222
Nursing Home Administration and Leadership, 226
Primary Care Providers, 234
Licensed Nurses, 237
Nurse Staffing, Regulation, and Quality of Care, 240
Infection Prevention and Control Leadership, 245
Psychosocial and Spiritual Care Providers, 247
Other Clinical Staff, 252
Direct-Care Workers, 256
Family Caregivers, 265

Volunteers, 268
Equity and the Workforce, 269
Factors That Influence the Relationship Between
  Staffing and Quality, 271
COVID-19 and Nursing Home Staffing, 273
Key Findings and Conclusions, 278
References, 281

6 NURSING HOME ENVIRONMENT AND
   RESIDENT SAFETY   303
   Ensuring the Safety of Nursing Home Residents, 303
   Nursing Home Emergency Planning,
     Preparedness, and Response, 324
   The Physical Environment, 329
   Key Findings and Conclusions, 341
   References, 342

7 PAYMENT AND FINANCING   357
   Paying for Nursing Home Care, 357
   Variability between Medicare and Medicaid Payments, 364
   Value-Based Payment Models and the Impact on
     Quality of Care, 366
   Financing Nursing Home Care, 380
   Key Findings and Conclusions, 385
   References, 388

8 QUALITY ASSURANCE: OVERSIGHT AND
   REGULATION   399
   History of Quality Assurance in Nursing Homes, 399
   Omnibus Budget Reconciliation Act of 1987, 401
   Federal and State Regulation, 403
   Private Accreditation, 415
   Enforcement and Penalties, 415
   CMS Oversight and Performance of the State Survey and
     Certification Processes, 420
   Long-Term Care Ombudsman Programs, 423
   Resident and Family Councils, 427
   Effectiveness of Quality Assurance for Improving the
     Quality of Care, 428
   Transparency and Accountability, 429
   Nursing Home Oversight During COVID-19, 434
   Key Findings and Conclusions, 437
   References, 440

9 HEALTH INFORMATION TECHNOLOGY — 453
Evolution of Health Information Technology in
   Nursing Homes, 455
Role of HIT in Quality Care in Nursing Homes, 457
Challenges of HIT Adoption and Use in Nursing Homes, 468
HIT and the COVID-19 Pandemic, 473
Other HIT Considerations for Quality Improvement, 478
Key Findings and Conclusions, 481
References, 482

10 RECOMMENDATIONS — 495
Committee Vision and Guiding Principles, 497
Overarching Goals and Recommendations, 499
Goal 1: Deliver Comprehensive, Person-Centered,
   Equitable Care that Ensures Residents' Health,
   Quality of Life, and Safety; Promotes Autonomy;
   and Manages Risks, 501
Goal 2: Ensure a Well-Prepared, Empowered,
   and Appropriately Compensated Workforce, 508
Goal 3: Increase Transparency and Accountability
   of Finances, Operations, and Ownership, 518
Goal 4: Create a More Rational and Robust
   Financing System, 519
Goal 5: Design a More Effective and Responsive System of
   Quality Assurance, 525
Goal 6: Expand and Enhance Quality Measurement and
   Continuous Quality Improvement, 530
Goal 7: Adopt Health Information Technology in All
   Nursing Homes, 535
What Would Quality Nursing Home Care Look Like?, 538
Conclusion, 541

APPENDIXES
A Biographic Sketches — 543
B Examples from the Initiative to Reduce Avoidable
    Hospitalizations Among Nursing Facility Residents — 555
C Recommendations by Area of Measurement and by Area
    of Research — 561
D Recommendations by Responsible Partners — 565
E Recommendations Timeline — 573

Preface

The Committee on the Quality of Care in Nursing Homes began their work in the fall of 2020 at a pivotal time when a bright light had been cast on care delivered in nursing homes because of the COVID-19 pandemic. While much of society previously had little awareness of the care delivered in nursing homes, the evening news channels and social media projected daily images of the pandemic's impact and of the inadequate care that put the safety of both residents and staff at risk while distraught family members watched from afar as their frail older loved ones were kept in isolation. The committee worked to describe the care being delivered in nursing homes before the pandemic, now made manifest by the crisis.

The committee was given a substantial task of examining how the United States "delivers, finances, measures, and regulates the quality of nursing home care." The challenge was enormous, but as reflected in the final recommendations, real change in nursing home care will require bold action in each of these domains. In the report chapters that follow, the committee presents the evidence of the need for change followed by specific recommendations. The final chapter concludes that "the way the United States finances, delivers, and regulates care in nursing home settings is ineffective, inefficient, fragmented, and unsustainable."

The discussions of the committee often centered around core values of a society that truly cares for the most vulnerable. We began our work with creating a word map of key words and phrases that described what we all hoped for in nursing home care. Words such as safety, equity, peaceful, joyous, integrity, and comfort were often shared as we all imagined what care in a nursing home should be. The committee members were constantly aware of the data, literature, and daily news stories of the travesties in nursing home care as they wrote this report. The committee also recognized the many examples of outstanding care being provided in nursing homes and realized that across the United States nursing home staff representing all disciplines are each day providing wonderful care to residents who they consider as beloved family members. Sadly, these staff have put their own lives at risk and are often not well trained, supported, or compensated. This report and the committee's recommendations assert strongly that residents of nursing homes need better care—and the people caring for them also need better care. The committee report is clear that we will not realize good-quality care of residents until we invest in the bedside staff who care for them.

The committee often reflected on the 1986 Institute of Medicine report *Improving the Quality of Care in Nursing Homes*, which was a critical milestone yet whose recommendations were not fully realized. As a nation we have made promises for better care in nursing homes, and those promises have not been kept. Our hope is that commitment and promises for quality nursing home care that were voiced throughout the pandemic will become promises kept. The recommendations from the committee are thoughtful and strategic. Perhaps the committee's biggest challenges came when we tried to balance the need for very aggressive, overdue change with the reality of limited resources, competing priorities, and the complexity of systems change. We believe the recommendations in this report achieve that balance of what is possible and what is desperately needed.

Is it too much to ask that each and every resident in every nursing home receives care that includes high-quality physical care, behavioral health, safety, and psychological support? Is it too much to ask for a plan of care to establish what is most needed for each resident to receive high-quality care that is truly person centered? Are we too bold to recommend on-site registered nurse coverage in nursing homes, a social worker, and an infection control specialist? After all that we have witnessed during the COVID-19 pandemic, is it too much to ask that nursing assistants are better trained to deliver care to often frail people with limited social support or resources in the last years of their lives? It is not too much to ask that all residents receive good-quality care regardless of race, ethnicity, or geographic location? In fact, the recommendations in this report are no more than what any one of us would want for ourselves or for those we love if we or they were in a nursing home. How can we not accept the committee's recommendations and profoundly change the delivery of care in U.S. nursing homes?

As with the evaluation of most areas of significant importance to our society, adopting and implementing the recommendations of this report will require more than funding, organizational commitment, education, and changing health policy—it will require moral courage. Improving the quality of care in nursing homes for the decades ahead will be a continuing process requiring research to strengthen our knowledge of best care, test models to deliver that care, and investment in the education and training of all of those who work in nursing homes. The recommended approach is bold, but it is possible. But most importantly, it is right. Indeed, improving nursing home care is a moral imperative because it is clearly the right thing to do. It is also a national imperative because it represents society's commitment to caring for those who cannot care for themselves.

It has been a great privilege to have served as chair of this committee. This report will be published as I celebrate my 45th year as a nurse, and I consider it one of the highlights of my career to have devoted over a year to working with this committee of some of the most dedicated colleagues I have known. Most have devoted their careers to advocating for improved care in nursing homes—a pursuit that has not been well funded, often recognized, or rewarded. These members each brought their knowledge and their passion for improved care to the table.

We are in great debt to the staff of the National Academies for their commitment to this work. Laurie Graig and Tracy Lustig as senior program staff led the project with the greatest integrity and vision. The entire staff of the National Academies, including Kaitlyn Friedman, Nikita Varman, and Rukshana Gupta, offered their dedication, organization, and energy to a task that at times seemed overwhelming.

As a nation, we will hopefully see the COVID-19 pandemic resolve in the months that will follow the release of this report. It will be too easy to turn our eyes away from the reform needed in nursing home care. This is the moment; this is the time to keep the promise of better care for those who are the most vulnerable in our society. The committee has delivered the blueprint to build a system of care that honors those who call the nursing home their home and the dedicated staff who care for them. Improving care in nursing homes is possible. It can be done. It must be done.

Betty Ferrell, Ph.D., FAAN, FPCN, CHPN, *Chair*
Committee on the Quality of Care in Nursing Homes

Acronyms and Abbreviations

AADNS	American Association of Directors of Nursing Services
ABPLM	American Board of Post-Acute and Long-Term Care Medicine
ACA	Patient Protection and Affordable Care Act
ACL	Administration for Community Living
ACO	accountable care organization
ACP	advance care planning
ADE	adverse drug event
ADL	activity of daily living
ADRD	Alzheimer's disease and related dementias
AHCA	American Health Care Association
AHRQ	Agency for Healthcare Research and Quality
AMDA	Society for Post-Acute and Long-Term Care Medicine
AONL	American Organization for Nursing Leadership
APM	alternative payment model
APRN	advanced practice registered nurse
APS	adult protective services
ATOP	Nevada Admissions and Transitions Optimization Program
BIPOC	Black, Indigenous, and other people of color
BPCI	Bundled Payments for Care Improvement Initiative
BSW	bachelor's degree in social work
CAH	critical access hospital
CAHPS	Consumer Assessment of Healthcare Providers and Systems
CASPER	Certification and Survey Provider Enhanced Reporting

CDC	Centers for Disease Control and Prevention
CE	continuing education
CHIP	Children's Health Insurance Program
CJR	Comprehensive Care for Joint Replacement Model
CLASS Act	Community Living Assistance Services and Supports Act
CMMI	Center for Medicare and Medicaid Innovation
CMS	Centers for Medicare & Medicaid Services
CNA	certified nursing assistant
COVID-19	severe acute respiratory syndrome coronavirus-19 (SARS-CoV-2)
CRB	care-resistant behavior
C-SNP	chronic condition special needs plan
CSWE	Council on Social Work Education
DHS	U.S. Department of Homeland Security
DNR	do not resuscitate
DOJ	U.S. Department of Justice
D-SNP	dual special needs plan
ECHO	Extension for Community Healthcare Outcomes
ED	emergency department
EHR	electronic health record
eMAR	electronic medication management system
EMR	electronic medical record
ESF	emergency support function
FEMA	Federal Emergency Management Agency
FFS	fee-for-service
FIDE	fully integrated dual eligible
FY	fiscal year
GAO	U.S. Government Accountability Office
HAI	health care–associated infection
HHS	U.S. Department of Health and Human Services
HIE	health information exchange
HIT	health information technology
HITECH	Health Information Technology for Economic and Clinical Health Act of 2009
HRSA	Health Resources and Services Administration
HUD	U.S. Department of Housing and Urban Development
IHI	Institute for Healthcare Improvement
INTERACT	Interventions to Reduce Acute Care Transfers

IOM	Institute of Medicine
I-SNP	institutional special needs plan
LGBTQ+	lesbian, gay, bisexual, transgender, queer (or questioning), and others
LPN	licensed practical nurse
LTC	long-term care
LTSS	long-term services and supports
LVN	licensed vocational nurse
MA	Medicare Advantage
MCWB	Mouth Care Without a Battle
MDS	Minimum Data Set
MedPAC	Medicare Payment Advisory Commission
MIPS	Merit-Based Incentive Payment System
MOQI	Missouri Quality Initiative
MSW	master's degree in social work
NAICS	North American Industry Classification System
NASW	National Association of Social Workers
NCAL	National Center for Assisted Living
NIH	National Institutes of Health
NNHI	National Nursing Home Initiative
NP	nurse practitioner
NQF	National Quality Forum
NRF	National Response Framework
NY–RAH	New York–Reducing Avoidable Hospitalizations
OBRA 87	Omnibus Budget Reconciliation Act of 1987
OIG	U.S. Office of the Inspector General
ONC	Office of the National Coordinator for Health Information Technology
OPTIMISTIC	Optimizing Patient Transfers, Impacting Medical Quality, and Improving Symptoms: Transforming Institutional Care
OTC	over the counter
P4P	pay-for-performance
PA	physician assistant
PASRR	preadmission screening and annual resident review
PDPM	patient-driven payment model
PIPP	Minnesota Performance-Based Incentive Payment Program
POLST	physician's order for life-sustaining treatment
PPE	personal protective equipment

QAPI	quality assurance and performance improvement
QIO	Quality Improvement Organization
QIPMO	Quality Improvement Program for Missouri
QOL	quality of life
RAI	Resident Assessment Instrument
RAVEN	Reduce Avoidable Hospitalizations using Evidence-Based Interventions for Nursing Facilities
REIT	real estate investment trust
RN	registered nurse
SAPO	state-authorized portable order
SCTT	Systems Change Tracking Tool
SFF	Special Focus Facility
SMI	serious mental illness
SNF	skilled nursing facility
SNFist	skilled nursing facility specialist
SNP	special needs plan
VA	U.S. Department of Veterans Affairs
VBP	value-based payment
VHA	Veterans Health Administration
WISH Act	Well-Being Insurance for Seniors to be at Home Act

Abstract

Nursing homes play a unique dual role in the nation's long-term care continuum, serving both as a place where people receive needed health care and a place they call home. Although long-term care is increasingly being provided in home- and community-based settings, nursing homes will likely always be needed for individuals who cannot get the level of care they require in those settings. The 1986 Institute of Medicine[1] report *Improving the Quality of Care in Nursing Homes* described numerous concerns, including neglect and abuse of nursing home residents, poor quality of life, excessive cost, inconsistent (or lack of) oversight, and the need for high-quality data. While many improvements have been made since then, the enormous toll that the COVID-19 pandemic had on nursing home residents, their families, and staff has brought new attention to the long-standing shortfalls that continue to plague nursing homes.

This report identifies critical opportunities to improve the quality of care in nursing homes through both short- and long-term actions across a wide variety of domains. Many recommendations will require dedicated coordination among federal and state governments, nursing homes, health care and social care providers, payers, regulators, researchers, and others as well as the active engagement of residents and their families. The nursing home sector urgently needs to be strengthened so that it can

---

[1] As of March 2016 the Health and Medicine Division of the National Academies of Sciences, Engineering and Medicine (National Academies) continues the consensus studies and convening activities previously carried out by the Institute of Medicine (IOM). The IOM name is used to refer to reports issued prior to July 2015.

respond effectively to the next public health emergency as well as drive critically important and urgently needed innovations to improve the quality of nursing home care. Implementation of the committee's integrated set of recommendations will move the nation closer to making high-quality, person-centered, and equitable care a reality for all nursing home residents, their chosen families, and the nursing home staff who provide care and support them in achieving their goals.

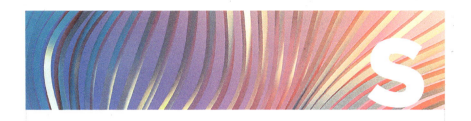

Summary

> "The pandemic has lifted the veil on what has been an invisible social ill for decades."
>
> —Daughter and caregiver of two parents with dementia who needed nursing home care.

Nursing homes play a unique dual role in the nation's long-term care continuum, serving as a place where people receive needed health care as well as a place they call home. Nearly 1.3 million Americans reside in more than 15,000 certified nursing homes in the United States. Although long-term care is increasingly provided in home and community-based settings, nursing homes will likely always be needed for individuals who have complex care needs, are without family or friends able to assist with their care, or lack the resources to be cared for at home.

The 1986 Institute of Medicine[1] report *Improving the Quality of Care in Nursing Homes* identified a variety of significant problems, including neglect and abuse of residents, poor quality of life, excessive cost, inconsistent (or lack of) oversight, and the need for high-quality outcomes data. The Omnibus Budget Reconciliation Act of 1987 (OBRA 87) established more stringent standards for nursing homes in a wide range of areas. While many important quality improvements have been made over the past four decades, ineffective responses to these complex challenges combined with

---

[1] As of March 2016, the Health and Medicine Division of the National Academies of Sciences, Engineering, and Medicine (National Academies) continues the consensus studies and convening activities previously carried out by the Institute of Medicine (IOM). The IOM name is used to refer to reports issued prior to July 2015.

the challenges associated with caring for a heterogeneous nursing home population have resulted in a system of nursing home care that often fails to provide the supports and care necessary to ensure the well-being and safety of nursing home residents—an unacceptable situation that has long been apparent to those who study, work in, or have loved ones in nursing homes.

The COVID-19 pandemic "lifted the veil," revealing and amplifying long-existing shortcomings in nursing home care such as inadequate staffing levels, poor infection control, failures in oversight and regulation, and deficiencies that result in actual patient harm. The pandemic also highlighted nursing home residents' vulnerability and the pervasive ageism evident in undervaluing the lives of older adults. The COVID-19 virus is particularly dangerous for individuals with serious underlying health conditions, which are common among nursing home residents. As a result, nursing home residents suffered disproportionately high rates of cases, hospitalizations, and deaths compared to the general population. For example, despite making up less than one-half of 1 percent of the U.S. population, as of October 2021, nursing home residents accounted for approximately 19 percent of all COVID-19 deaths. As of February 2022, more than 149,000 nursing home residents and more than 2,200 staff members had died of COVID-19. The ubiquity of COVID-19 cases and deaths in nursing homes of all types (across facilities with high and low quality ratings) is indicative of a more systemic problem, one that will require systemic solutions.

The pandemic's enormous toll on nursing home residents and staff drew renewed attention to the long-standing weaknesses that continue to impede the provision of high-quality nursing home care. In this context, the National Academies of Sciences, Engineering, and Medicine, with support from a coalition of sponsors, formed the Committee on the Quality of Care in Nursing Homes in 2020 to examine how the United States delivers, finances, regulates, and measures the quality of nursing home care.[2]

OVERARCHING CONCLUSIONS

After an extensive review of the evidence, the committee arrived at seven overarching conclusions.

First, **the way in which the United States finances, delivers, and regulates care in nursing home settings is ineffective, inefficient, fragmented, and unsustainable.** Despite significant measures to improve the quality of nursing home care in OBRA 87, the current system often fails to provide high-quality care and underappreciates and underprepares nursing home staff for their critical responsibilities.

Second, **immediate action to initiate fundamental change is necessary.** Even prior to the pandemic, nursing home care was neither consistently

---

[2] The complete statement of task is presented in Chapter 1 of this report.

comprehensive nor of high quality; such shortcomings jeopardized the health and well-being of nursing home residents. Regulations in place for 35 years have not been fully enforced, further amplifying residents' risk of harm. Those same shortcomings rendered nursing homes, their residents, and staff unprepared to respond to the COVID-19 pandemic.

Third, federal and state governments, nursing homes, health care and social care providers, payers, regulators, researchers, and others need to **make clear a shared commitment to the care of nursing home residents.** Fully realizing the committee's vision will depend upon the collaboration of multiple partners to honor this commitment to nursing home residents, their chosen families, and the staff who strive to provide the high-quality care every resident deserves.

Fourth, extreme care needs to be taken to ensure that quality-improvement initiatives are implemented using strategies that **do not exacerbate disparities in resource allocation, quality of care, or resident outcomes** (including racial and ethnic disparities), which are all too common in nursing home settings.

Fifth, high-quality research is needed to advance the quality of care in nursing homes. Much of the available research relies on retrospective cohort designs and is constrained by limited available data. This lack of evidence presents challenges to determining the best approaches that will improve quality of care in several areas.[3]

Sixth, **the nursing home sector has suffered for many decades from both underinvestment in ensuring the quality of care and a lack of accountability for how resources are allocated.** For example:

- Low staff salaries and benefits combined with inadequate training has made the nursing home a highly undesirable place of employment.
- Inadequate support for oversight and regulatory activities has contributed to the failure of state survey agencies to meet standards in a timely manner.
- Quality measurement and improvement efforts have largely ignored the voice of residents and their chosen families.
- Lack of transparency regarding nursing home finances, operations, and ownership impedes the ability to fully understand how current resources are allocated.

Implementing the committee's recommendations will likely require a significant investment of financial resources at the federal and state levels and from nursing homes themselves. However, this investment should not be viewed as simply adding more resources to the nursing home sector as it

---

[3] Appendix C includes tables for priority areas of measurement and research and data collection among the committee's recommendations.

currently operates, because that alone would not likely result in significant improvements. Rather, the committee calls for targeted investments (combined with current funding) that would be inextricably linked to requirements for transparency. Such transparency will enable stronger and more effective oversight to ensure resources are properly allocated to improving the quality of care.

Finally, key partners, such as the Centers for Medicare & Medicaid Services (CMS) and other federal agencies, may not currently have the full authority or resources to carry out the actions recommended. Therefore, as a final overarching conclusion, the committee notes that **all relevant federal agencies need to be granted the authority and resources from the U.S. Congress to implement the recommendations of this report.**

COMMITTEE VISION AND GUIDING PRINCIPLES

As the committee began its extensive review of the literature, a first step was to develop an overarching framework for this study, which clearly laid out the vision and guiding principles for high-quality nursing home care. These in turn, helped identify the committee's goals and recommendations (see Box S-1).

While the committee's vision identifies what high-quality nursing home care should look like, the guiding principles serve as a strong reminder that existing regulations *require* nursing homes to provide comprehensive, person-centered care. Using these guiding principles as a foundation, the committee developed seven goals (with associated recommendations) that represent an integrated approach to improving the quality of nursing home care.

The following sections provide a high-level overview of the committee's extensive set of recommendations, which can be found in full detail in Chapter 10.[4] Though the recommendations focus on diverse areas for improvement, they all share a common underlying premise: the challenges facing nursing homes are complex and multifaceted and require immediate attention on multiple fronts by many stakeholders. Some recommendations are intentionally broad, allowing flexibility in how they are implemented, while others are more targeted, with specific details on how to achieve the objectives. Some can be implemented immediately, while others will require a longer time line to be fully operational (but still require immediate initiation); some should be relatively straightforward to operationalize, while others are more aspirational and will require coordinated efforts to create significant long-term changes.[5] Importantly, the committee's

---

[4] Appendix D includes a table of the committee's recommendations organized by the key partners responsible for implementation.

[5] Appendix E includes the committee's estimated implementation time line.

> **BOX S-1**
> **Committee Vision and Guiding Principles
> for High-Quality Nursing Home Care**
>
> **COMMITTEE VISION:**
> Nursing home residents receive care in a safe environment that honors their values and preferences, addresses goals of care, promotes equity, and assesses the benefits and risks of care and treatments.
>
> **GUIDING PRINCIPLES:**
> To achieve this vision, nursing homes should deliver comprehensive, person-centered, interdisciplinary team-based care that meets or exceeds established quality standards and supports strong connections to health care and social service systems and resources, family, friends, and the community more broadly.
> High-quality nursing home care provides an environment that promotes quality of life; aligns with residents' medical, behavioral, and social care needs; reflects residents' values and preferences; promotes autonomy; and manages risks to ensure residents' safety. Such comprehensive, high-quality care includes the following, as appropriate:
>
> - Physical health care
> - Behavioral health care
> - Psychosocial care
> - Oral health care
> - Hearing and vision care
> - Rehabilitative care
> - Dementia care
> - Palliative care
> - End-of-life care
>
> Furthermore, it is the right of every nursing home resident to have equitable access to high-quality comprehensive, person-centered, and culturally sensitive nursing home care.

recommendations should be viewed and implemented as an interrelated package of reform measures.

GOAL 1: DELIVER COMPREHENSIVE, PERSON-CENTERED, EQUITABLE CARE THAT ENSURES THE HEALTH, QUALITY OF LIFE, AND SAFETY OF NURSING HOME RESIDENTS; PROMOTES RESIDENT AUTONOMY; AND MANAGES RISKS.

While person-centered care (as described by the principles in Box S-1) is foundational to the basic requirements specified in federal regulations for nursing home care, such care is not yet a reality to many nursing home residents. Significant gaps and shortcomings exist in the quality of services in areas ranging from the development of a comprehensive care plan for each resident to behavioral health, psychosocial care, oral health, and end-of-life care. Moreover, significant disparities in the quality of care also exist across nursing homes.

Care Planning

The resident care planning process has a central role in the full realization of person-centered, comprehensive, high-quality, and equitable care in the nursing home setting. This process encompasses four critical components: (1) creating the care plan, (2) reviewing it, (3) implementing it and evaluating its effectiveness, and (4) regularly revisiting it. Ideally, all components of the process are implemented, but this has yet to become a reality in all nursing homes. As a foundation to operationalizing person-centered care, Recommendation 1A[6] calls for immediate and consistent compliance with existing regulations, including the following:

- Identification of care preferences of residents and their chosen families using structured, shared decision-making approaches; and
- Documentation, review, and evaluation of the resident's care plan and its implementation.

Models of Care

Nursing homes provide an array of services to both short-stay (post-acute) and long-stay residents of all ages with a wide range of health conditions. Yet research on best practices related to clinical, behavioral, and psychosocial care delivery in nursing homes is scarce. Moreover, nursing homes are often not well integrated into the communities in which they are located nor with the broader health care system. Finally, little is known about how specific factors (e.g., staffing, environment, financing, technology, leadership) affect innovative models of care or how to ensure the sustainability of these approaches. To address these gaps, Recommendation 1B proposes a series of actions including

- Translational research and demonstration projects for the most effective care delivery models in nursing home settings;
- Prioritization of models that reduce disparities and strengthen connections to the community and broader health care systems; and
- Evaluation of innovations in all aspects of care.

---

[6] The numbers of the recommendations are provided here and can be found in their full detail in Chapter 10.

Emergency Preparedness and Response

Prior to the COVID-19 pandemic, there were numerous examples of nursing homes being unprepared to respond to emergencies and natural disasters. For example, in 2016, the top deficiency cited in nursing homes was infection control (45.4 percent of citations). The COVID-19 pandemic provided undeniable evidence of the pernicious impact of this lack of planning and preparedness. To be better positioned to respond to emergencies of all types, nursing homes need to be included as integral partners in emergency management planning, preparedness, and response on the national, state, and local levels. Moreover, as demonstrated by the prohibition against friends and family members visiting during the COVID-19 pandemic and the resultant harm of loneliness and social isolation, it is imperative to strike a careful balance between residents' safety and their behavioral and psychosocial health needs. To safeguard nursing home residents and staff against a broad range of potential public health emergencies and natural disasters, Recommendations 1C and 1D call for the following:

- Reinforcement and clarification of the emergency support functions of the National Response Framework;
- Formal relationships between nursing homes and local, county, and state-level public health and emergency management departments;
- The representation of nursing homes in emergency and disaster planning and management sessions and drills;
- Ready access to personal protective equipment;
- Enforcement of existing regulations; and
- Inclusion of measures related to emergency planning in Care Compare.

Physical Environment

Although the nursing home's physical environment is critical to residents' quality of life, the nursing home infrastructure is aging, and most nursing homes resemble institutions more than homes. Smaller, home-like environments play key roles in infection control and enhancing the quality of life for residents as well as staff. Recommendation 1E calls for the following:

- Creating incentives for new construction and renovation of nursing homes to provide smaller, more home-like environments and smaller units within larger nursing homes;
- Ensuring that new designs include private bedrooms and bathrooms; and
- Allowing flexibility to address a range of resident care and rehabilitation needs.

GOAL 2: ENSURE A WELL-PREPARED, EMPOWERED, AND APPROPRIATELY COMPENSATED WORKFORCE

Workers in nursing homes are often underappreciated, undercompensated, and underprepared for their roles in providing increasingly complex care. Decades of evidence support the need to enhance their training, salaries, and working conditions, yet little progress has been made to improve the quality of these jobs. The committee recommends increasing both the numbers and the qualifications of virtually all types of nursing home workers, which can exacerbate the challenges of recruitment. The committee recognizes that such a recommendation is particularly concerning given the current dire staffing situations for many nursing homes, largely due to the impact of the COVID-19 pandemic. However, robust evidence demonstrates the positive impact of enhanced staffing and training requirements on the quality of care. Enhanced requirements will further professionalize the nursing home workforce, which, when accompanied by improvements in the working environment, will contribute to the desirability of working in a nursing home. Nursing home leaders need to drive culture change, because high-quality care cannot be delivered without a complete transformation of workers' training and stature.

Compensation

Nursing home workers earn significantly less income than if they chose to work in other care settings. For example, the annual mean wage for registered nurses (RNs) in nursing homes is approximately $10,000 less (more than 10 percent less) than RNs in acute-care hospitals, and certified nursing assistants (CNAs) may earn little more than workers in other comparable entry-level jobs, such as cashier, food service worker, and warehouse worker. Successfully recruiting and retaining a high-quality nursing home workforce depends on more than "adequate" compensation—rather, competitive compensation is needed (in comparison to other job opportunities) in conjunction with a variety of incentives and supports to improve the desirability of these jobs. Recommendation 2A calls for the following:

- **Ensuring competitive wages and benefits through a variety of mechanisms.**

Providing benefits may encourage some nursing homes to reduce staffing levels or hire part-time rather than full-time staff. Thus, the committee emphasizes that nursing homes need to offer full-time, consistently assigned work whenever possible and desired by the workers in order to ensure high-quality care.

Staffing Standards and Expertise

Minimum staffing standards in nursing homes, particularly for licensed nursing staff, have been evaluated for decades. Despite substantial evidence demonstrating the relationship between nurse staffing and the quality of care in nursing homes, and 24-hour RN coverage being recommended for decades, today's nurse staffing requirements remain vague. Furthermore, CMS has not established minimum staffing requirements for certain key members of the interdisciplinary team. For example, despite social workers' key role in resident care, current federal regulations require only those nursing homes with 120 or more beds to hire a "qualified social worker" on a full-time basis. Moreover, this individual does not need to have a social work degree. Nursing homes are required to designate an infection prevention and control specialist, yet regulations did not fully prepare them for the impact of the COVID-19 pandemic. Recommendation 2B calls for the immediate implementation of the following requirements in nursing homes:

- Direct-care RN coverage (in addition to the director of nursing) at a minimum of a 24-hour, 7-days-per-week basis, with additional RN coverage as needed;
- Full-time social worker with a minimum of bachelor's degree in social work from an accredited program and 1 year of supervised experience in a health care setting; and
- An infection prevention and control specialist who is an RN, advanced practice RN (APRN), or a physician, at a level of dedicated time sufficient to meet the needs of the size and case mix of the nursing home.

There have been numerous calls over the years to increase nurse staffing in an effort to improve the quality of care in nursing homes. However, the same federal staffing regulations have been in place for decades, even though the types of residents and the complexity of their needs have changed dramatically. To inform future staffing requirements, Recommendation 2C calls for the following:

- Research on minimum and optimal staffing standards for all direct-care staff, including weekend and holiday staffing, based on resident case mix and type of staff needed for the care of specific populations; and
- Updated regulatory requirements based on findings from this research.

While nursing homes may meet current minimum staffing standards, additional expertise is often needed for the development of complex clinical care plans, staff training, and overall planning for care systems and quality improvement. Not every facility will have the ability or need to keep such expertise on staff; those who do not will need to develop ongoing relationships with a variety of professionals for consultation as needed. Recommendation 2D calls for the following:

- Establishing consulting or employment relationships with qualified licensed clinical social workers at the master's or doctoral level, APRNs, clinical psychologists, psychiatrists, pharmacists, and others; and
- Creating incentives for the direct hire of qualified licensed clinical social workers at the master's or doctoral level as well as APRNs for clinical care, including Medicare billing and reimbursement for these services.

Empowerment of Certified Nursing Assistants

Direct-care workers (primarily CNAs) provide the majority of hands-on care to nursing home residents. The demand for CNAs is increasing, yet nursing homes have persistent challenges in recruiting and retaining them. Furthermore, CNAs often have little opportunity for advancement. Because of the crucial role of this position in nursing homes, significantly improving the quality of care for nursing home residents requires investing in quality jobs for CNAs and enabling more workers to enter the CNA pipeline. To advance the role of and empower the CNA, Recommendation 2E calls for the following:

- Career advancement opportunities and peer mentoring;
- Free entry-level training and continuing education;
- Coverage of time for completing education and training programs;
- Expansion of the role of the CNA; and
- New models of care that take greater advantage of the role of the CNA as a member of the interdisciplinary team.

Education and Training

The education and training requirements for a variety of nursing home staff are inadequate or nonexistent. For CNAs, existing training curricula tend to focus on basic tasks rather than on achieving competencies to meet the complex care needs of nursing home residents. Minimum education and competency requirements need to be enhanced (or established) for a variety of nursing home workers and made standard at the national level. Current workers may need assistance in achieving these standards.

Finally, a key issue underlying the preparation of all types of workers for nursing home care is the inadequate foundation for a variety of geriatrics-related topics provided in their education and training programs. Recommendation 2F calls for the following:

- Minimum education and national competency requirements for nursing home administrators, medical directors, directors of nursing, and directors of social services;
- Increased minimum training hours and competency-based training for CNAs;
- Pathways to achieve baseline requirements for current staff; and
- Inclusion of content on gerontology, geriatrics assessment, long-term care, and palliative care in education programs for all health care professionals working in nursing homes.

Competency-based training for CNAs needs to include specific instruction related to health conditions and topics relevant to nursing home populations, such as dementia, infection prevention and control, behavioral health, chronic diseases, the use of assistive and medical devices, and cultural sensitivity and humility.

Beyond these enhanced baseline requirements, the education, training, and competency of the nursing home workforce need to be augmented on an ongoing basis. For example, workforce roles differ substantially in racial and ethnic makeup, and residents are increasingly diverse in terms of racial and ethnic, LGBTQ+, and younger populations. Additionally, the committee recognizes that family caregivers are an essential and valued part of the nursing home workforce and need support and training to be effective members of the care team. To enhance the education and training of the entire nursing home workforce, Recommendation 2G calls for the following:

- Annual continuing education for all nursing home staff;
- Ongoing diversity, equity, and inclusion training for all staff (including leadership), tailored to the unique community and worker needs;
- Resources and training for family caregivers; and
- Participation of chosen family as part of the caregiving team (in the manner and to the extent desired).

Data Collection and Research

In addition to enhanced requirements for nursing home staff, a greater number of more highly trained professionals need to be involved in the delivery of care in nursing homes. However, data are limited on the prevalence of these types of workers in nursing homes and on the extent of their training and expertise. Similarly, limited data exist for the contract and agency staff providing care in nursing homes. While evidence exists on the association between APRNs and the quality of care in nursing homes, baseline data are needed for other professionals to more fully assess their impact on the quality of care. Recommendation 2H calls for the following:

- Routine collection and reporting of data regarding
  - Baseline demographic information of medical directors, administrators, and directors of nursing;
  - The training, expertise, and staffing patterns of medical directors, APRNs, social workers, physicians, and physician assistants; and
  - Numbers and staffing patterns for all contract and agency staff.

While many of the barriers to recruitment and retention of nursing home workers are well known, more research is needed to understand persistent systemic barriers, including the influence of systemic and structural racism that has created and sustained racial and ethnic disparities among long-term care workers. Recommendation 2I calls for the following:

- Research on systemic barriers and opportunities to improve recruitment, training, and advancement of all nursing home workers; and
- Collection of gender, ethnicity, and race-related outcomes of job quality indicators.

GOAL 3: INCREASE TRANSPARENCY AND ACCOUNTABILITY OF FINANCES, OPERATIONS, AND OWNERSHIP

A key barrier to effective nursing home oversight has been lack of transparency related to nursing home finances, operations, and ownership. CMS makes some ownership information available, but these data are incomplete; often difficult to use (by researchers, consumers, and others); and do not allow for determining the corporate structure, finances, and operations of individual nursing homes or assessing quality across facilities owned or operated by the same entity. Moreover, there is little transparency regarding the practice of some nursing homes to contract with related-party organizations (those also owned by the nursing home owner) for services such as management, nursing, or therapy.

Increased transparency of and accountability regarding data on the finances, operations, and ownership of all nursing homes are needed for multiple purposes, including to more fully evaluate both how Medicare and Medicaid payments are spent and how ownership models and spending patterns impact the quality of care. Recommendations 3A and 3B call for the following:

- Collecting, auditing, and making detailed facility-level data on the finances, operations, and ownership of all nursing homes publicly available;
- Making data available in a real time, making the data readily usable, and maintaining the data in a searchable database;
- Ensuring the ability to assess data by common owner (i.e., owners of nursing home chains or of multiple nursing homes) or management company;
- Evaluating and the tracking quality of care by owner or management company; and
- Assessing the impact of ownership models and related-party transactions.

GOAL 4: CREATE A MORE RATIONAL AND ROBUST FINANCING SYSTEM

The current approach to financing nursing home care in the United States is highly fragmented. The federal-state Medicaid program plays a dominant role as a payer of long-stay nursing home care, but is constantly subject to state budget constraints. The federal Medicare program only covers short-stay post-acute care in nursing homes. Services such as hospice care are paid separately and not well integrated into standard nursing home care. Private insurance coverage for long-term care is limited, and relatively few people can afford to pay out of pocket for an extended nursing home stay. Eligibility rules also differ across states and sites of care. Such payment and eligibility differences can lead to unintended consequences. The separation of financing and payment systems for home- and community-based care from those for institutional care presents barriers to the rational cross-setting allocation of resources that would take into account costs as well as individuals' needs and preferences.

The committee's vision of improving the quality of nursing home care as well as expanding access, enhancing efficiency, and advancing equity will require a more stable system of financing over the long term and will likely require a federal benefit. While the committee acknowledges that enacting a new long-term care benefit will be politically challenging, a federal benefit has the most potential to achieve the following:

- Increase access to long-term care services and reduce unmet need,
- Reduce arbitrary barriers between sites of care,
- Reduce inequities in access to high-quality care,

- Reduce differences in resources across nursing homes, and
- Guarantee that payment rates are adequate to cover the expected level of quality.

To expand access and advance equity for all adults who need long-term care, including nursing home care, Recommendation 4A[7] calls for the following:

- Moving toward a federal long-term care benefit by studying how to design such a benefit and then implementing state demonstration programs to test the model prior to national implementation.

Ensuring Adequacy of Medicaid Payments

Nursing homes rely on higher payments for Medicare services to cross-subsidize lower Medicaid payments—an inefficient and unsustainable arrangement. Many nursing homes have a high number of Medicaid recipients and therefore receive relatively little benefit from higher Medicare payments. Lower Medicaid rates encourage nursing homes to prefer short-stay patients (covered by Medicare) to long-stay residents (covered by Medicaid), resulting in selective admission practices and unnecessary hospitalization of long-stay residents in order to have their post-acute care paid for by Medicare upon their return to the nursing home.

In general, the law requires states to provide assurances (and sometimes evidence) that their Medicaid programs' payments are adequate to provide access to high-quality care. Nursing home payment rates, however, are not subject to this requirement. To ensure adequate investment in caring for long-stay nursing home residents, Recommendation 4B calls for the following:

- Use of detailed and accurate nursing home financial information to ensure that Medicaid (or, eventually, federal) payments are at a level adequate to cover the delivery of nursing home care across all domains of care (as specified in Box S-1).

Paying for Direct-Care Services

An extensive body of research supports a strong connection between spending on direct care for residents and the quality of that care. The Patient Protection and Affordable Care Act required CMS to develop new Medicare cost reports to capture specific information on nursing home

---

[7] One committee member declined to endorse this recommendation.

costs in four categories: (1) direct and indirect care, (2) housekeeping and dietary services, (3) capital expenses, and (4) administrative services. However, nursing homes are not required by law to devote a specific portion of their payment to direct care. This results in great variability among nursing homes in terms of the actual dollar amount devoted to direct care as opposed to non-care costs (e.g., monitoring fees, lease payments). Recommendation 4C calls for the following:

- Designation of a specific percentage Medicare and Medicaid payments for direct-care services for nursing home residents, including staffing (including both the number of staff and their wages and benefits), behavioral health, and clinical care.

Value-Based Payment for Nursing Home Care

Nursing homes are one of the most common sites of post-acute care. To control rising post-acute care costs, Medicare joined the prevailing trend toward value-based payment and more strongly linking payment to value and quality of care rather than to the quantity of services. Medicare has implemented alternative payment models (APMs), such as accountable care organizations and bundled payments that hold care providers accountable for total costs of care. Research on Medicare APMs reveals that they are associated with reductions in both costs and service use without adverse consequences on patient outcomes.

Given the importance of controlling costs for post-acute care in nursing homes while maintaining or improving the quality of care, Medicare needs to build on the experience of existing value-based payment demonstrations. In contrast to the current bundled payments made to nursing homes for a limited number of conditions, however, such arrangements will need to be extended to cover all the costs of care for all conditions, including both acute care in the hospital and post-acute care in the nursing home setting. Bundled payments will shift financial accountability, and thus risk, for nursing home post-acute care to hospitals. Importantly, hospitals and other clinicians need to work collaboratively during an episode of care and be held financially accountable by linking payment to quality metrics. As bundled payments are expanded to all conditions, close monitoring and rigorous study of the impact on patient outcomes will be required to mitigate any unintended consequences. Thus, to improve the value of and accountability for Medicare payments for short-stay post-acute care in nursing homes, Recommendation 4D calls for the following:

- Extending the existing bundled payment initiatives to all conditions; and

- Holding hospitals financially accountable for Medicare post-acute care spending and outcomes.

The impact of APMs for long-stay nursing home care is unknown, but their use warrants exploration and testing in real-world situations. Given the uncertainty surrounding their impact, the committee emphasizes the critical importance of tying such payments to value through quality metrics on staffing, resident experience, functional status, and end-of-life care to ensure that APMs maintain quality of care. Equally important is the need for a targeted focus on reducing health disparities. To eliminate the current financial misalignment for long-stay residents created by having Medicaid coverage for nursing home services and Medicare coverage for health care services, Recommendation 4E calls for the following:

- Demonstration projects to explore the use of APMs for long-term nursing home care, separate from bundled payment initiatives for post-acute care, including
  - Use of global capitated budgets,
  - Making care provider organizations or health plans accountable for the total costs of care,
  - Inclusion of post-acute and hospice care in the capitated rate, and
  - Tying payments to broad-based quality metrics.

GOAL 5: DESIGN A MORE EFFECTIVE AND RESPONSIVE SYSTEM OF QUALITY ASSURANCE

Despite substantial changes in nursing home care since the implementation of OBRA 87, the general standards for oversight have largely remained the same.

State Surveys and CMS Oversight

States assist with the assessment of nursing homes' compliance with CMS requirements of participation through regular inspections and, as necessary, the investigation of complaints. Although federal oversight standards and processes are uniform across states, considerable variation exists in the implementation of routine inspection responsibilities, in the imposition of sanctions, and in the investigation of complaints. The survey process often fails to properly identify serious care problems, fully correct and prevent recurrence of identified problems, and investigate complaints in a timely manner. Moreover, CMS does not provide sufficient oversight of or transparency in the state survey process or adequately enforce existing sanctions for states' failures to perform these duties consistently. Recommendation 5A calls for the following:

- Ensuring that state survey agencies have adequate capacity, organizational structure, and resources for their responsibilities including monitoring, investigation of complaints, and enforcement;
- Refining, expanding, and publicly reporting oversight performance metrics of state survey agencies; and
- Using existing strategies of enforcement when states consistently fall short of expected standards.

Despite the prominent role of nursing home oversight and regulation, the evidence base for its effectiveness in ensuring a minimum standard of quality is relatively modest. The current quality assurance process is largely a standardized enterprise. Although a range of enforcement options are available, civil monetary penalties have been the most common sanction. The regulatory model needs significant improvement, particularly in relation to uneven enforcement, but there is little consensus (or evidence) to suggest which approaches would ultimately lead to improvement in the quality of care for nursing home residents. Recommendation 5B calls for the following:

- Developing and evaluating strategies to improve quality assurance efforts, including
  - Enhanced data monitoring to track performance and triage inspections;
  - Oversight across a broader segment of poorly performing facilities;
  - Modified formal oversight activities for high-performing facilities, provided adequate safeguards are in place; and
- Greater use of enforcement options beyond civil monetary penalties.

The committee notes that specific concerns have been raised pertaining to whether oversight can be reduced in some manner (e.g., less frequent or intense surveys) for high performers given that substantial safety risks or markers of decreases in quality (e.g., significant changes in staffing patterns) might occur between surveys. Therefore, the committee emphasizes the importance of using real-time quality metrics as an "early warning system" in conjunction with testing new approaches to ensure ongoing monitoring of safety and quality and enable rapid intervention if problems arise.

The Long-Term Care Ombudsman Program

The Long-Term Care Ombudsman Program is the only entity within the nursing home system whose sole mission is to be an advocate for the residents to ensure that they receive the care to which they are entitled. In general, limited funding affects a program's ability to reliably meet federal and state requirements and fully provide residents and their families with the strongest support possible. Recommendation 5C calls for the following:

- Increased funding for the Long-Term Care Ombudsman Program to
  - Hire additional paid staff,
  - Train staff and volunteers,
  - Bolster programmatic infrastructure,
  - Make data on programs and activities publicly available,
  - Develop metrics to document the effectiveness of the programs, and
  - Eliminate cross-state variation in capacity.
- Developing plans for collaboration with other relevant state-based entities.

Quality Assurance, Transparency, and Accountability

As noted earlier, the committee concluded that increased transparency and accountability will help to improve the quality of care. For quality assurance, the availability of more accurate and complete data on the finances, operations, and ownership of nursing homes will enable regulators to assess the quality of care across facilities with a common owner and levy sanctions as appropriate. Recommendation 5D calls for the following:

- Implementing strengthened oversight across facilities with a common owner; and
- Denying licensure and imposing enforcement actions on owners with a pattern of poor-quality care across facilities.

Certificate-of-Need Regulations and Construction Moratoria

As part of quality assurance, some states maintain certificate-of-need requirements to regulate expansions in the health care market, purportedly to constrain health care spending. Additionally, construction moratoria prohibit building any new health care facilities. However, these policies do not have much impact on overall Medicaid nursing home spending. Instead, they have been found to limit choice and reduce access, especially in rural areas; decrease the quality of care for some measures of quality; and discourage innovation. Recommendation 5E calls for the following:

- **Elimination of certificate-of-need requirements and construction moratoria.**

Eliminating such restrictive policies is not intended as a mechanism to increase the use of nursing homes or invest in nursing homes in lieu of other settings for long-term care. Rather, the committee seeks to expand consumer choice for those who need and choose nursing home care.

GOAL 6: EXPAND AND ENHANCE QUALITY MEASUREMENT AND CONTINUOUS QUALITY IMPROVEMENT

The primary purpose of quality measurement is to improve the quality of care and outcomes. Effective quality measures can be used for continuous quality improvement activities.

Quality Measurement

The CMS website Care Compare provides public reporting of quality measures for nursing homes. However, it does not directly report on a key domain of high-quality care—resident and family satisfaction and experience. Many other key indicators of high-quality care are also omitted, and several improvements are needed to enhance the quality of the publicly reported data. Care Compare needs to be enhanced and expanded to more fully reflect the quality of care in nursing homes. Recommendations 6A and 6B call for the following:

- **Addition of measures to Care Compare related to**
  - **Resident and family experience, and**
  - **Weekend staffing and staff turnover by role;**
- **Increased weight of staffing measures within the five-star composite rating;**
- **Facilitation of the ability to examine quality performance across facilities with common ownership or management company;**
- **Improvement in the validity of Minimum Data Set–based clinical quality; and**
- **Additional testing to improve differentiation in the five-star composite rating.**

Finally, several other key domains of high-quality care are not reflected among the measures in Care Compare, and more work is needed to develop valid measures for these domains. Recommendation 6C calls for the following:

- Developing and adopting new measures for Care Compare related to
  - Palliative care and end-of-life care;
  - Implementation of the resident's care plan;
  - Receipt of care that aligns with resident's goals, and the attainment of those goals;
  - Staff well-being and satisfaction;
  - Psychosocial and behavioral health; and
  - Various structural measures (e.g., health information technology adoption and interoperability, emergency preparedness and response, financial performance, staff employment arrangements).

Health Equity

The quality of nursing home care is particularly concerning for several high-risk populations who experience significant disparities in care, including racial and ethnic minorities and LGBTQ+ populations. However, the lack of robust data specific to race and ethnicity in nursing homes makes it difficult to document the true extent and impact of disparities in care. While developing measures of disparities in nursing home care is needed, doing so needs to be based on an overall health equity strategy for nursing homes. Recommendation 6D calls for developing the following:

- An overall health equity strategy for nursing homes;
- A minimum data set to identify and describe disparities;
- Measures of disparities to be included in a national report card;
- Culturally tailored interventions and policies; and
- Strategies to identify the types and degree of disparities in order to prioritize when action is needed, and promising pathways to reduce or eliminate those disparities.

Quality Improvement

Quality measures help guide quality-improvement efforts, but the extent to which individual nursing homes engage in quality improvement (and the effectiveness of such activities) is unknown. Many facilities lack adequate expertise and resources for effective quality improvement. The committee recognizes the role of CMS' Quality Improvement Organization (QIO) program in providing technical assistance to improve the quality of health care in general. However, the focus of the QIO program varies by scope of work, and attention to nursing homes specifically has been inconsistent. State and local programs providing onsite assistance by expert clinical staff have been shown to be effective in improving care quality, and nursing homes widely accept their help. Such programs have been effective at building trusting relationships, modifying technical assistance approaches to meet local needs and skills, and keeping up to date with scientific content.

The committee concluded that nursing homes would benefit from the availability of technical assistance from individuals at the state (or even local) level who are most familiar with their specific communities and challenges and have specific expertise in nursing home quality and a consistent and ongoing focus on nursing homes. Recommendation 6E calls for the following:

- Developing state-based, nonprofit, confidential technical assistance programs with an ongoing and consistent focus on nursing homes that include
  - Standards to promote comparable programs across states,
  - Ongoing analysis and reporting of the effectiveness of services,
  - Coordination with state surveyors and ombudsmen, and
  - Partnerships with relevant academic institutions of higher education.

GOAL 7: ADOPT HEALTH INFORMATION TECHNOLOGY IN ALL NURSING HOMES

Health information technology (HIT) has the potential to contribute to increased efficiency in care delivery, enhanced care coordination, improved staff productivity, the promotion of patient safety, and reduced health disparities. HIT includes a range of applications, including telehealth, videoconferencing, and electronic health records (EHRs). The COVID-19 pandemic underscored the critical importance of HIT applications, which provided vitally important means of connectivity and communication when nursing home lockdowns led to limited access to in-person clinical visits and residents' isolation from friends and family members.

Nursing home residents often have complex medical conditions that require care coordination among specialists in hospitals and other care settings, further underscoring the need for nursing homes to have EHRs that communicate with other systems to ensure smooth and safe care transitions as patients move from one health care setting to another. While federal programs provided incentives to eligible health care professionals and hospitals to support EHR adoption, nursing homes were not designated as eligible for such incentives. The long-term care sector, and nursing homes in particular, has been slower to adopt EHRs, due in part to the associated costs. Recommendation 7A calls for the following:

- Identifying pathways to provide financial incentives to nursing homes for certified EHR adoption.

As more nursing homes adopt HIT, it will be critical to monitor and track HIT adoption and interoperability (ability to communicate with other EHRs). The level of HIT adoption varies among nursing homes, so a baseline measure of adoption needs to be developed. Furthermore, it is vital to understand the various barriers and facilitators to HIT use in nursing homes in order to improve the efficiency, effectiveness of, and satisfaction with HIT—for staff as well as residents and their families. Recommendation 7B calls for the following:

- Developing and reporting measures of HIT adoption and interoperability; and
- Measuring and reporting nursing home staff, resident, and family perceptions of HIT usability.

If HIT is to realize its potential to improve the quality of care and increase staff productivity, it will require training nursing home leadership and staff, among other factors. However, despite evidence that training is a key contributor to staff satisfaction with HIT, most nursing homes do not provide adequate training. Recommendation 7C calls for the following:

- Development and ongoing implementation of training in core HIT competencies for nursing home leadership and staff.

To create an environment of continuous quality improvement, ongoing evaluation studies will be needed to assess the impact of HIT on resident outcomes, examine innovative ways to use HIT to improve resident care, and understand the key challenges of HIT adoption. Moreover, studies will need to explore the disparities in HIT adoption and use across nursing homes, paying particular attention to differences in geographic location, ownership status, the size of the nursing homes, and specific patient populations. Recommendation 7D calls for the following:

- Rigorous evaluation studies of HIT use, disparities in HIT adoption and use, innovative HIT applications, and assessment of perceptions of HIT usability.

CONCLUSION

The urgency to reform how care is financed, delivered, and regulated in nursing home settings is undeniable. Failure to act will guarantee the continuation of many shortcomings that prevent the delivery of high-quality care in all nursing homes. The COVID-19 pandemic provided powerful evidence of the deleterious impact of inaction and inattention to long-standing quality problems on residents, families, and staff. The pandemic, however, also serves as a stark reminder that nursing homes need to be better prepared to respond effectively to the next public health emergency, and serves as an impetus to drive critically important and urgently needed innovations to improve the quality of nursing home care. Implementing the committee's integrated set of recommendations will move the nation closer to making high-quality, person-centered, and equitable care a reality.

It has been 35 years since the passage of OBRA 87 and landmark nursing home reform measures. It is of the utmost importance that all nursing home partners work together to ensure that residents, their chosen families, and staff will no longer have to wait for needed improvements to the quality of care in nursing homes. The time to act is now.

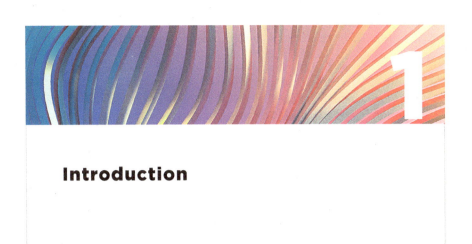

Introduction

Nursing homes, as their very name implies, play a unique dual role in the nation's long-term care continuum, serving as a place where people can receive needed health care and assistance with activities of daily living as well as a place they call home. For some, nursing homes serve as a temporary residence where they can recover after a hospitalization or illness. For others, it serves as their permanent home, a place where they receive care and services that should enable them to live a safe and fulfilled life. Currently, nearly 1.3 million Americans reside in more than 15,000 certified nursing homes (CDC, 2020; KFF, 2020a). Nearly 85 percent of nursing home residents are age 65 or older, and more than 40 percent are over age 85 (CMS, 2015). Aside from those nursing home residents who live there temporarily while rehabilitating from surgery or illness, most nursing home residents require assistance with activities of daily living because of chronic medical conditions or behavioral challenges, including dementia. About half of nursing home residents have Alzheimer's or other dementias (Harris-Kojetin et al., 2019). The heterogeneity of the nursing home population contributes to persistent challenges for achieving optimal care, including the ability to provide the appropriate environment, high-quality staff training, and comprehensive quality measurement.

Long-term care is increasingly being provided in home and community-based settings (Fashaw et al., 2020), and nursing home occupancy rates are decreasing (CDC, 2017; Harrington et al., 2018; KFF, 2020b). For example, occupancy rates declined from 83.7 percent in 2009 to 80.8 percent in 2016 (Harrington et al., 2018). Occupancy rates further declined during the first year of the COVID-19 pandemic (decreasing by nearly 20 percent from 2020 to the beginning of 2021) (NIC, 2021; Paulin, 2021; Taylor and Wilson, 2021). While occupancy rates rose during 2021, they have not yet returned to pre-pandemic rates (Berklan, 2021). In spite of this shift to community-based settings, nursing homes will likely always be needed for many reasons, including for individuals who have complex care needs, are without family or friends able to assist with care, or lack the resources to be cared for at home.

STUDY CONTEXT

Given the vulnerable state of many, if not most, nursing home residents and the large and growing number of older Americans, one would expect that the United States as a nation would ensure that nursing homes provide comprehensive, high-quality, person-centered care for the country's aging parents, aunts and uncles, brothers and sisters, friends, and loved ones. However, the current system of nursing home care in the United States often fails to provide the supports and quality of care necessary to ensure the well-being and safety of nursing home residents—an unacceptable situation that has long been apparent to those who research, work in, or have loved ones in nursing homes. Indeed, the 1986 Institute of Medicine[1] (IOM) report *Improving the Quality of Care in Nursing Homes* (IOM, 1986) addressed a variety of concerns related to the quality of care in nursing homes, including neglect and abuse of residents, poor quality of life, excessive cost, lack of or inconsistent regulatory oversight, lack of personal advocates for residents, and poor and unstandardized information. Thirty-five years ago, the Nursing Home Reform Act was enacted as part of the Omnibus Budget Reconciliation Act of 1987 (OBRA 87).[2] As a result, the Health Care Finance Administration (now the Centers for Medicare & Medicaid Services) issued comprehensive regulations and survey processes to "ensure that residents of nursing homes receive quality care that will result in their highest practicable physical, mental, and social wellbeing."[3] Studies since the enactment of OBRA 87 have noted improvements in information on resident status, a decreased use of physical and chemical restraints, and increases in direct-care staffing (Fashaw et al., 2020; Wiener et al., 2007). However, while not all nursing homes provide substandard, unsafe, or depersonalized care, many of the concerns raised in the 1986 IOM report remain problematic today.

---

[1] As of March 2016, the Health and Medicine Division of the National Academies of Sciences, Engineering and Medicine (National Academies) continues the consensus studies and convening activities previously carried out by the Institute of Medicine (IOM). The IOM name is used to refer to reports issued prior to July 2015.

[2] Omnibus Budget Reconciliation Act of 1987, Public Law 100-203; 100th Cong., 1st Sess., (December 22, 1987).

[3] Omnibus Budget Reconciliation Act of 1987, Public Law 100-203; 42 USC 1396r, 100th Cong., 1st Sess., (December 22, 1987).

The COVID-19 Pandemic

The COVID-19 pandemic and its devastating impact on nursing home residents and staff brought to the forefront the long-standing challenges in the nursing home system, such as inadequate staffing levels, poor infection control, and deficiencies that resulted in actual harm (GAO, 2003; Harrington et al., 2016, 2018; Kramer, 2021). In 2020, 42 percent of U.S. nursing homes received citations for deficiencies in infection control (KFF, 2020c), and 15 percent received citations for serious deficiencies that resulted in actual harm to a resident or put the resident at immediate risk for harm (KFF, 2020d).

Importantly, workers in nursing homes are often underappreciated, undercompensated, and underprepared for their roles in providing increasingly complex care. Robust data support the need to enhance training, salaries, and working conditions for nursing home workers, yet little progress has been made to improve the quality of these jobs (AHCA/NCAL, 2021). Again, the COVID-19 pandemic further exacerbated these preexisting shortcomings. For example, while the work of the direct-care workforce (e.g., certified nursing assistants) has commonly been referred to as physically demanding, in 2020 during the midst of the COVID-19 pandemic, the role of the nursing home worker was deemed among the most dangerous jobs in the country (Lewis, 2021). Burnout and turnover among the nursing home workforce due to the COVID-19 pandemic (which were prevalent even before the pandemic) are projected to exacerbate existing staff shortages across the country (Gandhi et al., 2021; Manchha et al., 2021).

The pandemic also highlighted the vulnerability of nursing home residents in general. The virus that causes COVID-19 (SARS-CoV-2) is particularly dangerous for individuals with underlying health conditions, especially conditions that are typical of nursing home residents. As a result, nursing home residents suffered disproportionately high rates of cases, hospitalizations, and deaths relative to the general population. For example, early in the pandemic, nursing home residents and staff accounted for 12 percent of all COVID-19 cases in the United States (Grabowski, 2020). Moreover, as of October 2021, despite nursing home residents making up less than one-half of 1 percent of the population (CDC, 2020; KFF, 2020a; U.S. Census Bureau, 2021) and just under 1.6 percent of all COVID-19 cases, they accounted for approximately 19 percent of all COVID-19 deaths (CDC, 2021a,b). The ubiquity of COVID-19 cases and deaths in nursing homes of all types (across facilities with high and low quality ratings) is indicative of a more systemic problem, one that will require systemic solutions.

Finally, the response to the COVID-19 pandemic shone a harsh light on pervasive ageism, or the undervaluing of the lives of older adults (Aronson, 2020; Carbonaro, 2020; Kendall-Taylor et al., 2020; Kilaru and Gee, 2020).

Kilaru and Gee (2020) reflected on structural ageism and noted that "complacency to the ongoing loss of life during the [COVID-19] pandemic may be the most unfortunate consequence of ageism [. . .] Ultimately, the pandemic has forced us to see how we value or devalue the lives of older adults." Fraser and colleagues (2020) asked, "Did a pre-pandemic lack of resources for residents of [long-term care] homes exacerbate this looming crisis and our slow response?" Tied to this undervaluing of older adults is the stigma that can be associated with working in a nursing home, which contributes to persistent staffing shortages (even before the pandemic) (Beynon et al., 2020; Danilovich, 2017; Manchha et al., 2021, 2022). For family members' perspectives, see Box 1-1.

BOX 1-1
Family Member Perspectives

"The pandemic has lifted the veil on what has been an invisible social ill for decades."

— Daughter and caregiver of two parents
with dementia who needed nursing home care

"I so wish our society valued more highly the lives of those who are elderly and vulnerable and those who serve them. I do not know how to solve that problem."

— M.K.

"These are not just our veterans, grandparents, parents, friends, siblings. This is us as well. We must do better. It is shameful that we do not."

— Family Member and Concerned Citizen

"These are the most needy, fragile members of society and it is sadly telling how poorly they're treated in this country."

— K.R.

"I honestly cannot express how it is. You have to experience it yourself. Being a resident with no dignity, no privacy, no connection to staff, being told what time to eat and shower, at mercy of staff. Or after you have a family member in a [long-term care] facility, when it is too late to make the impact of change. Hopefully hearing the stories you are going to get inundated with, you will begin to understand what is being requested from you to fix the system- it is broken, it is not going away, you may be there someday. Please do what is needed to change staffing ratios at the very least, because no matter how we speak up, we cannot do it on our own."

— M.K.

These quotes were collected from the committee's online call for resident, family, and nursing home staff perspectives.

Overall, the COVID-19 pandemic's enormous toll on nursing home residents, families, and nursing home staff drew renewed and urgent attention to the shortfalls that continue to plague the nursing home industry, while highlighting the opportunities to ensure high-quality care for nursing home residents.

STUDY ORIGIN AND STATEMENT OF TASK

With support from a coalition of sponsors, including The John A. Hartford Foundation, The Commonwealth Fund, the Jewish Healthcare Foundation, The Sephardic Foundation on Aging, and The Fan Fox & Leslie R. Samuels Foundation, the National Academies of Sciences, Engineering, and Medicine (National Academies) formed the Committee on the Quality of Care in Nursing Homes in the fall of 2020. The sponsors charged the committee to examine how the United States delivers, finances, regulates, and measures the quality of nursing home care (see Box 1-2).

PREVIOUS WORK OF THE NATIONAL ACADEMIES

Building upon the 1986 study *Improving the Quality of Care in Nursing Homes*, the 2001 IOM report *Improving the Quality of Long-Term Care* provided a comprehensive look at the quality of care and quality of life in long-term care broadly (including nursing homes, home and community-based settings, and residential care facilities) (IOM, 2001a). The report once again raised continuing concerns about the quality, cost, and accessibility of care and the adequacy of oversight in long-term care settings, especially nursing homes. Overall, the report provided recommendations for improving external oversight, strengthening the caregiving workforce, building organizational capacity, and improving reimbursement. The report concluded:

> [L]ong-term care should be consumer-centered focusing on the needs, circumstances, and preferences of people using care and involving them, to the extent possible, in planning, delivering, and evaluating care. (IOM, 2001a, pp. 248–249)

Several IOM studies focused specifically on the health care workforce. The 1996 report *Nursing Staff in Hospitals and Nursing Homes* made specific recommendations related to the numbers and types of nursing staff that should be present in nursing homes, key areas for training (e.g., geriatrics, occupational health and safety measures, culturally sensitive care, conflict management), and research needs (IOM, 1996). The report also examined work-related injury and stress for workers in nursing homes and

> **BOX 1-2**
> **Statement of Task**
>
> An ad hoc committee of the National Academies of Sciences, Engineering, and Medicine will examine how our nation delivers, finances, regulates, and measures the quality of nursing home care with particular emphasis on challenges that have arisen in light of the COVID-19 pandemic. The committee will consider a broad range of issues such as
>
> - ways to generate and assess the evidence base for interventions, structures, policies, and care models to promote care innovation while assuring quality of care;
> - the impact of current oversight and regulatory structures (including enforcement and penalties) on care quality and outcomes, which may include examination of the meaningfulness of the current five-star rating system and how it is interpreted by consumers and clinicians; and/or the validity, efficiency, and effectiveness of the current survey and certification structures and methods, including inspection standards, training of surveyors, and their adherence to standards;
> - the appropriateness of current emergency preparedness regulations and strategies for nursing homes in light of different environmental and pandemic threats to residents;
> - the influence of current nursing home real estate ownership and payment models on the delivery of high-quality care and regulatory compliance;
> - the role of the facility medical director as the clinical leader in nursing homes;
> - strategies to attract, train, and retain a more skilled workforce to nursing homes and survey agencies; and
> - the role of nursing homes in the continuum of post-acute and long-term care.
>
> The committee will develop a set of findings and recommendations to delineate a framework and general principles for improving the quality of care in today's nursing homes, delivering high-quality care in a consistent manner, and ensuring the safety and well-being of residents and staff in nursing homes. The committee may also consider the relevance of their findings and recommendations to other long-term care settings, if applicable.

recommended screening of workers for a history of abuse and criminal records. The 2004 study *Keeping Patients Safe: Transforming the Work Environment for Nurses* focused on the connection between the work environment for nurses and patient safety, with a particular focus on nursing hours (IOM, 2004). The report called for improvements in nurse staffing, specifically calling for 24/7 registered nurse presence in nursing homes along with specific hours per resident day for different types of nurses. The 2008 report

Retooling for an Aging America provided recommendations to build the capacity of the health care workforce overall to care for older adults (IOM, 2008). The committee recommended education and training to enhance the competence of all types of workers in the care of older adults, including training medical residents in nursing home settings and enhancing the competence of direct-care workers. The report also called for redesigning models of care to provide comprehensive care to older adults, noting the small-home approach to nursing home care as an example of person-centered care.

More recently, the 2020 National Academies study *Social Isolation and Loneliness in Older Adults* found that housing status can affect levels of social isolation and loneliness (NASEM, 2020). It noted that while long-term care providers may strive to provide home-like accommodations and person-centered care, long-term care may increase social isolation and loneliness, particularly for individuals who are living far away from their loved ones, are unable to engage in meaningful social interactions, or need to share a room with someone with whom they are not compatible.

STUDY APPROACH AND SCOPE

The Committee on the Quality of Care in Nursing Homes consisted of 17 members with a broad range of expertise, including public health, gerontology/geriatrics, public policy, health care and social care providers, health equity, health information technology, health care financing and administration, nursing home regulation, nursing home quality, emergency preparedness and response, and legal issues. Appendix A provides brief biographies of the committee members and staff.

The committee deliberated during five 2- to 3-day virtual meetings and many conference calls and ad hoc meetings between November 2020 and November 2021. Additionally, the committee held six virtual public webinars and invited speakers to offer comments or make presentations to inform the committee's deliberations. The speakers provided valuable input on a broad range of topics, including conceptualizing quality; family, resident, and clinical perspectives; industry, oversight, and regulatory perspectives (including the state survey process); issues related to staffing, culture change, equity, and nursing home leadership and ownership; quality improvement programs; and nursing home financing. The committee also established an online system for collecting narratives on resident, family, and nursing home staff experiences. Fifty-six sets of comments were submitted, and most came from the family members of nursing home residents. Quotes from these narratives are included in boxes throughout this report. Additionally, the committee completed an extensive search of the peer-reviewed literature and reviewed the gray literature, including publications by private organizations, advocacy groups, and government entities.

Overall Approach

The significant challenges to providing high-quality care in nursing homes are complex and pervasive and often extend past nursing homes themselves, reflecting challenges for long-term care in general as well as the broader health care system. Many experts have called for an entirely new system of nursing home care, which would go beyond the current realities of care delivery, regulation, financing, and quality measurement. Rebuilding an entirely new system is appealing, but the committee ultimately concluded that substantial and sustainable improvements in the quality of nursing home care require a realistic and intentional strategy that will in some areas necessitate incremental changes within the current system. Especially in areas with data and research gaps, for example, an incremental approach enables the time required to gather evidence for the best approach to achieving the committee's vision, while at the same time increases the likelihood that unintentional consequences for nursing home residents will be identified and mitigated. Focusing only on short-term "quick fixes" also would likely not achieve the sustainable changes needed to dramatically improve the quality of care provided in nursing homes over the long term. Therefore, the committee sought to ensure that its goals and recommendations represent a coherent and integrated plan of action to achieve both short-term improvements as well as long-term objectives. The committee's approach aligns with the statement of task, which specifically called on the committee to "develop a set of findings and recommendations to delineate a framework and general principles for improving the quality of care in today's nursing homes" (see Box 1-2). Many of the committee's recommendations aim to address high-level goals while allowing flexibility in how they should be implemented, while others contain greater detail about how to effectively implement the recommendations are specified. (See Chapter 10 for more on the committee's approach to implementing its recommendations.)

Definitions and Terminology

The report uses a number of terms that absent further clarification may lead to misinterpretation. Below are some important definitions and distinctions in terminology.

Nursing Homes

While the terms "nursing home" and "skilled nursing facility" are often used interchangeably, skilled nursing facilities are designed to focus on the provision of short-term medical care after a hospital stay (although they may also provide long-term care for people with chronic illnesses). Most nursing homes are licensed and serve as both long-term care and skilled nursing facilities. For the purposes of this report, unless otherwise noted, the committee uses the term *nursing home* to refer to both types of facility.

Nursing Home Residents

Nursing homes provide care to two different groups of people who have distinct care needs: short-stay individuals who require post-acute care after a hospital stay, and long-stay residents who have a more diverse range of care needs. For the purposes of this report, unless the distinction is important, the committee refers to all individuals within nursing homes as *residents,* while acknowledging the heterogeneity of the typical population in a nursing home that serves as both a long-term care facility and skilled nursing facility (i.e., long-stay "residents" and short-stay "patients").

Person-Centered Care versus Person-Directed Care

Person-centered care has been defined in many ways, has no single agreed-upon definition, and is often used interchangeably with other terms such as person-directed care and patient-centered care. The 2001 IOM report *Crossing the Quality Chasm* defined patient-centered care as "respectful of and responsive to individual patient preferences, needs, and values and [ensures] that patient values guide all clinical decisions" (IOM, 2001b, p. 40). A 2016 literature review found 15 different descriptions of person-centered care for older adults that addressed 17 central principles or values, mostly in the domains of whole-person care, respect and value, choice, dignity, self-determination, and purposeful living (Kogan et al., 2016). Person-centered care focuses on the recipient of care and their values, preferences, goals, and abilities, rather than the efficiency and convenience of care delivery for staff (Fazio et al., 2018). In nursing home regulations, the Centers for Medicare & Medicaid Services (CMS) has specified that person-centered care means to "focus on the resident as the locus of control, and support the resident in making their own choices and having control over their daily lives."[4] Person-centered care requires, at a minimum, knowledge of the range and types of needs of nursing home residents and an assessment and care planning model that identifies, prioritizes, and addresses those needs in the context of their goals, preferences, and values.

Whereas person-centered care recognizes the goals, values, and preferences of individuals in the development of a care plan, *person-directed care* involves including individuals and their chosen family members as co-creators in the development of their care plans. This may be particularly

---

[4] CMS Requirements for Long-Term Care Facilities—Definitions, 42 CFR § 483.5 (2017).

important in nursing homes where "care plans inform nearly all aspects of life" (Scales et al., 2017, p. 185). The committee recognizes person-directed care as an integral element of person-centered care in nursing homes. For the purposes of this report, the term person-centered care is used with the assumption that residents and their chosen family members are fully engaged.

Family Caregivers and Chosen Family

A variety of terms are used to describe the friends and family members who support the care of their loved one including family caregivers, informal caregivers, caregivers, and care partners. For the purposes of this report, the committee uses the term *family caregiver* with the understanding that family caregivers include both family members and non-family care partners (who the committee refers to as *chosen family*). The committee further recognizes that family caregivers may not actually provide hands-on care, but may provide support in other ways such as providing emotional support, representing the resident's perspective and history, acting as a surrogate decision maker, and advocating for the resident's safety and security (see more in Chapter 5). In the 2016 IOM report *Families Caring for an Aging America* it was said that

> The term "family caregiver" should be used to reflect the diverse nature of older adults' family and helping relationships. Some caregivers do not have a family kinship or legally defined relationship with the care recipient, but are instead partners, neighbors, or friends. Many older adults receive care from more than one family caregiver, and some caregivers may help more than one older adult. The circumstances of individual caregivers and the caregiver context are extremely variable. Family caregivers may live with, nearby, or far away from the person receiving care. Regardless, the family caregiver's involvement is determined primarily by a personal relationship rather than by financial remuneration. The care they provide may be episodic, daily, occasional, or of short or long duration. (IOM, 2016)

Health Equity Terms

The term *disparities* refers to differences in care, but the term *inequities* recognizes "health differences that are avoidable, unnecessary, unfair and unjust" (AMA and AAMC, 2021, p. 11). Furthermore, instead of referring to cultural competence, the committee has chosen to focus on cultural humility and cultural sensitivity. *Cultural competence* implies a finite concept that has an end point that can be attained (largely based on the learner's confidence and comfort, and mastery of specific knowledge) (AMA and AAMC, 2021). *Cultural humility*, on the other hand, recognizes the need for lifelong learning and self-reflection to redress power imbalances and develop mutually beneficial partnerships (Tervalon and Murray-Garcia, 1998). *Cultural sensitivity* means that cultural norms, values, and practices are understood, respected, and accommodated in the planning and implementation of care practices (Mahmood et al., 2021; Meydanlioglu et al., 2015).

Approach to the Continuum of Long-Term Care Services

Long-term care typically refers to the provision of a wide range of services for varying lengths of time to promote healthy well-being and independence. Most long-term care facilities serve older adults and individuals with disabilities or severe/chronic illnesses (NIA, 2017). Settings for long-term care include private homes, independent living facilities, assisted living facilities, nursing homes, and skilled nursing facilities. While individuals may move among these settings during their lifetime, this committee's charge was to focus only on the nursing home setting. However, in accordance with the statement of task, the committee does address the larger long-term care system as a contextual factor when appropriate.

Approach to Different Nursing Home Populations

Many different populations, with different care needs, goals, and lived experiences, reside in nursing homes. In particular, a significant and growing number of people under the age of 65 reside in nursing homes. Specific information about the characteristics of this population, however, is extremely limited, or outdated (see Chapter 2). For the purposes of this study, the committee primarily focused on older adults in nursing homes but asserts that its conclusions and recommendations are equally applicable for these populations, given the committee's focus on person-centered care.

Approach to Health Equity and Disparities

Systemic failings such as neighborhood segregation, racism, and ageism have long been present in health care. These failings contribute to the poor health outcomes consistently shown for racial/ethnic minorities and those with low socioeconomic status (e.g., low household income, educational attainment), which are exacerbated by reduced access to health care and compromised quality of care. The health disadvantages due to these systemic failings and the resultant health and health care–related disparities accumulate over the life course to create inequities in patient outcomes in the long-term care system (Dannefer, 2003). The 2017 National Academies report *Communities in Action: Pathways to Health Equity* stated:

> Health equity is the state in which everyone has the opportunity to attain full health potential and no one is disadvantaged from achieving this potential because of social position or any other socially defined circumstance. Health equity and opportunity are inextricably linked. Currently in the United States, the burdens of disease and poor health and the benefits of well-being and good health are inequitably distributed. This inequitable distribution is caused by social, environmental, economic, and structural factors that shape health and are themselves distributed unequally, with pronounced differences in opportunities for health. (NASEM, 2017, p. 1)

Health equity is generally aspirational and raises a wide range of questions. What does an equitable nursing home system generally—and a nursing home specifically—look like? What processes are needed for residents to receive care in an "equitable nursing home"? What are the barriers to an equitable nursing home system? Can we address those barriers, especially those related historical and structural racism? Do we define health equity in this context as a system where disparities across specific demographic categories (e.g., race, ethnicity, geographic location) are reduced, or a system where a demographic category does not predict poor quality nursing home care?

The committee determined early in the study process that health equity is a fundamental component of high-quality care. Rather than isolating the topic in an individual chapter, the committee decided that health equity would serve as a lens for all the topics discussed throughout the report. When an individual enters a nursing home, he or she should have the same expectations of high-quality care as any other regardless of race or ethnicity, language, gender, gender identity, or socioeconomic status. Importantly, the health equity lens was critical as the committee developed its recommendations focused on the goal of reducing disparities. That is, the committee considered how the implementation of each recommendation could affect sociodemographic groups differently or in ways that exacerbate disparities across groups.

Approach to the COVID-19 Pandemic

As noted above, the committee's charge was to undertake a broad assessment of the quality of care in nursing homes and the factors that affect that care. While this was not a study focused on the impact of the COVID-19 pandemic on nursing homes, the committee recognized that the pandemic itself served to reveal and amplify the long-standing challenges and serious problems that exist in nursing home settings and have a direct impact on the quality of care provided. Thus, the COVID-19 pandemic served as another lens through which the committee explored the wide range of issues affecting the quality of care in nursing homes. This report presents examples specific to the context of the COVID-19 pandemic, which serve to exemplify the challenges to providing quality, person-centered care to all nursing home residents.

Challenges of the Evidence Base

As the committee undertook the challenge of assessing the way the nation delivers, finances, regulates, and measures the quality of care in nursing homes, it quickly became evident that there were significant shortcomings in the evidence base on nursing home quality. First, the committee found a significant lack of data in many key areas, with many of the available data sources and studies quite dated; in many instances, the most recent studies on a specific topic had been conducted years or even decades earlier. Furthermore, much of the available research relies on retrospective cohort designs and is constrained by the limitations in data. Second, many sources did not distinguish among the populations studied. For example, in some studies, short-stay residents were not distinguished from long-stay residents, and studies of younger populations did not distinguish among the age groups below age 65. Moreover, many studies do not distinguish long-term care residents by setting of care (e.g., nursing home versus assisted living facility). Finally, given that this study was conducted in the midst of the COVID-19 pandemic, the committee was challenged to keep up with the inundation of information released on a daily basis—both in the popular press and the peer-reviewed literature. The committee sought to examine all sources and to prioritize the most salient research in order to inform its deliberations.

CONCEPTUAL MODEL OF NURSING HOME QUALITY

Given that the committee's charge was to examine the quality of care in nursing homes, the committee members sought to develop a framework to help guide them in their work. Over time, scholars and professional health care organizations have developed a variety of conceptual models in an attempt to concisely define and measure nursing home quality, and, as a framework for this study, the committee created an original conceptual model of the quality of care in nursing homes based on a content analysis of existing conceptual models (or approaches) of health care quality or quality of care in nursing homes (see Box 1-3). Committee members performed multiple iterative rounds of analysis on this model, with the committee refining the model throughout the study process.

As the model depicts (see Figure 1-1), the committee's vision of nursing home quality is that *residents of nursing homes receive care in a safe*

> **BOX 1-3**
> **Conceptual Models of Quality Reviewed by the Committee**
>
> - IOM Six Domains of Health Care Quality (IOM, 2001b)
> - IHI Triple Aim to optimizing health system performance (IHI, 2021a)
> - The 4M's Framework (Fulmer, 2018; IHI, 2021b)
> - National Quality Forum (NQF, 2021)
> - Donabedian (structure, process, and outcomes) (Donabedian, 1988)
> - CAHPS AHRQ Composite measures (Rauch et al., 2019)
> - Principles of Culture Change (see Chapter 4, Box 4-1)
> - Observable Indicators of Quality (Rantz et al., 2006)
> - Good Quality and Poor Quality of Care Model (Rantz et al., 1998)
> - Integrated Multidimensional Model of Quality Nursing Home Care (consumers/providers combined) (Rantz et al., 1999)

environment that honors their values and preferences, addresses goals of care, promotes equity, and assesses benefits and risks of care and treatments. However, as the committee's evaluation of the evidence in the following chapters demonstrates, this model of quality care is not the reality in many nursing homes; rather, huge gaps in the quality of care remain despite years of research, advocacy, and regulation.

The conceptual model has three major components—inputs, nursing home care, and outcomes—and the model's elements and the evidence supporting them are discussed throughout this report in greater detail. The model presents high-quality nursing home care as having a central focus on the nursing home residents that is person centered, culturally sensitive, respectful, and sensitive to social determinants of health. Additional core aspects of the model include that it is person directed; resident needs are met; and that it maintains dignity, maximizes independence, balances autonomy and safety, and allows for meaningful relationships.

Inputs to Nursing Home Quality

Inputs that affect nursing home care include payment and financing, national and state policy, market trends, consumer expectations, workforce, ownership and operators, the surrounding community, referring health systems, and external quality improvement supports. The committee emphasizes that equity transcends all key categories of nursing home care;

INTRODUCTION

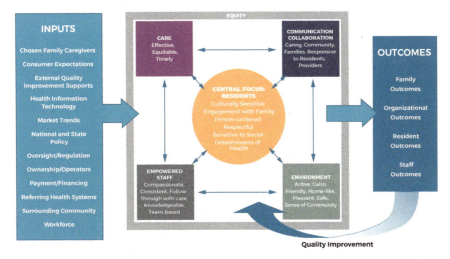

FIGURE 1-1 Conceptual model of the quality of care in nursing homes.

therefore, the model positions equity as surrounding nursing home care and envisioned that it must influence each of the categories.

Categories of Nursing Home Care

In addition to the central focus on residents, four other key categories in the conceptualization of high-quality nursing home care are

- Care that is effective, timely, and equitable;
- Communication that is caring and responsive to residents, families, providers, and community;
- Empowered staff who are knowledgeable, consistent, compassionate, and team based and who follow through with care; and
- An environment that is calm and active (in a way that aligns with residents' needs), friendly, and pleasant; that has community involvement; and that is home-like.

Care

The committee envisions the "care" category to encompass elements such as addressing basic human needs, including

- Physiological needs (e.g., food, water, and rest and safety and security needs, such as being free of illness and injury);
- Social needs (e.g., companionship, family, affection); and
- Self-esteem needs (e.g., independence, meaningful activities, self-worth; and the ability to reach one's full potential, including having optimal quality of life and meeting spiritual needs).

Care should also address individual care needs, including serious illness and end-of-life care, chronic disease, and behavioral health management (e.g., medication, treatment) with health restoration and preservation of function and comfort.

Communication

The communication category encompasses both relationships and communication. Thus the category includes fostering close relationships among residents, staff, and families; positive communication (verbal and nonverbal) with residents; staff who are open and listen to families; staff who take the time to really talk with residents; collaboration, communication, and shared decision making and care planning among staff, families, and health care providers. The category also includes coordination of care with internal and outside entities and the integration of health information technology.

Empowered Staff

The empowered staff category refers to having an effective, stable leadership involved in care. This ranges from registered nurses involved in planning and care delivery and knowledgeable, interdisciplinary staff who can meet resident basic human and behavioral health needs, to having all staff and leaders working as a team. The category also includes sensitivity to the culture of all staff, residents, and families; respect for residents' needs, likes, and dislikes; collaboration among staff and families in working with residents; and the involvement of staff and families in care plans. This category also includes having staff in adequate numbers and consistent staff to care for residents (staff who know them well and help meet their needs); adequate supervision and training; and low staff turnover and low staff burnout.

Environment

The environment category involves issues such as a physical environment for residents and staff that is designed to be safe and secure; is odor

INTRODUCTION

free and clean, with pleasant smells and sounds; and is well maintained and natural, with good lighting. Outdoor access is important, as is having community involvement; having interaction with volunteers, animals, and children; having residents engaged in age and functionally appropriate activities; and the nursing home feeling like a home, not a warehouse. Evidence of emergency preparedness is also a critical element of this category.

Outcomes of High-Quality Care

Outcomes of nursing home care include resident, family, staff, and organizational outcomes as well as outcomes related to regulation and oversight. Resident outcomes include quality of life, experience with care, satisfaction, nursing home quality measures (for both long-stay and short-stay residents), hospital admissions, health equity, and goal attainment. Family outcomes include experience with care, satisfaction, burden, and social connectedness. Staff outcomes include staff turnover and retention, staff satisfaction, and staff knowledge and competence. Organizational outcomes include publicly reported quality measures, occupancy rate, financial performance and reserves, community representation and connections, and health information technology connectivity. Oversight and regulatory outcomes include the results seen in state surveys.

Continuous Quality Improvement

Quality improvement is an important action step within the committee's conceptual model. The nursing home setting, as is the case in all sectors of health care, has a long history of using quality improvement methods to measure the quality of care. Facilities use the results of those measurements to strive to continuously improve care by engaging with the nursing home staff, residents, and families to develop and implement improvement plans. If successful, quality improvement efforts result in anticipated improvements documented in the outcomes. If the results are not as anticipated, the iterative problem-solving process for new solutions begins.

ORGANIZATION OF THE REPORT

The committee structured its report around the components of the conceptual model. This introductory chapter has described the study context, charge to the committee, scope and methods of the study, and the conceptual model. Chapter 2 provides additional information on the landscape of the nursing home sector today. Chapter 3 examines issues related to quality measurement and quality improvement. Chapter 4 focuses on care delivery in nursing homes, while Chapter 5 examines the workforce that supports nursing home residents. Chapter 6 addresses issues related to the safety and environment. Chapter 7 explores the financing of nursing home care. Chapter 8 addresses issues related to quality assurance, specifically, the oversight and regulation of nursing homes. Chapter 9 provides information on health information technology. Finally, Chapter 10 presents the committee's recommendations for improving the quality of care in nursing homes.

In addition to the main report, there are five appendixes. Appendix A contains committee and staff biographies. Appendix B provides examples of successful demonstration projects in the Initiative to Reduce Avoidable Hospitalizations among Nursing Facility Residents. Appendix C contains an overview of the areas of measurement and priority areas for research included among the committee's recommendations, and Appendix D provides a table of the committee's recommendations organized by responsible partner. Appendix E includes a categorization of the committee's recommendations according to an estimated implementation timeline.

CONCLUSION

Though nursing homes vary in size, type, and layout, in general they can be viewed as "complex social systems that consist of different participants, including staff, leaders, residents, and families in constantly shifting interactions" (Myhre et al., 2020). The following chapters present the evidence base for the current quality of care in nursing homes and, ultimately, the committee's integrated set of recommendations to move the nation closer to achieving high-quality, person-centered, and equitable care for all nursing home residents, their families, and the staff who provide care for and support residents' choices and goals.

REFERENCES

AHCA/NCAL (American Health Care Association and National Center for Assisted Living). 2021. *State of the long term care industry: Survey of nursing home and assisted living providers show industry facing significant workforce crisis.* https://www.ahcancal.org/News-and-Communications/Fact-Sheets/FactSheets/Workforce-Survey-September 2021.pdf (accessed October 7, 2021).

AMA and AAMC (American Medical Association and Association of American Medical Colleges). 2021. *Advancing health equity: Guide on language, narrative and concepts.* https://www.ama-assn.org/system/files/ama-aamc-equity-guide.pdf (accessed February 6, 2022).

Aronson, L. 2020. *Ageism is making the pandemic worse.* https://www.theatlantic.com/culture/archive/2020/03/american-ageism-crisis-is-helping-the-coronavirus/608905 (accessed February 7, 2022).

Berklan, J. M. 2021. *Nursing home occupancy woes worse than popularly reported, industry expert says.* https://www.mcknights.com/news/nursing-home-occupancy-woes-worse-than-popularly-reported-industry-expert-says (accessed February 5, 2022).

Beynon, C., R. Perkins, and L. Edelman. 2020. Breaking down stigma: Honoring nursing home staff during COVID-19. *Journal of Gerontological Nursing* 46(8):5.

Carbonaro, G. 2020. 'Every life matters': WHO chief warns against COVID-19 age discrimination. https://newseu.cgtn.com/news/2020-03-11/-Every-life-matters-WHO-warns-against-COVID-19-age-discrimination-OKDSHuH0gU/index.html (accessed February 14, 2022).

CDC (Centers for Disease Control and Prevention). 2017. *Table 92. Nursing homes, beds, residents, and occupancy rates, by state: United States, selected years 1995–2016*. https://www.cdc.gov/nchs/data/hus/2017/092.pdf (accessed November 19, 2021).

CDC. 2020. *National Center for Health Statistics—Nursing home care*. https://www.cdc.gov/nchs/fastats/nursing-home-care.htm (accessed October 16, 2020).

CDC. 2021a. *COVID data tracker*. https://covid.cdc.gov/covid-data-tracker/#datatracker-home (accessed June 7, 2021).

CDC. 2021b. *COVID data tracker weekly review*. https://www.cdc.gov/coronavirus/2019-ncov/covid-data/covidview/index.html (accessed November 12, 2021).

CMS (Centers for Medicare & Medicaid Services). 2015. *Nursing home data compendium*. Baltimore, MD: Centers for Medicare & Medicaid Services.

Danilovich, M. 2017. *Crisis of recruitment: Stereotypes hinder staffing in geriatric service*. https://medium.com/thrive-global/how-stereotypes-about-nursing-homes-can-make-aging-harder-for-everyone-51ff2d53fefd (accessed February 15, 2022).

Dannefer, D. 2003. Cumulative advantage/disadvantage and the life course: Cross-fertilizing age and social science theory. *Journals of Gerontology Series B: Psychological Sciences and Social Sciences* 58(6):S327–S337.

Donabedian, A. 1988. The quality of care. How can it be assessed? *JAMA* 260(12):1743–1948.

Fashaw, S. A., K. S. Thomas, E. McCreedy, and V. Mor. 2020. 30-year trends in nursing home composition and quality since the passage of OBRA. *Journal of the American Medical Directors Association* 21(2):233–239.

Fazio, S., D. Pace, J. Flinner, and B. Kallmyer. 2018. The fundamentals of person-centered care for individuals with dementia. *The Gerontologist* 58(S1):S10–S19.

Fraser, S., M. Lagace, B. Bongue, N. Ndeye, J. Guyot, L. Bechard, L. Garcia, V. Taler, CCNA Social Inclusion and Stigma Working Group, S. Adam, M. Beaulieu, C. D. Bergeron, V. Boudjemadi, D. Desmette, A. R. Doizzetti, S. Ethier, S. Garon, M. Gillis, M. Levasseur, M. Lortie-Lussier, P. Marier, A. Robitaille, K. Sawchuk, C. Lafontaine, and F. Tougas. 2020. Ageism and COVID-19: What does our society's response say about us? *Age Ageing* 49(5):692–695.

Fulmer, T. 2018. *Discovering the 4Ms: A framework for creating age-friendly health systems*. https://www.johnahartford.org/blog/view/discovering-the-4ms-a-framework-for-creating-age-friendly-health-systems (accessed February 25, 2021).

Gandhi, A., H. Yu, and D. C. Grabowski. 2021. High nursing staff turnover in nursing homes offers important quality information. *Health Affairs* 40(3):384–391.

GAO (U.S. Government Accountability Office). 2003. *Nursing home quality: Prevalence of serious problems, while declining, reinforces importance of enhanced oversight*. Washington, DC: U.S. Government Accountability Office.

Grabowski, D. C. 2020. *Strengthening nursing home policy for the postpandemic world: How can we improve residents' health outcomes and experiences?* New York: The Commonwealth Fund.

Harrington, C., J. F. Schnelle, M. McGregor, and S. F. Simmons. 2016. The need for higher minimum staffing standards in U.S. Nursing homes. *Health services insights* 9:13-19.

Harrington, C., H. Carrillo, R. Garfield, M. Musumeci, and E. Squires. 2018. *Nursing facilities, staffing, residents and facility deficiencies, 2009 through 2016*. https://files.kff.org/attachment/REPORT-Nursing-Facilities-Staffing-Residents-and-Facility-Deficiencies-2009-2016 (accessed February 5, 2022).

Harris-Kojetin, L., M. Sengupta, J. P. Lendon, V. Rome, R. Valverde, and C. Caffrey. 2019. *Long-term care providers and services users in the United States, 2015–2016.* Vital and Health Statistics, series 3, no. 43. Washington, DC: U.S. Government Publishing Office. https://www.cdc.gov/nchs/data/series/sr_03/sr03_43-508.pdf (accessed November 22, 2021).

IHI (Institute for Healthcare Improvement). 2021a. *The IHI Triple Aim.* http://www.ihi.org/Engage/Initiatives/TripleAim/Pages/default.aspx (accessed January 12, 2021).

IHI. 2021b. *What is an age-friendly health system?* http://www.ihi.org/Engage/Initiatives/Age-Friendly-Health-Systems/Pages/default.aspx (accessed November 18, 2021).

IOM (Institute of Medicine). 1986. *Improving the quality of care in nursing homes.* Washington, DC: National Academy Press.

IOM. 1996. *Nursing staff in hospitals and nursing homes: Is it adequate?* Washington, DC: National Academy Press.

IOM. 2001a. *Improving the quality of long-term care.* Washington, DC: National Academy Press.

IOM. 2001b. *Crossing the quality chasm: A new health system for the 21st century.* Washington, DC: National Academy Press.

IOM. 2004. *Keeping patients safe: Transforming the work environment of nurses.* Washington, DC: The National Academies Press.

IOM. 2008. *Retooling for an aging America: Building the health care workforce.* Washington, DC: The National Academies Press.

IOM. 2016. *Families caring for an aging America.* Washington, DC: The National Academies Press.

Kendall-Taylor, N., A. Neumann, and J. Schoen. 2020. *Advocating for age in an age of uncertainty.* https://ssir.org/articles/entry/advocating_for_age_in_an_age_of_uncertainty (accessed February 14, 2022).

KFF (Kaiser Family Foundation). 2020a. *Total number of residents in certified nursing facilities.* https://www.kff.org/other/state-indicator/number-of-nursing-facility-residents (accessed September 30, 2021).

KFF. 2020b. *Certified nursing facility occupancy rate.* https://www.kff.org/other/state-indicator/nursing-facility-occupancy-rates (accessed January 6, 2022).

KFF. 2020c. *Percent of certified nursing facilities with top ten deficiencies.* https://www.kff.org/other/state-indicator/percent-of-certified-nursing-facilities-with-top-ten-deficiencies-2014 (accessed September 30, 2021).

KFF. 2020d. *Percent of certified nursing facilities receiving a deficiency for actual harm or jeopardy.* https://www.kff.org/other/state-indicator/of-facilities-w-serious-deficiencies (accessed September 30, 2021).

Kilaru, A. S., and R. E. Gee. 2020. Structural ageism and the health of older adults. *JAMA Health Forum* 1(10):e201249.

Kogan, A. C., K. Wilber, and L. Mosqueda. 2016. Person-centered care for older adults with chronic conditions and functional impairment: A systematic literature review. *Journal of the American Geriatrics Society* 64(1):e1–e7.

Kramer, R. G. 2021. *Fixing nursing homes: A fleeting opportunity.* https://www.healthaffairs.org/do/10.1377/forefront.20210407.717832/full (accessed February 16, 2022).

Lewis, T. 2021. *Nursing home workers had one of the deadliest jobs of 2020.* https://www.scientificamerican.com/article/nursing-home-workers-had-one-of-the-deadliest-jobs-of-2020 (accessed January 6, 2022).

Mahmood, M. A., K. S. Khan, and J. R. Moss. 2021. Applying public health principles to better manage the COVID-19 pandemic: "Community participation," "equity," and "cultural sensitivity." *Asia Pacific Journal of Public Health* 33(8):951–952.

Manchha, A. V., N. Walker, K. A. Way, D. Dawson, K. Tann, and M. Thai. 2021. Deeply discrediting: A systematic review examining the conceptualizations and consequences of the stigma of working in aged care. *The Gerontologist* 61(4):e129–e146.

Manchha, A. V., K. A. Way, K. Tann, and M. Thai. 2022. The social construction of stigma in aged-care work: Implications for health professionals' work intentions. *The Gerontologist.* https://doi.org/10.1093/geront/gnac002.

Meydanlioglu, A., F. Arikan, and S. Gozum. 2015. Cultural sensitivity levels of university students in receiving education in health disciplines. *Advances in Health Sciences Education* 20:1195–1204.

Myhre, J., S. Saga, W. Malmedal, J. Ostaszkiewicz, and S. Nakrem. 2020. Elder abuse and neglect: An overlooked patient safety issue. A focus group study of nursing home leaders' perceptions of elder abuse and neglect. *BMC Health Services Research* 20(1):199.

NASEM (National Academies of Sciences, Engineering, and Medicine). 2017. *Communities in action: Pathways to health equity.* Washington, DC: The National Academies Press.

NASEM. 2020. *Social isolation and loneliness in older adults: Opportunities for the health care system.* Washington, DC: The National Academies Press.

NIA (National Institute on Aging). 2017. *What is long-term care?* https://www.nia.nih.gov/health/what-long-term-care (accessed April 20, 2021).

NIC (National Investment Center for Seniors Housing & Care). 2021. *Occupancy at U.S. skilled nursing facilities hits new low.* https://www.nic.org/news-press/occupancy-at-u-s-skilled-nursing-facilities-hits-new-low (accessed January 6, 2022).

NQF (National Quality Forum). 2021. *NQF.* http://www.qualityforum.org (accessed February 2, 2021).

Paulin, E. 2021. *Nursing homes are filled with empty beds, raising more concerns about care.* https://www.aarp.org/caregiving/nursing-homes/info-2021/nursing-home-low-occupancy.html (accessed January 6, 2022).

Rantz, M. J., D. R. Mehr, L. Popejoy, M. Zwygart-Stauffacher, L. L. Hicks, V. Grando, V. S. Conn, R. Porter, J. Scott, and M. Maas. 1998. Nursing home care quality: A multidimensional theoretical model. *Journal of Nursing Care Quality* 12(3):30–46.

Rantz, M. J., M. Zwygart-Stauffacher, L. Popejoy, V. T. Grando, D. R. Mehr, L. L. Hicks, V. S. Conn, D. Wipke-Tevis, R. Porter, J. Bostick, M. Maas, and J. Scott. 1999. Nursing home care quality: A multidimensional theoretical model integrating the views of consumers and providers. *Journal of Nursing Care Quality* 14(1):16–37; quiz 85–87.

Rantz, M. J., M. Zwygart-Stauffacher, D. R. Mehr, G. F. Petroski, S. V. Owen, R. W. Madsen, M. Flesner, V. Conn, J. Bostick, R. Smith, and M. Maas. 2006. Field testing, refinement, and psychometric evaluation of a new measure of nursing home care quality. *Journal of Nursing Measurement* 14(2):129–148.

Rauch, J., M. Baxter, D. Quave, N. Yount, and D. Shaller. 2019. *2019 CAHPS health plan survey database, 2019 chartbook: What consumers say about their experiences with their health plans and medical care.* https://cahpsdatabase.ahrq.gov/files/2019CAHPSHealthPlanChartbook.pdf (accessed February 25, 2021).

Scales, K., M. Lepore, R. A. Anderson, E. S. McConnell, Y. Song, B. Kang, K. Porter, T. Thach, and K. N. Corazzini. 2017. Person-directed care planning in nursing homes: Resident, family, and staff perspectives. *Journal of Applied Gerontology* 38(2):183–206.

Taylor, S., and S. Wilson. 2021. *Initial observations of SNF trends data illustrates COVID-19 challenges.* https://www.claconnect.com/resources/articles/2021/initial-observations-of-snf-trends-data-illustrates-covid-19-challenges (accessed January 20, 2022).

Tervalon, M., and J. Murray-Garcia. 1998. Cultural humility versus cultural competence: A critical distinction in defining physician training outcomes in multicultural education. *Journal of Health Care for the Poor and Underserved* 9(2):117–125.

U.S. Census Bureau. 2021. *U.S. and world population clock.* https://www.census.gov/popclock (accessed November 12, 2021).

Wiener, J. M., M. P. Freiman, D. Brown, and RTI International. 2007. *Nursing home care quality: Twenty years after the Omnibus Budget Reconciliation Act of 1987.* Durham, North Carolina: RTI International.

Evolution and Landscape of Nursing Home Care in the United States

The landscape of nursing home care has evolved significantly over the past few decades. When the Institute of Medicine (IOM) released *Improving the Quality of Care in Nursing Homes* in 1986, the contexts for policy, financing, program, research, and quality were vastly different. For example, the capacity to measure quality in long-term care settings was quite limited. Assisted living facilities did not exist, continuing care retirement communities were just being introduced, and home and community-based services were newly developed features of long-term services and supports. Personal computers were gradually coming on the market, electronic health records were in their infancy, and the Internet did not yet exist on a broad scale. This chapter documents the history, evolution, and current landscape of nursing home care in the United States and sets the stage for the report's subsequent chapters, which provide the evidence base for the committee's recommendations for delivering high-quality nursing home care.

BRIEF HISTORY OF NURSING HOMES

Historically, families were responsible for the majority of care for older adults or people with disabilities. Dating back to medieval times, poorhouses (also known as "almshouses") provided care in congregate settings for individuals with disabilities, orphans, and older adults (Ogden and Adams, 2019). Poorhouses were created based on principles of hospitality and shelter for the poor and individuals experiencing homelessness, but they soon became the only option for widows, orphans, older adults, and poor people with mental illnesses, physical ailments, such as epilepsy or blindness, and infectious diseases, such as tuberculosis (Gillick, 2018; Watson, 2012). Such poorhouses were known for nonexistent safety and sanitation standards and poor-quality care that was not customized to an individual's needs. Stigmatization of public assistance and of the populations of poorhouses perpetuated these harsh conditions and served as a barrier to improving care.

The first steps to improving care for older adults were taken with efforts in the early twentieth century to distinguish among the various populations residing within the poorhouses. Some individuals were transitioned out of poorhouses into state-sponsored, specialized institutions and other acute care facilities (Gillick, 2018; Watson, 2012). Despite such efforts, many older adults had no choice but to remain in poorhouses (Wagner, 2005).

The watershed moment for modern-day nursing home care in the United States was the passage of the Social Security Act in 1935, which prohibited providing federal assistance to residents of poorhouses (IOM, 1986a; Watson, 2012). With this ban, older adults were forced to seek long-term care in private institutions. However, amendments to the act in 1950 allowed payment for care in licensed public institutions, which led to a rapid growth of the current system of nursing homes (both public and private). As a result, "[by] shutting the almshouse door, policymakers gave birth to the modern nursing home industry" (FATE, 2020).

The demographics of residents in nursing homes have evolved over time, as has the proportion of the U.S. population seeking care in nursing homes. Today, alternative long-term care settings exist, and nursing home residents' level of acuity and case mix have shifted due to the availability of post-acute care, palliative care, and hospice options. While older adults are increasingly seeking care in alternate long-term care settings, such as assisted living facilities and at home, the number of short stays in nursing homes has also increased significantly (Yurkofsky and Ouslander, 2021a). As a result, nursing homes are generally admitting residents with higher acuity and nursing needs (Fry et al., 2018) and need to adapt to continue delivering high-quality care. Changes in the availability of care and disparities in access to care services are discussed below and in Chapter 4. Moreover, advances in health information technology (HIT) such as the development of electronic health records and health information exchanges, have transformed the way care is delivered. As of 2016, nearly 15,600 U.S. nursing homes containing 1.7 million beds cared for over 1.3 million residents (CDC, 2020a).

Care delivery in nursing homes has long mirrored an acute care model with a medical focus. The reconfiguration of hospitals after World War II to include rehabilitative care and extended recuperative care placed more of a formal medical focus on the role of nursing homes (IOM, 1986b). The 1946

Hospital Survey and Construction Act,[1] also known as the "Hill-Burton Act," formulated and financed the construction and staffing patterns of health care facilities, further transforming nursing homes into medical settings. The demand for nursing home care grew quickly—because of both an increase in the number of individuals who needed it and the expansion of coverage for care in this setting by Medicare and Medicaid. As a result, the industry embraced larger facilities with more beds and chain ownership (IOM, 1986b).

Over time, because nursing homes are also a place of residence, many stakeholders began to recognize the need to balance the delivery of clinical care with quality of life in order to make them feel more like homes. The culture change movement in nursing homes, which dates back to the 1980s, strives to fundamentally alter beliefs and practices among all stakeholders, including residents, staff, and communities, away from a medicalized, institutionalized model toward a person-centered care model (Koren, 2010). Resident choice is a core value of this movement, with an overarching goal of enhancing both quality of life and quality of care. (See Chapter 4 for further discussion about culture change in nursing homes.)

Most recently, the need for a more balanced approach between clinical care and ensuring quality of life in a home-like setting became even more evident by the catastrophic impact the COVID-19 pandemic had on nursing home care, residents, and staff. The scope of that impact became apparent early in the pandemic, generating widespread media attention and significant public alarm. The virus that causes COVID-19 (SARS-CoV-2) is particularly dangerous for older adults with underlying health issues. Thus, nursing home residents suffered disproportionately high rates of cases, hospitalizations, and deaths relative to the general population. The consequences of COVID-19 and efforts to address these are discussed throughout the report.

CURRENT NURSING HOME POPULATION

Over 1.3 million people in the United States live in nursing homes (CDC, 2020a). The demographic characteristics of this population vary greatly, as discussed below.

Age

The majority (83.5 percent) of nursing home residents are 65 and older. More than one-third (38.6 percent) are 85 and older (Harris-Kojetin et al., 2019) (see Figure 2-1).

---

[1] Hospital Survey and Construction Act of 1946, Public Law 79-725, 79th Cong., 2nd Sess. (August 13, 1946).

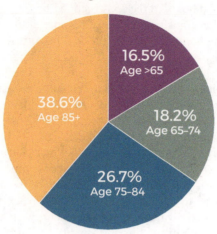

FIGURE 2-1 Age of residents in nursing homes.
SOURCE: Harris-Kojetin et al., 2019.

Residents under 65 are the most rapidly growing age group in nursing homes, despite the Healthy People 2010 and 2020 goals of shifting care of children and young adults out of nursing homes and into home- and community-based settings (Jin and Agrawal, 2017). Despite the increasing numbers of younger residents, very little is known about them (Shieu et al., 2021). The limited data available rarely distinguish by age group under 65, and most of it is not up to date. For example, a 2009 study of nursing home residents revealed that younger residents are often male, single, and with low levels of education and typically admitted from acute, psychiatric, or rehabilitation hospitals (Persson and Ostwald, 2009). In 2012, the prevalence of residents 30 years old or younger in nursing homes was approximately 5.5 out of 100,000 (Jin and Agrawal, 2017). New Jersey had the highest prevalence, at 14 out of 100,000 (Jin and Agrawal, 2017). A study found that between 2000 and 2017, the percentage of the nursing home population younger than 65 increased by nearly 6 percent and the average age fell by over 2 years (from 81.1 to 78.8) (Laws et al., 2021).

Both older and younger nursing home residents value autonomy, identity, socialization, and privacy. Younger residents in particular identify age-appropriate activities and environments, freedom and expression, and opportunities to interact with peers as important components of their quality of life (Muenchberger et al., 2012; Shieu et al., 2021).

Medicaid covers the cost of nursing home care for a large majority of younger nursing home residents (Miller, 2011). State Medicaid policies and programs vary widely, however, which may result in unequal nursing home use by younger residents from state to state. The expansion of Medicaid eligibility (as a result of the Affordable Care Act[2]) facilitated access to post-acute nursing home care for individuals under age 65 (Ritter et al., 2021).

The limited data available indicate that younger adult nursing home residents typically have a higher prevalence of psychiatric conditions, including anxiety, depression, bipolar disorder, and schizophrenia, than older adults (Miller et al., 2012). Middle-aged adults (31–64 years old) commonly present to nursing homes with chronic conditions (e.g., diabetes, chronic obstructive pulmonary disease, asthma, renal failure, or circulatory/heart conditions). From 2000 to 2008, the proportion of Black and Latinx middle-aged residents increased. Black middle-aged residents were also overrepresented compared with their proportion in the general population (Miller et al., 2012).

Gender Identity and Sexual Orientation

A significant lack of evidence about the lesbian, gay, bisexual, transgender, queer or questioning, and others (LGBTQ+) population in nursing homes is due, in part, to the overall lack of data on the LGBTQ+ population (Choi and Meyer, 2016; Fredriksen Goldsen et al., 2019). Measures of the LGBTQ+ population have never been included in the U.S. census, but approximately 3 million LGBTQ+ adults 55 or older live in the United States, which is projected to double in the next two decades (Espinoza, 2014; SAGE, 2021). LGBTQ+ older adults tend to be single and living alone without children, which makes it more likely that they will need to rely on families of choice or long-term care facilities as they age (SAGE, 2021).

LGBTQ+ older adults face unique challenges when seeking long-term care services. These include discrimination and harassment, inappropriate or neglectful care, a lack of LGBTQ+-specific resources, and anticipatory stress related to concealing their identities (Caceres et al., 2020; Putney et al., 2018). Approximately 20 percent of LGBTQ+ individuals have not shared their sexual orientation or gender identity with their health care providers because they are afraid of receiving substandard care (Caceres et al., 2020).

LGBTQ+ people who seek nursing home care may have unique health care and social care needs. For example, compared with cisgender and

---

[2] For more information, see https://www.hhs.gov/healthcare/about-the-aca/index.html (accessed October 4, 2021).

heterosexual[3] older adults, older members of the LGBTQ+ community are more likely to have poor physical or mental health, delay or avoid seeking health care, report having a disability, be socially isolated, smoke or engage in alcohol or substance use, report suicidal thoughts, have lower incomes, and experience poverty or homelessness (Candrian et al., 2021; SAGE, 2021).

Members of the LGBTQ+ community may face harassment and abuse in nursing homes. Nearly one-quarter of LGBTQ+ report experiencing verbal or physical harassment, or both, from other residents, and approximately 14 percent report experiencing verbal or physical harassment, or both, from staff (Justice in Aging et al., 2015). Significant percentages of LGBTQ+ adults report fearing neglect (67 percent), abuse (62 percent), limited access to services (61 percent), and verbal or physical harassment (60 percent) in long-term care settings (Houghton, 2018). Efforts to improve the quality of care for this population of nursing home residents include enhanced staff training in LGBTQ+-affirming care (Putney et al., 2018).

Race and Ethnicity

In 2018, 23 percent of all adults over 65 in the United States identified as part of racial and ethnic minority populations (about 9 percent were non-Hispanic Black, 6 percent were non-Hispanic other, and 8 percent were Hispanic) (AoA, 2020). Similarly, the majority of nursing home residents are non-Hispanic White, with smaller percentages identifying as non-Hispanic Black, Hispanic, or non-Hispanic other (see Figure 2-2) (Bowblis et al., 2021; Harris-Kojetin et al., 2019). Minority residents make up less than 2 percent of a facility's population in nearly half (43 percent) of all U.S. nursing homes (Sloane et al., 2021). However, the nursing home population (like the United States itself) is becoming more diverse. (See Chapter 5, Figure 5-3, for racial and ethnic diversity among nursing home staff.)

Disparities

A myriad of factors contribute to resident racial and ethnic disparities within and between nursing homes, including (1) limited clinical resources, (2) limited financial resources, (3) limited community resources, (4) lower levels of direct care, (5) limited or no bilingual staff or ombudsmen, and (6) larger staffing shortages (Lee et al., 2021). As a result, residents of racial or

---

[3] Cisgender is defined as "having or relating to a gender identity that corresponds to the culturally determined gender roles for one's birth sex (i.e., the biological sex one was born with)"; heterosexuality is defined as "sexual attraction to or activity between members of the opposite sex" (APA, 2020a,b).

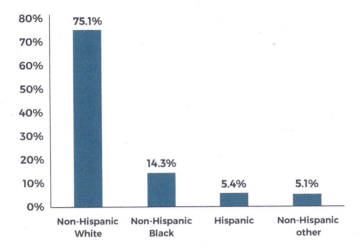

FIGURE 2-2 Race and ethnicity of nursing home residents.
SOURCE: Harris-Kojetin et al., 2019.

ethnic minority groups receive lower-quality care, which may result in higher rehospitalization rates and greater difficulties being discharged into their community as compared with non-Hispanic White residents (Lee et al., 2021).

For example, White nursing home residents with Alzheimer's disease and related dementias (ADRD) are more likely than Black or Hispanic residents to receive care in nursing homes with Alzheimer's special care units, which results in better health outcomes (Rivera-Hernandez et al., 2019). White nursing home residents with ADRD are also less likely to

- receive care in for-profit facilities, which typically demonstrate lower levels of quality than nonprofit facilities (see Chapter 8); and
- be enrolled in Medicare Advantage plans (which may be less willing to cover high use) (see Chapter 7) (Rivera-Hernandez et al., 2019).

White residents with ADRD are also less likely to be cognitively, functionally, or physically impaired compared to Hispanic and African American residents with ADRD, which suggests that the latter may be admitted to a nursing home at a later stage in their ADRD disease progression and receive delayed and inadequate care, although more research is needed to understand these characteristics' impact on access to services (Rivera-Hernandez et al., 2019).

One study in Minnesota used a resident-level dataset of long-stay residents to measure general quality of life and six simplified domain scores for resident quality of life in facility environment, attention from staff, food enjoyment, engagement, negative mood, and positive mood (Bowblis et al., 2021). In this study, the overall summary score reflected that Black, Indigenous, and other people of color (BIPOC) report lower quality of life than White nursing home residents (Bowblis et al., 2021). Previous studies found that disparities in quality of life for BIPOC residents, which was mostly explained by the racial composition of the facility itself (i.e., a higher percentage of BIPOC residents) (Bowblis et al., 2021; Shippee et al., 2016, 2020). Bowblis and colleagues (2021) concluded that "efforts need to focus on addressing systemic disparities for [nursing homes] with a high proportion of residents who are BIPOC" (p. 1051). Additionally, facilities with a higher concentration of racial and ethnic minority residents are more likely to have lower staffing levels, increasing their risk of poor-quality care (Li et al., 2015a,b). Another study found that Black residents were more likely than White residents to be dually eligible for Medicare and Medicaid and less likely to be admitted to nursing homes with four- or five-star ratings (Yan et al., 2021; see also Sharma et al., 2020). (See Chapter 3 for more on the five-star rating system.) Dual-eligible residents are more likely to be discharged to nursing homes with low staffing ratios and so more likely to become long-stay residents than Medicare-only beneficiaries (Rahman et al., 2014).

Research also reveals disparities in care, such as lower flu vaccination rates (Travers et al., 2018a,b), higher hospital readmission rates, and greater feelings of social isolation among racial and ethnic minorities than White residents in the same facility (Lee et al., 2021). According to reports by ombudsmen, racial and ethnic minority residents may avoid filing complaints about the quality of nursing home care out of fear of retaliation (Lee et al., 2021).

State surveyors are not required to collect data on race and ethnicity, nor are ombudsmen required to evaluate the quality of care and quality of life based on racial and ethnic differences. Other factors, such as privacy-related data constraints and small numbers of populations, also increase the difficulty in collecting and reporting data related to the race and ethnicity of nursing home residents (e.g., the Centers for Medicare & Medicaid Services [CMS] cannot publish data containing individual identifiers for a population of fewer than 10 individuals) (CMS, 2020). Moreover, racial and ethnic bias and sensitivity training is not currently required for nursing home staff (Mauldin et al., 2020). The lack of robust data specific to race and ethnicity in nursing homes makes it difficult to document the true extent and impact of disparities in care.

Systemic Issues

Systemic failings, such as neighborhood segregation, racism, and ageism, have had a long-standing impact on health care practices and policies, including those involved with nursing home care (Bowblis et al., 2021; Sloane et al., 2021). A systematic review of racial and ethnic disparities found that most are among long-term care facilities rather than within facilities, reflecting inequities in resources and infrastructure associated with residential segregation (Konetzka and Werner, 2009). Other studies have shown extensive racial segregation among nursing homes (Mack et al., 2020; Mauldin et al., 2020) and described the key factors driving it: (1) race-based facility preferences, (2) systemic racism, (3) disparities in funding, and (4) unequal distributions of staff (Mack et al., 2020).

This segregation contributes to consistently worse health outcomes in nursing homes for racial and ethnic minority populations, particularly if they are of lower socioeconomic status (Bowblis et al., 2021; Travers et al., 2021). For example, nursing homes located in an urban setting are at higher risk for having residents with low social engagement, which can contribute to worse physical health and low life satisfaction, increased social isolation and loneliness, higher mortality, poorer quality of life, cognitive decline, and visual or communication impairment (Bliss et al., 2017). These poor outcomes are exacerbated by reduced access to quality health care. These health and health care disparities accumulate over the life course to create and sustain inequities in resident outcomes (Bowblis et al., 2021).

Short-Stay and Long-Stay Residents

Nursing home residents comprise two distinct populations. Post-acute patients typically are admitted after a hospital stay and represent 43 percent of the nursing home population. Long-stay residents typically require care for chronic medical conditions and/or assistance with activities of daily living and represent 57 percent of the patient population (Harris-Kojetin et al., 2019). The average length of stay for a long-stay resident is 2.3 years, compared to 28 days for short-stay patients (Sifuentes and Lapane, 2020). The majority of the current long-stay population is White, but it is becoming more diverse (as discussed) (Bowblis et al., 2021). Figure 2-3 describes the common types of short- and long-stay residents.

Compared with short-stay residents, long-stay residents are more often women, more likely to be over the age of 65, and have higher rates of mental and chronic illnesses (Harris-Kojetin et al., 2019).

Residents under 65 account for 18.6 percent of the short-stay and 14.9 percent of the long-stay population (Harris-Kojetin et al., 2019). Recent findings indicate that a higher proportion of short-stay residents (23.8 percent) required an overnight hospital stay while living in a nursing home than long-stay residents (8.7 percent) (Harris-Kojetin et al., 2019).[4]

---

[4] This report used overnight hospitalization rates as measures of adverse and potentially avoidable events, but the data could also be the result of short-stay residents requiring hospitalization for acute illnesses or reflect differences in care preferences, as long-stay residents may prefer comfort care over hospitalization.

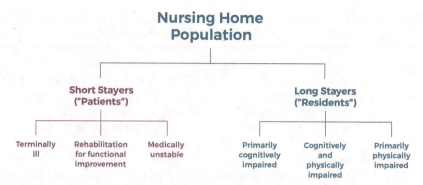

FIGURE 2-3 Types of short-stay and long-stay residents of nursing homes.
SOURCE: Ouslander and Grabowski, 2019.

Common Health Conditions

About 14.9 percent of people living in nursing homes require help with at least five activities of daily living (ADLs)[5] (CMS, 2015). Most have more than one chronic condition (such as arthritis, hypertension, diabetes, heart disease, or osteoporosis), and some also experience cognitive impairments or behavioral health conditions. The health of the nursing home population often differs between short- and long-stay residents (see Table 2-1).

Younger nursing home residents may have a wide range of care conditions, including depression, young-onset dementia, schizophrenia, seizure disorders, intellectual disabilities, traumatic injury, or hemi-quadriplegia, and many have little family or community support (Persson and Ostwald, 2009). Road traffic injuries, violence, and combat or sport injuries are common causes of traumatic brain injury and hemi-quadriplegia in this population (Shieu et al., 2021). Residents under 65 often experience higher rates of obesity, intellectual disabilities, and hemiplegia and quadriplegia than older adults in nursing homes (Persson and Ostwald, 2009).

Care Needs and Services Provided

To care for people with a variety of conditions, nursing homes provide a spectrum of services, including skilled nursing and medical care, 24-hour supervision, hospice and end-of-life care, treatments related to bladder or bowel incontinence, and assistance with ADLs.

---

[5] Activities of daily living are skills required to manage one's needs and can include basic ADLs (e.g., walking, feeding, dressing, personal hygiene, continence, and toileting) and instrumental ADLs (e.g., transportation, shopping, managing finances, meal preparation, housecleaning, and managing medications) (Edemekong et al., 2021).

TABLE 2-1 Common Conditions Among Nursing Home Residents

Condition	Percent of Nursing Home Residents
Arthritis	25.1% of short-stay residents
	29.7% of long-stay residents
Hypertension	71.5% of all residents
Diabetes	32.0% of all residents
Heart disease	38.1% of all residents
Osteoporosis	12.3% of all residents
Alzheimer's and related dementias	47.8% of all residents
	36.7% of short-stay residents
	58.9% of long-stay residents
Mild/no cognitive impairment	38.7% of all residents
Moderate cognitive impairment	24.8% of all residents
Severe cognitive impairment	36.6% of all residents
Significant mental health disorder*	65–91% of all residents
Depression	42.6% of short-stay residents
	53% of long-stay residents
Pain	33% of all residents
Fall resulting in no injury	11% of all residents
Fall resulting in injury	5.3% of all residents

SOURCES: CMS, 2015; Grabowski et al., 2010; Harris-Kojetin et al., 2019; Hunnicutt et al., 2017.
NOTE: Grabowski et al. (2010) uses the phrase "significant mental health disorder" to capture the various definitions used in other sources. The three studies define their variables differently to include psychiatric diagnoses, psychiatric morbidity, perceived mental health status, and any other mental health diagnosis.

As noted above, most nursing home residents need assistance with one or more ADLs, most frequently for the following:

- Bathing (96.7 percent),
- Dressing (92.7 percent),
- Toileting (89.3 percent),
- Walking or locomotion (92.0 percent),
- Transferring in and out of bed (86.8 percent), and
- Eating (59.9 percent) (Harris-Kojetin et al., 2019).

The majority of nursing homes provide both short-term rehabilitation and subacute care.[6] Individuals receiving subacute care have variations in the intensity of their care needs and the stability of their conditions.

---

[6] Subacute care is defined as intensive care typically provided in skilled nursing facilities for those with a critical illness, such as cancer or injury. It is less intensive than acute care, which is more typically provided in hospitals for debilitating illnesses, such as strokes and heart attacks, or recovery after a major surgery (Martel, 2019).

In contrast, the long-stay residents who need long-term care services and support typically have many chronic conditions (including one or more geriatric syndromes[7]) that require professional nursing surveillance to identify subtle changes in condition that could lead to hospitalization and potentially death. Some nursing homes have further diversified by providing specialty care focusing on, for example, dementia care and hospice or end-of-life care (Sherman and Touhy, 2017).

Nursing homes commonly deliver rehabilitation services, such as physical, occupational, or speech therapy for both long-stay and post-acute residents (NIA, 2021). Overall, about 32 percent of residents received rehabilitation services in 2016 (Harrington et al., 2018).

Nursing homes provide care through the end of life, and most (80.7 percent) offer hospice services (Harris-Kojetin et al., 2019).[8] From 1999 to 2019 (before the COVID-19 pandemic), an average of 21 percent of all deaths and 27 percent of all deaths among individuals at least 65 years old in the United States occurred in nursing homes or long-term care facilities (CDC, 2020b).

Chapter 4 provides an in-depth discussion of resident care needs and the services provided in nursing homes.

NURSING HOME CHARACTERISTICS

The broader continuum of long-term care facilities and services includes the following:

- independent living,
- outpatient therapy,
- inpatient therapy,
- home-based primary care,
- in-home services and supports,
- medical foster homes,
- residential care communities,[9]

---

[7] Geriatric syndromes are common health conditions among older adults. Four shared risk factors—older age, baseline cognitive impairment, baseline functional impairment, and impaired mobility—have been identified across five common geriatric syndromes (pressure ulcers, incontinence, falls, functional decline, and delirium). Geriatric syndromes do not fit into typical discrete conditions and are often assessed more holistically as multifactorial health conditions (Inouye et al., 2007).

[8] Calculated by the National Center for Health Statistics as the number of beds in a unit identified and dedicated by a facility for residents needing hospice services and/or the number of residents receiving hospice care benefit (Harris-Kojetin et al., 2019).

[9] Residential care communities cover a variety of residential settings, including assisted living facilities.

- adult day care,
- nursing homes, and
- hospice care (see Chapter 4 for more discussion on hospice services).

The various care settings in this continuum have different funding streams, ownership, and regulations, which can complicate care coordination and communication as individuals move across these settings (Goldberg, 2014).

Size, Type, and Location

The United States has 1.7 million nursing home beds, the vast majority of which (97.5 percent) are Medicare certified (CDC, 2020a; Harris-Kojetin et al., 2019). The number of certified beds in an individual nursing home ranges from 2 to 1,389, with an average of 106. The South has the largest share (34.8 percent) of nursing homes, while the Midwest has the largest share of nursing home beds. Metropolitan areas account for the large majority of nursing homes (71.5 percent), with 13.9 percent in micropolitan areas and 14.6 percent in other areas of the country[10] (Harris-Kojetin et al., 2019).

Nursing homes can be characterized according to their own unique design elements, the considerations for resident and staff well-being, and the type of care delivered. Common examples of the various types of nursing homes are listed below (Table 2-2).

The U.S. Department of Veterans Affairs

The Veterans Health Administration (VHA), an operating unit within the U.S. Department of Veterans Affairs (VA), is the largest integrated health care network in the United States, providing care to more than 9 million veterans per year.[11] In 2015, the VHA spent $7.4 billion (13 percent of health care expenditures) for long-term care services (Colello and Panangala, 2017). The VA provides long-term care in three settings classified as nursing homes: approximately 134 community living centers (VA owned and operated), approximately 1,769 community nursing homes (VA-contracted non-VA nursing homes), and approximately 148 state veterans homes (state-owned and -managed centers providing full-time care) (GAO, 2019). VA nursing homes can provide both post-acute and long-term care (VA, 2021).

---

[10] "Each metropolitan statistical area must have at least one urbanized area of 50,000 or more inhabitants. Each micropolitan statistical area must have at least one urban cluster of at least 10,000 but less than 50,000 population" (Census Bureau, 2021a).

[11] For more information, see https://www.va.gov/ (accessed November 3, 2021).

TABLE 2-2 Common Types of Nursing Homes

Nursing Home Type	Description	Design Elements
Traditional nursing home	- ≥20 residents on the ward - Differentiated tasks for staff - Routines and rules of the organization determining daily life - Care required by a resident's care plan covered by Medicaid; eligibility varies by state	- Large building - Long corridors - Shared rooms - Hospital-like atmosphere - Separate kitchen - Facilities, such as a restaurant and activity areas, attached to the ward
Small-scale living facility within a larger nursing home	- Typically 8–20 residents - Joint household - Meals (including dinner) prepared inside the home three times a day - Integrated tasks for staff - Small team of caregivers - Residents and informal caregivers determining daily life	- Home-like situation - Single rooms - Familiar interior - Common living room attached to kitchen - Outdoor area accessible
Stand-alone small-scale living facility	- Same characteristics as a small-scale living facility on the terrain of a larger nursing home - Situated in a neighborhood - Aims at close connections with the community and opportunities to maintain a social network	- Archetype house - Single rooms - Familiar interior - Common living room attached to kitchen - No direct access to facilities at a larger nursing home - Outdoor area accessible
Greenhouses	- A small campus of residences for 10–12 older and/or disabled persons - Medicaid coverage allowable	- Household-size kitchens - Dining areas - Activity space - Outdoor access

SOURCES: Adapted from CMS, 2021a; Cohen et al., 2016; de Boer et al., 2018.

Compared with the general nursing home population in the United States, the veteran nursing home population tends to be younger, more likely to be male, and more likely to suffer from disability, illness, chronic pain and injuries, and mental illnesses (NCVAS, 2020; VA-OIG, 2020). In 2019, the U.S. Government Accountability Office projected that the percentage of veterans requiring nursing home care would increase significantly (by 16 percent) between 2017 and 2022 (GAO, 2019).

Pediatric Nursing Homes

Pediatric nursing homes are also available for those under the age of 21. Data from 2015 identify about 29,000 children residing in 100 U.S. pediatric long-term care facilities (Hessels et al., 2017). That number has decreased in recent years due to an increased emphasis on home- and community-based settings (Friedman and Kalichman, 2014). An overwhelming majority (90 percent) of children with complex care needs[12] rely on Medicaid; their cost of care is expected to continue rising dramatically (PCCA, 2016). This population commonly includes children who

- are medically fragile;
- need brief, acute care after hospitalization;
- have complex medical needs;
- have functional impairments;
- have developmental or cognitive disabilities;
- require ventilator support;
- have more than one chronic condition; or
- have life-limiting conditions.

Similar to adult nursing homes, pediatric nursing homes typically provide skilled nursing care, occupational therapy, and recreational therapy (Children's National Hospital, 2021; Hessels et al., 2017; Nursing Home Law Center, 2010; Stein, 2001). Unlike adult nursing homes, pediatric facilities typically also coordinate with the local education system and provide other resident and family educational services (Children's National Hospital, 2021; Hessels et al., 2017; Stein, 2001). Children with complex care needs often need advanced medical devices, such as tracheostomies, gastric feeding tubes, or ventilators (PCCA, 2016). The length of stay in a nursing home varies significantly within this population: some children stay briefly after birth due to difficulty breathing, some stay for brief periods when their caregivers are unavailable, and some remain long term, eventually transitioning to adult facilities. At age 18 or 21, most "age out" of pediatric nursing homes (Children's National Hospital, 2021; HealthCarePathway.com, 2022; PCCA, 2016, 2020; Stein, 2001). This transition can be extremely confusing and labor intensive for families, as only about 40 percent of families receive transition services, funding streams often end and change, and adult nursing home providers often are not expert in caring for these individuals (PCCA, 2016; Stein, 2001). Additionally, no facilities specialize in caring for a population transitioning out of pediatric care, so

---

[12] Children with complex care needs most often have conditions in four categories: (1) chronic, severe health conditions, (2) substantial health service needs, (3) functional limitations, which are often severe, or (4) high health resource use. More technically, these children are classified under Clinical Risk Group of 5b or higher (PCCA, 2016). Examples of typical diagnoses include chronic lung disease, congenital heart disorders, orthopedic and respiratory conditions, spina bifida, traumatic brain injury, and congenital anatomical malformations; "these diagnoses are often accompanied by one or several comorbidities, and many also present with some form of developmental delays and intellectual disabilities" (PCCA, 2016).

most young adults enter traditional nursing facilities. This can be particularly difficult for residents aged 22–35 who may be socially isolated and not receive the care they need in typical nursing home settings (Ansberry, 2007; Marselas, 2019; Stein, 2001). Children and young adults living in adult nursing homes can be vulnerable to a variety of forms of mistreatment or abuse, including sexual abuse, physical abuse, neglect, molestation, and medication errors (Nursing Home Law Center, 2010). Additional challenges include the lack of pediatric-specific state regulations, unfamiliarity with the pediatric population on the part of surveyors, staffing shortages, and a lack of pediatric quality indicators or assessment tools (PCCA, 2016).

Critical Access Hospitals

CMS-designated critical access hospitals (CAHs) aim to improve access to essential services in rural locations. Some CAHs have extended care units that are licensed as nursing homes, as rural areas are less likely to have stand-alone facilities. This allows CAHs to use inpatient beds for acute care or nursing home–level care as needed, most often for older adults requiring post-acute care (RHIH, 2019). Overall, CAHs receive benefits to reduce the financial vulnerability of rural hospitals due to low census and are also eligible for Medicare cost-based reimbursement instead of payment by Medicare's Prospective Payment System (RHIH, 2019). However, CAH swing beds for post-acute nursing home care are not eligible for cost-based reimbursement (RHIH, 2019).[13] About 1,352 small rural hospitals are designated as CAHs in 45 states, and approximately 22 percent of them own a nursing home (Castellucci, 2020; Flex Monitoring Team, 2020). These hospitals have an overall occupancy rate of about 36 percent when including both observational and post-acute swing beds (MedPAC, 2021). In 2018, Medicare paid over $11 billion in total cost-based payments to CAHs, with an average payment of $8 million per CAH for all hospital care. This represents approximately 5 percent of all Medicare payments for inpatient and outpatient hospitals (MedPAC, 2020).

FACTORS THAT INFLUENCE THE QUALITY OF CARE IN NURSING HOMES

A variety of factors influence the quality of care in nursing homes. The following sections give a high-level overview for several key factors, including quality measurement and quality improvement, the workforce, the environment and safety, financing and payment, ownership, quality

---

[13] 42 CFR § 413.114(c); see: https://www.ecfr.gov/current/title-42/chapter-IV/subchapter-B/part-413 (accessed February 15, 2022).

Quality Measurement and Quality Improvement

Ensuring and improving the quality of care in nursing homes requires measuring it in order to inform consumers, hold providers and organizations accountable, and support evidence-based treatments and interventions. The current system for quality measurement in nursing homes is the CMS Five-Star Rating System, which establishes a score based on health inspections, staffing levels, and clinical outcomes. However, these measures do not include the resident and family experience. Chapter 3 further explores issues related to quality measurement and improvement.

Nursing Home Workforce

Nursing homes rely on 1.2 million individuals to provide care and maintain facilities (Denny-Brown et al., 2020). They typically use a variety of workers, including nursing staff (e.g., registered nurses, certified nursing assistants), administrators, housekeeping staff, dietary staff, and medical and social care providers. The vast majority of direct care is provided by low-paid, racially diverse, primarily female workers (Sloane et al., 2021). The number and types of staff may depend on the number of residents and the scope of services provided. Some of the workers may be contracted through agencies rather than hired as employees.

Nursing homes have historically struggled with workforce shortages and high rates of turnover—both exacerbated by the COVID-19 pandemic. Facility-level data from the Long-Term Care Facility Staffing Payroll-Based Journal shows that daily staffing levels varied greatly by facility and are often below CMS recommended levels; for example, 75 percent of nursing homes were almost never in compliance with registered nurse (RN) staffing levels (Geng et al., 2019). Similarly, turnover rates also varied but were well over 100 percent for RNs, licensed practical nurses, and certified nursing assistants (Gandhi et al., 2021). Between September and October 2021, over 30 percent of facilities reported staffing shortages (Paulin, 2021). Chapter 5 discusses the nursing home workforce and issues related to staffing.

Nursing Home Environment and Safety

The physical environment of nursing homes has a significant effect on resident well-being and quality of life. Most were built in the 1960s and 1970s, mirror the design of a hospital, and are not fully equipped to provide high-quality care (see Chapter 4 for more discussion) (Eijkelenboom et al., 2017; Kramer, 2021; Schwarz, 1997). Certain features of the environment can decrease quality of life, hinder infection control, and create barriers for staff caring for residents, including large buildings and units (Waters, 2021), shared rooms (Nygaard et al., 2020), poor air flow and filtration (Lynch and Goring, 2020), poor lighting (Wu et al., 2015), unwanted noise (Sloane et al., 2002), and limited outdoor access (Sandvoll et al., 2020). Ensuring resident safety requires addressing issues such as infection control, medication safety, physical injury prevention, and emergency preparedness. Chapter 6 further explores the environment and safety of nursing homes.

Financing and Payment

In 2020, Medicaid covered the majority of nursing home residents (62 percent); Medicare Part A was the primary payer for 12 percent of residents, and 26 percent had private insurance (KFF, 2020a). Medicare is the predominant payment source for post-acute care (typically associated with short-stay residents), while the federal-state Medicaid program primarily pays for long-term care in nursing homes (KFF, 2007, 2017; Sifuentes and Lapane, 2020).

Given that state Medicaid programs play a large role in paying for long-term nursing home care, competition among nursing homes is limited, which can limit incentives to improve quality. Additionally, Medicaid must provide long-term care to eligible individuals, but it is only required to do so in nursing home facilities. Many people prefer alternatives to nursing homes, but the availability of home and community-based care varies by state and may impact a resident's decision to enter a nursing home if no other options are available (Reaves and Musumeci, 2015). In 2018, for instance, 185,774 Medicaid beneficiaries were on a waitlist for home-based care (KFF, 2018). Facilities with higher proportions of Medicaid residents are often underresourced, understaffed, and located in poor and minority communities (Li et al., 2015a; Mack et al., 2020; Mor et al., 2004; Taylor et al., 2020).

According to industry surveys, the average cost of nursing home care has risen significantly over the past few years; this is projected to continue (Witt and Hoyt, 2021) and will likely create issues of access as the age and proportion of the U.S. population needing long-term care also rises (Johnson et al., 2021). According to one estimate, in 2016, the annual cost for a semi-private nursing home room was $82,128, and the annual cost for a private nursing home room was $92,376 (Witt and Hoyt, 2021). By 2030, costs are projected to rise to $125,085 and $142,254, respectively. Another study estimates approximately 7.8 million seniors (54 percent) will not qualify for Medicaid even after spending down their housing assets and will not be able afford nursing home care in 2029 (Pearson et al., 2019). Chapter 7 further explores the financing and payment of nursing home care.

Ownership

The majority of nursing homes (69.3 percent) are for profit, with nearly one-quarter nonprofit and 7.2 percent government owned (Harris-Kojetin et al., 2019). Private equity firms own approximately 11 percent of nursing homes (Gupta et al., 2021; Spanko, 2020). Nearly 60 percent of nursing homes are affiliated with a chain—defined as corporations that own or run two or more such facilities (Harris-Kojetin et al., 2019; Stevenson et al., 2013). State-level trends have demonstrated that the ownership of nursing homes by large national chains is declining and the number of smaller, regional, private investment-owned facilities is increasing (Stevenson et al., 2013). Researchers and policy makers have an increasing interest in determining the relationships between ownership type and quality outcomes; historically, quality has been lower in for-profit nursing homes (Comondore et al., 2009; GAO, 2011; Grabowski and Stevenson, 2008; Harrington et al., 2012; You et al., 2016) and those owned by private equity firms (Gupta et al., 2021; Harrington et al., 2012).

Some private equity investment firms have purchased publicly held chains. There is some evidence that private-equity–owned nursing homes also have lower staffing, poorer resident outcomes, and more deficiencies than nonprofit or public nursing homes (Gupta et al., 2021; Harrington et al., 2001; Pradhan et al., 2014; Stevenson and Grabowski, 2008). (See Chapter 8 for more on nursing home ownership.)

Quality Assurance (Oversight and Regulation)

CMS is ultimately responsible for the regulatory oversight of nursing homes at the federal level, but states assist with conducting inspections to certify compliance with federal regulations. To enforce standards of care, state survey agencies can levy sanctions against poorly performing nursing homes. In 2016, the top deficiencies cited were the following:

1. Infection control (45.4 percent),
2. Food sanitation (42.6 percent),
3. Accident environment (39.8 percent),
4. Quality of care (34.3 percent),
5. Pharmacy consultation (26.8 percent),
6. Unnecessary drugs (24.9 percent),
7. Comprehensive care plan (24.9 percent),
8. Clinical records (22.6 percent),

9. Dignity (20.6 percent), and
10. Qualified personnel (18.3 percent) (Harrington et al., 2018).

Chapter 8 further addresses the oversight and regulation of nursing homes.

Health Information Technology

HIT systems, such as electronic health records designed to facilitate health care delivery, management, and payment, have spread throughout the U.S. health care system. HIT capabilities in effectively promoting patient safety, enhancing the effectiveness of patient care delivery, facilitating the management of chronic conditions, and improving the efficiency of health care professionals are particularly important in nursing home settings, given the characteristics of the population. Residents typically have complex conditions, take multiple medications, and frequently undergo transitions in care (e.g., visits to the emergency department and hospital admissions) (Vest et al., 2019). Moreover, stays tend to be extended rather than episodic, with care typically lasting years rather than weeks or months. This requires more extensive ongoing communication, care coordination activities, and different HIT reporting mechanisms that can support staff in identifying, monitoring, and responding to changes in condition over an extended period (Rantz et al., 2010a,b). Other health technologies, such as telehealth, videoconferencing, and personal monitoring devices, are also effective tools in nursing homes. The importance of these technologies was made clear during the COVID-19 pandemic, when measures such as locking down facilities to protect vulnerable residents from infection limited access to in-person clinical services and residents' contact with friends and family members (Whitelaw et al., 2020). Chapter 9 explores the role of HIT in and barriers to its widespread adoption by nursing homes.

CRITICAL IMPACT OF COVID-19 ON NURSING HOMES

As of August 2020, nearly half (42 percent) of COVID-related deaths in the United States since the beginning of the pandemic had occurred in nursing homes and assisted living facilities (AP, 2020). By October 2021, that number was 1 in 5, despite residents accounting for only 1.6 percent of cases (CDC, 2021a,b) and less than one-half of 1 percent of the population (CDC, 2020a; KFF, 2020b; U.S. Census Bureau, 2021b). As of February 2022, more than 149,000 residents and more than 2,200 staff members had died of COVID-19 (CDC, 2022).

Population and Environmental Challenges

The nursing home population was especially vulnerable to the severe impacts of COVID-19 due to a variety of factors that increased their risk of infection, including the following:

- the age and health status of many nursing home residents,
- the high number of resident-to-resident interactions that occur as a result of the congregate care setting of nursing homes (including shared rooms), and
- the high number of staff-to-resident interactions among the dozens or sometimes hundreds of residents who require hours of direct care on a daily basis (Abrams et al., 2020; Coe and Van Houtven, 2020; Fallon et al., 2020; Konetzka et al., 2021; Thompson et al., 2020).

Other factors include the challenges of protecting residents with dementia who have difficulty adhering to social distancing and universal masking policies; inadequate and unavailable testing or personal protective equipment; preexisting staffing shortages exacerbated by infections among the staff; the number of low-wage staff who work in more than one facility; and contradictory federal, state, and county guidance and regulations (Konetzka et al., 2021; Ouslander and Grabowski, 2020; Thompson et al., 2020). These factors resulted in a large number of resident hospitalizations and deaths both in the United States and internationally.

Infection Prevention and Control Challenges

Another factor shaping the COVID-19 pandemic's effect was that nursing homes did not have adequate expertise and experience in the infection prevention and control practices necessary to limit the introduction and transmission of the virus within facilities (Grabowski and Mor, 2020). In 2020, a U.S. Government Accountability Office (GAO) report concluded that "infection control deficiencies were widespread and persistent in nursing homes prior to the pandemic and contributed to rapid spread of COVID-19 in facilities" (GAO, 2020). The entire health care system was struggling to address these issues due to an overall lack of prioritization, action, and support from the larger emergency response community and federal government.

While CMS requires that each nursing home have a staff member who is responsible for infection prevention and control,[14] this is not usually a

---

[14] CMS Requirements for Long Term Care Facilities—Infection Control, 42 CFR § 483.80 (2016).

full-time position, and such persons also have many other responsibilities. Efforts to isolate or cohort[15] those infected or quarantine those exposed were often delayed or inadequate and sometimes nonexistent, resulting in spread of the virus throughout facilities. Additionally, a lack of testing and consequent underestimate of COVID-19 prevalence resulted in delays in implementing limits on congregate activities, such as dining and group activities. Combined with a lack of personal protective equipment (PPE), these delays also facilitated spread of infection. Although CMS, CDC, state departments of health, and others issued infection control guidance, its volume and frequent changes posed significant challenges to nursing homes, which struggled to interpret, keep up with, and adapt to the latest guidance.

Adequate supplies of PPE, testing, and resources were not available in the early days of the pandemic and varied greatly by state. Staff were not adequately trained in infection prevention and control practices, including the appropriate use of PPE. Staff had not been fit tested for N95 respirators or trained in their use (Denny-Brown et al., 2020; GAO, 2020).

Recognizing the importance of asymptomatic infection in disease transmission was also delayed, with early reports claiming that it was not a major factor (CNBC, 2020). It has now been well documented that asymptomatic or pre-symptomatic infection was often how COVID-19 was introduced into, and spread within, nursing homes. Access to testing for COVID-19 was inadequate to identify those infected, either residents or staff, whether symptomatic or asymptomatic (Ouslander and Grabowski, 2020). Early on, when the availability of testing was very limited, nursing homes had to depend on symptom screening of staff and residents to protect residents, which did not identify many who were infected and able to transmit the virus. Testing staff was as important as testing residents. Moreover, appropriate public health measures, such as having staff work with only infected or uninfected residents if at all possible, were not put in place quickly (Konetzka et al., 2021; Ouslander and Grabowski, 2020).

Communication Challenges

Poor communications and the lack of integration between nursing homes and public health departments resulted in the failure to identify and address COVID-19 outbreaks promptly and implement appropriate recommendations and requirements. As noted, the changing nature of

---

[15] Cohorting, as defined by the Centers for Disease Control and Prevention (CDC), is the infection prevention and control practice "of grouping patients infected or colonized with the same infectious agent together to confine their care to one area and prevent contact with susceptible patients" (CDC, 2015). CDC guidance instructed facilities to identify a separate space to monitor and care for residents with confirmed COVID-19 infections (CDC, 2021d).

what was known about the virus itself and its transmission meant that recommendations from local, state, and federal public health agencies were changing frequently (CDC, 2021e; Espinosa, 2020). Nursing homes had difficulty monitoring these recommendations and often depended on local public health agencies to provide ongoing recommendations and requirements; this included recommendations for the duration of isolation and quarantine, diagnostic testing, monitoring of outbreaks (and determination of when outbreaks ended), requirements for PPE, and ongoing symptom monitoring for residents and staff (CDC, 2021d; Yurkofsky and Ouslander, 2021b).

Additionally, public health guidance contributed to fragmentation across the larger health care system, placing additional burdens on nursing homes. For example, nursing homes were required to accept hospital admissions who tested positive to relieve the overburdened hospitals (Altimari and Carlesso, 2022; CTDPH, 2022; Gleckman, 2020; Khimm, 2020; Sapien and Sexton, 2020). Lack of communication and resource sharing across the different health care sectors also contributed to the devastating impact in nursing homes (see Chapter 6 for more discussion on these issues).

Disparities Among Nursing Home Residents During COVID-19

In the first 6–8 months of the pandemic, nursing homes serving more than 40 percent non-White residents experienced more than three times as many COVID-19 cases and deaths as those serving primarily White residents (Gorges and Konetzka, 2021). These nursing homes tended to receive fewer quality rating stars, have higher concentrations of residents, and be located in urban areas (Abrams et al., 2020; Garcia et al., 2020). However, neither differences in the quality ratings nor the residents' prior underlying health appeared to explain COVID-19 disparities; rather, much of the difference was explained by high-minority facilities being larger and located in areas of higher COVID-19 prevalence (Gorges and Konetzka, 2021).

The pandemic had a greater impact on the nursing homes with a higher number of Black and Latinx residents (Gebeloff et al., 2020; Li et al., 2020a,b). Often such nursing homes are in communities with larger Black and Latinx populations, in areas with higher community rates of COVID-19 infection, or both (Garcia et al., 2020). Facilities with higher proportions of Black and Latinx residents also typically have limited resources, which negatively affects their access to PPE or infection prevention and control expertise (Sloane et al., 2021; Taylor et al., 2020). Moreover, Black and Latinx individuals are more likely to suffer serious consequences from COVID-19 infection because of deeply ingrained inequalities that make them more likely than White adults to have greater physiological dysregulation and accelerated biological aging (Garcia et al., 2020).

Later in the pandemic, the disproportionate effect on racial and ethnic minorities dissipated and reversed; by fall 2020 and winter 2021, nursing homes with more White residents had higher case and death rates (Gilman and Bassett, 2021; Kumar et al., 2021). This shift was consistent with where the virus was most prevalent during that time—states in the West and Upper Midwest with smaller non-White populations.

Some sources indicate that LGBTQ+ older adults may be more vulnerable to COVID-19 infection (SAGE and the Human Rights Campaign Foundation, 2020), but detailed data are not yet available.

The pandemic also had a significant impact on Medicare beneficiaries; about 42 percent of the 3.1 million nursing home residents who were Medicare beneficiaries had (or probably had) COVID-19 in 2020 (OIG, 2021). Furthermore, dually eligible beneficiaries were even more likely than Medicare-only beneficiaries to contract and die from COVID-19 (OIG, 2021).

Social Isolation and Loneliness

Nearly one-quarter of Americans 65 or older are considered socially isolated, and 43 percent of adults over 60 years old report feeling lonely (Anderson and Thayer, 2018; Cudjoe and Kotwal, 2020; Perissinotto et al., 2012). Residing in a nursing home can exacerbate feelings of loneliness (Trybusińska and Saracen, 2019). The majority (76 percent) of nursing home residents in a study of 365 people reported feeling lonelier than usual during the COVID-19 pandemic (Montgomery et al., 2020). More than half (64 percent) also indicated that they "no longer leave their rooms to socialize" with other residents (Montgomery et al., 2020).

The proportions of residents socializing with outside visitors, participating in activities, leaving their rooms, and eating communally all decreased sharply during the pandemic. In addition, nursing homes severely limited or prevented visitation by family members and loved ones to align with CMS directives, which exacerbated the impact of social isolation and loneliness. There were delays in identifying ways to address this isolation while also limiting residents' exposure to the virus (Montgomery et al., 2020). See Chapters 8 and 9 for more discussion on the impact of visitation restrictions.

Staffing Challenges

Multiple studies found that higher nurse staffing ratios mitigated the effect of an outbreak and resulted in fewer deaths (Gorges and Konetzka, 2020; Harrington et al., 2020; Konetzka et al., 2021; Li et al., 2020a). However, higher staffing ratios were not able to prevent an outbreak, given the role of staff traffic in COVID-19 into facilities. One study found that facilities with fewer unique staff members, defined as total staff size entering the facility each day, experienced fewer cases among residents than facilities with large numbers of distinct staff members, even after controlling for facility size, staff skill level, and direct care ratios (McGarry et al., 2021a). This issue was especially lethal when little was known about asymptomatic transmission and therefore widespread testing of asymptomatic individuals was uncommon. Nursing home workforce shortages intensified during the pandemic but varied by time and urban or rural location (Yang et al., 2021). A cross-sectional time-series study of over 15,000 nursing homes found that while urban nursing homes reported a relatively constant staffing shortage, rural nursing homes saw an increase in staffing shortages until November 2020 (Yang et al., 2021).

Vaccination Challenges

Introducing vaccines and prioritizing their distribution in long-term care facilities in late December 2020 greatly alleviated the impact of COVID-19 in nursing homes, whose vaccination rate is much higher than the national average (CDC, 2021c; CMS, 2021b). For example, new resident COVID-19 cases declined by 48 percent among vaccinated residents in the 3 weeks after a December 2020 vaccine clinic compared to a 21 percent decline in unvaccinated residents (Domi et al., 2021). As of December 1, 2021, U.S. nursing home staff had 677,173 COVID-19 cases and 2,152 COVID-19 deaths. Nationally, an average of 74.3 percent of staff members and 86.4 percent of residents were vaccinated per facility (CMS, 2021b).

Vaccination rates and COVID-19 cases and deaths varied by state; for example, Rhode Island had about 95 percent of residents and about 99 percent of staff vaccinated, whereas Nevada only had about 76 percent of residents and about 81 percent of staff vaccinated (CMS, 2021b). Organizational characteristics have also affected vaccine coverage. Nursing homes that are nonprofit and nonchain have higher rates of vaccine coverage (McGarry et al., 2021b; White et al., 2021). Race and ethnicity also influenced vaccination rates. A 2021 study found that Black residents are more likely to be in higher-risk facilities (which tend to be larger, for profit, and in the southern United States and in communities with high infection rates), where vaccination rates among both residents and staff are low (Reber and Kosar, 2021). One study of 27,000 employees found that vaccination rates varied by race and ethnicity (Feifer et al., 2021); they were highest for Asian (79.1 percent), followed by Pacific Islander (73.3 percent), White (70.3 percent), American Indian/Alaskan Native (61.8 percent), Hispanic (57.8 percent), and Black (50.9 percent) employees (those who did not specify race or ethnicity were 65 percent).

Overall, factors such as low vaccination rates among staff and new variants contributed to the continued serious impact of COVID-19 (McGarry et al., 2022; Nanduri et al., 2021). These staggering statistics are likely explained, in part, by the nursing home population being older, frailer, and more likely to be diagnosed with multiple chronic conditions compared to the general population.

Nursing Home Characteristics and COVID-19

A recent systematic review of the predictors of COVID-19 cases and deaths in nursing homes found that the two strongest and most consistent predictors were size—with larger facilities being at greater at risk—and COVID-19 prevalence in the surrounding community (Konetzka et al., 2021). Nursing homes with highest community prevalence had an average of five more deaths per facility than those with the lowest community transmission. Furthermore, the data showed no significant association between nursing home quality metrics (as assigned by Care Compare) and COVID-19 outcomes (Abrams et al., 2020; Chatterjee et al., 2020; Gorges and Konetzka, 2020). Beyond the star ratings, several studies examined specific and salient aspects of quality, such as prior infection control citations. These were also not associated with poor COVID-19 outcomes (Abrams et al., 2020; White et al., 2020).

Thus, the evidence reveals that the COVID-19 tragedy in nursing homes was not a "bad apples" problem. High-quality nursing homes were also at risk. This does not mean that quality and infection prevention and control are not important, but perhaps they are not sufficient. The ubiquity of COVID-19 cases and deaths within nursing homes is indicative of a more systemic problem, one that will require systemic solutions.

STRENGTHENING CONNECTIONS OF NURSING HOMES TO THE COMMUNITY AND BROADER HEALTH CARE SYSTEM

Nursing homes are often not well integrated into the local community or broader health care system, which has important implications for a range of issues from resident quality of care and quality of life to emergency planning, preparedness, and response. This apparent disconnect may be a historical artifact of the stigmatization of nursing homes and their residents based on their origins as "poorhouses" (described earlier). Another contributing factor may be community perception of nursing homes as businesses rather than health care institutions (OIG, 2006).

Research on the barriers and facilitators of effective care transitions highlights the importance of partnership among health care organizations, as well as coordination involving the broader health care community. Scott et al. (2017) point out, for example, that "as health care organizations seek to align their strategic priorities with federal incentives to reduce readmissions, it is becoming increasingly clear that no single health care organization" can provide all the necessary health care resources and services. They note that health care organizations "must engage in sustainable community health partnerships as key points of leverage for improving quality of care and reducing costs" (Scott et al., 2017, p. 444).

Forging effective relationships, strengthening communication, and creating partnerships between nursing homes and hospitals and academic medical centers are critical given that residents often require care in these settings for their often multiple complex medical conditions. Academic medical centers also have created partnerships to improve transitions for nursing home residents in their facilities (Balch, 2020). State and local technical assistance programs often involve academic–provider partnerships to improve the quality of care in nursing homes. Such programs may be particularly well suited to provide technical assistance due to familiarity with the local community and the ability to be seen as a trusted peer and as a result can facilitate the integration of nursing homes into their local communities and the broader health care system (see Chapter 3). Appropriately designed and implemented HIT can strengthen communications to ensure smooth transitions of care across health care settings (see Chapter 9).

Nursing homes are required by law to have their own emergency plans and procedures.[16] However, these plans are often incomplete and lack detail, making it difficult for administrators to execute them (OIG, 2012). It is imperative to explicitly include nursing homes in all elements of emergency planning, preparedness, and response at the federal, state, and local levels, as discussed further in Chapter 6. Moreover, as demonstrated during the pandemic, local academic medical centers can serve as sources of infection prevention and control expertise (Balch, 2020).

Community Engagement: Linking to Quality of Life and Care

Integrating the nursing home into the broader community is also critical on the level of the individual resident and family as well as staff members. Community engagement initiatives are emerging factors contributing to quality care and quality of life in nursing homes. These initiatives can strengthen civic ties and partnerships with external organizations. Community engagement, also referred to as "civic engagement," may involve residents volunteering at organizations or events, intergenerational interactions, mutual aid,[17] or the infusion of community events and activities

---

[16] CMS Requirements for Long Term Care Facilities—Emergency Preparedness, 42 CFR § 483.73 (2016).

[17] Mutual aid societies or networks date back to the early nineteenth century, refer to people cooperating to meet shared needs or face shared challenges, and are viewed as a way to build solidarity and connection between members of the community.

within the nursing home. Community engagement is an important component of person-centered care in that it emphasizes both meaningful engagement and social relationships, which are key constructs of this model of care (Hirdes et al., 2020). Increased community engagement activities are linked to strong culture change practices (Anderson and Dabelko-Schoeny, 2010; Duan and Mueller, 2019; Miller et al., 2018), increased resident psychological well-being and life satisfaction (Buedo-Guirado et al., 2020; Yuen et al., 2008), quality of life (Van Malderen et al., 2013), and positive effects on resident mental and functional health (Leedahl et al., 2015).

In one study that examined the typology of culture change implementation across nursing homes, findings linked higher frequencies of family and community engagement with facilities that strongly embraced culture change practices (Duan and Mueller, 2019). Another study found that in populations of older adults with extensive physical disabilities, social networks influenced social engagement, which increased quality of life (Jang et al., 2004).

Increased collaborative efforts with community organizations may also propel positive change in nursing homes and act as a supportive resource for improvement. One model, the Seniors Quality Leap Initiative, drives positive change in quality of care and quality of life practices in nursing homes. This model is composed of 11 organizations in Canada and the United States that meet with participating nursing homes through virtual and in-person meetings. Quality improvement initiatives include using evidence-based clinical quality of care indicators and quality of life metrics to establish common change initiatives (Hirdes et al., 2020).

THE FUTURE OF NURSING HOME CARE

Nursing homes within the long-term care continuum in the United States are characterized by a disjointed system with a lack of data, different funding streams, variable oversight, and insufficient communication—all of which combine to make quality improvement extremely difficult (Goldberg, 2014). Despite decades of improvement efforts, nursing homes still face many long-standing challenges in delivering quality care, many of which were revealed and exacerbated by the COVID-19 pandemic. Several additional challenges are imminent. The United States, like much of the world, has an aging population. Half of today's 65-year-olds will need some paid long-term care services before they die. By 2030, one in four Americans will be age 65 or older. The fastest growing group will be those over age 85; this group is expected to grow from 6.5 million to 11.8 million by 2035 and 19 million by 2060 (Vespa et al., 2020). Marriage and fertility rates have declined, while life expectancy has increased, meaning fewer family caregivers will be available. Additionally, climate change poses a threat to facilities located in areas where severe weather events are becoming more common.

To bolster nursing homes in the wake of the COVID-19 pandemic, the Nursing Home Improvement and Accountability Act[18] was introduced in August 2021 and is in committees in Congress as of the writing of this report. Designed to improve the quality of care through significant changes in key areas, including workforce, regulation, financial transparency, and accountability, the proposed legislation, if enacted, would

- Increase the federal Medicaid payment to states for the next 6 years,
- Require that funds allocated are used to increase staff pay and expand staffing in order to support and improve resident care,
- Require a registered nurse on duty 24/7,
- Require a full-time infection control specialist,
- Require nursing facilities to report more accurate quality and staffing data to the government,
- Fund a study to determine whether the government should set minimum staffing ratios at nursing homes,
- Ban facilities from mandating that residents sign pre-dispute arbitration agreements, and
- Create a $1.3 billion demonstration program to encourage the construction of facilities that house 5–14 residents.

This legislation addresses many changes necessary to improve quality of care, such as increasing funding, enforcing staffing requirements, and creating smaller facilities. Improving quality is of critical importance as the number of older people and people with disabilities needing long-term care is expected to grow.

Furthermore, the COVID-19 pandemic serves as a powerful impetus for addressing long-standing issues in nursing home care. The John A. Hartford Foundation surveyed more than 1,000 older adults about their preferences for long-term care, and the results underscore the urgency of implementing significant reform measures to improve the quality of care:

- 71 percent say they are unwilling to live in a nursing home in the future,
- 57 percent say COVID-19 influenced whether they would be willing to live in a nursing home,

---

[18] Nursing Home Improvement and Accountability Act of 2021, S.782, H.R. 1985; 117th Cong., 1st sess., (March 16, 2021). For more information, see https://www.finance.senate.gov/imo/media/doc/Nursing%20Home%20Improvement%20and%20Accountability%20Act_Sec-by-Sec_Final.pdf (accessed August 20, 2021).

- Nearly 90 percent say changes are needed to make nursing homes appealing to them, and
- Black and Hispanic older adults are more likely to say nursing homes are unsafe (JAHF, 2021).

These findings highlight the need for immediate change to improve the quality of care and quality of life in nursing homes. Achieving this change will require assessing key challenges and opportunities in the areas of quality measurement and improvement, care delivery, the workforce, the environment and safety, the use of HIT, payment and financing, ownership, and quality assurance.

REFERENCES

Abrams, H. R., L. Loomer, A. Gandhi, and D. C. Grabowski. 2020. Characteristics of U.S. nursing homes with COVID-19 cases. *Journal of the American Geriatrics Society* 68(8):1653–1656.

Altimari, D., and J. Carlesso. 2022. *CT asks nursing homes to accept COVID-positive admissions from hospitals*. https://ctmirror.org/2022/01/06/ct-orders-nursing-homes-to-accept-covid-positive-admissions-from-hospitals (accessed February 15, 2022).

Anderson, G. O., and C. Thayer. 2018. *Loneliness and social connections: A national survey of adults 45 and older*. https://www.aarp.org/research/topics/life/info-2018/loneliness-social-connections (accessed December 30, 2021).

Anderson, K. A., and H. I. Dabelko-Schoeny. 2010. Civic engagement for nursing home residents: A call for social work action. *Journal of Gerontological Social Work* 53(3):270–282.

Ansberry, C. 2007. *Babes among elders: Nursing-home kids*. https://www.wsj.com/articles/SB118298182684050679 (accessed January 6, 2022).

AoA (Administration on Aging). 2020. *2019 profile on older Americans*. https://acl.gov/sites/default/files/Aging%20and%20Disability%20in%20America/2019ProfileOlderAmericans508.pdf (accessed January 4, 2022).

AP (Associated Press). 2020. *DOJ seeks data on nursing home deaths in four Democratic-led states*. https://www.modernhealthcare.com/post-acute-care/doj-seeks-data-nursing-home-deaths-four-democratic-led-states (accessed August 31, 2020).

APA (American Psychological Association). 2020a. *APA dictionary of psychology: Cisgender*. https://dictionary.apa.org/cisgender (accessed November 20, 2021).

APA. 2020b. *APA dictionary of psychology: Heterosexuality*. https://dictionary.apa.org/heterosexuality (accessed November 20, 2021).

Balch, B. 2020. *Hospitals partner with nursing homes to prevent and fight outbreaks*. https://www.aamc.org/news-insights/hospitals-partner-nursing-homes-prevent-and-fight-outbreaks (accessed February 10, 2022).

Bliss, D., S. Harms, L. E. Eberly, K. Savik, O. Gurvich, C. Mueller, J. F. Wyman, and B. Virnig. 2017. Social engagement after nursing home admission: Racial and ethnic disparities and risk factors. *Journal of Applied Gerontology* 36(11):1306–1326.

Bowblis, J. R., W. Ng, O. Akosionu, and T. P. Shippee. 2021. Decomposing racial and ethnic disparities in nursing home quality of life. *Journal of Applied Gerontology* 40(9):1051–1061.

Buedo-Guirado, C., L. Rubio Rubio, C. G. Dumitrache Dumitrache, and J. Romero Coronado. 2019. Active aging program in nursing homes: Effects on psychological well-being and life satisfaction. *Psychosocial Intervention* 29:49–57.

Caceres, B. A., J. Travers, J. E. Primiano, R. E. Luscombe, and C. Dorsen. 2020. Provider and LGBT individuals' perspectives on LGBT issues in long-term care: A systematic review. *The Gerontologist* 60(3):e169–e183.

Candrian, C., J. Sills, and J. Lowers. 2021. LGBT seniors in the pandemic: Silenced and vulnerable. *Annals of LGBTQ Public and Population Health* 1(4):277–281.

Castellucci, M. 2020. *Critical-access hospitals with long-term care units face more COVID-19 dangers*. https://www.modernhealthcare.com/critical-access-hospitals/critical-access-hospitals-long-term-care-units-face-more-COVID-19-dangers (accessed May 21, 2021).

CDC (Centers for Disease Control and Prevention). 2015. *Multidrug-resistant organisms (MDRO) management glossary*. https://www.cdc.gov/infectioncontrol/guidelines/mdro/glossary.html (accessed January 7, 2022).

CDC. 2020a. *National Center for Health Statistics—Nursing home care*. https://www.cdc.gov/nchs/fastats/nursing-home-care.htm (accessed October 16, 2020).

CDC. 2020b. *Underlying cause of death 1999–2018*. https://wonder.cdc.gov/controller/datarequest/D76;jsessionid=DAF37CC1A927ECD997AE74CA476A (accessed November 18, 2020).

CDC. 2021a. *COVID data tracker*. https://covid.cdc.gov/covid-data-tracker/#datatracker-home (accessed June 7, 2021).

CDC. 2021b. *COVID data tracker weekly review*. https://www.cdc.gov/coronavirus/2019-ncov/covid-data/covidview/index.html (accessed November 12, 2021).

CDC. 2021c. *COVID data tracker: COVID-19 vaccinations in the United States*. https://covid.cdc.gov/covid-data-tracker/#vaccinations_vacc-people-onedose-pop-5yr (accessed December 11, 2022).

CDC. 2021d. *Interim infection prevention and control recommendations to prevent SARS-CoV-2 spread in nursing homes*. https://www.cdc.gov/coronavirus/2019-ncov/hcp/long-term-care.html (accessed September 15, 2021).

CDC. 2021e. *COVID-19: What's new & updated*. https://www.cdc.gov/coronavirus/2019-ncov/whats-new-all.html (accessed July 8, 2021).

CDC. 2022. *COVID-19 nursing home data*. https://data.cms.gov/covid-19/covid-19-nursing-home-data (accessed February 17, 2022).

Chatterjee, P., S. Kelly, M. Qi, and R. M. Werner. 2020. Characteristics and quality of U.S. nursing homes reporting cases of coronavirus disease 2019 (COVID-19). *JAMA Network Open* 3(7):e2016930.

Children's National Hospital. 2021. *Skilled nursing: The HSC pediatric skilled nursing facility*. https://childrensnational.org/hsc/hsc-pediatric-center/medical-programs/inpatient-programs/skilled-nursing#:~:text=The%20HSC%20Pediatric%20Skilled%20Nursing%20Facility%20(SNF)%20is%20a%20nursing,from%20birth%20through%20age%2021 (accessed January 3, 2022).

Choi, S. K., and I. H. Meyer. 2016. *LGBT aging: A review of research findings, needs, and policy implications*. https://www.lgbtagingcenter.org/resources/pdfs/LGBT-Aging-A-Review.pdf (accessed September 23, 2021).

CMS (Centers for Medicare & Medicaid Services). 2015. *Nursing home data compendium*. Baltimore, MD: Centers for Medicare & Medicaid Services.

CMS. 2020. *Data use agreement (DUA) (agreement for use of centers for Medicare and Medicaid services (CMS) data containing individual-specific information*. https://www.cms.gov/Medicare/CMS-Forms/CMS-Forms/CMS-Forms-Items/CMS045932 (accessed January 6, 2022).

CMS. 2021a. *Nursing facilities.* https://www.medicaid.gov/medicaid/long-term-services-supports/institutional-long-term-care/nursing-facilities/index.html (accessed January 6, 2022).

CMS. 2021b. *COVID-19 nursing home data.* https://data.cms.gov/COVID-19/COVID-19-nursing-home-data (accessed September 15, 2021).

CNBC. 2020. *WHO: Coronavirus patients who don't show symptoms aren't driving the spread of the virus.* https://www.cnbc.com/video/2020/06/08/who-coronavirus-patients-who-dont-show-symptoms-arent-spreading-new-infections.html (accessed April 27, 2021).

Coe, N. B., and C. H. Van Houtven. 2020. Living arrangements of older adults and COVID-19 risk: It is not just nursing homes. *Journal of the American Geriatrics Society* 68(7):1398–1399.

Cohen, L. W., S. Zimmerman, D. Reed, P. Brown, B. J. Bowers, K. Nolet, S. Hudak, S. Horn, and the THRIVE Research Collaborative. 2016. The Green House model of nursing home care in design and implementation. *Health Services Research* 51(Suppl 1):352–377.

Colello, K. J., and S. V. Panangala. 2017. *Long-term care services for veterans.* https://fas.org/sgp/crs/misc/R44697.pdf (accessed August 23, 2021).

Comondore V. R., P. J. Devereaux, Q. Zhou, S. B. Stone, J. W. Busse, N. C. Ravindran, K. E. Burns, T. Haines, B. Stringer, D. J. Cook, S. D. Walter, T. Sullivan, O. Berwanger, M. Bhandari, S. Banglawala, J. N. Lavis, B. Patrisor, H. Schunemann, K. Walsh, N. Bhatnager, and G. H. Guyatt. 2009. Quality of care in for-profit and not-for-profit nursing homes: Systematic review and meta-analysis. *BMJ* 339:b2732.

CTDPH (State of Connecticut Department of Public Health). 2022. *Hospital discharges to post-acute care during the COVID-19 pandemic.* https://interactive.fox61.com/pdfs/ACH-to-PAC-transfer-guidance-6Jan22.pdf (accessed February 14, 2022).

Cudjoe, T. K. M., and A. A. Kotwal. 2020. "Social distancing" amid a crisis in social isolation and loneliness. *Journal of the American Geriatrics Society* 68(6):E27–E29.

de Boer, B., H. C. Beerens, M. A. Katterbach, M. Viduka, B. M. Willemse, and H. Verbeek. 2018. The physical environment of nursing homes for people with dementia: Traditional nursing homes, small-scale living facilities, and green care farms. *Healthcare* 6(4):137.

Denny-Brown, N., D. Stone, B. Hays, and D. Gallaghe. 2020. *COVID-19 intensifies nursing home workforce challenges.* Washington, DC: Office of the Assistant Secretary for Planning and Evaluation.

Domi, M., M. Leitson, D. Gifford, and K. Sreenivas. 2021. *Nursing home resident and staff COVID-19 cases after the first vaccination clinic.* https://www.ahcancal.org/Data-and-Research/Center-for-HPE/Documents/CHPE-Report-Vaccine-Effectiveness-Feb2021.pdf (accessed January 6, 2022).

Duan, Y., and C. Mueller. 2019. An empirical typology of culture change implementation in nursing homes. *Innovation in Aging* 3(Supplement_1):S801-S802.

Edemekong, P. F., D. L. Bomgaars, S. Sukumaran, and S. B. Levy. 2021. Activities of daily living. In *StatPearls [internet].* Treasure Island, FL: StatPearls Publishing.

Eijkelenboom, A., H. Verbeek, E. Felix, and J. van Hoof. 2017. Architectural factors influencing the sense of home in nursing homes: An operationalization for practice. *Frontiers of Architectural Research* 6(2):111–122.

Espinosa, E. 2020. *Why does the CDC keep changing COVID guidelines?* https://buckhead medicine.com/cdc-keep-changing-COVID-guidelines (accessed July 8, 2021).

Espinoza, R. 2014. *Out and visible: The experiences and attitudes of lesbian, gay, bisexual and transgender older adults, ages 45–75.* https://www.sageusa.org/wp-content/uploads/2018/05/sageusa-out-visible-lgbt-market-research-full-report.pdf (accessed September 23, 2021).

Fallon, A., T. Dukelow, S. P. Kennelly, and D. O'Neill. 2020. COVID-19 in nursing homes. *QJM: An International Journal of Medicine* 113(6):391–392.

FATE (Foundation Aiding the Elderly). 2020. *The history of nursing homes.* https://www.4fate.org/history.pdf (accessed September 30, 2020).

Feifer, R. A., L. Bethea, and E. M. White. 2021. Racial disparities in COVID-19 vaccine acceptance: Building trust to protect nursing home staff and residents. *Journal of the American Medical Directors Association* 22(9):1853–1855.e1851.

Flex Monitoring Team. 2020. *Critical access hospital locations list.* https://www.flexmonitoring.org/critical-access-hospital-locations-list (accessed May 21, 2021).

Fredriksen Goldsen, K., H.-J. Kim, H. Jung, and J. Goldsen. 2019. The evolution of aging with pride—National Health, Aging, and Sexuality/Gender Study: Illuminating the iridescent life course of LGBTQ adults aged 80 years and older in the United States. *International Journal of Aging and Human Development* 88(4):380–404.

Friedman, S. L., and M. A. Kalichman. 2014. Out-of-home placement for children and adolescents with disabilities. *Pediatrics* 134(4):836–846.

Fry, L., L. Fry, A. Philip, T. Mackenzie, L. Von Der Ahe, E. Doan, and F. Ahmed. 2018. High acuity unit in SNF: Novel program to improve quality of care for post-acute patients. *Journal of the American Medical Directors Association* 19(3):B18.

Gandhi, A., H. Yu, and D. C. Grabowski. 2021. High nursing staff turnover in nursing homes offers important quality information. *Health Affairs* 40(3):384–391.

GAO (U.S. Government Accountability Office). 2011. *Nursing homes: Private investment homes sometimes differed from others in deficiencies, staffing, and financial performance.* Washington, DC: U.S. Government Accountability Office.

GAO. 2019. *VA nursing home care: VA has opportunities to enhance its oversight and provide more comprehensive information on its website.* Washington, DC: U.S. Government Accountability Office.

GAO. 2020. *Infection control deficiencies were widespread and persistent in nursing homes prior to COVID-19 pandemic.* Washington, DC: U.S. Government Accountability Office.

Garcia, M. A., P. A. Homan, C. Garcia, and T. H. Brown. 2020. The color of COVID-19: Structural racism and the disproportionate impact of the pandemic on older Black and Latinx adults. *Journals of Gerontology, Series B: Psychological Sciences and Social Sciences* 76(3):e75–e80.

Gebeloff, R., D. Ivory, M. Richtel, M. Smith, K. Yourish, S. Dance, J. Fortiér, E. Yu, and M. Parker. 2020. *The striking racial divide in how COVID-19 has hit nursing homes.* https://www.nytimes.com/article/coronavirus-nursing-homes-racial-disparity.html (accessed October 16, 2020).

Geng, F., D. G. Stevenson, and D. C. Grabowski. 2019. Daily nursing home staffing levels highly variable, often below CMS expectations. *Health Affairs* 38(7):1095–1100.

Gillick, M. R. 2018. *The evolution of the nursing home.* https://www.americanscientist.org/article/the-evolution-of-the-nursing-home (accessed February 25, 2021).

Gilman, M., and M. T. Bassett. 2021. Trends in COVID-19 death rates by racial composition of nursing homes. *Journal of the American Geriatrics Society* 69(9):2442–2444.

Gleckman, H. 2020. *States are beginning to move COVID-19 patients from hospitals to nursing facilities.* https://www.forbes.com/sites/howardgleckman/2020/03/31/states-are-beginning-to-move-covid-19-patients-from-hospitals-to-nursing-facilities/?sh=7ace9a7b4401 (accessed November 8, 2021).

Goldberg, T. H. 2014. The long-term and post-acute care continuum. *West Virginia Medical Journal* 110(6):24–30.

Gorges, R. J., and R. T. Konetzka. 2020. Staffing levels and COVID-19 cases and outbreaks in U.S. nursing homes. *Journal of the American Geriatrics Society* 68(11):2462–2466.

Gorges, R. J., and R. T. Konetzka. 2021. Factors associated with racial differences in deaths among nursing home residents with COVID-19 infection in the US. *JAMA Network Open* 4(2):1–10.

Grabowski, D. C., and V. Mor. 2020. Nursing home care in crisis in the wake of COVID-19. *JAMA* 324(1):23–24.

Grabowski, D. C., and D. G. Stevenson. 2008. Ownership conversions and nursing home performance. *Health Services Research* 43(4):1184–1203.

Grabowski, D. C., K. A. Aschbrenner, V. F. Rome, and S. J. Bartels. 2010. Quality of mental health care for nursing home residents: A literature review. *Medical Care Research and Review* 67(6):627–656.

Gupta, A., S. T. Howell, C. Yannelis, and A. Gupta. 2021. *Does private equity investment in healthcare benefit patients? Evidence from nursing homes.* Working Paper 28474. https://www.nber.org/papers/w28474 (accessed February 25, 2021).

Harrington, C., S. Wollhandler, J. Mullan, H. Carrilo, and D. U. Himmelstein. 2001. Does investor ownership of nursing homes compromise the quality of care? *American Journal of Public Health* 91(9):1452–1455.

Harrington, C., B. Olney, H. Carrillo, and T. Kang. 2012. Nurse staffing and deficiencies in the largest for-profit nursing home chains and chains owned by private equity companies. *Health Services Research* 47(1 Pt 1):106–128.

Harrington, C., H. Carrillo, R. Garfield, and E. Squires. 2018. *Nursing facilities, staffing, residents and facility deficiencies, 2009 through 2016.* https://www.kff.org/medicaid/report/nursing-facilities-staffing-residents-and-facility-deficiencies-2009-through-2016 (accessed October 22, 2020).

Harrington, C., L. Ross, S. Chapman, E. Halifax, B. Spurlock, and D. Bakerjian. 2020. Nurse staffing and coronavirus infections in California nursing homes. *Policy Politics & Nursing Practice* 21(3):174-186.

Harris-Kojetin, L., M. Sengupta, J. P. Lendon, V. Rome, R. Valverde, and C. Caffrey. 2019. *Long-term care providers and services users in the United States, 2015–2016.* https://www.cdc.gov/nchs/data/series/sr_03/sr03_43-508.pdf (accessed April 2, 2021).

HealthCarePathway.com. 2022. *Pediatric extended care and long-term care facilities.* https://www.healthcarepathway.com/pediatric-extended-care-and-long-term-care-facilities/ (accessed January 3, 2022).

Hessels, A. J., S. W. Darby, E. Simpser, L. Saiman, and E. L. Larson. 2017. National testing of the Nursing-Kids Intensity of Care Survey for pediatric long-term care. *Journal of Pediatric Nursing* 37:86–90.

Hirdes, J. P., A. Declercq, H. Finne-Soveri, B. F. Fries, L. Geffen, G. Heckman, T. Lum, B. Meehan, N. Millar, and J. N. Morris. 2020. The long-term care pandemic: International perspectives on COVID-19 and the future of nursing homes. *Balsillie Papers* 2(4).

Houghton, A. 2018. *Maintaining dignity: Understanding and responding to the challenges facing older LGBT Americans.* Washington, DC: AARP Research.

Hunnicutt, J. N., C. M. Ulbricht, J. Tjia, and K. L. Lapane. 2017. Pain and pharmacologic pain management in long-stay nursing home residents. *Pain* 158(6):1091–1099.

Inouye, S. K., S. Studenski, M. E. Tinetti, and G. A. Kuchel. 2007. Geriatric syndromes: Clinical, research, and policy implications of a core geriatric concept. *Journal of the American Geriatrics Society* 55(5):780–791.

IOM (Institute of Medicine). 1986a. *Improving the quality of care in nursing homes.* Washington, DC: National Academy Press.

IOM. 1986b. *For-profit enterprise in health care.* Washington, DC: National Academy Press.

JAHF (The John A Hartford Foundation). 2021. *Age-friendly insights: Poll reveals how older adults feel about nursing homes.* https://www.johnahartford.org/dissemination-center/view/age-friendly-insights-how-do-older-adults-feel-about-nursing-homes (accessed January 7, 2022).

Jang, Y., J. A. Mortimer, W. E. Haley, and A. R. B. Graves. 2004. The role of social engagement in life satisfaction: Its significance among older individuals with disease and disability. *Journal of Applied Gerontology* 23(3):266–278.

Jin, E., and R. Agrawal. 2017. State-by-state variation in the number of children and young adults in nursing homes, 2005–2012. *Maternal and Child Health Journal* 21(12):2149–2152.

Johnson, R. W., M. M. Favreault, J. Dey, W. Marton, and L. Anderson. 2021. *Most older adults are likely to need and use long-term services and supports.* https://aspe.hhs.gov/reports/most-older-adults-are-likely-need-use-long-term-services-supports-issue-brief (accessed January 6, 2022).

Justice in Aging, National Gay and Lesbian Task Force, Services & Advocacy for LGBT Elders (SAGE), Lambda Legal, National Center for Lesbian Rights, and National Center for Transgender Equality. 2015. *LGBT older adults in long-term care facilities: Stories from the field.* Washington, DC: Justice in Aging.

KFF (Kaiser Family Foundation). 2007. *Changes in characteristics, needs, and payment for care of elderly nursing home residents: 1999 to 2004.* https://www.kff.org/medicaid/report/changes-in-characteristics-needs-and-payment-for/ (accessed June 21, 2021).

KFF. 2017. *Medicaid's role in nursing home care.* https://files.kff.org/attachment/Infographic-Medicaids-Role-in-Nursing-Home-Care (accessed January 7, 2022).

KFF. 2018. *Waiting list enrollment for Medicaid section 1915(c) home and community-based services waivers.* https://www.kff.org/health-reform/state-indicator/waiting-lists-for-hcbs-waivers/ (accessed May 25, 2021).

KFF. 2020a. *Distribution of certified nursing facility residents by primary payer source.* https://www.kff.org/other/state-indicator/distribution-of-certified-nursing-facilities-by-primary-payer-source/ (accessed April 29, 2021).

KFF. 2020b. *Total number of residents in certified nursing facilities.* https://www.kff.org/other/state-indicator/number-of-nursing-facility-residents (accessed September 30, 2021).

Khimm, S. 2020. *Coronavirus spreads in a New York nursing home forced to take recovering patients.* https://www.nbcnews.com/news/us-news/coronavirus-spreads-new-york-nursing-home-forced-take-recovering-patients-n1191811 (accessed February 15, 2020).

Konetzka, R. T., and R. M. Werner. 2009. Review: Disparities in long-term care: Building equity into market-based reforms. *Medical Care Research and Review* 66(5):491–521.

Konetzka, R. T., E. M. White, A. Pralea, D. C. Grabowski, and V. Mor. 2021. A systematic review of long-term care facility characteristics associated with COVID-19 outcomes. *Journal of the American Geriatrics Society* 69(10):2766–2777.

Koren, M. J. 2010. Person-centered care for nursing home residents: The culture-change movement. *Health Affairs (Millwood)* 29(2):312–317.

Kramer, R. G. 2021. *Fixing nursing homes: A fleeting opportunity.* https://www.healthaffairs.org/do/10.1377/hblog20210407.717832/full (accessed April 13, 2021).

Kumar, A., I. Roy, A. M. Karmarkar, K. S. Erler, J. L. Rudolph, J. A. Baldwin, and M. Rivera-Hernandez. 2021. Shifting U.S. patterns of COVID-19 mortality by race and ethnicity from June–December 2020. *Journal of the American Medical Directors Association* 22(5):966–970.e963.

Laws, M. B., A. Beeman, S. Haigh, I. B. Wilson, and R. R. Shield. 2021. Prevalence of serious mental illness and under 65 population in nursing homes continues to grow. *Journal of the American Medical Directors Association* S1525-8610(21):00941-00945. https://doi.org/10.1016/j.jamda.2021.10.020.

Lee, K., R. L. Mauldin, W. Tang, J. Connolly, J. Harwerth, and K. Magruder. 2021. Examining racial and ethnic disparities among older adults in long-term care facilities. *Gerontologist* 61(6):858–869.

Leedahl, S. N., R. K. Chapin, and T. D. Little. 2015. Multilevel examination of facility characteristics, social integration, and health for older adults living in nursing homes. *The Journals of Gerontology: Series B* 70(1):111–122.

Li, Y., C. Harrington, H. Temkin-Greener, K. You, X. Cai, X. Cen, and D. B. Mukamel. 2015a. Deficiencies in care at nursing homes and racial/ethnic disparities across homes fell, 2006–11. *Health Affairs* 34(7):1139–1146.

Li, Y., C. Harrington, D. B. Mukamel, X. Cen, X. Cai, and H. Temkin-Greener. 2015b. Nurse staffing hours at nursing homes with high concentrations of minority residents, 2001-11. *Health Affairs (Project Hope)* 34(12):2129–2137.

Li, Y., H. Temkin-Greener, G. Shan, and X. Cai. 2020a. COVID-19 infections and deaths among Connecticut nursing home residents: Facility correlates. *Journal of the American Geriatrics Society* 68(9):1899–1906.

Li, Y., X. Cen, X. Cai, and H. Temkin-Greener. 2020b. Racial and ethnic disparities in COVID-19 infections and deaths across S.S. Nursing homes. *Journal of the American Geriatrics Society* 68(11):2454–2461.

Lynch, R. M., and R. Goring. 2020. Practical steps to improve air flow in long-term care resident rooms to reduce COVID-19 infection risk. *Journal of the American Medical Directors Association* 21(7):893–894.

Mack, D. S., B. M. Jesdale, C. M. Ulbricht, S. N. Forrester, P. S. Michener, and K. L. Lapane. 2020. Racial segregation across U.S. nursing homes: A systematic review of measurement and outcomes. *The Gerontologist* 60(3):e218–e231.

Marselas, K. 2019. *Pediatric nursing home looks to create new kind of long-term care facility for young adults as numbers grow.* https://www.mcknights.com/news/pediatric-nursing-home-looks-to-create-new-kind-of-long-term-care-facility-for-young-adults-as-numbers-grow (accessed July 23, 2021).

Martel, P. 2019. *What is the difference between acute and sub-acute care?* https://www.knollwoodnursingcenter.com/difference-between-acute-sub-acute-care (accessed December 28, 2021).

Mauldin, R. L., K. Lee, W. Tang, S. Herrera, and A. Williams. 2020. Supports and gaps in federal policy for addressing racial and ethnic disparities among long-term care facility residents. *Journal of Gerontological Social Work* 63(4):354–370.

McGarry, B. E., A. D. Gandhi, D. C. Grabowski, and M. L. Barnett. 2021a. Larger nursing home staff size linked to higher number of COVID-19 cases in 2020. *Health Affairs* 40(8). https://doi.org/10.1377/hlthaff.2021.00323.

McGarry, B. E., K. Shen, M. L. Barnett, D. C. Grabowski, and A. D. Gandhi. 2021b. Association of nursing home characteristics with staff and resident COVID-19 vaccination coverage. *JAMA Internal Medicine* 181(12):1670–1672.

McGarry, B. E., M. L. Barnett, D. C. Grabowski, and A. D. Gandhi. 2022. Nursing home staff vaccination and COVID-19 outcomes. *New England Journal of Medicine* 386(4):397-398.

MedPAC (Medicare Payment Advisory Commission). 2020. *Critical access hospitals payment system.* http://www.medpac.gov/docs/default-source/payment-basics/medpac_payment_basics_20_cah_final_sec.pdf?sfvrsn=0 (accessed August 23, 2021).

MedPAC. 2021. *March report to Congress: Medicare and the health care delivery system.* http://medpac.gov/docs/default-source/reports/mar21_medpac_report_to_the_congress_sec.pdf (accessed August 16, 2021) (accessed August 16, 2021).

Miller, N. A. 2011. Relations among home- and community-based services investment and nursing home rates of use for working-age and older adults: A state-level analysis. *American Journal of Public Health* 101(9):1735–1741.

Miller, N. A., L. M. Pinet-Peralta, and K. T. Elder. 2012. A profile of middle-aged and older adults admitted to nursing homes: 2000–2008. *Journal of Aging and Social Policy* 24(3):271–290.

Miller, S. C., M. L. Schwartz, J. C. Lima, R. R. Shield, D. A. Tyler, C. W. Berridge, P. L. Gozalo, M. J. Lepore, and M. A. Clark. 2018. The prevalence of culture change practice in US nursing homes: Findings from a 2016/2017 nationwide survey. *Medical Care* 56(12):985–993.

Montgomery, A., S. Slocum, and C. Stanik. 2020. *Experiences of nursing home residents during the pandemic.* https://altarum.org/sites/default/files/uploaded-publication-files/Nursing-Home-Resident-Survey_Altarum-Special-Report_FINAL.pdf (accessed February 25, 2021).

Mor, V., J. Zinn, J. Angelelli, J. M. Teno, and S. C. Miller. 2004. Driven to tiers: Socioeconomic and racial disparities in the quality of nursing home care. *The Milbank Quarterly* 82(2):227–256.

Muenchberger, H., C. Ehrlich, E. Kendall, and M. Vit. 2012. Experience of place for young adults under 65 years with complex disabilities moving into purpose-built residential care. *Social Science and Medicine* 75(12):2151–2159.

Nanduri, S., T. Pilishvili, G. Derado, M. M. Soe, P. Dollard, H. Wu, Q. Li, S. Bagchi, H. Dubendris, R. Link-Gelles, J. A. Jernigan, D. S. Budnitz, J. Bell, A. L. Benin, N. Shang, J. R. Edwards, J. R. Verani, and S. J. Schrag. 2021. Effectiveness of Pfizer-Biontech and Moderna vaccines in preventing SARS-CoV-2 infection among nursing home residents before and during widespread circulation of the SARS-CoV-2 b.1.617.2 (delta) variant—National Healthcare Safety Network, March 1–August 1, 2021. *Morbidity and Mortality Weekly Report* 70:1163–1166.

NCVAS (National Center for Veterans Analysis and Statistics). 2020. *Veteran population.* https://www.va.gov/vetdata/veteran_population.asp (accessed January 8, 2021).

NIA (National Institute on Aging). 2021. *Residential facilities, assisted living, and nursing homes.* https://www.nia.nih.gov/health/residential-facilities-assisted-living-and-nursing-homes (accessed April 19, 2021).

Nursing Home Law Center. 2010. *Children in nursing homes: Truly the most vulnerable.* https://www.nursinghomelawcenter.org/news/nursing-home-abuse/children-in-nursing-homes-truly-the-most-vulnerable (accessed July 23, 2021).

Nygaard, A., L. Halvorsrud, E. K. Grov, and A. Bergland. 2020. What matters to you when the nursing is your home: A qualitative study on the views of residents with dementia living in nursing homes. *BMC Geriatrics* 20(1):227.

OIG (Office of the Inspector General). 2006. *Nursing home emergency preparedness and response during recent hurricanes.* Washington, DC: Office of the Inspector General, U.S. Department of Health and Human Services.

OIG. 2012. *Gaps continue to exist in nursing home emergency preparedness and response during disasters: 2007–2010.* Washington, DC: Office of the Inspector General, U.S. Department of Health and Human Services.

OIG. 2021. *COVID-19 had a devastating impact on Medicare beneficiaries in nursing homes during 2020.* Washington, DC: Office of the Inspector General, U.S. Department of Health and Human Services.

Ogden, L. L., and K. Adams. 2009. Poorhouse to warehouse: Institutional long-term care in the United States. *Publius* 39(1):138–163.

Ouslander, J. G., and D. C. Grabowski. 2019. Rehabbed to death reframed: In response to "rehabbed to death: Breaking the cycle". *Journal of the American Geriatrics Society* 67(11):2225–2228.

Ouslander, J. G., and D. C. Grabowski. 2020. COVID-19 in nursing homes: Calming the perfect storm. *Journal of the American Geriatrics Society* 58(10):2153–2162.

Paulin, E. 2021. *Worker shortages in nursing homes hit pandemic peak as COVID-19 deaths continue.* https://www.aarp.org/caregiving/health/info-2021/nursing-home-covid-19-report-november.html (accessed February 14, 2022).

PCCA (Pediatric Complex Care Association). 2016. *Children and young adults with medical complexity: Serving an emerging population. A white paper prepared for the Centers for Medicare & Medicaid Services.* https://pediatriccomplexcare.org/wp-content/uploads/2016/03/PCCA-CMSWhitePaper012716.pdf (accessed July 23, 2021).

PCCA. 2020. *PCCA quality benchmark: Data from 2015 Q2 to 2019 Q4.* https://pediatric-complexcare.org/pdf/PCCA-Quality-Benchmark-Report-2015-Q2-2019-Q4_6-26-2020.pdf (accessed January 4, 2022).

Pearson, C. F., C. C. Quinn, S. Loganathan, A. R. Datta, B. B. Mace, and D. C. Grabowski. 2019. The forgotten middle: Many middle-income seniors will have insufficient resources for housing and health care. *Health Affairs* 38(5). https://doi.org/10.1377/hlthaff.2018.05233.

Perissinotto, C. M., I. Stijacic Cenzer, and K. E. Covinsky. 2012. Loneliness in older persons: A predictor of functional decline and death. *Archives of Internal Medicine* 172(14):1078–1083.

Persson, D. I., and S. K. Ostwald. 2009. Younger residents in nursing homes. *Journal of Gerontological Nursing* 35(10):22–31.

Pradhan, R., R. Weech-Maldonado, J. S. Harman, M. Al-Amin, and K. Hyer. 2014. Private equity ownership of nursing homes: Implications for quality. *Journal of Health Care Finance* 42(2).

Putney, J. M., S. Keary, N. Hebert, L. Krinsky, and R. Halmo. 2018. "Fear runs deep": The anticipated needs of LGBT older adults in long-term care. *Journal of Gerontological Social Work* 61(8):887–907.

Rahman, M., P. Gozalo, D. Tyler, D. C. Grabowski, A. Trivedi, and V. Mor. 2014. Dual eligibility, selection of skilled nursing facility, and length of Medicare paid post-acute stay. *Medical Care Research and Review* 71(4):384–401.

Rantz, M. J., M. Skubic, G. Alexander, M. A. Aud, B. J. Wakefield, C. Galambos, R. J. Koopman, and S. J. Miller. 2010a. Improving nurse care coordination with technology. *Computers, Informatics, Nursing* 28(6):325–332.

Rantz, M. J., L. Hicks, G. F. Petroski, R. W. Madsen, G. Alexander, C. Galambos, V. Conn, J. Scott-Cawiezell, M. Zwygart-Stauffacher, and L. Greenwald. 2010b. Cost, staffing and quality impact of bedside electronic medical record (EMR) in nursing homes. *Journal of the American Medical Directors Association* 11(7):485–493.

Reaves, E. L., and M. Musumeci. 2015. *Medicaid and long-term services and supports: A primer.* https://www.kff.org/medicaid/report/medicaid-and-long-term-services-and-supports-a-primer (accessed January 4, 2022).

Reber, S., and C. Kosar. 2021. *Vaccine hesitancy in nursing homes isn't all politics.* https://www.brookings.edu/research/vaccine-hesitancy-in-nursing-homes-isnt-all-politics (accessed January 7, 2022).

RHIH (Rural Health Information Hub). 2019. *Critical access hospitals (CAHs).* https://www.ruralhealthinfo.org/topics/critical-access-hospitals (accessed May 21, 2021).

Ritter, A. Z., S. Freed, and N. B. Coe. 2021. Younger individuals increase their use of nursing homes following ACA Medicaid expansion. *Journal of the American Medical Directors Association.* S1525-8610(21)00742-8. Online ahead of print. https://doi.org/10.1016/j.jamda.2021.08.020.

Rivera-Hernandez, M., A. Kumar, G. Epstein-Lubow, and K. S. Thomas. 2019. Disparities in nursing home use and quality among African American, Hispanic, and white Medicare residents with Alzheimer's disease and related dementias. *Journal of Aging and Health* 31(7):1259–1277.

SAGE (Services & Advocacy for LGBT Elders). 2021. *Facts on LGBT aging.* https://www.sageusa.org/resource-posts/facts-on-lgbt-aging (accessed September 23, 2021).

SAGE and the Human Rights Campaign Foundation. 2020. *COVID-19 & LGBTQ older people.* https://www.sageusa.org/wp-content/uploads/2020/04/COVID19-elder-issuebrief-032720b-1-1.pdf (accessed September 23, 2021).

Sandvoll, A. M., E. K. Grov, and M. Simonsen. 2020. Nursing home residents' ADL status, institution-dwelling and association with outdoor activity: A cross-sectional study. *PeerJ* 8:e10202.

Sapien, J., and J. Sexton. 2020. *Andrew Cuomo's report on controversial nursing home policy for COVID patients prompts more controversy*. https://www.propublica.org/article/andrew-cuomos-report-on-controversial-nursing-home-policy-for-covid-patients-prompts-more-controversy (accessed February 15, 2022).

Schwarz, B. 1997. Nursing home design: A misguided architectural model. *Journal of Architectural and Planning Research* 14(4):343–359.

Scott, A. M., J. Li, S. Oyewole-Eletu, H. Q. Nguyen, B. Gass, K. B. Hirschman, S. Mitchell, S. M. Hudson, and M. V. Williams. 2017. Understanding facilitators and barriers to care transitions: Insights from Project ACHIEVE site visits. *Joint Commission Journal on Quality and Patient Safety* 43(9):433–447.

Sharma, H., M. C. Perraillon, R. M. Werner, D. C. Grabowski, and R. T. Konetzka. 2020. Medicaid and nursing home choice: Why do duals end up in low-quality facilities? *Journal of Applied Gerontology* 39(9):981–990.

Sherman, R. O., and T. Touhy. 2017. An exploratory descriptive study to evaluate Florida nurse leader challenges and opportunities in nursing homes settings. *SAGE Open Nursing*, January. https://doi.org/10.1177/2377960817718754.

Shieu, B. M., J. A. Almusajin, C. Dictus, A. S. Beeber, and R. A. Anderson. 2021. Younger nursing home residents: A scoping review of their lived experiences, needs, and quality of life. *Journal of the American Medical Directors Association* 22(11):2296–2312.

Shippee, T. P., C. Henning-Smith, T. G. Rhee, R. N. Held, and R. L. Kane. 2016. Racial differences in Minnesota nursing home residents' quality of life: The importance of looking beyond individual predictors. *Journal of Aging and Health* 28(2):199–224.

Shippee, T. P., W. Ng, and J. R. Bowblis. 2020. Does living in a higher proportion minority facility improve quality of life for racial/ethnic minority residents in nursing homes? *Innovation in Aging* 4(3):igaa014.

Sifuentes, A. M. F., and K. L. Lapane. 2020. Oral health in nursing homes: What we know and what we need to know. *The Journal of Nursing Home Research Sciences* 6:1–5.

Sloane, P. D., C. M. Mitchell, G. Weisman, S. Zimmerman, K. M. Foley, M. Lynn, M. Calkins, M. P. Lawton, J. Teresi, L. Grant, D. Lindeman, and R. Montgomery. 2002. The Therapeutic Environment Screening Survey for Nursing Homes (TESS-RN): An observational instrument for assessing the physical environment of institutional settings for persons with dementia. *Journals of Gerontology, Series B: Psychological Sciences and Social Sciences* 57(2):S69–S78.

Sloane, P. D., R. Yearby, R. T. Konetzka, Y. Li, R. Espinoza, and S. Zimmerman. 2021. Addressing systemic racism in nursing homes: A time for action. *Journal of the American Medical Directors Association* 22(4):886–892.

Spanko, A. 2020. *COVID-19 brings private equity investment in nursing homes into the spotlight*. https://skillednursingnews.com/2020/03/COVID-19-brings-private-equity-investment-in-nursing-homes-into-the-spotlight (accessed January 8, 2021).

Stein, R. E. K. 2001. Challenges in long-term health care for children. *Ambulatory Pediatrics* 1(5):280–288.

Stevenson, D. G., and D.C. Grabowski. 2008. Private equity investment and nursing home care: Is it a big deal? *Health Affairs* 27(5):1399–1408.

Stevenson, D. G., J. S. Bramson, and D. C. Grabowski. 2013. Nursing home ownership trends and their impacts on quality of care: A study using detailed ownership data from Texas. *Journal of Aging & Social Policy* 25(1):30–47.

Taylor, J., J. Mishory, and O. Chan. 2020. *Even in nursing homes, COVID-19 racial disparities persist.* https://tcf.org/content/commentary/even-nursing-homes-COVID-19-racial-disparities-persist (accessed April 27, 2021).

Thompson, D.-C., M.-G. Barbu, C. Beiu, L. G. Popa, M. M. Mihai, M. Berteanu, and M. N. Popescu. 2020. The impact of COVID-19 pandemic on long-term care facilities worldwide: An overview on international issues. *BioMed Research International* 2020:8870249.

Travers, J. L., A. W. Dick, and P. W. Stone. 2018a. Racial/ethnic differences in receipt of influenza and pneumococcal vaccination among long-stay nursing home residents. *Health Services Research* 53(4):2203–2226.

Travers, J. L., K. L. Schroeder, T. E. Blaylock, and P. W. Stone. 2018b. Racial/ethnic disparities in influenza and pneumococcal vaccinations among nursing home residents: A systematic review. *The Gerontologist* 58(4):e205–e217.

Travers, J. L., M. Agarwal, L. V. Estrada, A. W. Dick, T. Gracner, B. Wu, and P. W. Stone. 2021. Assessment of coronavirus disease 2019 infection and mortality rates among nursing homes with different proportions of Black residents. *Journal of the American Medical Directors Association* 22(4):893–898.e892.

Trybusińska, D., and A. Saracen. 2019. Loneliness in the context of quality of life of nursing home residents. *Open Medicine* 14:354–361.

U.S. Census Bureau. 2021a. *About.* https://www.census.gov/programs-surveys/metro-micro/about.html (accessed October 29, 2021).

U.S. Census Bureau. 2021b. *U.S. and world population clock.* https://www.census.gov/popclock/ (accessed November 12, 2021).

VA (Department of Veterans Affairs). 2021. *Geriatrics and extended care: Residential settings and nursing homes.* https://www.va.gov/geriatrics/pages/Nursing_Home_and_Residential_Services.asp (accessed January 7, 2022).

VA-OIG (Department of Veterans Affairs, Office of the Inspector General). 2020. *Review of VHA community living centers and corresponding star ratings.* Washington, DC: Department of Veterans Affairs.

Van Malderen, L., T. Mets, and E. Gorus. 2013. Interventions to enhance the quality of life of older people in residential long-term care: A systematic review. *Ageing Research Reviews* 12(1):141–150.

Vespa, J., L. Medina, and Armstrong, D. M. 2020. *Demographic turning points for the United States: Population projections for 2020 to 2060.* https://www.census.gov/content/dam/Census/library/publications/2020/demo/p25-1144.pdf (accessed August 3, 2021).

Vest, J. R., H. Y. Jung, K. Wiley, Jr., H. Kooreman, L. Pettit, and M. A. Unruh. 2019. Adoption of health information technology among us nursing facilities. *Journal of the American Medical Directors Association* 20(8):995–1000.e1004.

Wagner, D. 2005. *The poorhouse: America's forgotten institution.* https://socialwelfare.library.vcu.edu/issues/poor-relief-almshouse (accessed October 2, 2020).

Waters, R. 2021. The big idea behind a new model of small nursing homes. *Health Affairs* 40(3):378–383.

Watson, S. D. 2012. From almshouses to nursing homes and community care: Lessons from Medicaid's history. *Georgia State University Law Review* 26(3):13.

White, E. M., C. M. Kosar, R. A. Feifer, C. Blackman, S. Gravenstein, J. Ouslander, and V. Mor. 2020. Variation in SARS-CoV-2 prevalence in U.S. skilled nursing facilities. *Journal of the American Geriatrics Society* 68(10):2167–2173.

White, E. M., T. F. Wetle, A. Reddy, and R. R. Baier. 2021. Front-line nursing home staff experiences during the COVID-19 pandemic. *Journal of the American Medical Directors Association* 22(1):199–203.

Whitelaw, S., M. A. Mamas, E. Topol, and H. G. C. Van Spall. 2020. Applications of digital technology in COVID-19 pandemic planning and response. *The Lancet Digital Health* 2(8):e435–e440.

Witt, S., and J. Hoyt. 2021. *Nursing home costs.* https://www.seniorliving.org/nursing-homes/costs (accessed September 15, 2021).

Wu, M. C., H. C. Sung, W. L. Lee, and G. D. Smith. 2015. The effects of light therapy on depression and sleep disruption in older adults in a long-term care facility. *International Journal of Nursing Practice* 21(5):653–659.

Yan, D., S. Wang, H. Temkin-Greener, and S. Cai. 2021. Admissions to high-quality nursing homes from community: Racial differences and Medicaid policy effects. *Health Services Research* 56(S2):16–17.

Yang, B. K., M. Carter, and W. Nelson. 2021. Trends in COVID-19 cases, related deaths, and staffing shortage in nursing homes by rural and urban status. *Geriatric Nursing* 42(6):1356–1361.

You, K., Y. Li, O. Intrator, D. Stevenson, R. Hirth, D. Grabowski, and J. Banaszak-Holl. 2016. Do nursing home chain size and proprietary status affect experiences with care? *Medical Care* 54(3):229–234.

Yuen, H. K., P. Huang, J. K. Burik, and T. G. Smith. 2008. Impact of participating in volunteer activities for residents living in long-term-care facilities. *American Journal of Occupational Therapy* 62(1):71–76.

Yurkofsky, M., and J. G. Ouslander. 2021a. *Medical care in skilled nursing facilities (SNFs) in the United States.* https://www.uptodate.com/contents/medical-care-in-skilled-nursing-facilities-snfs-in-the-united-states (accessed July 16, 2021).

Yurkofsky, M., and J. G. Ouslander. 2021b. *COVID-19: Management in nursing homes.* https://www.uptodate.com/contents/COVID-19-management-in-nursing-homes (accessed July 8, 2021).

Quality Measurement and Quality Improvement

Quality measurement has been characterized as "fundamental to systematic improvement of the healthcare system" (Burstin et al., 2016). In the early 2000s, two notable reports from the Institute of Medicine (IOM), *To Err is Human* (2000) and *Crossing the Quality Chasm* (2001a), fostered a national conversation about the quality of health care. At that time, the IOM defined the six aims of quality improvement in health care—i.e., to make health care more safe, timely, equitable, efficient, effective, and patient centered (IOM, 2001a). This chapter provides an overview of quality measurement in the nursing home setting and describes how such measures can, in turn, be used to improve the quality of care for residents of nursing homes.

THE PURPOSE OF QUALITY MEASUREMENT

The primary purpose of quality measurement is to support work aimed at improving the quality of care and outcomes (Conway et al., 2013; Rantz et al., 2002). The Agency for Healthcare Research and Quality (AHRQ) defines quality improvement as

> The framework we use to systematically improve the ways care is delivered to patients. Processes have characteristics that can be measured, analyzed, improved, and controlled. [Quality improvement] entails continuous efforts to achieve stable and predictable process results, that is, to reduce process variation and improve the outcomes of these processes both for patients and the health care organization and system. Achieving sustained [quality improvement] requires commitment from the entire organization, particularly from top-level management. (AHRQ, 2013)

In addition to this overarching goal of quality improvement, quality measurement serves several other distinct purposes, including

- assisting consumers in making choices about providers and facilities;
- ensuring care providers' accountability for outcomes, including through public reporting, value-based purchasing programs, and accreditation or certification;
- providing evidence to inform treatment decisions, optimize clinical interventions, and elucidate the effectiveness of interventions on patient and family outcomes;
- guiding quality improvement activities; and
- producing new knowledge through clinical and health services research to guide policy (AHRQ, 2012; Basch et al., 2013; Conway et al., 2013; Landrum et al., 2019).

Accurate and interpretable information on nursing home quality needs to be readily available to all those seeking nursing home care as well as to the friends or family that may help with nursing home decisions. Faced with a determination concerning the need for nursing home care, people may feel overwhelmed with anxiety and questions, such as: How do I choose? How can I be sure the care will be what I need? Will the care be of good quality, and how will I know if the quality is good? How can I get the best possible care that I want and now need? In addition, such information needs to be available to public and private payers for nursing home care, namely the Medicare and Medicaid state and federal payers, private insurance companies, and individuals who have the resources to pay privately. Payers want to know that they are paying for high-quality care.

State and federal regulators of nursing homes are charged with the responsibility of ensuring a level of quality of care that "protects" the public (IOM, 2001b). This protection is a basic assurance that the quality of care meets a fundamental level so that, when needed, safe nursing home care is available in a community. However, people often say that they want "high-quality care" or the "best care" instead of care that meets a minimal, fundamentally safe level. This desire to know when nursing homes actually provide high-quality care underlies the need for good measures of quality in nursing homes.

Nursing homes in the United States and around the world face unprecedented times, as the COVID-19 pandemic has had a disproportionate impact on nursing homes where the most vulnerable older adults live and receive care (Cockburn, 2020). Friends and family who were barred from entry to places they had been visiting frequently struggle with the loss of family members and loved ones they could not visit and comfort during the end of life. With thousands dying in a short period of time, the public sentiment has been that the "protections with basic assurance of quality" have been lost to widespread poor care in nursing homes where fundamental basic needs go unmet for days or weeks on end (Cockburn, 2020; Karlawish et al., 2020; Simpson, 2020). The tragedy of the pandemic provides an opportunity for re-envisioning nursing home care using quality measurements to guide those changes.

PRINCIPLES AND DEFINITIONS

The Centers for Medicare & Medicaid Services (CMS) defines quality measures as "tools that help us measure or quantify healthcare processes, outcomes, patient perceptions, and organizational structure and/or systems that are associated with the ability to provide high-quality health care and/or that relate to one or more quality goals for health care. These goals include effective, safe, efficient, patient-centered, equitable, and timely care" (CMS, 2020a). Measuring the quality of care relies on comparing that care against recognized standards of care (NQF, 2021). Therefore, individual quality measures facilitate consistent comparisons against those standards. Donabedian's framework is commonly used to categorize quality measures as measures of structure, process, or outcome (Donabedian, 1988). Structural measures include the size of the nursing home, the types and numbers of staff, and the profit or not-for-profit status of the home. Process measures include the specific steps in the systematic delivery of care, such as assessments of clinical conditions, whether personal decisions about care (e.g., end of life) are discussed and recorded for all staff to honor, or if personal care is actually completed. Outcome measures include such things as mortality rates, infection types and rates, and satisfaction with care. Many issues need to be considered when developing quality measures (see Table 3-1).

TABLE 3-1 Criteria to Develop and Evaluate/Measure Quality

Importance to measure	Evaluates the evidence to support a measure and the potential variation in performance across providers
Scientific acceptability	Assesses the reliability and validity of the measure
Feasibility	Assesses the burden involved with collecting the measure information
Usability and use	Evaluates if a measure can be appropriately used in an accountability program
Related and competing measures	Assesses if the measure is duplicative of other measures; requests harmonization or selection of best in class

SOURCE: Landrum et al., 2019.

Quality measurement in nursing homes can range from simple care measures to complex care management measures. For example, "The resident's face is clean and free from food particles" or "The resident's breath is fresh and free from odor" would be examples of simple care measures (Rantz et al., 2002). Complex care management measures include such things as documentation that the advanced directive form was discussed and completed with (a) items checked related to antibiotics, hydration, tube feedings, and hospitalizations; (b) other feelings and beliefs documented; and (c) the signature of the resident or responsible person and the primary care provider's signature, with dates, obtained. Extracting simple measures of everyday care from records and observations of workflow can be an easy method to rapidly collect data, compare to past performance, develop plans to improve performance, and implement those plans (Rantz et al., 2002). Discoveries of new and better ways to treat health conditions occur regularly, and continuous measurement is essential to ensuring that such improvements are incorporated into care delivery in a timely manner. More importantly, quality data will show if those changes have produced measurable improvements for the residents of nursing homes and their families or significant others in areas that are important to them.

Any system of quality measurement needs to support quality improvement through comparative reports, often designed as feedback reports. These reports need to be easily visualized and understood so that care staff can see how making changes in clinical care will lead to improvements in quality. To be most effective, these feedback reports need to be available in as close to real time as possible and emphasized quickly at the point of care. In addition to measurement and feedback, the implementation of quality improvement efforts can benefit from other approaches, including learning collaboratives and coaching (Ivers et al., 2012, 2014; Powell et al., 2015).

Ensuring that a nursing home makes lasting quality improvement changes requires systematic follow-up and reinforcement by organizational leaders sustained over many months, if not years (Norton et al., 2018; Rantz et al., 2012a,b, 2013; Vogelsmeier et al., 2021). Quality assurance and quality improvement are therefore related in that quality assurance "involves assessing or evaluating quality; identifying problems or issues with care delivery and designing quality improvement activities to overcome them; and follow-up monitoring to make sure the activities did what they were supposed to" (Jevaji, 2016). (See Chapter 8 for more on oversight and regulatory approaches to quality assurance.)

EVOLUTION OF QUALITY MEASUREMENT IN NURSING HOMES

In the 1800s, following the Crimean War, Florence Nightingale developed multiple standards for nursing care and called for change in the profession to achieve higher standards (Nightingale, 1859). She initiated a process to set standards for care, and then measured the care that was actually delivered in order to improve the quality of care delivered (Burstin et al., 2016; Rantz et al., 2002). This process was prompted by the appalling death rates and poor infection control practices in the Crimean War, strikingly similar to what has happened during the pandemic of COVID-19 in nursing homes in the United States and throughout the world.

The 1986 IOM report *Improving the Quality of Care in Nursing Homes* laid the foundation for the evolution of quality measurement based on resident assessment information, noting that a "system to obtain standardized data on residents is essential" (IOM, 1986, p. 24). That report envisioned that this assessment system would have "multiple uses both for nursing home management and for government regulatory agencies" (IOM, 1986, p. 24) and that a registered nurse would perform the assessments "upon admission, periodically, and whenever there is a change in resident status" (IOM, 1986, p. 26).

These assessments, part of the Resident Assessment Instrument process, included the Minimum Data Set (MDS)[1] for ongoing assessment of resident needs and conditions (Morris et al., 1990). In 1989, the Health Care Finance Administration (the predecessor to CMS) sponsored the multistate Nursing Home Casemix and Quality demonstration project to develop a quality measurement system using MDS data (Abt Associates Inc., 2002). These quality indicators, developed and tested during the late 1980s and 1990s and publicly reported in 2002, were the forerunners of today's quality measures that staff use for quality improvement and that regulators use in the survey process.

National Quality Forum

In 1999, the Strategic Framework Board, a precursor to the National Quality Forum (NQF),[2] was created to design a strategy for national quality measurement and reporting, to articulate guiding principles and priorities for the system, and identify barriers and solutions for implementing quality measurement systems. The guiding principles were

(1) There should be a single level of quality available to all Americans;
(2) Quality should not be determined by where someone lives or receives care, or by type of insurance;

---

[1] The Minimum Data Set "is part of the federally mandated process for clinical assessment of all residents in Medicare and Medicaid certified nursing homes. This process provides a comprehensive assessment of each resident's functional capabilities and helps nursing home staff identify health problems" (CMS, 2012).

[2] For more information, see www.qualityforum.org (accessed November 1, 2021).

(3) Quality measurement systems should include focused actions with single sets of priorities that are translated through the local health care delivery system; and
(4) National standards are needed to ensure consistency in measurement requirements imposed by different stakeholders across the health care system (McGlynn, 2003).

Finally, the board developed a framework for selecting national goals that were linked with the IOM's aims for improving safety, effectiveness, patient-centered systems, timeliness, efficiency, and equitable service delivery in the health care system (IOM, 2001a).

Today, the NQF uses a consensus-based process to endorse quality measures. At the time that NQF was created, the science of quality measurement was still developing and, for the most part, measures were not widely available for many health care settings and clinical environments. As a result, most measures were developed and adopted through individual health care organizations, which resulted in nonstandard measures across organizations and competing measurement systems across settings. Furthermore, because of a lack of oversight, regulation, and enforcement, there was insufficient stakeholder engagement (e.g., among health care workers and patients) in quality measurement processes and reporting.

The NQF's Measures Application Panel for Post-Acute Care/Long-Term Care Workgroup provides multistakeholder, pre-rulemaking input to CMS. In 2020, the panel identified measures of care coordination, interoperability, and patient-reported outcomes as being among the most important measures in health care settings (NQF, 2020).

CARE COMPARE[3] AND THE CMS FIVE-STAR RATING SYSTEM

In the late 1990s, federally mandated public reporting began for nursing homes on Nursing Home Compare, a web-based report card for certified nursing homes. The hope was that, as with other types of public reporting, consumers could use the information to help inform their choices and providers could use the information for quality improvement. Originally the website was not widely promoted, and it limited its information to regulatory deficiencies; a decade later, it expanded to include nurse staffing data (Konetzka et al., 2020). In 2002, through the Nursing Home Quality Initiative, the website added 10 clinical quality measures based on aggregated assessment data from the MDS (CMS, 2003). At this time, the

---

[3] Formerly known as Nursing Home Compare, CMS changed the name to Care Compare in fall 2020 (CMS, 2021a).

website was more broadly promoted and allowed consumers to compare quality measures across nursing homes nationwide (CMS, 2003; Harris and Clauser, 2002). In 2008, Nursing Home Compare began publishing a five-star composite rating for each nursing home, ranging from one to five stars. The five-star rating is based on quality in three domains: inspections (based on deficiencies and effort needed to correct those deficiencies), staffing, and quality measures (Konetzka et al., 2020). Each of these domains is translated into a composite star rating, which the website also reports.

Calculation of the Star Rating

Calculating the overall star rating begins with assigning ratings in the inspections domain, based on the in-state distribution of inspection scores, divided into percentiles. Nursing homes can then gain one or two extra stars by performing well in the staffing or quality measures domains, or they can lose up to two stars by performing poorly in them. Thus, the inspections domain is weighted most heavily (CMS, 2021a,b). CMS regularly updates the rating system and website, not only by updating the reported scores on a quarterly basis (CMS, 2021a), but also by creating new measures, amending the list of included measures, and improving the interface. Although calculating the inspections score has changed little over the years, substantial changes have been made to the staffing and quality measures domains (CMS, 2020b; RTI International, 2012).

Staffing Domain

The staffing component of the rating system underwent a significant change when the underlying data source was changed. From Nursing Home Compare's inception, staffing data were based on the Online Survey Certification and Reporting system (later replaced by the Certification and Survey Provider Enhanced Reporting system) data reflecting facility-reported staffing hours for the 2 weeks prior to the annual Medicaid recertification inspection. Thus, if nursing homes anticipated their survey dates and increased their staffing numbers prior to the survey, the data would not reflect actual staffing ratios throughout the year (Sharma et al., 2019). Furthermore, nuances of staffing, such as weekday versus weekend staffing, could not be examined. There were also concerns that facilities might inflate their numbers, given that the data were not audited. In 2016, CMS began requiring nursing facilities to submit ongoing data on staffing which are audited in the new Payroll-Based Journal system (CMS, 2018; Geng et al., 2019; OIG, 2021), and in April 2018, CMS began using these new staffing data in Care Compare. The reported measures did not change, but the underlying data were presumed to be more valid. Concerns remain that average staffing ratios do not fully reflect all of the aspects of staffing that contribute to quality, such as expertise among staff (Snyder et al., 2019).

Quality Measures Domain

The quality measures domain has undergone changes in both data source and content. CMS has removed some measures, particularly those whose validity became more doubtful over time (e.g., "improvement in walking") and added other newly established measures (e.g., the percent of residents who received influenza vaccinations, hospital readmission). Prior to the use of the five-star system, all quality measures were based on the MDS. Starting in 2018, CMS added several measures based on Medicare claims. These claims-based measures have the advantage that they are not based on facility-reported data and therefore may be more valid, as concerns have been raised about gaming of the MDS-based measures (Davila et al., 2021; Perraillon et al., 2019a,b). However, these newer measures have the disadvantage of being based only on data for Medicare fee-for-service beneficiaries, leaving out those in Medicare Advantage plans and the under-65 population that may not be on Medicare,[4] which could raise concerns regarding the adequate measurement of quality for facilities that have disproportionate numbers of these types of residents. Table 3-2 shows the specific quality measures (both MDS-based measures and claims-based measures) for short-stay and long-stay residents used in the calculation of the five-star rating.

The weight or possible points assigned to each measure used in the five-star rating has also changed over time. Measures on which most facilities have improved (so that there is very little variation left to distinguish performance) receive fewer points than those with more potential for improvement. There have also been multiple changes in how the total quality measure scores are assigned to star ratings, as keeping constant thresholds would result in an increasing number of nursing homes receiving four or five stars in this domain. Finally, average star ratings vary by state; for example, average ratings range from 2.48 in Louisiana to 4.02 in Hawaii (CMS, 2021c).

---

[4] The most current list of measures and the technical specifications for calculating them can be found on the CMS website: https://www.cms.gov/Medicare/Provider-Enrollment-and-Certification/CertificationandComplianc/Downloads/APPENDIX-New-Claims-based-Measures-Technical-Specifications-January-2020.pdf (accessed November 1, 2021).

TABLE 3-2 Quality Measures Used in the Five-Star Rating

Quality Measure Label	Data Source
SHORT-STAY QUALITY MEASURES	
Percentage of residents who improved in their ability to move around on their own	MDS
Percentage of skilled nursing facility (SNF) residents with pressure ulcers/pressure injuries that are new or worsened	MDS
Percentage of residents who take antipsychotic medication for the first time	MDS
Percentage of short-stay residents who were rehospitalized after a nursing home admission	Claims
Percentage of short-stay residents who have had an outpatient emergency department (ED) visit	Claims
Rate of successful return to home and community from a SNF	Claims
LONG-STAY QUALITY MEASURES	
Percentage of residents whose ability to move independently worsened	MDS
Percentage of residents whose need for help with daily activities has increased	MDS
Percentage of high-risk residents with pressure ulcers	MDS
Percentage of residents who have/had a catheter inserted and left in their bladder	MDS
Percentage of residents with a urinary tract infection	MDS
Percentage of residents experiencing one or more falls with major injury	MDS
Percentage of residents who got an antipsychotic medication	MDS
Number of hospitalizations per 1,000 resident days	Claims
Number of outpatient ED visits per 1,000 long-stay resident days	Claims

SOURCE: CMS, 2021a.
NOTE: Additional quality measures are reported and available, but are not included in the calculation of the five-star rating.

Overall Star Rating

Star ratings increased over the first five years (2009–2013) of use of the five-star rating system (see Table 3-3), particularly in the quality measures and staffing domains (Abt Associates Inc., 2014). In 2019, CMS announced updates to the five-star rating system, including new thresholds for staffing and quality measurement domains, and the use of payroll-based data for staffing data (CMS, 2019). As shown in Table 3-3, many nursing homes' subsequent ratings fell (Bose and Wilson, 2019; Reape, 2019). (See later in this chapter for more on self-reported data and the five-star system.)

TABLE 3-3 Nursing Homes' Five-Star Ratings, 2009–2019

	2009	2013	2019
One star	22.7%	10.5%	19.1%
Two stars	20.7%	20.8%	19.2%
Three stars	21.5%	18.2%	18.9%
Four stars	23.4%	26.5%	21.9%
Five stars	11.8%	24.1%	20.8%

SOURCES: Abt Associates Inc., 2014; Reape, 2019.

Risk Adjustment and Validity of Care Compare Measures

One systematic review of the effectiveness of Care Compare included an assessment of evidence on the risk adjustment, correlation, and validity of the included quality metrics (Konetzka et al., 2020). The findings of this review are summarized below.

Risk Adjustment

One concern regarding the measures included in Care Compare is inadequate risk adjustment—that is, a failure to account for the fact that some nursing homes serve a sicker population than others, which makes it difficult to perform as well on measures of quality. Many providers believe their facilities' ratings misrepresent the quality of the care they provide due inadequate risk adjustment (Kim et al., 2014; Perraillon et al., 2019a). Many measures in Care Compare do incorporate some risk adjustment. For example, among staffing measures expected staffing ratios adjust for resident severity, and among clinical quality measures the hospitalization measures are adjusted for resident age, sex, and comorbidities, among other factors. Despite substantial research and testing of measures of clinical quality, risk adjustment remains imperfect because of "inherent tradeoffs between the desire for validity and the desire to avoid complexity" (Konetzka et al., 2020, p. 304; see also Zimmerman et al., 1995). For example, Konetzka and colleagues (2020) noted specific findings from the following studies:

- Resident case-mix[5] accounts for half of the variation in measures that have not been adjusted for risk (Li et al., 2010);
- False negative rates are high among unadjusted measures (Li et al., 2009); and
- The introduction of appropriate risk-adjustment approaches would significantly change overall facility rankings (Arling et al., 2007; Mukamel et al., 2008).

---

[5] Case mix refers to the diversity and complexity of care needs for a given population.

Konetzka and colleagues (2020) concluded that adding fairly simple risk variables, such as a regression adjustment for resident comorbidities, could greatly improve the validity of nursing home rankings.

Correlation of Measures

The validity of measures can be assessed by examining either the correlation among reported measures or the correlation of reported measures with broader, unreported measures. Konetzka and colleagues (2020) noted that a lack of correlation among reported measures could be due to the fact that an individual provider truly excels in one domain (e.g., staffing) but not in another (e.g., a specific clinical measure). However, they added that very low correlations may signal that the measures themselves have poor validity. Some studies have demonstrated low correlations among reported measures (Brauner et al., 2018; Saliba et al., 2018), while others show little correlation between reported measures and quality of life (QOL) (Kim et al., 2014) and resident or family satisfaction (Çalıkoğlu et al., 2012; Williams et al., 2016). Two broad measures of quality, the rate of admissions or readmissions to the hospital and mortality, have mixed evidence for their correlation with the individual measures reported in Care Compare (Fuller et al., 2019; Neuman et al., 2014; Saliba et al., 2018; Snyder et al., 2019; Unroe et al., 2012; Xu et al., 2019).

Validity of the Composite Five-Star Rating

Despite limited evidence on the validity of the overall five-star composite rating, Konetzka and colleagues (2020) concluded that the star ratings capture insightful information about the extremes regarding nursing home quality. First, the overall star rating appears to accurately reflect the nursing home characteristics commonly associated with low or high quality (e.g., nonprofit status, percentage of Medicaid residents, ownership status, socioeconomic characteristics of the residents) (Konetzka and Gray, 2017; Perraillon et al., 2019b; Unroe et al., 2012). Second, nursing homes with higher star ratings have lower rates of hospital admissions or readmissions and mortality (Cornell et al., 2019; Unroe et al., 2012).

Another important consideration is whether the ratings accurately reflect differences in levels of quality between facilities and how likely families are to use them to select a nursing home. Qualitative studies suggest that only ratings of the extremes (facilities with five stars versus facilities with one star) are predictive of rehospitalization for heart failure (Unroe et al., 2012), patient safety outcomes (Brauner et al., 2018), and resident and family satisfaction (Williams et al., 2016). Such studies have not found significant differences among nursing homes rated two, three, or four stars. However, Cornell and colleagues (2019) conducted a rigorous study and found stronger negative relationships between star rating and outcomes such as mortality and long-term nursing home admission, but not for hospital readmissions. While Konetzka and colleagues (2020) concluded that the five-star composite rating appears valid at the extremes, they questioned "whether the star ratings are helpful to consumers choosing among nursing homes that are closer to average" (Konetzka et al., 2020). Other findings conclude that star ratings could be improved by adding consumers' assessments of their quality of care experience (Mukamel et al., 2021). Although the five-star composite measure seems to have face validity and predictive validity at the extremes, the evidence is mixed as to whether the star ratings are helpful to consumers choosing among nursing homes that are closer to average. (See below for more on the usefulness of the five-star rating system for consumers.)

Summary

The validity of Care Compare appears to have improved overall with the additions of the five-star composite measure, claims-based quality measures, and the use of payroll-based staffing data. However, more work is needed in regards to the individual measures including better approaches to risk adjustment, improved correlation among measures that should be correlated, and refinement of the composite measure to better distinguish modest increments in quality.

Relationship between the Five-Star Rating and COVID-19

Limited, but mixed, evidence exists on the relationship between COVID-19 cases among residents in nursing homes and the home's quality ratings. For example, several studies suggest that nursing homes with higher quality ratings are associated with lower rates of COVID-19 cases and deaths (Khairat et al., 2021; Ouslander and Grabowski, 2020; Williams et al., 2021). However, "this relationship, particularly with regard to case rates, can be partially attributed to external factors: lower-rated nursing homes are often located in areas with greater COVID-19 community spread and serve more socioeconomically vulnerable residents than higher-rated nursing homes" (Khairat et al., 2021, p. 2025).

In contrast, a literature review by Ochieng and colleagues (2021) of studies between April 2020 and January 2021 found that 8 of 12 studies did not find an association between quality ratings and COVID-19 cases or deaths (Abrams et al., 2020; Chatterjee et al., 2020; Chen et al., 2020; Figueroa et al., 2020; New York State Department of Health, 2021; Rowan et al., 2020; Sugg et al., 2021; White et al., 2020a). All four studies that demonstrated associations between quality ratings and COVID-19 cases or deaths examined data from single states (Bui et al., 2020; He et al., 2020; Li et al., 2020a; Rau and Almendrala, 2020).

Evidence on Gaming of the Data

Konetzka and colleagues (2020) questioned whether the improved performance shown by providers on Care Compare measures truly reflects improvements in residents' outcomes. Part of the challenge of the current rating system is that both staffing and quality measures are based on self-reported data from nursing homes, which could allow for "gaming" where nursing homes could falsify their data or use questionable strategies to improve scores.

Efforts to assess gaming in Care Compare "have used a common, if indirect, strategy . . . based on the assumption that 'real' improvement should be at least somewhat correlated either with the mechanisms to improve quality or with related (untargeted) measures of quality where spillovers from true quality improvement would be expected" (Konetzka et al., 2020, p. 303). Several studies have shown a lack of correlation between self-reported measures of improvement (e.g., outcomes, staffing ratios) and associated process or structural measures as well as a decrease in correlations after public reporting was initiated (Han et al., 2016; Werner et al., 2013; Zinn et al., 2008). Furthermore, several studies have shown decreases in these correlations along with changes in documentation and coding patterns after Care Compare began publicly reporting quality measures (Konetzka et al., 2015; Ryskina et al., 2018; Werner et al., 2011). Furthermore, a 2020 analysis by Integra Med Analytics found that the self-reported nursing home data are often underreported and uncorrelated to hospital-based measures (Integra Med Analytics, 2020)

Additionally, qualitative evidence also suggests that nursing home staff may be changing data or using other strategies to improve their scores without necessarily improving care (Davila et al., 2021; Perraillon et al., 2019a). Nursing home staff "reported substantial coding-related efforts to improve scores on the clinical quality measures, often led by a centralized director of clinical operations in the case of chain facilities" (Konetzka et al., 2020, p. 303). Examples included a staff member asking a resident about pain level[6] only after the resident had received pain medications or counting inappropriate staff types among reports of staffing ratios.

---

[6] The committee recognizes that pain is no longer a quality measure as of October 2019 (CMS, 2019).

Investigative journalism has also drawn attention to the issue of gaming of self-reported data (Silver-Greenberg and Gebeloff, 2021; Thomas, 2014, 2015). For example, a 2014 article in the *New York Times* found that two-thirds of nursing homes being monitored for quality held four or five stars in the staffing and quality measures domains (which are largely based on self-reported data), but more than 95 percent had only one or two stars in the inspection domain (based on the findings of state surveyors). (Thomas, 2014). Similarly, a study of the early years of the five-star rating system showed that 71 percent of nursing homes had four or five stars in the quality measures domain while only 34.1 percent of nursing homes had four or five stars in the inspections domain (Abt Associates Inc., 2014). A 2021 article in the *New York Times* noted that "in one sign of the problems with self-reported data, nursing homes that earn five stars for their quality of care are nearly as likely to flunk in-person inspections as to ace them" (Silver-Greenberg and Gebeloff, 2021). The article further noted that auditing of self-reported data is rare, even when nursing homes are cited for misreporting such data (Silver-Greenberg and Gebeloff, 2021). In 2015, the U.S. Government Accountability Office (GAO) recommended auditing of self-reported data to ensure quality and reliability (GAO, 2015).

Usefulness of Five-Star Rating and Care Compare for Consumers

As noted earlier, concerns have been raised about the ability of the five-star rating system to provide useful information to consumers (Edelman, 2015; Konetzka et al., 2020; LeadingAge, 2015). In 2007, Phillips and colleagues questioned the ability of performance measurement systems (in general) "to truly help consumers differentiate among homes providing different levels of quality" adding that "for consumers, performance measurement models are better at identifying problem facilities than potentially good homes" (Phillips et al., 2007). In 2016, the GAO issued a report highlighting challenges to the usefulness of the five-star rating system and Care Compare for consumers (GAO, 2016). First, they noted difficulty in understanding and comparing overall star rating, given the complexity of the calculation and potentially "masking the importance of the component ratings" (GAO, 2016, p. 16). GAO noted, as discussed previously, concerns about the ability to distinguish among nursing homes with two, three, or four stars. They stated, "for example, in one state, 28 percent of homes with a 3-star overall rating had a better health inspection score than the average health inspection score for homes with an overall 4-star rating" (GAO, 2016, p. 17). GAO also noted the inability of consumers to compare the quality of nursing homes across states (as ratings are relative only to other nursing homes in the same state). Finally, GAO noted the lack of information about consumer satisfaction, stating "many stakeholders told us that they would like to see resident satisfaction included in the five-star system" (GAO, 2016, p. 23). They further concluded that "until consumer satisfaction information is included in the rating system, consumers will continue to make nursing home decisions without the benefit of this key performance measure and may not be choosing the home that would best meet their needs" (GAO, 2016, p. 24). (See later in this chapter for more on resident and family satisfaction and experience surveys.)

What is Missing from Care Compare?

Care Compare does not include several aspects of high-quality care that are important for consumers to consider when seeking nursing home care that best meets their needs. These areas include resident and family satisfaction and experience of care (discussed later in this chapter), palliative and end-of-life care, implementation of the resident's care plan, psychosocial and behavioral health services, safety indicators (e.g., emergency preparedness and response, infection prevention and control), staff satisfaction, staff employment arrangements, health information technology adoption and interoperability, and the nursing home's financial performance.

Palliative and End-of-Life Care Measures

Nursing homes often serve as the final home for many residents prior to death; currently, about 25 percent of Medicare beneficiaries die in a nursing home (Teno et al., 2018). Furthermore, over one-third of older Americans have a nursing home stay in the last 90 days of life (Teno et al., 2018). Thus, measuring the quality of palliative and end-of-life care for people receiving care in nursing homes is important. Measures of palliative and end-of-life care parallel, and in some cases overlap, those in other settings (e.g., hospital, home) and other patient populations (e.g., care of older adults). Areas of particular focus for palliative and end-of-life care include the assessment and management of common end-of-life symptoms, open and empathetic communication with patients and families, elicitation and documentation of patients' preferences for life-sustaining treatments, mitigation of psychosocial and spiritual/existential distress, and grief and bereavement support (NQF, 2012a). Specific measures also include bereaved family evaluations of care at the end of life (NQF, 2012a) and concordance between patient preferences for care at the end of life and care received (Sanders et al., 2018).

Few palliative care measures have been developed specifically for use in the nursing home setting, and these tools have limited psychometric support and no single measure is widely used (Steel et al., 2003; Thompson et al., 2011). Some have proposed using existing administrative data such as MDS pain measures and Medicare claims to measure rates of potentially burdensome treatments and transitions (e.g., end-of-life hospitalizations, intensive care unit admissions) and hospice use for long-term care residents (Gozalo et al., 2011; Mukamel et al., 2012, 2016; Temkin-Greener et al., 2016).

To date, the quality of end-of-life care in nursing homes is consistently measured and reported by the Veterans Health Administration's community living centers. The key measure that the Veterans Health Administration uses is the Bereaved Family Survey, an NQF-endorsed measure administered to next of kin for all veterans dying in an inpatient Veterans Health Administration facility, including community living centers (NQF, 2012b; Thorpe et al., 2016). Family evaluations of overall end-of-life care for "veterans who died in Community Living Centers were better than those of veterans dying in acute or intensive care units but worse than those dying in hospice or palliative care units" (Ersek et al., 2015).

Other Measures

In the committee's judgment, several other measures or areas could also be better represented on Care Compare. For example, the committee identified the implementation of residents' plans of care and psychosocial and behavioral health services provided by each nursing home as important topics to consumers who are looking for specific services that they need and that are important to them (provided that the data can be validated). For example, consumers may be interested in information about costs and specialized services (Konetzka and Perraillon, 2016), and measures of patient safety can be difficult to elucidate (Brauner et al., 2018). Other safety indicators are likely important for consumers, especially following the pandemic, such as emergency preparedness, emergency response management, and infection prevention and control. Finally, consumers often value aspects of quality other than those reported in Care Compare (Mukamel et al., 2020), including staff satisfaction and staff employment arrangements (e.g., full-time, part-time, contract, and agency staff), both of which have been demonstrated to affect the quality of care (White et al., 2020b,c). Consumers also are likely interested in the availability of single-occupancy rooms (Grabowski, 2020; Silow-Carroll et al., 2021), health information technology adoption and interoperability (Vest et al., 2019), and financial performance (Weech-Maldonado et al., 2019), which can reflect the long-term stability and availability of the services they are seeking. Some of these measures can be readily reported from data already collected by CMS, but others will need to be further developed and tested before being publicly reported.

RESIDENT- AND FAMILY-REPORTED OUTCOMES: QUALITY OF LIFE, EXPERIENCE OF CARE, AND SATISFACTION

Measures of resident and family satisfaction represent an aspect of quality that is not currently reflected in the five-star rating (Williams et al., 2016), and consumers want to be able to see resident and family satisfaction on Care Compare (Konetzka and Perraillon, 2016; Schapira et al., 2016). As noted by Castle and colleagues, "measuring and reporting satisfaction with care may be important in helping seniors and their families choose a nursing home and also may be important in helping facilities improve some aspects of quality" (Castle et al., 2018).

The committee's vision of quality, as emanating from the nursing home resident's valuation of the benefits and harms of care, makes the resident's voice central to achieving and measuring quality. This vision, rooted in principles of autonomy and self-determination, centers on an assessment of the quality of care for the nursing home resident by

- Establishing advance care plans (Fleuren et al., 2020);
- Ascertaining goals (Glazier et al., 2004);
- Identifying needs and symptoms (Saliba and Buchanan, 2012);
- Identifying preferences for residential care and activities (Housen et al., 2009; Roberts et al., 2018; Saliba and Schnelle, 2002);
- Measuring outcomes (Edelen and Saliba, 2010; NQF, 2013; Saliba et al., 2012); and
- Assigning relative values to quality measures (Weimer et al., 2019).

This section focuses on the assessment of quality by nursing home residents and their families, which is typically not included in national quality reports (Sangl et al., 2005). For a nursing home worker's perspective on measuring quality of life, see Box 3-1.

BOX 3-1
Nursing Home Worker Perspective

"Metrics for quality of life or wellbeing—this is critical. There need to be incentives to push care towards what matters to older adults and nursing home residents."

– Physician and researcher from Amherst, MA
who has worked in long-term care facilities

This quote was collected from the committee's online call for resident, family, and nursing home staff perspectives.

Consumer assessment of quality can be of three types: (1) observation of the care, staff, and environment; (2) evaluation of the experience of care; and (3) satisfaction with the technical delivery and resulting outcomes of care. Observations can be guided by validated measures which can be scored to interpret quality and, in turn, help with choosing a facility (Rantz et al., 2006). The experience of care includes how the consumer perceives the way care is delivered, communication with providers, and characteristics of the care environment (e.g., cleanliness, odors, amenities). Technical measures of care processes and outcomes are only moderately correlated with resident and family reports of the experience of care (Kane et al., 2003; Li et al., 2016). Obtaining residents' assessment of their care experience becomes even more important in the nursing home setting, where residents have high levels of support needs and rely on the nursing home staff and environment to meet their needs on a continuing basis for weeks, months, or even years (IOM, 2001a; Katz and Akpom, 1976; Saliba and Schnelle, 2002).

Design Considerations

Several important design principles need to be considered in efforts to systematically assess and report on the experience of residents in nursing homes. The science for developing reliable and valid consumer surveys related to health care is well established (Bolarinwa, 2015; Cleary and McNeil, 1988; CMS, 2020c). The process begins with extensive literature reviews and intensive interviews with patients, families, and other stakeholders to identify those aspects of care that are most important to measure. Survey methodology also delineates methods to quantify and minimize the bias that can be introduced by aspects such as the mode of interview, interviewer type, concerns about recrimination, and the ordering and wording of questions (Krosnick, 1999). Several of these considerations are particularly important for nursing home settings. Anonymity of survey responses is critical to obtaining unfiltered answers to questions, particularly if a person is in an ongoing, dependent relationship with the nursing home being evaluated. The wording of items and responses needs to be clear and written to match the cognitive steps the respondent employs to arrive at an answer. For example, a response option of yes/no may not be appropriate when the actual answer varies depending on conditions or frequency. Care needs to be taken to create items that are worded in a neutral manner and not in a way that encourages a desired response. The recall of multiple episodes can be challenging, particularly if a respondent is being asked to identify a single defining characteristic despite variation that occurs either day to day or over time.

Interacting with these design principles are the characteristics of the nursing home setting and the resident. Although residents with moderate cognitive impairment can answer questions about their symptoms and preferences (Saliba and Buchanan, 2008), these questions need to be carefully worded and tested for clarity and message (Housen et al., 2008; Sangl et al., 2007). For those residents unable to self-report or to reliably report on their care experiences, proxy respondents might be used. While family evaluations of care are not interchangeable with residents' evaluations, proxy reports are widely used in evaluating care for patients who cannot speak for themselves (e.g., individuals with disabilities, very young children and infants, individuals at the end of life) and where family members are involved in the care to the degree that they are considered as the recipients of care (i.e., the patient-family as a unit of care, such as that which occurs in hospice or for pediatric patients). Thus including families' evaluations and experiences is warranted (Frentzel et al., 2012; Kane et al., 2005; Li et al., 2016).

There will be discord when the assessment is about events experienced by the resident but not the proxy. Additionally, because of the ongoing nature of care and number of encounters, the care experience may have day-to-day variation. Most importantly, as noted above, residents in the nursing home are reliant on the staff, who essentially control most elements of their environment and daily activities. This may interfere with resident evaluation of the care experience in two ways. First, residents and families may accommodate themselves to the shortcomings of the environment or care delivery, and, second, given the interaction of dependence and staff control, they may hesitate to criticize out of fear of recrimination.

Quality of Life

QOL is a multidimensional construct comprised of behavioral competence, objective environment, perceived QOL, and psychological well-being (Lawton, 1991). Although some models include objective and subjective components, generally the emphasis is on a person's own assessment of his or her QOL, based on the person's values and goals. While QOL is influenced by the quality of care (Kane et al., 2003), it encompasses broader concepts of psychological, social, spiritual, and existential well-being.

Under a contract from CMS, researchers developed and tested a survey to measure nursing home resident-reported QOL in order to determine the psychosocial domains that were absent or not sufficiently emphasized in the MDS (Kane et al., 2003, 2004). The resulting instrument contained 54 items covering resident satisfaction in 10 domains: autonomy, comfort, security, meaningful activity, relationships, functional competence, enjoyment, privacy, dignity, and spiritual well-being. A shortened 34-item version was also developed. The testing of the related items showed only modest correlation with a general satisfaction score, suggesting that the measures of experience addressed different constructs from satisfaction. The survey developers acknowledged that the survey was not a full assessment of QOL, as it did not include measures of affect, functional status, or health. Evaluating QOL (and the impact of care on QOL) is particularly important for long-term care residents because the nursing home is their permanent home, the place they will spend the final weeks, months, or years of their lives. As such, QOL was folded into the resident and family experience measures described in the following sections.

CAHPS Measures

AHRQ sponsored the development of the Consumer Assessment of Healthcare Providers and Systems (CAHPS®) program.[7] This suite of surveys captures reliable and valid data to assess some elements of patients' experience with various aspects of the health system and providers, and CAHPS survey data are used to provide publicly reported quality scores for Medicare and Medicaid. CMS mandates the collection of CAHPS surveys in several settings or populations (e.g., hospitals, Medicare Advantage, home health care, hospice care) by independent, credentialed survey vendors, and AHRQ supports the ongoing evaluation of item performance and association of ratings with patient characteristics (Klein et al., 2011; Martino et al., 2016).

Nursing Home CAHPS

CAHPS, with support from CMS, developed three "experience of care" surveys, available in English and Spanish, for nursing homes: the Long-Stay Resident Survey, the Discharged Resident Survey (for short-stay patients), and the Family Member Survey. The three surveys serve different purposes. "The [Long-Stay Resident Survey] provides the perspective from residents able to respond about their care; the [Discharged Resident Survey] presents a view from persons receiving rehabilitation. [The Family Member Survey] represents the experiences of those residents receiving the most days of care and who would otherwise be unable to voice their experiences" (Frentzel et al., 2012, p. S26). Furthermore, "measures based on consumer feedbacks offer unique insights into care quality and residents' quality of life because, by construction, they may largely reflect the varied aspects of interpersonal care experiences of residents and their family members, which are likely not well captured by clinical measures" (Li et al., 2016, p. 10).

The Long-Stay Resident Survey is the only CAHPS survey administered in person, with the sample consisting of residents in the facility of more

---

[7] For more information about CAHPS, see https://www.ahrq.gov/cahps/about-cahps/index.html (accessed November 5, 2021).

than 100 days (AHRQ, 2020; Sangl et al., 2007). Items ask about environment, care, communication and respect, autonomy, and activities. The Discharged Resident Survey is mailed by an independent vendor to nursing home residents who have been discharged after short stay (defined as less than 100 days) and differs from the long-stay version by including questions about therapy services. The Family Member Survey is also administered by mail and asks about the facility staff's meeting of resident's basic needs (e.g., eating, drinking, toileting), staff kindness and respect toward resident, nursing home provision of information and encouragement of family involvement, nursing home staffing, care of belongings, cleanliness, and an overall rating of quality (AHRQ, 2020; Frentzel et al., 2012). Nursing home CAHPS is the first CAHPS survey to include items for both quality of care and quality of life (Sangl et al., 2007).

While CMS mandates the collection of CAHPS surveys in other health care settings, the collection of the Nursing Home CAHPS survey is not required. This situation has been attributed to the resource requirements for in-person interviews in the long-stay version, concerns about the exclusion of persons with cognitive impairment, industry resistance to public reporting of detailed measures of resident experience, and concerns about whether family or proxy reports fairly capture the experience of residents (Frentzel et al., 2012; MedPAC, 2021). However, not implementing CAHPS in nursing homes when the surveys are carried out in other health care settings disadvantages nursing home residents and families in preventing their ability to provide feedback about their care experiences, and to use such information to make informed decisions when choosing a nursing home. Nursing homes are also disadvantaged by not having consumer reports of their experiences to improve services and care delivery.

Reliability and Validity of Nursing Home CAHPS

While many nursing home administrators report using resident satisfaction surveys, and satisfaction information is reported as being useful, the surveys being used vary widely and may not be adequately validated (Castle, 2007; Castle et al., 2004, 2018). Comparatively, Nursing Home CAHPS measures had extensive item development (described in the previous section on "design considerations") and testing for reliability and validity (AHRQ, 2018, 2019; Castle et al., 2018; Frentzel et al., 2012; Sangl et al., 2007). Development of Nursing Home CAHPS resident surveys was based on a literature review, the use of focus groups with nursing home residents and their families about what topics and measures were important to them, cognitive testing to ensure residents could understand and answer the questions, field testing, and testing to develop composites and transition items (AHRQ, 2018). Similarly, the Family Member Survey was developed based on a literature review, focus groups with residents and their families about what topics and measures were important to them, a public call for measures, cognitive testing with people who have family members in nursing homes, input from a technical expert panel regarding the use and value of a family member survey, field testing, and psychometric testing (AHRQ, 2019).

A 2018 analysis of the Discharged Resident Survey concluded that "the standardization and reliability that [it] provides could facilitate the same benefits we have seen in other industries for the CAHPS family of instruments (i.e., quality improvement, reimbursement, public reporting, and benchmarking)" (Castle et al., 2018, pp. 1241–1242). However, as most of this survey's question domains are the same as the Long-Stay Resident Survey, and considering that most discharged residents are short stay, testing is needed to determined necessary adjustments for the Discharged Resident Survey (Baskin et al., 2012; Castle et al., 2018). A 2012 analysis of the Family Member Survey found that "the final family member survey, using formative research to develop the draft, cognitive testing to refine the items, psychometric analyses, and technical expert input, represents a well tested, valid, and reliable survey" (Frentzel et al., 2012, p. S26). Higher family ratings on nursing home care are associated with better care, resident outcomes, and several risk-adjusted quality measures (e.g., lower rates of pressure ulcers, hospital admission, and mortality) (Li et al., 2016). These reflect similar findings of psychometric testing for Family Member Surveys conducted in hospital-based CAHPS surveys (Li et al., 2016).

State-Based Surveys of Resident and Family Experience and Satisfaction

Some states have supported surveys of resident experience and satisfaction. In Michigan, nursing homes can receive incentive payments for submitting resident satisfaction surveys, though the exact design and content of those surveys is determined by the facility or chain (Michigan DHHS, 2021a). A few states have created their own surveys which combine satisfaction and experience items, and some have required nursing homes to collect these for over a decade. For example, the Ohio Long-Term Care Ombudsman Program began conducting nursing home resident and family surveys in 2002 (Ejaz et al., 2003; Straker et al., 2016). Posted surveys show variation in scores across facilities and across domains (Pyle, 2017). Similarly, evaluations of consumer experience surveys in Maryland have shown disparities in ratings of all care domains that persist over time (Li et al., 2014) as well as differences in experiences of care that are associated with proprietary status and nursing home chain size (You et al., 2016).

Since 2006, Minnesota has posted a report card that includes long-stay resident and family QOL and short-stay resident experience survey results (Minnesota DHHS, 2021). These surveys are administered annually and are also part of the Minnesota Performance-Based Incentive Program for nursing home quality improvement (Kane et al., 2007). The Long-Stay Resident Survey is conducted in person by an independent research firm; the other surveys are completed by mail (Kane et al., 2007; Minnesota DHHS, 2021).

Industry Measures of Resident and Family Experience and Satisfaction

In parallel with federal and state efforts, the nursing home industry has developed and implemented its own measures of resident and family satisfaction. For example, CoreQ, endorsed by the American Health Care Association, has three versions: long-term care residents, long-term care family, and short-stay discharged patients (Castle et al., 2020; CoreQ, 2019; Schwartz, 2021). Each version consists of three or four general questions that focus less on rating the quality of resident experience and more on summative satisfaction ratings. Another example of an industry-developed tool is NRC Health's My Inner View Customer Satisfaction Survey (NRC Health, 2021). Many nursing homes promote and advertise high scores from self-designed and administered surveys of their residents. However, consumer advocates and survey methodologists have raised concerns that item wording and the choice of response formats may increase the tendency of respondents to provide socially appropriate response choices and thus provide only minimal variation in the scale (Bowling, 2005; Dillman et al., 2014; Nadash et al., 2019).

OVERVIEW OF QUALITY IMPROVEMENT

In his remarks to this committee, Donald Berwick, the president emeritus and a senior fellow at the Institute for Healthcare Improvement, said that "most improvement agendas [have] excessive reliance on control, metrics, accountability, and fixing damage, with little energy left over for learning and not much energy left over for invention." Technical assistance is one of the primary mechanisms of quality improvement. The role of technical assistance depends in part upon the nursing home recognizing its need for additional knowledge and expertise. Without the motivation to improve quality, little change may occur. The following sections highlight key historical and current efforts to improve the quality of care in nursing homes. (See Appendix B for more details on some of the quality improvement programs discussed below.)

History of National Quality Improvement Efforts

The Joint Commission, founded in 1951, accredits and certifies health care organizations and programs in the United States (Joint Commission, 2021). In 1966, The Joint Commission initiated the Long-Term Care Accreditation Program that stimulated interest from nurses and other leaders in nursing homes to examine the quality of care delivered in their organizations (Rantz et al., 2002). In 1973, the American Nurses Association and the American Hospital Association sponsored a conference that challenged nurses to take responsibility for quality assurance activities within their health care organizations (Lang and Clinton, 1983).

In 1972, the federal government mandated professional standards review organizations (later called peer-review organizations) to oversee the quality of care delivered by health care organizations to Medicare beneficiaries, including those in nursing homes. In 2002, these programs were renamed as Quality Improvement Organizations (QIOs) and are currently overseen by CMS. The 2006 IOM report *Medicare's Quality Improvement Organization Program: Maximizing Potential* (IOM, 2006) was prepared in response to a request from the U.S. Congress for an evaluation of the QIO program. The IOM committee recommended that CMS should assess the QIO program in several ways, including (1) the program as a whole, (2) individual QIOs, and (3) selected quality improvement interventions implemented by QIOs. Additionally, the committee recommended independent, external evaluations of the QIO program's overall contributions and effectiveness.

As the QIO core contract concluded in 2006, CMS staff conducted a national evaluation of the improvements achieved by QIOs working with nursing homes, home health, and physician offices. While there were some measurable improvements, the evaluation's conclusions were limited because of design flaws in the analysis (Rollow et al., 2006; Shortell and Peck, 2006). Congress continued to question the effectiveness of the QIOs, noting documented problems with the program (Freedland, 2009; Reichard, 2007). The QIO program's 9th Scope of Work (2008–2011) targeted poorly performing nursing homes, but an independent evaluation highlighted the limited accuracy of the targeting methods used to select nursing homes to work with and the specific performance measures selected for improvement (Stevenson and Mor, 2009).

A 25-year review of external evaluations of the QIO program, including the internal monitoring and evaluation protocols, found that all such evaluations have found the impact of the QIO program to be small or difficult to interpret; additionally, the review found that inconsistencies in data collection and measurement create difficulties in monitoring and evaluations of effectiveness (Shaw-Taylor, 2014). This review also noted that the QIO program cost at that time was about $200 million per year and that the ninth scope of work cost more than $1 billion. These costs and continued questions about the effectiveness of the program prompted the Office of the Inspector General to examine the duplicative efforts of QIOs with other CMS quality improvement efforts and the relative contribution of each effort (OIG, 2015). To date, the effectiveness and relative contributions of the QIO program have not been fully determined.

Standardized CMS quality measures have been used to guide quality improvement, in large part because of their prominent use in payment, policy, consumer choice, and accountability. The extent to which individual facilities engage in quality improvement and the effectiveness of such activities are unknown. Furthermore, many facilities lack adequate expertise and resources to engage in effective quality improvement. Various groups have established quality improvement coalitions and initiatives to support these efforts. Coalitions may involve the QIOs, academic partnerships, and state-level initiatives. The following sections give a brief overview of some of the larger initiatives as examples.

FEDERAL INITIATIVES FOR QUALITY IMPROVEMENT

The federal government has played a key role in improving the quality of care in nursing homes. Notable efforts include implementation of quality assurance and performance improvement (QAPI) programs and various CMS-supported campaigns and interventions.

Quality Assurance Performance Improvement Program

Federal efforts to embed the use of quality improvement methods include regulations of the Omnibus Budget Reconciliation Act of 1987[8] that required facilities to have quarterly meetings to identify needed quality assurance activities and to develop and implement plans to correct quality deficiencies (Rantz et al., 2002). In 2016, the Patient Protection and Affordable Care Act[9] (ACA) required that all skilled nursing facilities implement QAPI programs as a condition of reimbursement by Medicare and Medicaid. The QAPI activities expand the team members to include representatives of all staff in the nursing home as well as residents and families or significant others in continuously identifying opportunities for improvement (AHCA and NCAL, 2021).

---

[8] Omnibus Budget Reconciliation Act of 1987, Public Law 100-203; 100th Cong., 1st sess. (December 22, 1987).

[9] Patient Protection and Affordable Care Act, Public Law 111-148; 111th Cong., 2nd sess. (March 23, 2010).

QAPI seeks to achieve two critical aspects of quality management: quality assurance (the enforcement of standards for the quality of services and outcomes) (see Chapter 8) and performance improvement through the continuous quality improvement process (CMS, 2016). CMS oversees several quality improvement initiatives for nursing homes, but QAPI is meant to be ongoing and more comprehensive, so enrolling in another initiative does not necessarily mean a nursing home is meeting QAPI regulations. QAPI identifies five key elements of quality management:

(1) The design and scope of the program address all systems of care, including clinical care, QOL, choice, and safety;
(2) Leadership is engaged and actively seeks input from all stakeholders including staff, residents, and their families;
(3) Facilities have a data collection and monitoring system;
(4) Facilities have performance-improvement projects to assess and address particular problem areas; and
(5) Facilities employ systemic analyses and approaches to identify and address issues, develop policies, and look toward sustainable improvement (CMS, 2016).

In spite of these regulations and efforts, the COVID-19 pandemic revealed an absence of QAPI practices in many nursing homes. Moreover, when a QAPI is absent during annual inspections, it is often not cited as a deficiency (Bonner, 2021).

CMS-Supported Campaigns and Interventions

CMS has supported and continues to support several nursing home quality improvement programs (CMS, 2017a). Despite the large investment, some of these large-scale CMS-supported initiatives have not been evaluated rigorously. The next section gives an overview to some of these initiatives.

Interventions to Reduce Acute Care Transfers

The Interventions to Reduce Acute Care Transfers (INTERACT) program was created by CMS to reduce transfers to hospitals through improved identification, evaluation, management, and communication about acute changes in nursing home resident conditions (Ouslander et al., 2014). The identification of common, nonspecific changes in condition may "help guide decisions about further evaluation of changes in resident condition, when to communicate with primary care clinicians, when to consider transfer to the hospital, and provide suggestions on how to manage some conditions in the facility without hospital transfer when it is safe and feasible" (Ouslander et al., 2014, p. 5). Studies of the impact of the INTERACT program have shown mixed results; however, measurable improvement has been demonstrated in avoidable hospitalizations, cost savings to Medicare, and care process improvements (Huckfeldt et al., 2018; Kane et al., 2017; Mochel et al., 2021; Ouslander et al., 2011, 2014; Vasilevskis et al., 2017).

The National Nursing Home Quality Improvement Campaign

The National Nursing Home Quality Improvement Campaign, which began in 2006 as the Advancing Excellence in America's Nursing Homes Campaign, provides long-term care providers, consumers, advocates, and quality improvement professionals with freely accessible, evidence-based resources to support quality improvement activities (National Consumer Voice, 2021). CMS funding for the campaign ended in 2019, but a group of nongovernmental stakeholders continues to support the website (Great Plains Quality Innovation Network, 2019; NNHQI, 2021).[10]

The National Nursing Home Quality Care Collaborative

Modeled after the Institute for Healthcare Improvement breakthrough series approach (IHI, 2003) and led by Quality Innovation Network–QIOs, the goal of the collaborative is to rapidly spread best practices that are identified from high-performing nursing homes to other facilities. The program has had limited evaluation, but one case study did report success in learning to apply quality improvement techniques (Gillespie et al., 2016).

National Partnership to Improve Dementia Care in Nursing Homes

Launched in 2012, the National Partnership to Improve Dementia Care in Nursing Homes has the mission of improving the quality of care provided to individuals with dementia living in nursing homes. Membership varies across states but often involves the Quality Innovation Network–QIO, the survey agency, and other related state offices (e.g., Department of Aging); industry (e.g., Leading Age, American Health Care Association affiliates); professional associations; resident advocacy groups; academic institutions; nursing homes; and others. The initial target of the partnership was to reduce antipsychotic use and has now expanded to promote the use of nonpharmacologic, person-centered dementia care practices (CMS, 2021d). The partnership met its initial goal of reducing the prevalence of antipsychotic use in long-stay nursing home residents by 30 percent by the

---

[10] See www.nhQualityCampaign.org (accessed November 1, 2021).

end of 2016 (CMS, 2017b). Overall, the rates of antipsychotic use among long-stay residents has decreased from 23.9 percent in 2011 to 15.7 percent in 2017 (CMS, 2017b).

Initiative to Reduce Avoidable Hospitalizations Among Nursing Facility Residents

CMS' Medicare–Medicaid Coordination Office, in collaboration with the Center for Medicare and Medicaid Innovation, ran the Initiative to Reduce Avoidable Hospitalizations Among Nursing Facility Residents from 2012 to 2020. Partnering programs and organizations included

- The Optimizing Patient Transfers, Impacting Medical Quality, and Improving Symptoms: Transforming Institutional Care (OPTIMISTIC) project;
- The Reduce Avoidable Hospitalizations using Evidence-Based Interventions for Nursing Facilities (RAVEN) program;
- The Missouri Quality Initiative (MOQI);
- The New York–Reducing Avoidable Hospitalizations (NY–RAH) project;
- The Nevada Admissions and Transitions Optimization Program initiative;
- CHI/Alegent Creighton Health (Nebraska); and
- The Alabama Quality Assurance Foundation's Nursing Facility Initiative.

Each of the seven participating sites was individually evaluated against key metrics and in aggregate (in comparison to a national comparison group) by an independent team that performed extensive quantitative and qualitative analyses. Phase One (2012–2016) involved the delivery of evidence-based practices to "improve the overall health and healthcare of participating long-stay nursing facility residents with the primary goals of reducing potentially avoidable hospitalizations, improving quality of care, and decreasing health care spending" (RTI International, 2017, p. 13). All partnering initiatives were "required to employ staff, such as registered nurses (RNs), or advanced practice registered nurses (APRNs) . . . to provide full- or part-time support" (RTI International, 2017, p. 13). Additionally, the nurses focused on improving care processes and communication among providers using INTERACT and assisted in training staff on how to use quality improvement methods to improve all key aspects of care delivery (e.g., nutrition, hydration, mobility, communication, end-of-life care planning). For the intervention period of 2014–2016, the evaluation team found "persuasive evidence of the Initiative's effectiveness in reducing hospital inpatient admissions, ED visits, and hospitalization-related Medicare expenditures" (RTI International, 2017, p. 223).

Phase Two of the initiative (2016–2020) addressed six key conditions: pneumonia, congestive heart failure, chronic obstructive pulmonary disease/asthma, skin infection, dehydration, and urinary tract infection. During this phase, CMS offered payment incentives for each of these conditions in an effort to reduce hospitalizations (RTI International, 2021, p. ES 3). Phase Two included two different intervention groups: one in which the payment intervention was added to the existing clinical supports (i.e., RN and APRN support) and the other a "payment only" intervention group, which did not have the RN and APRN supports. Overall, providing payment incentives to nursing facilities to reduce use and expenditures was not effective (RTI International, 2017).

Four of the participating sites (MOQI, NY–RAH, OPTIMISTIC, and RAVEN) had a strong clinical focus. Details of these programs, including their key components and outcomes, are provided in Appendix B.

STATE AND LOCAL INITIATIVES FOR QUALITY IMPROVEMENT

In addition to federal efforts, different approaches to quality improvement in nursing homes have been implemented at the state and local levels. These efforts include academic–provider partnerships and state-supported programs.

Academic–Provider Partnerships

Many targeted quality improvement efforts in nursing homes focus on such topics as pressure ulcers, falls, antibiotic use, pain, palliative care, and hospital transfers (Rantz et al., 2009, 2012a, 2012b; Sloane et al., 2020). These projects are often initiated by an academic research team and involve a single facility or smaller groups of facilities from a single geographic region. Funding for these projects comes from a variety of sources, including federal research grants, foundation grants, and government contracts, including those supported with civil monetary penalty funds. In general, the results of these studies have been mixed; however, the use of quality improvement methods to improve quality of care is well supported with significant results or trends in improvement. In addition to discrete quality improvement projects, academic researchers also have partnered with nursing homes and other stakeholders to form quality improvement programs. Two examples of this type of partnership are the Arkansas Coalition for Nursing Home Excellence and the Quality Improvement Program for Missouri (QIPMO) (Beck et al., 2014; Rantz et al., 2003, 2009). Another example of academic–provider partnerships is the model of a teaching nursing home wherein students, faculty, and health care workers collaborate to improve care for residents (Mezey et al., 2008).

The Arkansas Coalition for Nursing Home Excellence

The Arkansas program was a broad coalition of nursing home organizations, state survey representatives, academics specializing in geriatrics, the Arkansas ombudsman, and advocates, all focusing on efforts to improve quality and support culture change in the state's nursing homes. The program, which coincided in some years with the National Consumer's Voice Advancing Excellence Campaign (2006–2016), was active for 10 years (2004–2014) and reported success with improvement in pressure ulcers, physical restraints, chronic pain, acute pain, and complaints from 2004–2011 (Beck et al., 2014; National Consumer Voice, 2021).

The Quality Improvement Program for Missouri

Developed and tested in the 1990s, and adopted in 1999 (and still operating today), QIPMO is a cooperative project between the Missouri Department of Health and Senior Services and the University of Missouri Sinclair School of Nursing whose goal is to improve quality of care in Missouri nursing homes (Popejoy et al., 2000; Rantz et al., 2001, 2003). In the program, quality improvement nurses (nurses with graduate education in geriatric nursing) and leadership coaches (nursing home administrators) contact and offer free, confidential clinical and operational consultation to long-term care facilities. Every facility in the state is contacted at least annually with offers for site visits to help with quality improvement. In 2019, QIPMO nurses contacted 696 different facilities, organizations, and stakeholders and conducted 561 onsite visits in 342 different facilities to assist with the improvement of clinical systems and care. QIPMO leadership coaches contacted 605 different facilities, organizations, and stakeholders and conducted 258 onsite visits in 172 different facilities to assist with leadership quality improvement and education (Sinclair School of Nursing, 2021a,b). There were 527 active providers in Missouri in fiscal year 2019, which means the five QIPMO gerontological nurses and three leadership coaches reached, onsite, 71 and 63 percent, respectively, of active providers.[11]

---

[11] Quality Improvement Program for Missouri (QIPMO) testimony presented to the National Academies of Sciences, Engineering, and Medicine Committee on the Quality of Care in Nursing Homes; Nicky Martin, M.P.A., B.S., LNHA, CDP, IP, LTC leadership coach, program team leader; and Wendy Boren, B.S.N., R.N., IP, clinical educator/consultant; May 10, 2021.

QIPMO has been found to improve the quality of care outcomes of nursing home residents and to reduce the cost of care, including annual care cost savings of more than $4.7 million statewide, several times more than the program costs (Rantz et al., 2003, 2009; University of Missouri Interdisciplinary Center on Aging, 2008). A 2018 evaluation of the administrator coaching service for survey readiness assistance found that use of the service resulted in a reduction of severe citations from 52.3 percent pre-training to 39 percent post-training and a reduction of administrator turnover from 22.1 percent pre-training to 19.5 percent post-training (Phillips et al., 2018).

Academic–provider partnerships such as QIPMO offer several advantages. With the program being managed within the state, it is easier to build support for the use of the clinical and administrative services. Communication among the nursing home associations, the nursing homes (and other long-term care settings), and state agency staff can be facilitated more readily so that trusting relationships can be built. Working onsite with the QIPMO nurse or leadership coach, facility staff can improve care systems in ways that are not possible with their individual efforts alone. Affiliation with a well-recognized and respected state university adds credibility to the educational offerings and increases consultation acceptance (Popejoy et al., 2020; Rantz et al., 2009).

The statewide infrastructure and rapid communication network of QIPMO was critical during the COVID pandemic (Pool and Boren, 2020; Popejoy et al., 2020). QIPMO served as a communication network to get consistent, helpful, accurate information to all long-term care settings in the state, even helping with the distribution of personal protective equipment. Virtual support groups were held at least weekly for administrative and clinical staff to ask questions and seek clarification about rapidly changing guidance on best practices. With daily (or as often as needed) electronic communication to all long-term care facilities in the state it was possible to quickly distribute "condensed, practical" implementation guidelines and revisions of changing national guidelines (Pool and Boren, 2020; Popejoy et al., 2020).

While QIPMO has shown success, this specific model has not been adopted or tested in other states, and its success may be dependent on several factors that may not exist elsewhere, such as state support and the involvement of a strong nursing and health sciences school with substantial expertise and commitment to nursing homes.

Teaching Nursing Homes

In the 1980s the National Institute on Aging and the Robert Wood Johnson Foundation funded teaching nursing home models that linked nursing homes, nursing programs, and academic medicine (Mezey et al., 2008). The teaching nursing home was conceptualized as a way to increase research, improve resident health outcomes, expand staff training, and improve knowledge about geriatric care. The model was considered to be successful and has been shown to improve attitudes about nursing homes and working with older adults, decrease staff turnover rates, improve outcomes, and lower costs (Mezey and Lynaugh, 1989; Mezey et al., 1988; Shaughnessy et al., 1995).

In March 2005, a summit of experts in geriatrics endorsed the teaching nursing home model (with a reciprocal nature that encouraged a "culture of learning" for both nursing homes and the academic programs) over a more typical model of a nursing home collaboration with academia in which a student is simply placed into a nursing home for a clinical rotation (Mezey et al., 2008). The summit participants saw value in teaching nursing homes for interdisciplinary team training, faculty development, and enhancing the educating and credentialing of nursing home staff.

In 2021, the Jewish Healthcare Foundation, The John A. Hartford Foundation, and the Henry L. Hillman Foundation provided funding for the Pennsylvania Teaching Nursing Home project to test an updated version of the teaching nursing home in three different partnerships (Jewish Healthcare Foundation, 2021). In its announcement of the pilot project, the Jewish Healthcare Foundation stated:

> The partnerships will equip existing skilled nursing facility staff with clinical, training, research, and quality improvement support, creating a critical bridge between bedside care and academic innovation and clinical expertise. With increased opportunities to learn first-hand and in a real-life setting, students and staff will enhance their clinical skills while improving the functioning and health status of seniors. Project leaders anticipate the results of the pilot will inform a better model for ongoing clinical quality improvement and safety in long-term care. (Jewish Healthcare Foundation, 2021)

State-Supported Quality Improvement Programs

States may also take the initiative to develop or test quality improvement programs within their own borders.

Minnesota Performance-Based Incentive Payment Program

The Minnesota Performance-Based Incentive Payment Program (PIPP) uses an alternative approach to pay-for-performance to fund nursing home–initiated quality improvement projects (Arling et al., 2013, 2014). (See later in this chapter as well as Chapter 7 for more on market-based incentives to improve the quality of care in nursing homes.) Under a competitive process, nursing homes submit proposals that an expert panel evaluates. The program funds a select group of proposals, all of which must include clear and measurable performance targets. In addition to funding, the state offers technical assistance, particularly during the proposal development stage. Projects that do not meet their performance targets can lose up to 20 percent of the project funding.

From 2007 to 2010, PIPP supported 66 projects at 174 of the state's 373 nursing facilities (Arling et al., 2013, 2014). The projects had a broad range of goals, with many focused on clinical quality and technology and many targeting discrete areas such as culture change, art therapy, and resident psychological well-being. Only 3 of the 66 projects lost funding because they failed to meet performance improvement targets. Moreover, participating facilities demonstrated significantly greater gains than facilities not participating in PIPP according to a multidimensional composite measure of quality as well as in targeted areas during years 2008–2010 as compared with the baseline of 2006–2007. Finally, these facilities also maintained their quality advantage during years 2011–2013 after their quality improvement projects were completed. PIPP in Minnesota has not been adopted or tested in other states and may be dependent on factors that may not exist elsewhere. However, PIPP has been shown to be an effective example of a state-based quality improvement initiative (Arling et al., 2013, 2014).

The Systems Change Tracking Tool^{SM}

The Systems Change Tracking Tool (SCTT) was developed by Altarum to "capture the adoption of culture change practices over time" in nursing homes (Perry et al., 2021). The tool was based on the idea that culture change to prioritize person-centered care is fundamental to improving the quality of care. The tool seeks to track and measure improvements in person-centered care in order to determine the impact of culture change practices on quality of care.

SCTT was funded as a grant from the Michigan Department of Health and Human Services in 2019 using funds from civil monetary penalties; the project is expected to conclude in early 2022 (Perry et al., 2021). The project was implemented in six nursing homes in Michigan (with varying characteristics, including star rating) and provided culture change training and curriculum from The Eden Alternative[12] to nursing home staff as part of a quality improvement initiative. The participating nursing homes admitted

---

[12] For more information, see https://www.edenalt.org (accessed November 16, 2021).

that the COVID-19 pandemic affected their ability to fully implement culture change practices. However, "throughout 2020 and 2021, homes made steady progress towards re-establishing more person-centered care practices and unifying them with infection control protocols to better serve their residents" (Perry et al., 2021). Altarum plans to pilot a shortened version of the tool for nursing home residents in eight nursing homes in Tennessee. While these projects have not been fully evaluated, they may provide insight as to how focusing on person-centered care can lead to demonstrable changes in quality.

OTHER APPROACHES TO QUALITY IMPROVEMENT

In addition to specific efforts at the federal, state, and local levels, other approaches have been used to improve the quality of care in nursing homes. Specific examples include the use of market-based incentives (e.g., value-based purchasing) and the development of age-friendly health systems.

Market-Based Incentives to Improve Quality in Nursing Homes

Market-based incentives to improve care appear to have had positive impacts on quality measures. However, the gains have been largely confined to a narrow range of targeted measures and do not necessarily reflect overall better quality of care (Arling et al., 2020; Werner and Konetzka, 2010). Also, there are likely some unintended consequences affecting nursing homes that serve higher numbers of minority residents. For example, Hefele and colleagues (2019) found that "hospitals serving racial/ethnic minority groups and low-income people perform worse" under the value-based purchasing programs they studied (Hefele et al., 2019, p. 1130). Furthermore, they raised concerns about using incentive-based programs in nursing homes, particularly because "vulnerable populations may be disproportionately affected by penalties" (Hefele et al., 2019, p. 1130). Value-based purchasing, as a mechanism to improve quality of care, is discussed more fully in Chapter 7.

Age-Friendly Health Systems

The Age-Friendly Health System initiative represents a collaboration of the John A. Hartford Foundation, the Institute for Healthcare Improvement, the American Hospital Association, and the Catholic Health Association of the United States. The initiative uses a 4 M's framework—know what *matters* to the individual; prevent, identify, treat, and manage *mentation* (e.g., dementia, depression, delirium); encourage *mobility*; and use *medications* that do not interfere with preferences, mobility, or mentation)

(Fulmer, 2018; IHI, 2021). That is, the framework is designed to ensure that care follows evidence-based practices, does not cause harm, and aligns with older adults' (and their family caregivers') preferences.

The person-centeredness of the Age-Friendly Health System initiative aligns with the committee's vision of high-quality care (see Chapter 1). Furthermore, Edelman and colleagues (2021) suggested how the 4 M's framework could be applied to the nursing home setting in order to improve the quality of care. Such an approach could include the integration of what matters to the resident into QAPI monitoring and the care plan, the provision of activities and treatments that improve cognition and mobility, and medication management (Edelman et al., 2021). (See Chapter 4 for more on person-centered care.)

TECHNICAL ASSISTANCE FOR QUALITY IMPROVEMENT

Technical assistance can have different meanings but generally refers to the process by which an entity works with providers to build capacity, implement innovations, and enhance competence in order to improve outcomes (IOM, 2006; Wandersman et al., 2012). Technical assistance to implement advances in science originated in the land-grant universities established under the Morrill Act of 1862 to meet the growing need for people with expertise in science and agriculture. The Morrill Act of 1890 provided for regular appropriation to these institutions so they could continue to function in that capacity (Encyclopaedia Britannica, 2017). Technical assistance can help a provider to detect areas in need of improvement, identify root causes of problems, implement interventions and systems changes, teach process improvement methods, promote best practices, facilitate knowledge transfer, analyze performance data, and coordinate quality improvement efforts (IOM, 2006). In its 2006 evaluation of the QIO program, IOM concluded that the public sector needs to play a substantial role in improving care quality for all Americans, especially those who depend on Medicare and Medicaid, and "some level of technical assistance should be available through the federal government as a public good" (IOM, 2006, p. 63).

Technical assistance leading to successful implementation of quality improvement initiatives partly depends on an organization's willingness and readiness to change and capacity to implement change (Holt et al., 2010; Le et al., 2014; Weiner, 2009; Weiner et al., 2008). For example, one study of instituting quality improvement methods in nursing homes identified "readiness indicators" among those that were most likely to improve, including

- A leadership team (e.g., nursing home administrator, director of nursing) interested in learning about how to use quality reports to improve care,

- A change champion within the nursing home,
- Willingness to involve all staff in educational activities,
- Plans for continuous education of new staff, and
- Continuous involvement of all staff to encourage "ownership" of the process and responsibility for change (Rantz et al., 2012b).

However, Wandersman and colleagues (2012) discussed the importance of proactive technical assistance, which they describe as "a strategic approach to bringing specific knowledge and skills to recipients, and then helping recipients to adopt and use the information and skills effectively" (Wandersman et al., 2012, p. 451). They add that proactive technical assistance can be both anticipatory and responsive:

> In an anticipatory role, technical assistance providers catalyze the technical assistance process rather than wait for technical assistance requests to arrive, which is important because potential technical assistance recipients with lower capacity levels are less likely to make technical assistance requests. Technical assistance providers then continue to be proactive subsequent to the first contact in helping recipients to use the information and skills with quality. Proactive technical assistance providers are also responsive to recipients. They customize technical assistance so that it starts with and builds upon recipients' current capacities and moves toward an ideal level of capacity to use specific information and skills with quality. (Wandersman et al., 2012, p. 451)

The Value of Technical Assistance in Nursing Homes

The examples of national, state, and local approaches to quality improvement in nursing homes discussed earlier in this chapter all have their foundation in assisting workers to increase their knowledge, skills, and capacity to deliver up-to-date, necessary care. The examples do have positive outcome evaluations of their services to improve the quality of nursing home care. Furthermore, a 2010 analysis of the Special Focus Facility (SFF) program noted that "according to some states, the SFF Program is more effective when combined with state-based quality improvement activities," citing QIPMO as a noteworthy program (GAO, 2010). However, many of the specific state and local programs have not been replicated in other states. Consistent, regular funding has been shown to be necessary for them to be sustainable, effectively adopted, and consistently used.

Some features of effective technical assistance from the evidence of state and local programs include building a trusting relationship between the nursing home staff and people offering the technical assistance, modifying the assistance to best fit current needs and skills of each nursing home (it is not "one size fits all"), and making sure the scientific content (for example, specific care of complex residents with health, physical, mental, and social-behavioral needs) is the most up to date and accurate. State and local programs may be particularly well suited to provide technical assistance due to familiarity with the local community and the ability to be seen as a trusted peer. Such programs may also help integrate nursing homes into their local communities and the broader health care system. Additionally, technical assistance staff must assess each staff member's readiness to learn and successfully engage in quality improvement activities (Le et al., 2014; Rantz et al., 2012b; Wandersman et al., 2012). When some nursing homes are not ready to operationalize quality improvement initiatives but others are, technical assistance programs need to consider readiness in prioritizing their efforts.

QUALITY IMPROVEMENT AND DISPARITIES

Braverman and colleagues (2017) noted that "for the purposes of measurement, health equity means reducing and ultimately eliminating disparities in health and its determinants that adversely affect excluded or marginalized groups."

The existence of racial and socioeconomic disparities in nursing homes is well known. In 2004, it was reported that

> The nearly 15 percent of U.S. nonhospital-based nursing homes that serve predominantly Medicaid residents have fewer nurses, lower occupancy rates, and more health-related deficiencies. They are more likely to be terminated from the Medicaid/Medicare program, are disproportionately located in the poorest counties, and are more likely to serve African-American residents than are other facilities. (Mor et al., 2004, p. 227)

Today, this disparity still exists, as African American and other minority residents more often live in poorer-quality nursing homes with higher Medicaid populations than White nursing home residents (Gorges and Konetzka, 2021; Sharma et al., 2020). Early in the COVID-19 pandemic, nursing homes with greater percentages of African American and other minority residents were more likely to have COVID-19 cases (Abrams et al., 2020) and had two to four times the proportion of cases and deaths from COVID-19 than with higher proportions of White residents (Gorges and Konetzka, 2021; Li et al., 2020b). Nursing homes serving underserved populations (such as those with higher proportions of Hispanic or Latinx residents, Black residents, and people who are funded by Medicaid) are more likely to have been penalized under value-based purchasing (Hefele et al., 2019). Additionally, nursing homes with more residents with serious mental illness are more likely to have lower star ratings, lower direct-care staffing, and for-profit ownership than all other nursing homes (Jester et al., 2020). Clearly, with these sustained disparities there is a critical need to ensure that residents of diverse racial and ethnic backgrounds, as well as those with serious mental illness, can access and receive high-quality nursing home care when they need it.

Additionally, it is important that quality improvement initiatives carefully and intentionally include measurement and reporting of demographic variables as well as the structural factors that drive inequities. Data on sociodemographic characteristics need to be collected consistently so that quality improvement outcome measures can be evaluated on any differences across these characteristics. This would then enable the determination of when the degree of difference warrants action for targeted interventions for disparities. These interventions, "tailored to overcome barriers and meet the needs of populations" (Mutha et al., 2012), can ultimately address inequities and disparities in access to high-quality nursing home care (Green, 2017; Hirschhorn et al., 2021; Weinick and Hasnain-Wynia, 2011).

COORDINATED EFFORTS DURING THE COVID-19 PANDEMIC

While not framed as quality improvement efforts, several initiatives during the COVID-19 pandemic were intended to assist nursing homes with infection control and prevention issues. The state and federal resources in these efforts included strike teams that provided expertise, personal protective equipment, testing, vaccinations, and other resources important to nursing homes.

Rapid Response Network

The Rapid Response Network, supported and promoted by the Institute for Healthcare Improvement, The John A. Hartford Foundation, and Age-Friendly Health Systems, held 20-minute web-based "huddles" twice a week for 11 weeks (IHI, 2020). The topics presented included a range of pragmatic clinical and administrative issues such as screening and testing for COVID, infection control, advanced care planning during COVID, tending to the emotional well-being of residents and staff during the pandemic, and addressing pandemic-related staffing and workforce shortages. The series ran from August through October 2020 and has not yet been rigorously evaluated for its impact on the quality of care. Descriptive and participant reports summarized by the program sponsors concluded that the huddles were helpful to nursing home participants (Brandes et al., 2021).

Project ECHO®

Project ECHO (Extension for Community Healthcare Outcomes) uses teams of experts to mentor local clinicians virtually to help reduce health disparities affecting underserved areas. In response to the COVID-19 pandemic, Project ECHO was used to disseminate information quickly to nursing homes with just-in-time learning, short presentations, exemplars, and group discussion (Lingum et al., 2021). AHRQ and the Institute for Healthcare Improvement partnered with Project ECHO to create the AHRQ–ECHO National Nursing Home COVID-19 Action Network, which offers quality improvement training programs for CMS-certified nursing homes aimed at stopping the spread of COVID-19 (AHRQ, 2021). The effort was supported through a $237 million contract made to AHRQ under the Coronavirus Aid, Relief, and Economic Security (CARES) Act.[13] Key areas targeted by the initiative include keeping COVID-19 out of unaffected nursing homes, early identification of infections among residents and staff, prevention of spread, caring for residents with mild cases, sharing information on how to protect residents and staff, and reducing social isolation (Project ECHO, 2021).

Although Project ECHO has not been evaluated for its impact on facility and resident outcomes, the participation of nursing homes in the program during the COVID pandemic has been reported to be high. A systematic review of prior Project ECHO program evaluations concluded that the method is effective and potentially cost-saving, although this review did not include engaging nursing homes in ECHO (Zhou et al., 2016).

THE FUTURE OF QUALITY IMPROVEMENT IN NURSING HOMES

The science of quality improvement has been enhanced in part by recent trends in clinical trials, most notably the recognition that strictly controlled efficacy trials of complex interventions (such as quality improvement) require efforts to ensure that interventions can be tailored to the local site and that barriers to dissemination and implementation can be addressed. Commonly used methods in implementation science, such as the use of clinical champions, stakeholder engagement, feedback reports, action planning, and coaching, also are important quality improvement strategies. Ultimately, quality improvement has to involve all of the interdisciplinary team in nursing homes—leadership, direct-care workers, nurses, social workers, and all staff delivering service to residents. Quality improvement

---

[13] Coronavirus Aid, Relief, and Economic Security (CARES) Act, Public Law 116-136; 116th Cong., 2nd Sess., (March 27, 2020).

cannot be accomplished by making one or two staff members accountable for the process; it truly needs a team effort and a persistent, long-term commitment to examining all aspects of the nursing home operation—direct care, business practices, facility maintenance, infection control, and team and management practices.

KEY FINDINGS AND CONCLUSIONS

Quality Measurement

- Inspections receive the most weight in the calculation of the five-star rating.
- The staffing component of the five-star rating may not fully reflect the adequacy of staffing in nursing homes.
- Although the five-star composite measure appears to distinguish nursing homes at the extremes (five stars versus one star), the rating offers little to distinguish among nursing homes rated at two, three, or four stars.
- More work is needed in regards to the individual measures within Care Compare, including better approaches to risk adjustment and improved correlation among measures that should be correlated.
- Gaming of self-reported data needs to be minimized by strategies such as auditing and evaluating the data sources used in public reporting of the quality measures.
- Several key domains of high-quality care are not measured directly in Care Compare, including resident and family satisfaction and experience, effectiveness of behavior and mental health services, and the quality of palliative and end-of-life care.
- Obtaining residents' assessment of their care experience becomes even more important in the nursing home setting, where residents have high levels of support needs and rely on the nursing home staff and environment to meet their needs on a continuing basis for weeks, months, or even years.
- Not implementing surveys of resident and family satisfaction and experience in nursing homes disadvantages nursing home residents and families from providing feedback about their care experiences, and making informed decisions when choosing a nursing home. Nursing homes are also disadvantaged by not having consumer reports of their experiences to improve services and care delivery.
- While many nursing home administrators report using resident satisfaction surveys, and satisfaction information is reported as being useful, the surveys being used vary widely and may not be adequately validated.
- The nursing home CAHPS survey had extensive item development and testing for reliability and validity.

Quality Improvement

- Evidence about the effectiveness and relative contribution of QIOs to quality improvement in health care, particularly in nursing homes, is lacking.
- Technical assistance leading to successful implementation of quality improvement initiatives depends, in part, on an organization's willingness and readiness to change as well as having the capacity to implement change.
- State programs that focus on helping nursing home staff with quality improvement activities within nursing homes using onsite assistance by expert clinical staff and collaborating groups are effective in improving quality of care, and their help is widely accepted by nursing homes.
- Features of effective technical assistance from state and local programs include building a trusting relationship between the nursing home staff and people offering the technical assistance, modifying the assistance to best fit current needs and skills of each nursing home, and making sure the scientific content is the most up to date and accurate.
- Dedicated funding streams are needed to sustain initiatives shown to improve quality in demonstration projects.
- The COVID-19 pandemic revealed an absence of QAPI practices in many nursing homes.
- Quality improvement cannot be accomplished by making one or two staff members accountable for the process; effective quality improvement initiatives need team effort and a persistent, long-term commitment to examining all aspects of the nursing home operation.

Quality and Disparities

- Nursing homes in low-income neighborhoods, with high numbers of African American and other minority residents, and nursing homes primarily serve Medicaid residents have lower quality of care ratings and lower direct-care staffing.
- Early in the pandemic, nursing homes with greater percentages of racial and ethnic minority residents experienced higher probably of COVID-19 cases and two to four times the proportion of cases and deaths from COVID-19.
- Nursing homes with more residents with serious mental illness are more likely to have lower star ratings, lower direct-care staffing, and for-profit ownership than all other nursing homes.
- There is limited, but mixed, evidence on the relationship between COVID-19 cases among residents in nursing homes and the home's quality ratings.

- Quality improvement initiatives need to carefully and intentionally include measurement and reporting of the structural factors that drive inequities as well as demographic variables.

REFERENCES

Abrams, H. R., L. Loomer, A. Gandhi, and D. C. Grabowski. 2020. Characteristics of U.S. nursing homes with COVID-19 cases. *Journal of the American Geriatrics Society* 68(8):1653–1656.

Abt Associates Inc. 2002. *Evaluation of the Nursing Home Casemix and Quality demonstration.* https://www.cms.gov/Research-Statistics-Data-and-Systems/Statistics-Trends-and-Reports/Reports/downloads/Abt_2002_3.pdf (accessed October 29, 2021).

Abt Associates Inc. 2014. *Nursing home compare five-star quality rating system: Year five report [public version].* https://www.cms.gov/Medicare/Provider-Enrollment-and-Certification/CertificationandComplianc/Downloads/NHC-Year-Five-Report.pdf (accessed February 1, 2022).

AHCA and NCAL (Agency for Health Care Administration and National Center for Assisted Living). 2021. *Quality assurance/performance improvement (QAPI).* https://www.ahcancal.org/Survey-Regulatory-Legal/Pages/QAPI.aspx (accessed March 12, 2021).

AHRQ (Agency for Healthcare Research and Quality). 2012. *Uses of quality measurement.* https://www.ahrq.gov/patient-safety/quality-resources/tools/chtoolbx/uses/index.html (accessed February 2, 2021).

AHRQ. 2013. *Module 4. Approaches to quality improvement.* https://www.ahrq.gov/ncepcr/tools/pf-handbook/mod4.html (accessed April 26, 2021).

AHRQ. 2018. *Development of the CAHPS nursing home resident surveys.* https://www.ahrq.gov/cahps/surveys-guidance/nh/resident/Development-Resident-Surveys.html (accessed February 7, 2022).

AHRQ. 2019. *Development of the CAHPS nursing home Family Member Survey.* https://www.ahrq.gov/cahps/surveys-guidance/nh/family/development-family-member-survey.html (accessed February 7, 2022).

AHRQ. 2020. *CAHPS nursing home surveys.* https://www.ahrq.gov/cahps/surveys-guidance/nh/index.html (accessed August 16, 2021).

AHRQ. 2021. *About AHRQ's Nursing Home Network.* https://www.ahrq.gov/nursing-home/about/index.html (accessed November 1, 2021).

Arling, G., T. Lewis, R. L. Kane, C. Mueller, and S. Flood. 2007. Improving quality assessment through multilevel modeling: The case of nursing home compare. *Health Services Research* 42(3 Pt 1):1177–1199.

Arling, G., V. Cooke, T. Lewis, A. Perkins, D. C. Grabowski, and K. Abrahamson. 2013. Minnesota's provider-initiated approach yields care quality gains at participating nursing homes. *Health Affairs* 32(9):1631–1638.

Arling, G., K. Abrahamson, Z. Hass, and D. Xu. 2020. *Nursing facility quality of care and costs: Literature review and findings from a special analysis.* https://www.purdue.edu/hhs/nur/faculty/documents/VBR%20Report%20on%20NF%20Care%20Quality%20and%20Cost%2029-Jul-2020.pdf (accessed April 9, 2021).

Arling, P. A., K. Abrahamson, E. J. Miech, T. S. Inui, and G. Arling. 2014. Communication and effectiveness in a U.S. nursing home quality improvement collaborative. *Nursing & Health Sciences* 16(3):291–297.

Basch, E., P. Torda, and K. Adams. 2013. Standards for patient-reported outcome-based performance measures. *JAMA* 310(2):139–140.

Baskin, R. M., J. Sangl, and M. W. Zodet. 2012. *Effect of different imputation methods on factor analyses of CAHPS nursing home survey.* Rockville, MD: Agency for Healthcare, Research and Quality.

Beck, C., K. J. Gately, S. Lubin, P. Moody, and C. Beverly. 2014. Building a state coalition for nursing home excellence. *The Gerontologist* 54(Suppl 1):S87–S97.

Bolarinwa, O. A. 2015. Principles and methods of validity and reliability testing of questionnaires used in social and health science researches. *Nigerian Postgraduate Medical Journal* 22(4):195–201.

Bonner, A. 2021. Hope springs eternal: Can Project ECHO transform nursing homes? *Journal of the American Medical Directors Association* 22(2):225–227.

Bose, J., and S. Wilson. 2019. *Nursing homes' star ratings significantly impacted by new CMS updates.* https://www.claconnect.com/resources/articles/2019/nursing-homes-star-ratings-significantly-impacted-by-new-cms-updates (accessed February 1, 2022).

Bowling, A. 2005. Mode of questionnaire administration can have serious effects on data quality. *Journal of Public Health* 27(3):281–291.

Brandes, R., E. Miranda, A. Bonner, J. Baehrend, T. Fulmer, and J. Lenoci-Edwards. 2021. Leveraging national nursing home huddles for rapid COVID-19 response. *Geriatrics* 6(2):62.

Brauner, D., R. M. Werner, T. P. Shippee, J. Cursio, H. Sharma, and R. T. Konetzka. 2018. Does Nursing Home Compare reflect patient safety in nursing homes? *Health Affairs (Millwood)* 37(11):1770–1778.

Braverman, P., E. Arkin, T. Orleans, D. Proctor, and A. Plough. 2017. *What is health equity? And what difference does a definition make?* Princeton, NJ: Robert Wood Johnson Foundation.

Bui, D. P., I. See, E. M. Hesse, K. Varela, R. R. Harvey, E. M. August, A. Winquist, S. Mullins, S. McBee, E. Thomasson, and A. Atkins. 2020. Association between CMS quality ratings and COVID-19 outbreaks in nursing homes - West Virginia, March 17-June 11, 2020. *Morbidity and Mortality Weekly Report* 69(37):1300–1304.

Burstin, H., S. Leatherman, and D. Goldmann. 2016. The evolution of healthcare quality measurement in the United States. *Journal of Internal Medicine* 279(2):154–159.

Çalıkoğlu, Ş., C. S. Christmyer, and B. U. Kozlowski. 2012. My eyes, your eyes—the relationship between CMS five-star rating of nursing homes and family rating of experience of care in Maryland. *Journal for Healthcare Quality* 34(6):5–12.

Castle, N., J. Engberg, and A. Men. 2018. Satisfaction of discharged nursing home residents. *Journal of Applied Gerontology* 37(10):1225–1243.

Castle, N. G. 2007. A review of satisfaction instruments used in long-term care settings. *Journal of Aging & Social Policy* 19:9–41.

Castle, N. G., T. J. Lowe, J. Lucas, J. Robinson, and S. Crystal. 2004. Use of satisfaction surveys in New Jersey nursing homes and assisted living facilities. *Journal of Applied Gerontology* 34:156–171.

Castle, N. G., D. Gifford, and L. B. Schwartz. 2020. The CoreQ: Development and testing of a nursing facility resident satisfaction survey. *Journal of Applied Gerontology* 40(6):629–637. https://doi.org/10.1177/0733464820940871.

Chatterjee, P., S. Kelly, M. Qi, and R. M. Werner. 2020. Characteristics and quality of U.S. nursing homes reporting cases of coronavirus disease 2019 (COVID-19). *JAMA Network Open* 3(7):e2016930.

Chen, M. K., J. Chevalier, and E. Long. 2020. *Nursing home staff networks and COVID-19.* https://www.nber.org/papers/w27608 (accessed February 1, 2022).

Cleary, P. D., and B. J. McNeil. 1988. Patient satisfaction as an indicator of quality care. *Inquiry* 25(1):25–36.

CMS (Centers for Medicare & Medicaid Services). 2003. *Nursing Home Quality Initiative overview.* https://www.cms.gov/Medicare/Quality-Initiatives-Patient-Assessment-Instruments/NursingHomeQualityInits/Downloads/NHQIOverView20030731.pdf (accessed July 29, 2021).

CMS. 2012. *Minimum Data Set 3.0 public reports.* https://www.cms.gov/Research-Statistics-Data-and-Systems/Computer-Data-and-Systems/Minimum-Data-Set-3-0-Public-Reports (accessed November 1, 2021).

CMS. 2016. *QAPI description and background.* https://www.cms.gov/Medicare/Provider-Enrollment-and-Certification/QAPI/qapidefinition (accessed July 29, 2021).

CMS. 2017a. *Nursing home quality initiatives questions and answers.* https://www.cms.gov/Medicare/Provider-Enrollment-and-Certification/QAPI/Downloads/Nursing-Home-Quality-Initiatives-FAQ.pdf (accessed March 2, 2021).

CMS. 2017b. *Data show National Partnership to Improve Dementia care achieves goals to reduce unnecessary antipsychotic medications in nursing homes.* https://www.cms.gov/newsroom/fact-sheets/data-show-national-partnership-improve-dementia-care-achieves-goals-reduce-unnecessary-antipsychotic (accessed July 29, 2021).

CMS. 2018. *Transition to payroll-based journal (PBJ) staffing measures on the Nursing Home Compare tool on medicare.Gov and the five star quality rating system.* https://www.cms.gov/Medicare/Provider-Enrollment-and-Certification/SurveyCertificationGenInfo/downloads/QSO18-17-NH.pdf (accessed November 4, 2021).

CMS. 2019. *Updates to the Nursing Home Compare website and the five star quality rating system.* https://www.cms.gov/Medicare/Provider-Enrollment-and-Certification/SurveyCertificationGenInfo/Downloads/QSO-20-02-NH.pdf (accessed November 5, 2021).

CMS. 2020a. *Quality measures.* https://www.cms.gov/Medicare/Quality-Initiatives-Patient-Assessment-Instruments/QualityMeasures (accessed May 24, 2021).

CMS. 2020b. *MDS 3.0 quality measures user's manual (v14.0).* https://www.cms.gov/Medicare/Quality-Initiatives-Patient-Assessment-Instruments/NursingHomeQualityInits/NHQIQualityMeasures (accessed November 4, 2021).

CMS. 2020c. *Consumer Assessment of Healthcare Providers and Systems (CAHPS).* https://www.cms.gov/Research-Statistics-Data-and-Systems/Research/CAHPS (accessed August 16, 2021).

CMS. 2021a. *Design for care compare nursing home five-star quality rating system: Technical users' guide.* https://www.cms.gov/Medicare/Provider-Enrollment-and-Certification/CertificationandComplianc/Downloads/usersguide.pdf (accessed November 1, 2021).

CMS. 2021b. *Brief explanation of five star rating methodology.* https://www.cms.gov/medicare/provider-enrollment-and-certification/certificationandcomplianc/downloads/brieffivestartug.pdf (accessed November 1, 2021).

CMS. 2021c. *Provider information.* https://data.cms.gov/provider-data/dataset/4pq5-n9py (accessed October 8, 2021).

CMS. 2021d. *National Partnership to Improve Dementia Care in Nursing Homes.* https://www.cms.gov/Medicare/Provider-Enrollment-and-Certification/SurveyCertificationGenInfo/National-Partnership-to-Improve-Dementia-Care-in-Nursing-Homes (accessed April 8, 2021).

Cockburn, A. 2020. *Elder abuse: Nursing homes, the coronavirus, and the bottom line.* https://harpers.org/archive/2020/09/elder-abuse-nursing-homes-COVID-19 (accessed March 15, 2021).

Conway, P. H., F. Mostashari, and C. Clancy. 2013. The future of quality measurement for improvement and accountability. *JAMA* 309(21):2215–2216.

CoreQ. 2019. *CoreQ.* http://www.coreq.org (accessed March 28, 2021).

Cornell, P. Y., D. C. Grabowski, E. C. Norton, and M. Rahman. 2019. Do report cards predict future quality? The case of skilled nursing facilities. *Journal of Health Economics* 66:208–221.

Davila, H., T. P. Shippee, Y. S. Park, D. Brauner, R. M. Werner, and R. T. Konetzka. 2021. Inside the black box of improving on nursing home quality measures. *Medical Care Research and Review* 78(6):758–770.

Dillman, D. A., J. D. Smyth, and L. M. Christian. 2014. *Internet, phone, mail, and mixed-mode surveys: The tailored design method*, 4th ed. New York: John Wiley & Sons.

Donabedian, A. 1988. The quality of care: How can it be assessed? *JAMA* 260(12):1743–1748.

Edelen, M. O., and D. Saliba. 2010. Correspondence of verbal descriptor and numeric rating scales for pain intensity: An item response theory calibration. *Journals of Gerontology, Series A: Biological and Medical Sciences* 65(7):778–785.

Edelman, L. S., J. Drost, R. P. Moone, K. Owens, G. L. Towsley, G. Tucker-Roghi, and J. E. Morley. 2021. Editorial: Applying the age-friendly health system framework to long term care settings. *Journal of Nutrition, Health & Aging* 25(2):141–145.

Edelman, T. 2015. *Changes to nursing home compare and the five star quality rating system*. https://medicareadvocacy.org/changes-to-nursing-home-compare-and-the-five-star-quality-rating-system (accessed February 1, 2022).

Ejaz, F. K., J. K. Straker, K. Fox, and S. Swami. 2003. Developing a satisfaction survey for families of Ohio's nursing home residents. *The Gerontologist* 43(4):447–458.

Encyclopaedia Britannica. 2017. *Land-grant universities*. https://www.britannica.com/topic/land-grant-university (accessed February 7, 2022).

Ersek, M., J. Thorpe, H. Kim, A. Thomasson, and D. Smith. 2015. Exploring end-of-life care in Veterans Affairs community living centers. *Journal of the American Geriatrics Society* 63(4):644–650.

Figueroa, J. F., R. K. Wadhera, I. Papanicolas, K. Riley, J. Zheng, E. J. Orav, and A. K. Jha. 2020. Association of nursing home ratings on health inspections, quality of care, and nurse staffing with COVID-19 cases. *Journal of the American Medical Association* 324(11).

Fleuren, N., M. F. I. A. Depla, D. J. A. Janssen, M. Huisman, and C. M. P. M. Hertogh. 2020. Underlying goals of advance care planning (ACP): A qualitative analysis of the literature. *BMC Palliative Care* 19(1):27.

Freedland, S. 2009. Grassley questions CMS' use of Defense Audit Agency to oversee QIOs. *Inside CMS* 12(12):10–12.

Frentzel, E. M., J. A. Sangl, C. T. Evensen, C. Cosenza, J. A. Brown, S. Keller, and S. A. Garfinkel. 2012. Giving voice to the vulnerable: The development of a CAHPS nursing home survey measuring family members' experiences. *Medical Care* 50(Suppl):S20–S27.

Fuller, R. L., N. I. Goldfield, J. S. Hughes, and E. C. McCullough. 2019. Nursing Home Compare star rankings and the variation in potentially preventable emergency department visits and hospital admissions. *Population Health Management* 22(2):144–152.

Fulmer, T. 2018. *Discovering the 4Ms: A framework for creating age-friendly health systems*. https://www.johnahartford.org/blog/view/discovering-the-4ms-a-framework-for-creating-age-friendly-health-systems (accessed February 25, 2021).

GAO (U.S. Government Accountability Office). 2010. *Poorly performing nursing homes: Special focus facilities are often improving, but CMS's program could be strengthened*. Washington, DC: U.S. Government Accountability Office.

GAO. 2015. *Nursing home quality: CMS should continue to improve data and oversight*. Washington, DC: U.S. Government Accountability Office.

GAO. 2016. *Nursing homes: Consumers could benefit from improvements to the Nursing Home Compare website and five-star quality rating system*. Washington, DC: U.S. Government Accountability Office.

Geng, F., D. G. Stevenson, and D. C. Grabowski. 2019. Daily nursing home staffing levels highly variable, often below CMS expectations. *Health Affairs* 38(7):1095–1100.

Gillespie, S. M., T. Olsan, D. Liebel, X. Cai, R. Stewart, P. R. Katz, and J. Karuza. 2016. Pioneering a nursing home quality improvement learning collaborative: A case study of method and lessons learned. *Journal of the American Medical Directors Association* 17(2):136–141.

Glazier, S. R., J. Schuman, E. Keltz, A. Vally, and R. H. Glazier. 2004. Taking the next steps in goal ascertainment: A prospective study of patient, team, and family perspectives using a comprehensive standardized menu in a geriatric assessment and treatment unit. *Journal of the American Geriatrics Society* 52(2):284–289.

Gorges, R. J., and R. T. Konetzka. 2021. Factors associated with racial differences in deaths among nursing home residents with COVID-19 infection in the U.S. *JAMA Network Open* 4(2):1–10.

Gozalo, P., J. M. Teno, S. L. Mitchell, J. Skinner, J. Bynum, D. Tyler, and V. Mor. 2011. End-of-life transitions among nursing home residents with cognitive issues. *New England Journal of Medicine* 365(13):1212–1221.

Grabowski, D. C. 2020. *Strengthening nursing home policy for the postpandemic world: How can we improve residents' health outcomes and experiences?* https://www.commonwealthfund.org/publications/issue-briefs/2020/aug/strengthening-nursing-home-policy-postpandemic-world (accessed November 5, 2021).

Great Plains Quality Innovation Network. 2019. *National Nursing Home Quality Improvement Campaign changes.* https://greatplainsqin.org/blog/23950 (accessed November 30, 2021).

Green, A. R. 2017. Time for nursing homes to recognize and address disparities in care. *The Joint Commission Journal on Quality and Patient Safety* 43(11):551–553.

Han, X., N. Yaraghi, and R. Gopal. 2016. *Five-star ratings for sub-par service: Evidence of inflation in nursing home ratings.* https://www.brookings.edu/research/five-star-ratings-for-sub-par-service-evidence-of-inflation-in-nursing-home-ratings (accessed February 25, 2021).

Harris, Y., and S. B. Clauser. 2002. Achieving improvement through nursing home quality measurement. *Health Care Financing Review* 23(4):5–18.

He, M., Y. Li, and F. Fang. 2020. Is there a link between nursing home reported quality and COVID-19 cases? Evidence from California skilled nursing facilities. *Journal of the American Medical Directors Association* 21(7):905–908.

Hefele, J. G., X. J. Wang, and E. Lim. 2019. Fewer bonuses, more penalties at skilled nursing facilities serving vulnerable populations. *Health Affairs* 38(7):1127–1131.

Hirschhorn, L. R., H. Magge, and A. Kiflie. 2021. Aiming beyond equality to reach equity: The promise and challenge of quality improvement. *BMJ (Clinical Research Ed.)* 374:n939.

Holt, D. T., C. D. Helfrich, C. G. Hall, and B. J. Weiner. 2010. Are you ready? How health professionals can comprehensively conceptualize readiness for change. *Journal of General Internal Medicine* 25(Suppl 1):50–55.

Housen, P., G. R. Shannon, B. Simon, M. O. Edelen, M. P. Cadogan, L. Sohn, M. Jones, J. L. Buchanan, and D. Saliba. 2008. What the resident meant to say: Use of cognitive interviewing techniques to develop questionnaires for nursing home residents. *The Gerontologist* 48(2):158–169.

Housen, P., G. R. Shannon, B. Simon, M. O. Edelen, M. P. Cadogan, M. Jones, J. Buchanan, and D. Saliba. 2009. Why not just ask the resident? *Journal of Gerontological Nursing* 35(11):40–49.

Huckfeldt, P. J., R. L. Kane, Z. Yang, G. Engstrom, R. Tappen, C. Rojido, D. Newman, B. Reyes, and J. G. Ouslander. 2018. Degree of implementation of the Interventions to Reduce Acute Care Transfers (INTERACT) quality improvement program associated with number of hospitalizations. *Journal of the American Geriatrics Society* 66(9):1830–1837.

IHI (Institute for Healthcare Improvement). 2003. *The breakthrough series: IHI's collaborative model for achieving breakthrough improvement.* Boston MA: Institute for Healthcare Improvement.

IHI. 2020. *COVID-19 rapid response network for nursing homes: Tackling high-priority COVID-19 challenges for nursing homes.* http://www.ihi.org/Engage/Initiatives/COVID-19-Rapid-Response-Network-for-Nursing-Homes/Pages/default.aspx (accessed November 1, 2021).

IHI. 2021. *What is an age-friendly health system?* http://www.ihi.org/Engage/Initiatives/Age-Friendly-Health-Systems/Pages/default.aspx (accessed November 18, 2021).

Integra Med Analytics. 2020. *Underreporting in nursing home quality measures.* https://www.nursinghomereporting.com/post/underreporting-in-nursing-home-quality-measures (accessed February 5, 2022).

IOM (Institute of Medicine). 1986. *Improving the quality of care in nursing homes.* Washington, DC: National Academy Press.

IOM. 2000. *To err is human: Building a safer health systems.* Washington, DC: National Academy Press.

IOM. 2001a. *Crossing the quality chasm: A new health system for the 21st century.* Washington, DC: National Academy Press.

IOM. 2001b. *Improving the quality of long-term care.* Washington, DC: National Academy Press.

IOM. 2006. *Medicare's Quality Improvement Organization program: Maximizing potential.* Washington, DC: The National Academies Press.

Ivers, N., G. Jamtvedt, S. Flottorp, J. M. Young, J. Odgaard-Jensen, S. D. French, M. A. O'Brien, M. Johansen, J. Grimshaw, and A. D. Oxman. 2012. Audit and feedback: Effects on professional practice and healthcare outcomes. *Cochrane Database of Systematic Reviews* 2012(6):CD000259.

Ivers, N. M., A. Sales, H. Colquhoun, S. Michie, R. Foy, J. J. Francis, and J. M. Grimshaw. 2014. No more "business as usual" with audit and feedback interventions: Towards an agenda for a reinvigorated intervention. *Implementation Science* 9(1):14.

Jester, D. J., K. Hyer, and J. R. Bowblis. 2020. Quality concerns in nursing homes that serve large proportions of residents with serious mental illness. *The Gerontologist* 60(7):1312–1321.

Jevaji, S. 2016. *The Q series: What is health care quality assurance?* https://blog.ncqa.org/the-q-series-what-is-health-care-quality-assurance (accessed November 16, 2021).

Jewish Healthcare Foundation. 2021. *Pennsylvania teaching nursing home pilot aims to transform care model.* https://www.jhf.org/press-releases/entry/pennsylvania-teaching-nursing-home-pilot-aims-to-transform-care-model (accessed November 19, 2021).

Joint Commission. 2021. *Joint Commission FAQs.* https://www.jointcommission.org/about-us/facts-about-the-joint-commission/joint-commission-faqs (accessed November 1, 2021).

Kane, R. A., K. C. Kling, B. Bershadsky, R. L. Kane, K. Giles, H. B. Degenholtz, J. Liu, and L. J. Cutler. 2003. Quality of life measures for nursing home residents. *Journals of Gerontology: Series A, Biological and Medical Sciences* 58(3):240–248.

Kane, R. A., R. L. Kane, B. Bershadsky, L. J. Cutler, K. Giles, J. J. Liu, K. Kang, L. Zhang, K. C. Kling, and H. B. Degenholtz. 2004. *Measures, indicators, and improvement of quality of life in nursing homes (RFP: HCFA-98-002/PK).* https://www.cms.gov/Medicare/Quality-Initiatives-Patient-Assessment-Instruments/NursingHomeQualityInits/Downloads/NHQIVol2-ContentsPreface.pdf (accessed April 9, 2021).

Kane, R. L., R. A. Kane, B. Bershadsky, H. Degenholtz, K. Kling, A. Totten, and K. Jung. 2005. Proxy sources for information on nursing home residents' quality of life. *Journals of Gerontology, Series B* 60(6):S318–S325.

Kane, R. L., G. Arling, C. Mueller, R. Held, and V. Cooke. 2007. A quality-based payment strategy for nursing home care in Minnesota. *The Gerontologist* 47(1):108–115.

Kane, R. L., P. Huckfeldt, R. Tappen, G. Engstrom, C. Rojido, D. Newman, Z. Yang, and J. G. Ouslander. 2017. Effects of an intervention to reduce hospitalizations from nursing homes: A randomized implementation trial of the INTERACT program. *JAMA Internal Medicine* 177(9):1257–1264.

Karlawish, J., D. C. Grabowski, and A. K. Hoffman. 2020. Opinion: Continued bans on nursing home visitors are unhealthy and unethical. https://www.washingtonpost.com/opinions/2020/07/13/residents-good-nursing-homes-should-consider-re-allowing-visitors (accessed April 6, 2021).

Katz, S., and C. A. Akpom. 1976. A measure of primary sociobiological functions. *International Journal of Health Services* 6(3):493–508.

Khairat, S., L. C. Zalla, J. Adler-Milstein, and C. E. Kistler. 2021. U.S. nursing home quality ratings associated with COVID-19 cases and deaths. *Journal of the American Medical Directors Association* 22(10):2021–2025.

Kim, S. J., E. C. Park, S. Kim, S. Nakagawa, J. Lung, J. B. Choi, W. S. Ryu, T. J. Min, H. P. Shin, K. Kim, and J. W. Yoo. 2014. The association between quality of care and quality of life in long-stay nursing home residents with preserved cognition. *Journal of the American Medical Directors Association* 15(3):220–225.

Klein, D. J., M. N. Elliott, A. M. Haviland, D. Saliba, Q. Burkhart, C. Edwards, and A. M. Zaslavsky. 2011. Understanding nonresponse to the 2007 Medicare CAHPS survey. *The Gerontologist* 51(6):843–855.

Konetzka, R. T., and Z. S. Gray. 2017. The role of socioeconomic status in nursing home quality ratings. *Seniors Housing & Care Journal* 25(1):3–14.

Konetzka, R. T., and M. C. Perraillon. 2016. Use of Nursing Home Compare website appears limited by lack of awareness and initial mistrust of the data. *Health Affairs* 35(4):706–713.

Konetzka, R. T., D. J. Brauner, M. Coca Perraillon, and R. M. Werner. 2015. The role of severe dementia in nursing home report cards. *Medical Care Research and Review* 72(5):562–579.

Konetzka, R. T., K. Yan, and R. M. Werner. 2020. Two decades of Nursing Home Compare: What have we learned? *Medical Care Research and Review* 78(4):295–310.

Krosnick, J. A. 1999. Survey research. *Annual Review of Psychology* 50(1):537–567.

Landrum, M., C. Nguyen, and M. Chernew. 2019. *Measurement systems: A framework for next generation measurement of quality in healthcare*. National Quality Forum. http://www.qualityforum.org/Story/Measurement_Systems_White_Paper.aspx (accessed February 25, 2021).

Lang, N. M., and J. F. Clinton. 1983. Assessment and assurance of the quality of nursing care: A selected overview. *Evaluation & the Health Professions* 6(2):211–231.

Lawton, M. P. 1991. A multidimensional view of quality of life in frail elders. In J. Birren, J. Lubben, J. Rowe, and D. Deutchman (eds.), *The concept and measurement of quality of life in the frail elderly*. San Diego: Academic Press. Pp. 3–27.

Le, L. T., B. J. Anthony, S. M. Bronheim, C. M. Holland, and D. F. Perry. 2014. A technical assistance model for guiding service and systems change. *The Journal of Behavioral Health Sciences & Research* 43(3).

LeadingAge. 2015. *What the 5-star rating system changes mean for nursing homes.* https://leadingage.org/members/what-5-star-rating-system-changes-mean-nursing-homes (accessed February 1, 2022).

Li, Y., X. Cai, L. G. Glance, W. D. Spector, and D. B. Mukamel. 2009. National release of the nursing home quality report cards: Implications of statistical methodology for risk adjustment. *Health Services Research* 44(1):79–102.

Li, Y., J. Schnelle, W. D. Spector, L. G. Glance, and D. B. Mukamel. 2010. The "Nursing Home Compare" measure of urinary/fecal incontinence: Cross-sectional variation, stability over time, and the impact of case mix. *Health Services Research* 45(1):79–97.

Li, Y., Z. Ye, L. G. Glance, and H. Temkin-Greener. 2014. Trends in family ratings of experience with care and racial disparities among Maryland nursing homes. *Medical Care* 52(7):641–648.

Li, Y., Q. Li, and Y. Tang. 2016. Associations between family ratings on experience with care and clinical quality-of-care measures for nursing home residents. *Medical Care Research and Review* 73(1):62–84.

Li, Y., H. Temkin-Greener, G. Shan, and X. Cai. 2020a. COVID-19 infections and deaths among Connecticut nursing home residents: Facility correlates. *Journal of the American Geriatrics Society* 68(9):1899–1906.

Li, Y., X. Cen, X. Cai, and H. Temkin-Greener. 2020b. Racial and ethnic disparities in COVID-19 infections and deaths across U.S. nursing homes. *Journal of the American Geriatrics Society* 68(11):2454–2461.

Lingum, N. R., L. G. Sokoloff, R. M. Meyer, S. Gingrich, D. J. Sodums, A. T. Santiago, S. Feldman, S. Guy, A. Moser, S. Shaikh, C. J. Grief, and D. K. Conn. 2021. Building long-term care staff capacity during COVID-19 through just-in-time learning: Evaluation of a modified ECHO model. *Journal of the American Medical Directors Association* 22(2):238–244.e231.

Martino, S. C., M. N. Elliott, A. M. Haviland, D. Saliba, Q. Burkhart, and D. E. Kanouse. 2016. Comparing the health care experiences of Medicare beneficiaries with and without depressive symptoms in Medicare managed care versus fee-for-service. *Health Services Research* 51(3):1002–1020.

McGlynn, E. A. 2003. Introduction and overview of the conceptual framework for a national quality measurement and reporting system. *Medical Care* 41(1 Suppl):I1–I7.

MedPAC (Medicare Payment Advisory Commission). 2021. *Report to Congress: Medicare and the health care delivery system.* http://www.medpac.gov/docs/default-source/reports/jun21_medpac_report_to_congress_sec.pdf (accessed August 16, 2021).

Mezey, M. D., and J. E. Lynaugh. 1989. The teaching nursing home program. Outcomes of care. *The Nursing Clinics of North America* 24(3):769–780.

Mezey, M. D., J. E. Lynaugh, and M. M. Cartier. 1988. The teaching nursing home program, 1982–1987: A report card. *Nursing Outlook* 36:285–292.

Mezey, M. D., E. L. Mitty, and S. G. Burger. 2008. Rethinking teaching nursing homes: Potential for improving long-term care. *The Gerontologist* 48(1):8–15.

Michigan DHHS (Michigan Department of Health and Human Services). 2021a. *MDHHS—Nursing facility quality measure initiative.* https://www.michigan.gov/mdhhs (accessed February 2, 2021).

Minnesota DHHS (Minnesota Department of Health and Minnesota Department of Human Services). 2021. *Minnesota nursing home report card technical user guide.* https://nhreportcard.dhs.mn.gov/technicaluserguide.pdf (accessed July 6, 2021).

Mochel, A. L., C. L. Holle, J. L. Rudolph, J. G. Ouslander, D. Saliba, V. Mor, and B. S. Mittman. 2021. Influencing factors associated with implementation of INTERACT (Interventions to Reduce Acute Care Transfers) in VA community living centers (CLCs) using the consolidated framework. *Journal of Aging & Social Policy*, June 4:1–17.

Mor, V., J. Zinn, J. Angelelli, J. M. Teno, and S. C. Miller. 2004. Driven to tiers: Socioeconomic and racial disparities in the quality of nursing home care. *The Milbank Quarterly* 82(2):227–256.

Morris, J. N., C. Hawes, B. E. Fries, C. D. Phillips, V. Mor, S. Katz, K. Murphy, M. L. Drugovich, and A. S. Friedlob. 1990. Designing the national resident assessment instrument for nursing homes. *The Gerontologist* 30(3):293–307.

Mukamel, D. B., L. G. Glance, Y. Li, D. L. Weimer, W. D. Spector, J. S. Zinn, and L. Mosqueda. 2008. Does risk adjustment of the CMS quality measures for nursing homes matter? *Medical Care* 46(5):532–541.

Mukamel, D. B., T. Caprio, R. Ahn, N. T. Zheng, S. Norton, T. Quill, and H. Temkin-Greener. 2012. End-of-life quality-of-care measures for nursing homes: Place of death and hospice. *Journal of Palliative Medicine* 15(4):438–446.

Mukamel, D. B., H. Ladd, T. Caprio, and H. Temkin-Greener. 2016. Prototype end-of-life quality measures based on MDS 3 data. *Medical Care* 54(11):1024–1032.

Mukamel, D. B., D. L. Weimer, Y. Shi, H. Ladd, and D. Saliba. 2020. Comparison of consumer rankings with Centers for Medicare & Medicaid Services five-star rankings of nursing homes. *JAMA Network Open* 3(5):e204798.

Mukamel, D. B., D. Saliba, D. L. Weimer, and H. Ladd. 2021. Families' and residents' perspectives of the quality of nursing home care: Implications for composite quality measures. *Journal of the American Medical Directors Association* 22(8):1609–1614.e1601.

Mutha, S., A. Marks, I. Bau, and M. Regenstein. 2012. *Bringing equity into quality improvement: An overview and opportunities ahead.* https://healthforce.ucsf.edu/sites/healthforce.ucsf.edu/files/publication-pdf/6.1%20Part%201%20_Equity%20into%20QI.pdf (accessed November 11, 2021).

Nadash, P., J. G. Hefele, E. A. Miller, A. Barooah, and X. Wang. 2019. A national-level analysis of the relationship between nursing home satisfaction and quality. *Research on Aging* 41(3):215–240.

National Consumer Voice (National Consumer Voice for Quality Long-Term Care). 2021. *National Nursing Home Quality Improvement (NNHQI) campaign.* https://theconsumervoice.org/issues/recipients/nursing-home-residents/advancing-excellence (accessed May 13, 2021).

Neuman, M. D., C. Wirtalla, and R. M. Werner. 2014. Association between skilled nursing facility quality indicators and hospital readmissions. *JAMA* 312(15):1542–1551.

New York State Department of Health. 2021. *Factors associated with nursing home infections and fatalities in New York State during the COVID-19 global health crisis.* https://www.health.ny.gov/press/releases/2020/docs/nh_factors_report.pdf (accessed February 1, 2022).

Nightingale, F. 1859. *Notes on nursing: What it is, and what it is not.* London: Harrison. Reprint: New York: Dover Publications, 1969.

NNHQI (National Nursing Home Quality Improvement Campaign). 2021. *Resources & downloads.* https://nhqualitycampaign.org/resources-downloads/ (accessed November 30, 2021).

Norton, S. A., S. Ladwig, T. V. Caprio, T. E. Quill, and H. Temkin-Greener. 2018. Staff experiences forming and sustaining palliative care teams in nursing homes. *The Gerontologist* 58(4):e218–e225.

NQF (National Quality Forum). 2012a. *Palliative care and end-of-life care—A consensus report.* https://www.qualityforum.org/Publications/2012/04/Palliative_Care_and_End-of-Life_Care%e2%80%94A_Consensus_Report.aspx (accessed May 24, 2021).

NQF. 2012b. *Performance measurement coordination strategy for hospice and palliative care.* https://www.qualityforum.org/Publications/2012/06/Performance_Measurement_Coordination_Strategy_for_Hospice_and_Palliative_Care.aspx (accessed May 24, 2021).

NQF. 2013. *Patient-reported outcomes in performance measurement.* https://www.qualityforum.org/Publications/2012/12/Patient-Reported_Outcomes_in_Performance_Measurement.aspx (accessed February 25, 2021).

NQF. 2020. *Measure Applications Partnership 2020 considerations for implementing measures. Final report: Post-acute care and long-term care.* http://www.qualityforum.org/Publications/2020/02/MAP_2020_Considerations_for_Implementing_Measures_Final_Report_-_PAC_LTC.aspx (accessed February 25, 2021).

NQF. 2021. *The ABCs of measurement* https://www.qualityforum.org/Measuring_Performance/ABCs_of_Measurement.aspx (accessed December, 31, 2020).

NRC Health. 2021. *Post-acute customer experience*. https://nrchealth.com/solutions-old/post-acute-customer-experience (accessed November 1, 2021).

Ochieng, N., P. Chidambaram, R. Garfield, and T. Neuman. 2021. *Factors associated with COVID-19 cases and deaths in long-term care facilities: Findings from a literature review*. https://www.kff.org/coronavirus-covid-19/issue-brief/factors-associated-with-covid-19-cases-and-deaths-in-long-term-care-facilities-findings-from-a-literature-review (accessed February 1, 2022).

OIG (Office of the Inspector General). 2015. *Quality Improvement Organizations provide support to more than half of hospital but overlap with other programs*. Washington, DC: Department of Health and Human Services Office of the Inspector General.

OIG. 2021. *CMS use of data on nursing home staffing: Progress and opportunities to do more*. Washington, DC: Department of Health and Human Services Office of the Inspector General.

Ouslander, J. G., and D. C. Grabowski. 2020. COVID-19 in nursing homes: Calming the perfect storm. *Journal of the American Geriatrics Society* 68:2153–2162.

Ouslander, J. G., G. Lamb, R. Tappen, L. Herndon, S. Diaz, B. A. Roos, D. C. Grabowski, and A. Bonner. 2011. Interventions to reduce hospitalizations from nursing homes: Evaluation of the INTERACT II collaborative quality improvement project. *Journal of the American Geriatrics Society* 59(4):745–753.

Ouslander, J. G., A. Bonner, L. Herndon, and J. Shutes. 2014. The Interventions to Reduce Acute Care Transfers (INTERACT) quality improvement program: An overview for medical directors and primary care clinicians in long term care. *Journal of the American Medical Directors Association* 15(3):162–170.

Perraillon, M. C., D. J. Brauner, and R. T. Konetzka. 2019a. Nursing home response to Nursing Home Compare: The provider perspective. *Medical Care Research and Review* 76(4):425–443.

Perraillon, M. C., R. T. Konetzka, D. He, and R. M. Werner. 2019b. Consumer response to composite ratings of nursing home quality. *American Journal of Health Economics* 5(2):165–190.

Perry, M., C. Stanik, A. Montgomery, and S. Slocum. 2021. *Perspective: The case for person-centered residential long-term care in 2021: Measure it, move it forward*. https://altarum.org/news/case-person-centered-residential-long-term-care-2021-measure-it-move-it-forward (accessed November 16, 2021).

Phillips, C. D., C. Hawes, T. Lieberman, and M. J. Koren. 2007. Where should momma go? Current nursing home performance measurement strategies and a less ambitious approach. *BMC Health Services Research* 7:93–93.

Phillips, L., C. Oyewusi, N. Martin, L. Youse, and M. Rantz. 2018. Impact of survey readiness training on nursing home quality of care. *Innovation in Aging* 2(Suppl 1):723–723.

Pool, D., and W. Boren. 2020. *Second responders: Answering the call for help in long-term care*. https://www.mcknights.com/blogs/second-responders-answering-the-call-for-help-in-long-term-care (accessed April 15, 2021).

Popejoy, L. L., M. J. Rantz, V. Conn, D. Wipke-Tevis, V. T. Grando, and R. Porter. 2000. Improving quality of care in nursing facilities. Gerontological clinical nurse specialist as research nurse consultant. *Journal of Gerontological Nursing* 26(4):6–13.

Popejoy, L., A. Vogelsmeier, W. Boren, N. Martin, S. Kist, K. Canada, S. J. Miller, and M. Rantz. 2020. A coordinated response to the COVID-19 pandemic in Missouri nursing homes. *Journal of Nursing Care Quality* 35(4):287–292.

Powell, B. J., T. J. Waltz, M. J. Chinman, L. J. Damschroder, J. L. Smith, M. M. Matthieu, E. K. Proctor, and J. E. Kirchner. 2015. A refined compilation of implementation strategies: Results from the Expert Recommendations for Implementing Change (ERIC) project. *Implementation Science* 10(1):21.

Project ECHO. 2021. *Partnering with nursing homes: AHRQ ECHO national nursing home COVID-19 action network.* https://hsc.unm.edu/echo/institute-programs/nursing-home/pages/ (accessed May 12, 2021).

Pyle, E. 2017. *State website shows where Ohio nursing homes excel, fall short.* https://www.dispatch.com/news/20170611/state-website-shows-where-ohio-nursing-homes-excel-fall-short (accessed February 2, 2021).

Rantz, M. J., L. Popejoy, G. F. Petroski, R. W. Madsen, D. R. Mehr, M. Zwygart-Stauffacher, L. L. Hicks, V. Grando, D. D. Wipke-Tevis, J. Bostick, R. Porter, V. S. Conn, and M. Maas. 2001. Randomized clinical trial of a quality improvement intervention in nursing homes. *The Gerontologist* 41(4):525–538.

Rantz, M. J., T. V. Miller, L. L. Popejoy, and M. Zwygart-Stauffacher. 2002. *Outcome-based quality improvement for long-term care: Using MDS, process, and outcomes measures.* 2nd ed. New York: Aspen Publishers, Inc.

Rantz, M. J., A. Vogelsmeier, P. Manion, D. Minner, B. Markway, V. Conn, M. A. Aud, and D. R. Mehr. 2003. Statewide strategy to improve quality of care in nursing facilities. *The Gerontologist* 43(2):248–258.

Rantz, M. J., M. Zwygart-Stauffacher, D. R. Mehr, G. F. Petroski, S. V. Owen, R. W. Madsen, M. Flesner, V. Conn, J. Bostick, R. Smith, and M. Maas. 2006. Field testing, refinement, and psychometric evaluation of a new measure of nursing home care quality. *Journal of Nursing Measurement* 14(2):129–148.

Rantz, M. J., D. Cheshire, M. Flesner, G. F. Petroski, L. Hicks, G. Alexander, M. A. Aud, C. Siem, K. Nguyen, C. Boland, and S. Thomas. 2009. Helping nursing homes "at risk" for quality problems: A statewide evaluation. *Geriatric Nursing* 30(4):238–249.

Rantz, M. J., M. Zwygart-Stauffacher, L. Hicks, D. Mehr, M. Flesner, G. F. Petroski, R. W. Madsen, and J. Scott-Cawiezell. 2012a. Randomized multilevel intervention to improve outcomes of residents in nursing homes in need of improvement. *Journal of the American Medical Directors Association* 13(1):60–68.

Rantz, M. J., M. Zwygart-Stauffacher, M. Flesner, L. Hicks, D. Mehr, T. Russell, and D. Minner. 2012b. Challenges of using quality improvement methods in nursing homes that "need improvement." *Journal of the American Medical Directors Association* 13(8):732–738.

Rantz, M. J., M. Zwygart-Stauffacher, M. Flesner, L. Hicks, D. Mehr, T. Russell, and D. Minner. 2013. The influence of teams to sustain quality improvement in nursing homes that "need improvement." *Journal of the American Medical Directors Association* 14(1):48–52.

Rau, J., and A. Almendrala. 2020. *COVID-plagued California nursing homes often had problems in past.* https://khn.org/news/covid-plagued-california-nursing-homes-often-had-problems-in-past/ (accessed February 1, 2022).

Reape, P. 2019. *April 2019 five-star ratings decrease for 37% of nursing facilities.* https://hwco.cpa/april-2019-five-star-ratings-decrease-for-37-of-nursing-facilities/ (accessed February 1, 2022).

Reichard, J. 2007. *Medicare quality improvement stagnating, Senators complain.* https://www.commonwealthfund.org/publications/newsletter-article/medicare-quality-improvement-stagnating-senators-complain (accessed July 6, 2021).

Roberts, T. J., A. Gilmore-Bykovskyi, M. Lor, D. Liebzeit, C. J. Crnich, and D. Saliba. 2018. Important care and activity preferences in a nationally representative sample of nursing home residents. *Journal of the American Medical Directors Association* 19(1):25–32.

Rollow, W., T. R. Lied, P. McGann, J. Poyer, L. LaVoie, R. T. Kambic, D. W. Bratzler, A. Ma, E. D. Huff, and L. D. Ramunno. 2006. Assessment of the Medicare Quality Improvement Organization Program. *Annals of Internal Medicine* 145(5):342–353.

Rowan, P., R. Gupta, and R. S. Lester. 2020. *A study of the COVID-19 outbreak and response in Connecticut long-term care facilities: Final report*. Princeton, NJ: Mathematica.

RTI International. 2012. *MDS 3.0 quality measures user's manual (v5.0)*. https://www.cms.gov/medicare/quality-initiatives-patient-assessment-instruments/nursinghomequalityinits/downloads/mds30qm-manual.pdf (accessed November 4, 2021).

RTI International. 2017. *Evaluation of the Initiative to Reduce Avoidable Hospitalizations among Nursing Facility Residents: Final report*. Waltham, MA: RTI International.

RTI International. 2021. *Evaluation of the Initiative to Reduce Avoidable Hospitalizations among Nursing Facility Residents—Payment reform: Fourth annual report*. Baltimore, MD: RTI International.

Ryskina, K. L., R. T. Konetzka, and R. M. Werner. 2018. Association between 5-star nursing home report card ratings and potentially preventable hospitalizations. *Inquiry* 55:46958018787323.

Saliba, D., and J. Buchanan. 2008. *Development & validation of a revised nursing home assessment tool: MDS 3.0*. https://www.cms.gov/Medicare/Quality-Initiatives-Patient-Assessment-Instruments/NursingHomeQualityInits/downloads/MDS30FinalReport.pdf (accessed February 25, 2021).

Saliba, D., and J. Buchanan. 2012. Making the investment count: Revision of the Minimum Data Set for nursing homes, MDS 3.0. *Journal of the American Medical Directors Association* 13(7):602–610.

Saliba, D., and J. F. Schnelle. 2002. Indicators of the quality of nursing home residential care. *Journal of the American Geriatrics Society* 50(8):1421–1430.

Saliba, D., S. DiFilippo, M. O. Edelen, K. Kroenke, J. Buchanan, and J. Streim. 2012. Testing the PHQ-9 interview and observational versions (PHW-9 OV) for MDS 3.0. *Journal of the American Medical Directors Association* 13(7):618–625.

Saliba, D., D. L. Weimer, Y. Shi, and D. B. Mukamel. 2018. Examination of the new short-stay nursing home quality measures: Rehospitalizations, emergency department visits, and successful returns to the community. *Inquiry* 55:46958018786816.

Sanders, J. J., J. R. Curtis, and J. A. Tulsky. 2018. Achieving goal-concordant care: A conceptual model and approach to measuring serious illness communication and its impact. *Journal of Palliative Medicine* 21(S2):S17–S27.

Sangl, J., D. Saliba, D. R. Gifford, and D. F. Hittle. 2005. Challenges in measuring nursing home and home health quality: Lessons from the first National Healthcare Quality Report. *Medical Care* 43(3):I-24–I-32.

Sangl, J., J. Buchanan, C. Cosenza, S. Bernard, S. Keller, N. Mitchell, J. Brown, N. Castle, E. Sekscenski, and D. Larwood. 2007. The development of a CAHPS instrument for nursing home residents (NHCAHPS). *Journal of Aging and Social Policy* 19(2):63–82.

Schapira, M. M., J. A. Shea, K. A. Duey, C. Kleiman, and R. M. Werner. 2016. The Nursing Home Compare report card: Perceptions of residents and caregivers regarding quality ratings and nursing home choice. *Health Services Research* 51(Suppl 2):1212–1228.

Schwartz, L. 2021. *CoreQ measures receive re-endorsement from the National Quality Forum (NQF)*. https://www.ahcancal.org/News-and-Communications/Blog/Pages/CoreQ-Measures-Receive-Re-Endorsement-from-the-National-Quality-Forum-(NQF)-.aspx (accessed July 29, 2021).

Sharma, H., R. T. Konetzka, and F. Smieliauskas. 2019. The relationship between reported staffing and expenditures in nursing homes. *Medical Care Research and Review* 76(6):758–783.

Sharma, H., M. C. Perraillon, R. M. Werner, D. C. Grabowski, and R. T. Konetzka. 2020. Medicaid and nursing home choice: Why do duals end up in low-quality facilities? *Journal of Applied Gerontology* 39(9):981–990.

Shaughnessy, P. W., A. M. Kramer, D. F. Hittle, and J. F. Steiner. 1995. Quality of care in teaching nursing homes: Findings and implications. *Health Care Financing Review* 16(4):55–83.

Shaw-Taylor, Y. 2014. Making quality improvement programs more effective. *International Journal of Health Care Quality Assurance* 27(4):264–270.

Shortell, S. M., and W. A. Peck. 2006. Enhancing the potential of Quality Improvement Organizations to improve quality of care. *Annals of Internal Medicine* 145(5):388–389.

Silow-Carroll, S., D. Peartree, S. Tucker, and A. Pham. 2021. *Fundamental nursing home reform: Evidence on single-resident rooms to improve personal experience and public health.* https://www.healthmanagement.com/wp-content/uploads/HMA.Single-Resident-Rooms-3.22.2021_final.pdf (accessed November 5, 2021).

Silver-Greenberg, J., and R. Gebeloff. 2021. Maggots, rape and yet five stars: How U.S. Ratings of nursing homes mislead the public. https://www.nytimes.com/2021/03/13/business/nursing-homes-ratings-medicare-covid.html?campaign_id=9&emc=edit_nn_20210313&instance_id=28051&nl=the-morning&regi_id=98348276&segment_id=53394&te=1&user_id=d3b6076e56d56335bd158430d6fd0d63 (accessed March 15, 2021).

Simpson, A. 2020. *Nursing home coronavirus rules provoke backlash.* https://www.pewtrusts.org/en/research-and-analysis/blogs/stateline/2020/04/10/nursing-home-coronavirus-rules-provoke-backlash (accessed April 6, 2021).

Sinclair School of Nursing University of Missouri. 2021a. *QIPMO program statistics.* https://nursinghomehelp.org/qipmo-program/statistics (accessed October 15, 2021).

Sinclair School of Nursing University of Missouri. 2021b. *Leadership coaching statistics.* https://nursinghomehelp.org/leadership-coaching/statistics (accessed October 15, 2021).

Sloane, P. D., S. Zimmerman, K. Ward, C. E. Kistler, D. Paone, D. J. Weber, C. J. Wretman, and J. S. Preisser. 2020. A 2-year pragmatic trial of antibiotic stewardship in 27 community nursing homes. *Journal of the American Geriatrics Society* 68(1):46–54.

Snyder, D. J., T. R. Kroshus, A. Keswani, E. B. Garden, K. M. Koenig, K. J. Bozic, D. S. Jevsevar, J. Poeran, and C. S. Moucha. 2019. Are Medicare's Nursing Home Compare ratings accurate predictors of 90-day complications, readmission, and bundle cost for patients undergoing primary total joint arthroplasty? *Journal of Arthroplasty* 34(4):613–618.

Steel, K., G. Ljunggren, E. Topinková, J. N. Morris, C. Vitale, J. Parzuchowski, S. Nonemaker, D. H. Frijters, T. Rabinowitz, K. M. Murphy, M. W. Ribbe, and B. E. Fries. 2003. The RAI-PC: An assessment instrument for palliative care in all settings. *American Journal of Hospice and Palliative Care* 20(3):211–219.

Stevenson, D. G., and V. Mor. 2009. Targeting nursing homes under the Quality Improvement Organization Program's 9th statement of work. *Journal of the American Geriatrics Society* 57(9):1678–1684.

Straker, J., K. McGrew, J. Dibert, C. Burch, and A. Raymore. 2016. *Ohio nursing home and residential care facility satisfaction: Survey testing and development for residents and families.* https://sc.lib.miamioh.edu/xmlui/bitstream/handle/2374.MIA/5925/Ohio%27s%20Nursing%20Homes%20and%20Residential%20Care%20Family%20Satisfaction.pdf (accessed February 25, 2021).

Sugg, M. M., T. J. Spaulding, S. J. Lane, J. D. Runkle, S. R. Harden, A. Hege, and L. S. Iyer. 2021. Mapping community-level determinants of COVID-19 transmission in nursing homes: A multi-scale approach. *Science of the Total Environment* 752:141946.

Temkin-Greener, H., Q. Li, Y. Li, M. Segelman, and D. B. Mukamel. 2016. End-of-life care in nursing homes: From care processes to quality. *Journal of Palliative Medicine* 19(12):1304–1311.

Teno, J. M., P. Gozalo, A. N. Trivedi, J. Bunker, J. Lima, J. Ogarek, and V. Mor. 2018. Site of death, place of care, and health care transitions among U.S. Medicare beneficiaries, 2000–2015. *JAMA* 320(3):264–271.

Thomas, K. 2014. *Medicare star ratings allow nursing homes to game the system.* https://www.nytimes.com/2014/08/25/business/medicare-star-ratings-allow-nursing-homes-to-game-the-system.html?searchResultPosition=1 (accessed February 1, 2022).

Thomas, K. 2015. *Government will change how it rates nursing homes.* https://www.nytimes.com/2015/02/13/business/government-will-change-how-it-rates-nursing-homes.html?searchResultPosition=2 (accessed February 1, 2022).

Thompson, S., M. Bott, D. Boyle, B. Gajewski, and V. P. Tilden. 2011. A measure of palliative care in nursing homes. *Journal of Pain and Symptom Management* 41(1):57–67.

Thorpe, J. M., D. Smith, N. Kuzla, L. Scott, and M. Ersek. 2016. Does mode of survey administration matter? Using measurement invariance to validate the mail and telephone versions of the Bereaved Family Survey. *Journal of Pain and Symptom Management* 51(3):546–556.

University of Missouri Interdisciplinary Center on Aging. 2008. *Improvements in Missouri nursing homes using QIPMO services.* https://agingmo.com/wp-content/uploads/2017/10/QIPMO08.pdf (accessed May 12, 2021).

Unroe, K. T., M. A. Greiner, C. Colón-Emeric, E. D. Peterson, and L. H. Curtis. 2012. Associations between published quality ratings of skilled nursing facilities and outcomes of Medicare beneficiaries with heart failure. *Journal of the American Medical Directors Association* 13(2):188.e1–e6.

Vasilevskis, E. E., J. G. Ouslander, A. S. Mixon, S. P. Bell, J. M. L. Jacobsen, A. A. Saraf, D. Markley, K. C. Sponsler, J. Shutes, E. A. Long, S. Kripalani, S. F. Simmons, and J. F. Schnelle. 2017. Potentially avoidable readmissions of patients discharged to post-acute care: Perspectives of hospital and skilled nursing facility staff. *Journal of the American Geriatrics Society* 65(2):269–276.

Vest, J. R., H. Y. Jung, K. Wiley, Jr., H. Kooreman, L. Pettit, and M. A. Unruh. 2019. Adoption of health information technology among U.S. nursing facilities. *Journal of the American Medical Directors Association* 20(8):995–1000.e1004.

Vogelsmeier, A., L. Popejoy, K. Canada, C. Galambos, G. Petroski, C. Crecelius, G. L. Alexander, and M. Rantz. 2021. Results of the Missouri Quality Initiative in sustaining changes in nursing home care: Six-year trends of reducing hospitalizations of nursing home residents. *Journal of Nutrition, Health, and Aging* 25(1):5–12.

Wandersman, A., V. H. Chien, and J. Katz. 2012. Toward an evidence-based system for innovation support for implementing innovations with quality tools: Tools, training, technical assistance, and quality assurance/quality improvement. *American Journal of Community Psychology* 50(3-4):445–459.

Weech-Maldonado, R., R. Pradhan, N. Dayama, J. Lord, and S. Gupta. 2019. Nursing home quality and financial performance: Is there a business case for quality? *Inquiry* 56:46958018825191.

Weimer, D. L., D. Saliba, H. Ladd, Y. Shi, and D. B. Mukamel. 2019. Using contingent valuation to develop consumer-based weights for health quality report cards. *Health Services Research* 54(4):947–956.

Weiner. B. J. 2009. A theory of organizational readiness for change. *Implementation Science* 4:67.

Weiner, B. J., H. Amick, and S. D. Lee. 2008. Conceptualization and measurement of organizational readiness for change. *Medical Care Research and Review* 65(4):379–436.

Weinick, R. M., and R. Hasnain-Wynia. 2011. Quality improvement efforts under health reform: How to ensure that they help reduce disparities—not increase them. *Health Affairs* 30(10):1837–1843.

Werner, R. M., and R. T. Konetzka. 2010. Advancing nursing home quality through quality improvement itself. *Health Affairs (Millwood)* 29(1):81–86.

Werner, R. M., R. T. Konetzka, E. A. Stuart, and D. Polsky. 2011. Changes in patient sorting to nursing homes under public reporting: Improved patient matching or provider gaming? *Health Services Research* 46(2):555–571.

Werner, R. M., R. T. Konetzka, and M. M. Kim. 2013. Quality improvement under Nursing Home Compare: The association between changes in process and outcome measures. *Medical Care* 51(7):582–588.

White, E. M., C. M. Kosar, R. A. Feifer, C. Blackman, S. Gravenstein, J. Ouslander, and V. Mor. 2020a. Variation in SARS-CoV-2 prevalence in U.S. Skilled nursing facilities. *Journal of the American Geriatrics Society* 68(10):2167–2173.

White, E. M., L. H. Aiken, D. M. Sloane, and M. D. McHugh. 2020b. Nursing home work environment, care quality, registered nurse burnout and job dissatisfaction. *Geriatric Nursing* 41(2):158–164.

White, E. M., C. M. Kosar, M. Rahman, and V. Mor. 2020c. Trends in hospitals and skilled nursing facilities sharing medical providers, 2008–16. *Health Affairs* 39(8):1312–1320.

Williams, A., J. K. Straker, and R. Applebaum. 2016. The nursing home five star rating: How does it compare to resident and family views of care? *The Gerontologist* 56(2):234–242.

Williams, C. S., Q. Zheng, A. J. White, A. I. Bengtsson, E. T. Shulman, K. R. Herzer, and L. A. Fleisher. 2021. The association of nursing home quality ratings and spread of COVID-19. *Journal of the American Geriatrics Society* 69(8):2070–2078.

Xu, D., R. Kane, and G. Arling. 2019. Relationship between nursing home quality indicators and potentially preventable hospitalisation. *BMJ Quality and Safety* 28(7):524–533.

Zhou, C., A. Crawford, E. Serhal, P. Kurdyak, and S. Sockalingam. 2016. The impact of Project ECHO on participant and patient outcomes: A systematic review. *Academic Medicine* 91(10):1439–1461.

Zimmerman, D. R., S. L. Karon, G. Arling, B. R. Clark, T. Collins, R. Ross, and F. Sainfort. 1995. Development and testing of nursing home quality indicators. *Health Care Financing Review* 16(4):107–127.

Zinn, J. S., W. D. Spector, D. L. Weimer, and D. B. Mukamel. 2008. Strategic orientation and nursing home response to public reporting of quality measures: An application of the Miles and Snow typology. *Health Services Research* 43(2):598–615.

4

Care Delivery

Nursing homes play a critical role in the continuum of care within the U.S. health care system, providing essential services ranging from assistance with basic needs to care for people with complex medical conditions to end-of-life care. The intensity of the medical condition and the associated care needs are as varied as each individual nursing home resident and require a broad range of resources and skills among nursing home staff (Harrington et al., 2018; Zweig et al., 2011). As discussed in Chapter 5, a diverse workforce—physicians, physician assistants, nurses, nursing assistants, nurse practitioners, social workers, activity personnel, rehabilitation specialists, dietary staff, and others—delivers the wide range of care in the nursing home setting. While the committee recognizes that care delivery is inextricably linked to those who provide the care, this chapter focuses specifically on the types of care provided to nursing home residents. Chapter 5 details the characteristics of the nursing home workforce, including challenges related to staffing, training, and retention.

Care provided by nursing homes is among the most heavily regulated sectors of the U.S. health care system (Koren, 2010). To be certified—and thus be eligible for Medicare and Medicaid payments—nursing homes are required by federal regulations[1] to provide "the necessary care and services to attain or maintain the highest practicable physical, mental, and psychosocial well-being in accordance with the comprehensive assessment and plan of care,"[2] and to "promote each resident's quality of life."[3] The broad

---

[1] The Nursing Home Reform Act incorporated into the Omnibus Budget Reconciliation Act (OBRA) of 1987 contained a sweeping set of reforms aimed at improving the quality of care in nursing homes.
[2] CMS Requirements for Long-Term Care Facilities—Quality of Life, 42 CFR § 483.24 (2016).
[3] CMS Requirements for Long-Term Care Facilities—Admission, transfer, and discharge rights, 42 CFR § 483.15 (2016).

range of services that nursing homes are required by law to provide are shown in Box S-1 in the Summary chapter of this report.

To meet the extensive statutory requirements nursing homes must discover and address each resident's individualized needs.[4] As Koren observed more than a decade ago, the nursing home reform measures contained in the Omnibus Budget Reconciliation Act of 1987 (OBRA 87) made nursing homes "the only sector of the entire health care industry to have an explicit statutory requirement for what is now known as 'patient-centered care'" (Koren, 2010). The committee's conceptual model sees comprehensive, person-centered, equitable care as the central characteristic of high-quality care in the nursing home setting. Such person-centered care requires, at a minimum, knowledge of the range and types of needs of nursing home residents and an assessment and care planning model that identifies, prioritizes, and addresses those needs.

NEEDS-BASED CARE FOR NURSING HOME RESIDENTS

The committee's conceptual model (Chapter 1) specifies care that meets the individual needs of each resident as the central focus of nursing homes. It is useful, therefore, to identify and categorize the various needs of nursing home residents—both individually and collectively—and the ways that quality care should address those needs. The work of Abraham Maslow, who developed an overall model of human needs (Figure 4-1), provides one starting point for understanding those needs. Maslow's model includes a five-category hierarchy, with each higher level depending on first satisfying the needs in the levels below. The most basic level includes physiological needs such as food, water, and rest; the second level involves safety and security; the third encompasses social needs such as friendship and intimate relationships; the fourth level addresses self-esteem needs that support self-worth and a feeling of accomplishment; and the fifth level entails self-actualization and achieving one's full potential (Maslow, 1943, 1954).[5]

Maslow's hierarchy of needs has been applied multiple times in health care settings (Abraham, 2011; Bayoumi, 2012; Nydén et al., 2003; Zalenski and Raspa, 2006), and the field of nursing has found the model particularly useful in promoting culture change and developing patient care plans (Reitman, 2010). Maslow's hierarchy has also been used in hospice and palliative care to guide efforts to provide effective and meaningful care to

---

[4] CMS Requirements for Long-Term Care Facilities—Quality of Life, 42 CFR § 483.24 (2016).
[5] Maslow's hierarchy is a visual representation of a theory put forth by psychologist Abraham Maslow in his 1943 paper for *Psychological Review*, "A Theory of Human Motivation." Maslow's concepts were more fully developed in his 1954 book, *Motivation and Personality*.

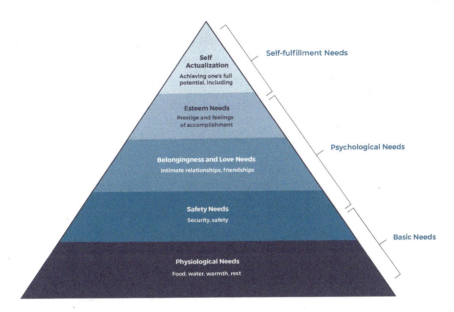

FIGURE 4-1 Maslow's hierarchy of needs.
SOURCE: Maslow, 1943; Maslow, 1954.

patients at the end of life (Zalenski and Raspa, 2006). Maslow's perspective provides an important conceptual framework for understanding the range of needs of nursing home residents and how comprehensive care can be delivered to meet those needs (Jackson et al., 2014).

Another lens with which to consider the range of needs of nursing home residents is provided by the Centers for Medicare & Medicaid Services (CMS) Resident Assessment Instrument (RAI)–Minimum Data Set (MDS). Introduced in the early 1990s as part of implementing OBRA 1987, the RAI–MDS is a standardized, needs-based resident assessment designed to inform care planning (Morris et al., 1990). CMS issued the most recent MDS 3.0 in 2010 (CMS, 2020b). All federally certified nursing homes are required to complete the full RAI–MDS upon an individual's admission to the nursing home and again on an annual basis. In addition, nursing homes must update a portion of the MDS quarterly and also after any significant change in the condition of a resident. Current needs-related domains covered by the MDS include basic functional activities (activities of daily living [ADLs] and continence), diagnosis-related medical care needs, symptoms (e.g., pain, shortness of breath), perception and communication (hearing, speech, vision), cognitive health and related assistance needs, nutrition (including swallowing/intake issues), and the maintenance of skin integrity.

Other MDS components are more treatment related and include medications, special treatments, procedures, and restraint use.[6]

A third perspective on identifying and categorizing the various needs of nursing home residents is provided by using quality-of-life measures applicable to nursing home residents. These measures include domains of quality such as physical comfort, functional competence, privacy, autonomy, dignity, meaningful activity, enjoyment, individuality, relationships, security and order, and spiritual well-being (Cutler and Kane, 2006; Travers et al., 2022).

Bringing these three frameworks together provides an overarching structure for understanding the full range of needs of nursing home residents as well as the types of care required to address those needs. The committee contends that planning and providing needs-based quality care in the nursing home setting should address, at minimum, the key elements outlined in the three frameworks (summarized in Table 4-1). The discussion in this chapter features all of the domains listed in Table 4-1, except safety and security. Key areas related to resident safety and security such as falls, medication management, resident abuse, and protecting the health and safety of residents and staff during a public emergency are all discussed in Chapter 6.

ASSESSING THE NEEDS OF NURSING HOME RESIDENTS

Federal regulation and advocacy efforts represent two of the more important factors that have pushed nursing home care delivery to meet residents' individualized needs. As noted above, federal regulations play a major role in shaping the delivery of nursing home care in the United States. Since first getting involved in nursing home care with the passage of the Social Security Act of 1935 (IOM, 1986), the federal government has revised its regulations and standards for nursing homes multiple times in response to studies and reports describing deficiencies in care (IOM, 1986, 2001). The most current regulations are codified in the 2016 update of the consolidated Medicare and Medicaid requirements for participation for long-term care facilities.[7]

Nursing home advocacy groups have also led efforts to improve nursing home care. In 1997, several of these organizations coalesced under the umbrella of the Pioneer Network, whose work led to what is known as the culture change movement. The culture change movement is a broad-based

---

[6] The current 45-page MDS 3.0 is available at https://www.cms.gov/Medicare/Quality-Initiatives-Patient-Assessment-Instruments/NursingHomeQualityInits/Downloads/Archive-Draft-of-the-MDS-30-Nursing-Home-Comprehensive-NC-Version-1140.pdf (accessed October 21, 2021).

[7] CMS Requirements for Long-Term Care Facilities—Quality of Life, 42 CFR Part 483, Subpart B (2016).

TABLE 4-1 The Needs of Nursing Home Residents

Domain*	Key Need Areas within Each Domain
Physiological Needs	Physical comfort; nutrition and hydration, warmth, sleep, personal hygiene (ADLs/continence); access to sunlight and fresh air; preservation of skin integrity; symptom management (e.g., pain, constipation, shortness of breath)
Safety and Security	Freedom from injury; provision of privacy; protection from development of and/or worsening of illness, including infection; security of personal possessions; freedom from noxious stimuli (e.g., noise, glare, odor); management of diagnosis-related medical issues and symptoms (including some aspects of rehabilitation); comfort with and sense of security regarding staff; certain aspects of support for mood and behavioral needs and expressions
Social	Companionship, affection, touch, family and other relationships, sense of inclusion, maximizing sensory perception and communication abilities, sexuality, support of cognitive needs
Self-Esteem	Functional competence, autonomy; dignity; self-expression; support for personal preferences, including customary routines, food and activity preferences, and engagement in activities that incur risk such as use of tobacco and alcohol; ability to initiate and engage in activities that are meaningful to the individual and that help maintain their identity; certain aspects of support for mood and behavioral needs and expressions
Achievement of Full Potential / Optimal Quality of Life	Enjoyment; participation in expressive/creative activities; maximization of physical, mental, and psychological function through ongoing opportunities, stimulation, and rehabilitation; absence or minimization of displeasure, anxiety, or boredom; opportunity for creation of legacies and life review; opportunity to express one's spirituality and participate in religious and spiritual practices.

SOURCE: Adapted from Bennett, 1980.
NOTE: * All domains are crucial to maximize quality of life; typically satisfying the first few areas listed in the table (physiological needs, safety, and security) is a prerequisite for satisfying the other areas (self-esteem and achievement of optimal quality of life).

effort to transform nursing homes from impersonal medical institutions into person-centered homes offering resident-directed long-term care services and supports, with the ultimate goal being the creation of vibrant communities of older adults and the people who care for and support them (Koren, 2010; Mitty, 2005; Pioneer Network, 2021; White-Chu et al., 2009). In order to achieve that goal, the culture change movement promotes a set of core principles (Box 4-1), many of which CMS has incorporated into its revised requirements for nursing homes requirements of participation.[8]

---

[8] For the full CMS Requirements of Participation, see https://www.cms.gov/Regulations-and-Guidance/Legislation/CFCsAndCoPs/LTC (accessed October 21, 2021).

> **BOX 4-1**
> **The Core Principles of Culture Change**
>
> - Holistic, resident-directed care
> - Home-like atmosphere
> - Close relationships among residents, family members, staff, and the community, including promoting consistent staff assignment to specific residents
> - Resident and staff (particularly certified nursing assistants) empowerment to become self-determining decision makers
> - Collaborative decision making among nursing home leadership and staff (flattening the hierarchy)
> - Integration of continuous quality improvement processes into care
>
> SOURCES: Koren, 2010; Mitty, 2005; Pioneer Network, 2021; White-Chu et al., 2009.

Early culture change efforts have included state-level efforts such as the development of the Promoting Excellent Alternatives in Kansas (PEAK) initiative that enabled the state to promote culture change through the survey process. State coalitions were formed in Arkansas and in other states such as Missouri, where a culture change coordinator was added to the survey agency to promote culture change adoption. These state-level efforts were incorporated into revisions of CMS's Interpretive Guidelines for nursing home surveyors, which featured a greater focus on resident choice and autonomy (Beck et al., 2014; Doll et al., 2017; Grabowski et al., 2014a,b).

One large-scale study evaluated the impact of culture change on the quality of care of nursing home residents. The study found that the adoption of culture change was associated with a nearly 15 percent decline in survey deficiencies related to health care. The researchers interpreted these results as indicating that culture change has the potential to improve nursing home resident care outcomes (Grabowski et al., 2014b). Importantly, research reveals that a nursing home's ability to implement culture change practices depends on the availability of financial and staff resources and that, as a result, nursing homes that are more heavily dependent on Medicaid financing may find it much more challenging to implement culture change practices (Miller et al., 2014; Shield et al., 2014). Such resource-limited nursing homes will likely require extra support, such as specialized training and assistance from experts from "high-performing nursing homes" (Chisholm et al., 2018).

A family member's perspective of culture change in the nursing home setting was provided to the committee during its first public webinar by Kathy Bradley, the founder and chief executive officer of Our Mother's Voice (see Box 4-2).

> **BOX 4-2**
> **Family Member Perspective**
>
> "[C]ulture change began to happen. For example, staff learned mama's nonverbal communication. . . . With this change, not just Mama's but everyone's quality of life improved. Another example: Mama went from having urinary tract infections and dehydration every 6 weeks to experiencing 2.5 years of good health. The facility implemented a hydration program, and everyone's health improved. So even at her late stage in dementia, a culture of person-centered care mattered to her. When culture change like this occurs, it's almost magic. Staff are happier, residents are happier, work is easier, and days are more enjoyable for everyone. Both staff and residents feel valued and empowered. Behavioral challenges decrease and the use of psychotropic and sedating medications decline. Quality of life improves."
>
> — **Kathy Bradley, Family Member and Founder, CEO, and Board President of Our Mother's Voice**
> *This quote was collected from the committee's public webinar on January 26, 2021.*

In addition to these various culture change initiatives, individual facilities and groups of facilities owned by the same organization or company have developed specific programs to deliver high-quality, resident-directed care in nursing home settings (Avila Institute, 2017; CAPC, 2008; Mead, 2013).[9]

Key Role of the Care Plan

The culture change movement counts resident-directed, person-centered care among its core tenets. In the nursing home setting, the care plan figures prominently in the provision of such care to residents. CMS requires that nursing homes develop and implement a comprehensive care plan for each person admitted to a nursing home either for post-acute care ("short-stay") or long-term care ("long-stay"). The care plan must be based on a comprehensive assessment, developed using the MDS, of the resident's goals and preferences, needs, and strengths. The comprehensive care plan is to include measurable goals and a timeframe in which the resident's physical and mental health and psychosocial needs are met. Framed by federal and state regulations and guided by culture change principles, these care plans

---

[9] An example of a culture change tool is the Artifacts of Culture Change 2.0. This is a recently updated self-assessment tool for nursing homes to determine the extent to which they have implemented culture change practices. For more information, see https://www.pioneernetwork.net/wp-content/uploads/2021/02/Artifacts_2.0_NH_Form_030521.pdf (accessed November 3, 2021).

are intended to address the residents' full range of needs and can shape the quality of care and the quality of life for nursing home residents (Dellefield et al., 2015; Lepore et al., 2018).

A care plan is integral to assessing a resident's individual needs, as discussed in the previous section of this chapter, and presents a plan to support each resident's care, interests, strengths, and preferences. Residents and family members are expected to be involved in the development of the care plan to ensure that accurate and complete information is included.[10] While the care planning process is focused on the individual resident, it is a shared effort in which the resident's chosen family members are viewed as "co-creators" of the resident's care plan (Chen et al., 2016; Scales et al., 2019). Ideally, the care plan should contain detailed documentation of "what matters" to the resident—defined as "knowing and aligning care with and older adult's health outcome goals and care preferences." Providing care that reflects "what matters" to the older adult is a key component of the age-friendly health system framework, and is compatible with—and facilitates—the provision of person-centered care (Adams-Wendling et al., 2008; Edelman et al., 2021; Koren, 2010). The comprehensive care plan is essential to ensure appropriate and adequate care delivery and improved resident health outcomes (Rantz et al., 2004). Health information technology, such as the use of an effective electronic health record, can play a key role in facilitating the nursing home resident care plan process, discussed in Chapter 9.

CMS 2016 regulatory updates require nursing homes to give residents the chance to become more directly engaged—or, as the revised regulation state, residents are to be the *locus of control*—in their own care planning. Residents work with nursing home staff to ensure that their goals and preferences are reflected in the plan and that, importantly, the plan is revised as the residents' needs and preferences change over time (Lepore et al., 2018).

In addition, the updated guidelines specify that an interdisciplinary team (detailed in Box 4-3) that includes the attending physician, a registered nurse with responsibility for the resident, a nursing assistant with responsibility for the resident, a member of the nutrition services staff, and others who would provide care to the resident must prepare, implement, review, and revise the care plan as appropriate.[11] In the case of services that the facility does not provide directly (e.g., laboratory, dialysis, dental, specialized behavioral health, pharmacy, hospice), the facility is responsible for managing those contracts and coordinating the associated services.[12] Specific roles and functions of the individual care team members are discussed further in Chapter 5.

---

[10] For more information, see https://theconsumervoice.org/uploads/files/issues/assessment_care_planning-final.pdf (accessed November 22, 2021).

[11] CMS Requirements for Long-Term Care Facilities—Comprehensive Person-Centered Care Planning, 42 CFR §483.21 (2016).

[12] Ibid.

> **BOX 4-3**
> **Nursing Home Interdisciplinary Care Teams**
>
> The 2016 nursing home regulations were the first significant revisions to federal nursing home regulations in nearly 25 years (discussed further in Chapter 8). As part of the revisions, CMS expanded the definition of the interdisciplinary care team in nursing homes to include, but not be limited to, the following[a]
>
> - Attending physician,
> - Registered nurse with responsibility for the resident,
> - Nurse aide with responsibility for the resident,
> - Member of food and nutrition services staff,
> - Resident and the resident's representative(s), and
> - Other appropriate staff or professionals in disciplines as determined by the resident's needs or as requested by the resident.
>
> Specifically, the 2016 regulations expanded the definition of the interdisciplinary care team to include certified nursing assistants and nurse aides, the dietary staff, and the resident and his or her representative(s). The interdisciplinary care team is responsible for conducting resident assessments to create and continually update comprehensive person-centered care plans for each resident.
>
> [a] CMS Requirements for Long-Term Care Facilities—Comprehensive Person-Centered Care Planning, 42 CFR §483.21 (2016).

The updated regulations specify that meetings of the interdisciplinary care team take place on a quarterly basis and include input from residents and their families. In addition, the care plan should be reviewed in the event of a significant change in a resident's status. These changes are detailed by CMS in the *Long-Term Care Resident Assessment Instrument User's Manual*.[13] The MDS assessment of residents' needs and the development and implementation of the care plan by the interdisciplinary care team are essential to providing high-quality, age-friendly care to nursing home residents (Edelman et al., 2021). Effective leadership at the RN level is critical to ensuring the accurate translation and integration of the care plan into nursing home operations (Dellefield, 2006; Forbes-Thompson et al., 2006). Taken as a whole, the updated care planning regulations help to advance nursing home care toward the goal of person-centered care (Lepore et al., 2018).

---

[13] See MDS 3.0 RAI Manual v1.17.1 Replacement Manual Pages and Change Tables, October 2019 (cms.gov).

Continuing to Improve Care Assessment and Planning

Given its central role in identifying residents' needs and developing an approach to address those needs, the resident care planning process is foundational to the provision of high-quality care in nursing homes. However, many nursing homes are not meeting care plan requirements. According to an analysis by the Department of Health and Human Services (HHS) Office of the Inspector General (OIG), the failure to develop comprehensive care plans represented the fifth most common nursing home deficiency type[14] cited by state survey agencies over the period 2013 to 2017. Such care plan deficiencies represented slightly less than 10 percent of the total top 10 deficiencies over that time period (OIG, 2019). Previous OIG inspections found that for more than one-quarter of resident stays, the nursing home did not develop care plans that met federal requirements (OIG, 2013).

In general, the care assessment and planning process has weaknesses in three key areas that warrant improvement. First, care plans often focus on basic physiologic, safety, and security needs, such as nutrition, personal hygiene, skin integrity, falls, and infection. While meeting these needs is important and contributes to quality of life, an overemphasis on those needs can detract from addressing equally critical social, self-esteem, and quality-of-life needs (Calkins and Brush, 2016). For example, nursing homes rarely address the need for affection and physical connection, including sexual needs (Roelofs et al., 2015), and even when they do, their focus is generally on the safety and protection of vulnerable persons.

Second, opportunities to engage in creative expression are limited, as are meaning-making activities such as reminiscence therapy, which involves the use of photographs or music to evoke memories or generate conversation (Woods et al., 2018), or dignity therapy, which is an approach to help patients as they face the end of life (Cuevas et al., 2021) by focusing on psychosocial or existential distress (Allen et al., 2014; Goddard et al., 2013; Hall et al., 2013). In addition residents may also have limited volunteer opportunities that can promote social interaction and self-esteem. Finally, addressing needs for spiritual and existential care in nursing homes is uneven and limited despite the importance of these concerns for many nursing home residents (Morley and Sanford, 2014).

Other challenges involve residents' rights related to choice and autonomy. Personal choice and autonomy are key components of self-esteem (see Table 4-1). The resident's right to self-determination was enacted into law as part of the Nursing Home Reform Law of 1987,[15] and as noted earlier,

---

[14] A nursing home's failure to meet a federal participation requirement is defined as a deficiency. Examples of deficiencies include a nursing home's failure to adhere to proper infection control measures and to provide necessary care and services (OIG, 2019).

[15] Nursing Home Reform Law of 1987, Public Law 100-203, 42 USC 1395i-3, 100th Cong., 1st Sess., (December 22, 1987).

updated CMS guidance reinforces and strengthens the rights of residents to exercise maximal choice and autonomy (Beck et al., 2014; Doll et al., 2017; Grabowski et al., 2014a). Despite the significant positive associations among residents' choice, sense of autonomy, and quality of life (Bhattacharyya et al., 2021; McCabe et al., 2021), residents often report limited choice and autonomy (Moilanen et al., 2021). Furthermore, observational studies of staff interactions with residents reveal that resident daily choices such as food, ambulation, and socializing often are curtailed, sometimes without staff awareness of the restrictions they impose (Bhattacharyya et al., 2021). Reasons for these limitations are multifactorial and include staff concerns about causing harm to residents; staff knowledge, attitudes, and habits; lack of time to offer choices; and fear of survey deficiencies, complaints, and legal action (Bekkema et al., 2021; Calkins and Brush, 2016).

Respecting resident autonomy is particularly challenging in situations where preferences clash with best clinical practices, safety, and the rights of other residents (Calkins and Brush, 2016; Sherwin and Winsby, 2011). These potential conflicts can be as seemingly mundane as keeping the volume on the TV too high because of hearing loss, thereby disturbing one's roommate or others in nearby rooms. These potential conflicts can, however, include more serious issues such as a resident's refusal to be vaccinated against the COVID-19 virus, for example, which could put other residents, staff, and families at risk. Another common dilemma is the resident's desire to ambulate independently, which may increase the chance of falling. A recent, poignant example is the imposition of visitation restrictions during the COVID-19 pandemic; residents' rights and need to socialize were severely curtailed to limit the spread of infection. Very often, mitigating risk is prioritized over residents' autonomy in nursing homes.

Efforts to address these issues have focused on using structured, shared decision-making approaches to balance autonomy and risk, although the nursing home sector has not adopted these approaches widely (Behrens et al., 2018; Calkins and Brush, 2016). Making progress toward honoring residents' choices will likely also require a recalibration and re-interpretation of quality indicators such as fall rates (Brauner et al., 2018; Davila et al., 2021).

Identifying and Addressing Unmet Needs

Unmet health care needs can be viewed as the gap between the care and services necessary to address a specific health issue or condition and the actual care that an individual receives (Herr et al., 2014). Research examining unmet needs from the perspective of nursing home residents is relatively rare; what is available focuses on the absence of care itself and on clinical outcomes that can result from inadequate care. Among the health outcomes most often attributed to inadequate care in nursing homes are avoidable hospitalizations, pressure ulcers, falls, infections, pain, malnutrition, and a higher risk of mortality and lower quality of life (Kalánková et al., 2020; Ogletree et al., 2020). Studies conducted in nursing homes in the United States and Europe indicate that the unmet needs that nursing home residents identify most commonly include timely assistance with ADLs (including mobility), meaningful daytime activities, sensory (vision, hearing) and communication issues, and accommodation for disabilities (Freedman and Spillman, 2014; Tobis et al., 2018; van den Brink et al., 2018). These unmet needs reflect a neglect of physical care, which is a serious ethical and clinical violation (Kalánková et al., 2020). Psychosocial needs (e.g., companionship, relief from distress) are ranked highly in most studies of unmet needs among nursing home residents, with residents having suffered even greater neglect with lockdowns and isolation during the COVID-19 pandemic (Kemp, 2021; Ruopp, 2020; Simard and Volicer, 2020). Addressing unmet needs is critical to residents' well-being and quality of life.

Residents with higher levels of disability tend to identify both more reported needs and more unmet needs. In contrast, persons with cognitive impairment report fewer needs and fewer unmet needs, which is not surprising since an awareness of need and the ability to communicate need verbally can be impaired in these individuals (Duan et al., 2020; van den Brink et al., 2018). There are two caveats to these findings; first, nursing home residents may hesitate to speak up when asked by staff about unmet needs, and second, persons in settings with fewer resources may identify fewer unmet needs, believing that expressing these needs is futile. As a result, it is important to include perspectives and sources beyond residents to identify gaps in care and unmet needs (Duan et al., 2020).

Certain subpopulations of nursing home residents appear to have particularly high levels of unmet needs. The key characteristics of these subpopulations include racial or ethnic minorities, individuals who lack fluency in English, individuals with moderate or advanced cognitive impairment, and those with aphasia or other communication challenges (Berridge and Mor, 2018; Cooper et al., 2018; Kalánková et al., 2020). In addition, certain facility factors appear to be associated with higher levels of unmet needs, including a large share of residents being on Medicaid; higher resident-to-staff ratios; poor-quality nursing leadership or high leadership turnover, or both; and high proportions of contracted staff relative to employed staff (Castle and Engberg, 2007; Mor et al., 2004). (See Chapter 5 for more discussion on issues related to employed and contracted nursing home staff.)

Subpopulations that may have high levels of unmet needs include residents who do not speak English and are in nursing homes that do not have staff members who speak their native language or English-speaking residents in homes where staff have limited English proficiency. Addressing language

> **BOX 4-4**
> **Family Member Perspective**
>
> "[T]he wait times for staff to respond to help (my mother) to the restroom or with other needs were so long that she had to hire additional caregivers in addition to the exorbitant cost of the residence. (She once timed an 80-minute wait.) Family members also had to take a lot of time off work just to be sure she was taken care of. Most people cannot afford that and just suffer through it."
>
> — Anonymous, Berkeley, California
>
> *This quote was collected from the committee's online call for resident, family, and nursing home staff perspectives.*

barriers between residents and staff takes on greater importance as residents' diversity increases, as discussed in Chapter 2. Language barriers and associated miscommunication can negatively impact health outcomes and lead to lower patient and staff satisfaction and care that is not aligned with an individual's preferences (Al Shamsi et al., 2020; Forsgren et al., 2016). Nursing homes are required by law to communicate medical information to residents in their native language.[16] A range of approaches can be used to address language barriers in health care settings, including professional interpreters (which increases costs), family members or friends as interpreters, or online translation tools (Al Shamsi et al., 2020).[17]

Despite the best intentions and efforts on the part of nursing home staff, however, some unmet needs will always exist. For example, some things that residents may want are either too detrimental to their well-being, such as smoking, refusing medications, or not bathing, or pose a risk to others in a congregate setting. Furthermore, nursing home staff will always have more things that they *could* be doing for residents than are possible, considering the realities of not being able to provide one-on-one care and not having all possible skills and techniques available in all nursing homes at all times. A key role of members of the nursing home leadership team is to help identify and prioritize the care needs of each individual resident. Box 4-4 provides a family member's perspective on identifying and addressing unmet needs.

---

[16] CMS Requirements for Long-Term Care Facilities—Resident Rights, 42 CFR § 483.10 (c)(1) (2016).

[17] One example is SEIU 1199's Training and Employment Fund's English for Speakers of Other Languages program (see: https://www.1199seiubenefits.org/esol) (accessed April 22, 2022).

PROVIDING CARE TO ADDRESS RESIDENTS' NEEDS

As discussed in the previous section of this chapter, the care plan documents the needs and preferences of each individual nursing home resident and serves to guide the provision of necessary health care services. The wide range of services to address the varied needs of nursing home residents are discussed in the sections that follow, organized according to Maslow's hierarchy of needs.

Physiological Care

This section examines the first level of Maslow's hierarchy—basic needs—exploring the ways in which nursing homes provide for the varied physiological care needs of nursing home residents. Nursing homes provide care to two different groups of people who have distinct physiological care needs: short-stay individuals who require post-acute care after a hospital stay of at least 3 days,[18] and long-stay residents who have a more diverse range of care needs. The broad diversity of clinical needs of nursing home patients combined with their vulnerability to adverse outcomes complicates the challenge of providing quality care in the nursing home setting (Yurkofsky and Ouslander, 2021).

Nursing homes serve as a place for recuperation that provides post-hospitalization therapies and supports. Twenty percent of all hospitalized Medicare beneficiaries are discharged to skilled nursing facilities for post-acute care (MedPAC, 2021). These short-stay patients receive physical, occupational, and speech therapy as required to make the gains in function necessary to be discharged from the nursing home (Yurkofsky and Ouslander, 2021).

As discussed further in Chapter 7, a new reimbursement method known as the patient-driven payment model (PDPM) took effect in late 2019, replacing the previous system based on resource utilization groups. The PDPM approach to payment, which is based on the complexity of patient care rather than minutes of therapy provided, has resulted in a decrease in the volume of therapy services provided in nursing homes (McGarry et al., 2021).

Long-stay residents tend to need assistance with ADLs, and to have high rates of medically complex conditions that often require multiple medications and skilled nursing care (Fashaw et al., 2020; Katz et al., 2021). The most common of the complex conditions faced by nursing home residents include Alzheimer's and related dementias (47.8 percent of residents), diabetes (32 percent), heart disease (38.1 percent), and hypertension (71.5 percent) (Harris-Kojetin et al., 2019).

---

[18] The medically necessary inpatient hospital stay of 3 consecutive days or more (CMS, 2019a) requirement was waived during the COVID-19 pandemic (CMS, 2021a).

Assistance with ADLs

Many nursing home residents require assistance with routine but essential ADLs such as eating, bathing, and mobility (Table 4-2). A person's ability to accomplish these activities independently determines his or her functional status and serves as a predictor of nursing home admission (Edemekong et al., 2021). Federal regulations require that nursing homes maintain the resident's condition or prevent or slow further deterioration of a resident's ability to perform these activities (CMS, 2019b) and that they provide the necessary services to enable residents to maintain good nutrition, grooming, and personal oral hygiene if they need assistance with those tasks. As noted in Chapter 2, most residents require assistance with one or more ADLs (Harris-Kojetin et al., 2019).

Ambulating Nursing home residents face ambulatory challenges ranging from difficulty walking to an inability to get out of bed by oneself. Nearly two-thirds of nursing home residents depend on a wheelchair or require extensive support from others to move around. According to data available from CMS,[19] an average of 3.7 percent of nursing home residents in 2016 were either in a bed or a recliner for 22 or more hours per day. More than one-fifth of nursing home residents suffered from contractures, which are limitations on the full range of motion of any joint resulting from deformity, lack of use, or pain (Harrington et al., 2018).

TABLE 4-2 Activities of Daily Living (ADLs)

ADL Category	Description
Ambulating	The extent of an individual's ability to move from one position to another and walk independently.
Feeding	The ability of a person to feed oneself.
Dressing	The ability to select appropriate clothes and to put the clothes on.
Personal hygiene	The ability to bathe and groom oneself and to maintain dental hygiene, nail and hair care.
Continence	The ability to control bladder and bowel function.
Toileting	The ability to get to and from the toilet, using it appropriately and cleaning oneself.

SOURCE: Edemekong et al., 2021.

---

[19] CMS has a national database of all data elements collected by state survey agencies during the annual Medicare and Medicaid certification inspection. The Online Survey, Certification and Reporting System (OSCAR) and the Certification and Survey Provider Enhanced Reporting (CASPER) system capture state-level nursing home information on characteristics of nursing home facilities, residents, staffing, and deficiencies.

Pressure injury A lack of mobility presents a danger to nursing home residents as it can result in pressure injuries (previously referred to as pressure ulcers and informally known as bedsores), localized damage to the skin and/or underlying tissue that results from pressure, friction, or a lack of proper blood flow when an individual remains in bed or in one position for long periods of time (Bhattacharya and Mishra, 2015; Mäki-Turja-Rostedt et al., 2018). Pressure injuries cause pain and create a vicious cycle in which the pain leads to reduced mobility, which leads to more pressure injuries and even more pain, and so on; at the same time, the reduced mobility and pressure injuries also heighten the resident's risk for infection and mortality. Both short- and long-term nursing home residents are at risk for pressure injuries due to factors such as a lack of mobility after surgery, cognitive impairment, incontinence, hip fracture, and strokes (Harrington et al., 2018). Other factors that increase the risk for pressure injuries include more severe illnesses upon admission, history of recent pressure injuries, nutritional challenges, and use of positioning equipment or catheters (Horn et al., 2004, 2010). Pressure injuries are considered among the most common medical errors across inpatient and outpatient settings in the United States (Van Den Bos et al., 2011).

Pressure injury is an important indicator of quality in the nursing home setting. More than 8 percent of active nursing home residents[20] had one or more unhealed pressure ulcers as of Q2 in 2021 according to MDS 3.0 frequency reports (CMS, 2021b). More than 75 percent of residents received special skin care to prevent or reduce such injuries (Harrington et al., 2018). Nursing homes are required to document all interventions to address pressure injury, including the use of devices to relieve pressure, protocols related to positioning and turning, and any wound treatments. Nursing home care team members have a key role to play in the identification of risk factors for pressure injury and in bringing in physical and occupational therapists, dieticians, and wound care specialists to implement care interventions (Yurkofsky and Ouslander, 2021). Specifically, research indicates that higher RN staffing hours per resident and higher nurse aide staffing hours per resident (certified nursing assistants or licensed practical nurses) were associated with fewer pressure ulcers (Castle and Anderson, 2011; Horn et al., 2004, 2005).

Nutrition and hydration CMS regulations require nursing homes to provide each resident with adequate food and liquids to maintain proper nutrition and hydration. Ensuring that each individual resident's eating needs are met

---

[20] "An active resident is a resident whose most recent assessment transaction is not a discharge and whose most recent transaction has a target date (assessment reference date for an assessment record or entry date for an entry record) less than 150 days old" (CMS, 2021b).

is challenging in the nursing home setting, given the large share of residents with eating difficulties and the variation in residents' degrees of dependency, preferences, and routines (Liu et al., 2014).

Dehydration In addition to nutritional challenges, nursing home residents are particularly vulnerable to dehydration because of age-related physiological changes, such as deteriorating kidney function, a reduced ability to sense thirst, and reduced muscle mass (which limits the amount of water that is typically stored in muscles). The risk of dehydration is especially acute for nursing home residents with cognitive impairments that make it difficult for them to communicate that they are thirsty, with conditions that reduce appetite and fluid intake, or with physical impairments that prevent them from obtaining sufficient fluids. Certain medications such as diuretics also increase the risk of dehydration. Interventions including offering fluids to residents on a regular basis have resulted in a lower prevalence of dehydration in nursing homes (Greene et al., 2019; Yurkofsky and Ouslander, 2021).

Weight loss The MDS quarterly reassessment process includes assessing for weight loss, which CMS views as a quality indicator for nursing home care. Cases in which a resident's weight changes 5 percent over a 30-day period or 10 percent over a 6-month period require nursing homes to review care plans. Research shows that an unintentional weight loss of 5 percent is associated with a significantly increased risk of mortality (Sullivan et al., 2004; Yurkofsky and Ouslander, 2021). Approximately 6 percent of active nursing home residents had weight loss (not physician prescribed) as of Q2 in 2021 according to MDS 3.0 frequency reports (CMS, 2021b).

Many nursing home residents face difficulties maintaining adequate nutrition and hydration. This is particularly true for individuals admitted to nursing homes after a hospital stay, where they may have been designated "nothing by mouth" or have been on a restricted diet, either because of surgery or the need to conduct imaging studies. Another factor is the difficulty of aligning food offerings in institutional settings such as nursing homes with each resident's individual preferences. Conditions such as gastrointestinal disorders, delirium, and pain can affect a resident's nutritional status and ability to maintain weight, as can a terminal illness, depression, medication side effects, and a chronic illness that affects appetite, chewing, swallowing, or digesting (Ahmed and Haboubi, 2010; Pilgrim et al., 2015; Wells and Dumbrell, 2006). Weight loss and reduced food intake commonly occur as people near the end of life (Agarwal, 2021; Pilgrim et al., 2015).

The multiple conditions and complex care regimens of nursing home residents make the clinical management of nutritional needs extremely challenging for those providing care for nursing home residents (Liu et al., 2014; Palese et al., 2018). Research has identified a number of factors that are critical to ensuring adequate nutritional care in the nursing home setting, including assessing the barriers to adequate nutrition; reducing risk factors; attending to specialized diets, altering food presentation, providing supplements when appropriate; being aware of the importance of psychosocial and environmental issues; and considering the role of medication both as a cause and therapeutic adjunct (Sloane et al., 2008). Given that a key issue for many nursing home residents is adequate nutritional intake, groups such as the American Diabetes Association have recommended minimizing the use of restrictive diets (Munshi et al., 2016).

Other nutritional and weight loss–related interventions in the nursing home setting include involving speech and occupational therapists and behavioral health clinicians to address the factors driving weight loss, which can range from the problems listed above to ill-fitting dentures. For example, for residents who have difficulty handling utensils as a result of reduced dexterity resulting from stroke, arthritis, or a fracture, nursing homes can provide special utensils with easier-to-grasp handles, while speech and occupational therapists can target difficulties swallowing. Moreover, registered dieticians can conduct nutritional assessments and specify dietary options, including providing nutritional supplements for residents facing weight loss (Yurkofsky and Ouslander, 2021).

Meeting residents' nutritional needs Meeting nursing home residents' nutritional needs often requires the provision of feeding assistance to those who cannot feed themselves (Batchelor-Murphy et al., 2019; Kilgore, 2014; Yurkofsky and Ouslander, 2021). Federal regulations mandate that each residents' nutritional needs and related care preferences be met with sufficient staff, including a qualified dietitian or other clinically qualified nutrition professional and support staff, which may also include feeding assistants.[21] Studies have found, however, that many nursing homes do not have sufficient staff to meet resident needs (Simmons and Bertrand, 2013; Simmons and Schnelle, 2004, 2006; Simmons et al., 2008). Weight loss and dehydration have been found to be associated with inadequate nursing care and lack of assistance with eating and drinking (Simmons and Schnelle, 2004, 2006; Simmons et al., 2008).

Nutritional challenges were further complicated by the COVID-19 pandemic, which disrupted communal dining and exacerbated existing staff shortages. Moreover, poor nutrition was found to increase older adults' risk of contracting COVID-19 as well as other chronic conditions (Keser et al., 2021).

---

[21] CMS Requirements for Long-Term Care Facilities—Food and nutrition services, 42 CFR § 483.60 (2016).

Continence and toileting The most common needs of nursing home residents are related to bladder or bowel incontinence. One study found that nearly 65 percent of residents had bladder incontinence and nearly 45 percent had bowel continence in 2016 (Harrington et al., 2018). Bladder or urinary incontinence is associated with increased risks of hospitalization, urinary tract infections, and pressure injuries, and it has a significant effect on quality of life. CMS uses the development of urinary incontinence as a quality indicator for long-term nursing home residents (Dubeau et al., 2006; Yurkofsky and Ouslander, 2021), and at least one analysis found associations between urinary incontinence and poorer self-reported quality of life in the domains of dignity, autonomy, and mood (Xu and Kane, 2013).

Interventions include developing toileting schedules and prompted voiding, which both require staff assistance to review the care plan and schedule, and also conducting regular check-ins with residents on their continence needs and abilities. Other interventions include exercises to improve mobility and control, dietary interventions such as increasing fluid and fiber intake, and supplementary interventions such as using laxatives or stool softeners (Leung and Schnelle, 2008). Regular review of all interventions is particularly important to maintain residents' safety (e.g., preventing from falls) and dignity, as continence care often goes beyond social norms of privacy and touch (Ostaszkiewicz et al., 2020). One study found that using an improved assessment tool reduced the rate of incontinence among nursing home residents without a toileting plan from 79 to 38 percent (Morgan et al., 2008). Use of clinical guidelines, standardized assessments, and regulatory enforcement as well as leveraging organizational culture change practices have been identified as ways to enable nursing homes to meet residents' continence and toileting needs (Lyons, 2010).

Post-Acute and Rehabilitation Care

Nursing homes provide rehabilitation services for two different groups of individuals—short-stay patients and long-term nursing home residents, with each having different care and rehabilitation needs. Approximately 1.5 million Medicare fee-for-service beneficiaries received such services in the nursing home setting in 2019 (MedPAC, 2021).

Short-stay patients Some patients require intensive rehabilitation services after surgery, an illness, or injury (MedPAC, 2020). Most nursing homes provide post-acute care, recuperation, and rehabilitation services, such as the continuation of intravenous antibiotics or a course of physical, occupational, or speech therapy. Nearly one-third of nursing home admissions in 2016 involved post-acute or rehabilitation services (Harrington et al., 2018). Medicare covers post-acute care in nursing home facilities, and ensures skilled services are covered to maintain a resident's condition or prevent or slow a decline or deterioration of the resident's condition (CMS, 2021c). Post-acute care in a skilled nursing facility is designed to be short term, a "bridge to home" (Flint et al., 2019).

Patients are most commonly referred to nursing homes for post-acute care for septicemia (sepsis), joint replacement, heart failure and shock, hip and femur procedures, and pneumonia (MedPAC, 2020). These patients are expected to make gains in function from continuing medical therapy and rehabilitation services, most often a combination of physical therapy focused on mobility (including wheelchair mobility), occupational therapy focused on self-care issues such as dressing and feeding, and speech therapy focused on eating, swallowing, and communication problems (Yurkofsky and Ouslander, 2021).

Rehabilitation care can either be active, involving the resident engaging in physical exercise, for example, or passive, involving the use of ultrasound or whole-body vibration. Rehabilitation care in the nursing home setting can be provided by a nurse, physiotherapist, kinesiologist, rehabilitation aide, or fitness instructor in a small group (up to six people) or on an individual basis (McArthur et al., 2015). As noted above, the new PDPM payment system has reduced the amount of therapy provided to nursing home residents.

In an effort to monitor the quality of rehabilitation care provided in the nursing home setting, CMS added new quality measures for short-stay patients to Nursing Home Compare in 2016. Previous star ratings did not distinguish between the quality of care for short-stay and for long-stay nursing home residents. The ratings for the quality of care for short-stay rehabilitation services include measures related to emergency room visits and rehospitalizations, control of pain and treatment of pressure injuries, and independent movement as an element of recovery (Graham, 2019). The new measures are important indicators of nursing home quality. Whereas discharge from nursing homes to the community after a short-term stay has been identified as a critical sign of person-centered care, rehospitalizations and transfers from nursing homes to emergency departments are viewed as potential signs of inappropriate or inadequate nursing home care that leave residents vulnerable to adverse health events while in the hospital. By providing additional information, these new measures enhance the nursing home five-star composite ranking. An early analysis of the measures revealed an association between improved performance on the new measures and nursing home characteristics such as fewer deficiencies, higher staffing and more skilled staffing, nonprofit ownership, and lower proportion of Medicaid residents. The study's authors emphasized the importance of better understanding of these measures, in light of CMS's plans to include the measure on rehospitalizations in the value-based purchasing program for nursing homes, discussed further in Chapter 7 (Saliba et al., 2018).

Long-stay patients Although the goal for short-term post-acute care patients is to regain functional independence, for long-term residents, the goal is to maintain functional abilities to maintain the best quality of life (Graham, 2019). A wide range of physical rehabilitation services are available in the nursing home setting to help residents maintain mobility, strength, and balance, or focus on a specific ADL.

In 2011, patient advocates filed a lawsuit, *Jimmo v. Sebelius*, arguing that Medicare was denying coverage for therapy based on a patient's lack of improvement or progress. The *Jimmo* settlement agreement specified that coverage of therapy services is not determined by the "presence or absence of a beneficiary's potential for improvement or restoration, but rather on the beneficiary's need for skilled care." The agreement clarified that rehabilitative care may be necessary to improve or maintain an individual's current condition or to prevent further deterioration. The agreement also provided that the Medicare benefit policy manual must include these clarifications (CMS, 2019b, 2021b).

Restorative Care for Long-Stay Residents

Nursing homes also provide restorative care programs to respond to the federal regulations to provide each resident with the "necessary care and services to attain or maintain the highest level of physical, mental, and psychosocial well-being in accordance with the comprehensive assessment and plan of care."[22]

Restorative care can be defined as an approach to care that focuses on evaluating residents' functional capabilities in areas such as walking, range of motion, bed mobility, dressing, eating, swallowing, and communicating. Restorative care reimbursed by Medicare is typically provided to residents who need to maintain functional gains after completing physical, occupational, or speech therapy, or for residents who experience a decrease in function. One study found that although 66 percent of nursing homes provided restorative care programs, less than one-third of long-stay nursing home residents participated in such programs. The study recommended considering implementing restorative care programs as a "philosophy of integrated care" rather than as discrete activities. Proponents of this approach emphasize the importance of training all nursing home staff to integrate activities that promote function and physical activity into all resident interactions (Talley et al., 2015).

---

[22] CMS Requirements for Long-Term Care Facilities—Quality of Care, 42 CFR § 483.25 (2016).

Pain and Symptom Management

Given that a significant share of nursing home residents have multiple chronic conditions, the management of pain and symptoms is a critical element of care that nursing homes deliver to their residents. Many nursing home residents experience pain, and the appropriate management of pain is critical to their quality of life. Studies that revealed extensive undertreatment or lack of treatment of pain in nursing homes led CMS to enact policy changes that included strengthening nursing home guidance on pain for surveyors in 2009 as well as enhanced measures of pain in MDS 3.0 (Yurkofsky and Ouslander, 2021).

A large share of all nursing home residents—up to 80 percent—experience persistent pain, such as that related to arthritis (Hunnicutt et al., 2017a; Nakashima et al., 2019). Others experience acute pain caused by a new medical or surgical condition, including post-operative pain. Finally, pain at the end of life is common among nursing home residents (Andersson et al., 2018; Teno et al., 2018). The provision of palliative care and hospice care in the nursing home setting is discussed in greater detail later in this chapter.

A study of more than 1.3 million long-stay nursing home residents from 2011 to 2012 found that nearly 39 percent experienced at least some pain and that nearly 20 percent had persistent pain. Of the residents with persistent pain, 6.4 percent received no pharmacologic pain management, and more than 30 percent were undertreated (received no scheduled analgesics for their pain). The study also revealed race and ethnicity disparities as higher rates of untreated and undertreated pain as non-Hispanic Black, Hispanic, and other race/ethnicity residents had higher rates of untreated and undertreated pain compared to White residents. The study concluded that although the prevalence of untreated pain had declined since the enactment of the policy changes and enhanced guidance referred to above, the overall prevalence of pain among nursing home residents is still high. The study called for further research on promoting equity in pain management as well improving overall pain management practices in nursing homes (Hunnicutt et al., 2017b).

Another study examined nursing home residents who required staff to assess their pain because of their inability to do so themselves. The study found that staff documented pain and its treatment less frequently in non-Hispanic Black residents and Hispanic residents than in non-Hispanic White residents. Researchers called for further study to further elucidate differential pain expression, explicit bias, and implicit bias. An enhanced understanding of these factors will enable the design of specific interventions to lessen existing disparities in pain management and treatment (Morrison et al., 2021).The awareness of factors related to differential expression of pain is particularly important in providing care for nursing home residents with dementia. Research indicates that 60 to 80 percent of nursing home residents with dementia experience pain on a regular basis (Corbett et al., 2012). It is challenging, however, to effectively assess and manage pain in residents with dementia given difficulty these residents typically have communicating about their pain to nursing home staff. As a result, residents with dementia often express pain through behavioral symptoms, such as agitation or wandering, which can then lead to mismanagement of pain (Achterberg et al., 2019). Improved understanding of the factors associated with differential expression of pain among nursing home residents will facilitate the development of specific interventions to lessen existing disparities in pain management and treatment (Morrison et al., 2021).

Oral Health Care

Oral health has a significant effect on an individual's physiological and social well-being. Poor oral health is associated with pain, reduced function, malnutrition, and a range of medical conditions including cardiovascular disease, pulmonary health issues, and aspirational pneumonia. In addition, research has identified associations between diabetes and periodontal disease, tooth loss, and oral cancer as well as an increased risk of cognitive impairment and dementia with gingivitis, dental caries, or tooth loss (Porter et al., 2015; Sifuentes and LaPane, 2020; Zimmerman et al., 2017). Moreover, symptoms related to poor oral health care, such as bad breath and altered speech, can affect self-esteem and quality of life (Hoben et al., 2016; Maramaldi et al., 2018). Key risk factors for poor oral health among nursing home residents include having Alzheimer's or other forms of dementia, receiving hospice care, and having a longer length of stay (Zimmerman et al., 2017).

Because of the critical role that oral health plays in overall health, federal regulations require nursing homes to provide services that enable residents to maintain good oral hygiene.[23] Specifically, regulations require nursing homes to

- Conduct an oral health assessment of each resident upon admission and quarterly and annually thereafter and record the information in the MDS;
- Meet residents' routine and emergency dental service needs using outside services;
- Make appointments for residents requesting dental care and arrange for transportation;

---

[23] CMS Requirements for Long-Term Care Facilities—Resident Assessment, 42 CFR § 483.20 (2016).

- Apply for dental service reimbursement; and
- Refer residents with lost or damaged dentures within 3 days.

Nonetheless, fewer than one in five nursing home residents receive daily assistance with oral health care, such as tooth brushing. Moreover, only 15 percent have very good or better oral hygiene (Coleman and Watson, 2006; Sifuentes and Lapane, 2020; Zimmerman et al., 2017).

One reason for this deficiency may be that the responsibility for conducting an oral health assessment typically falls on certified nursing assistants (CNAs), many of whom lack specific oral health training (Sifuentes and Lapane, 2020). Another reason may be that while nursing homes are required to conduct oral health assessments, they are not required to provide *routine* dental services for all residents. Medicaid is the primary payer for the large majority of long-stay nursing home residents; consequently nursing homes provide routine dental services only if the Medicaid plan of the particular state in which the nursing home is located covers such routine dental services. Given the high cost of dental health care services, Medicaid beneficiaries are typically unable to afford to pay out of pocket for such care. Compounding the problem is that many states have responded to fiscal pressures by trimming or eliminating Medicaid dental coverage. Additionally, even in states with Medicaid dental coverage, beneficiaries often face great difficulty locating dental providers who accept Medicaid, given that only 20 percent of all dentists participate in the Medicaid program (Northridge et al., 2020).

Providing oral health care in the nursing home setting Assistance with daily oral health care for nursing home residents is typically the responsibility of the CNAs, who do not receive necessary training to provide oral health care assistance and typically face significant competing demands on their time. Additional challenges include staff perceptions that oral health care is not a priority, staff hesitancy or unwillingness to perform the tasks, and resident resistance to staff assistance with their oral care. Further complicating the delivering of oral health care services to nursing home residents is the increasing prevalence among current nursing home residents of dental prostheses and bridges that require complex care to maintain. As noted earlier, a large share of nursing home residents have some form of dementia and typically require assistance with basic oral care, while at the same time often making it challenging to staff to provide such care. As a result, oral care practices in nursing homes tend to be of poor quality, characterized by insufficient or improper tooth brushing. For example, one study (Coleman and Watson, 2006) revealed that, on average, CNAs brush residents' teeth for 16 seconds, a significantly shorter timespan than the American Dental Association's recommended 2 minutes of brushing (Hoben et al., 2016; Porter et al., 2015; Sloane et al., 2013; Zimmerman et al., 2020).

Another important element of high-quality daily oral care is providing and using appropriate supplies. Toothbrushes should have soft bristles, be replaced every 3 months, and be stored in a manner that allows them to dry and that prevents infection. For individuals who have difficulty swallowing, toothpaste can cause choking, so for many residents an alcohol-free rinse is preferable. Cleaning between the teeth can be done safely with an interdental brush, which also should be changed every 3 months. Given the importance of infection control, steps such as hand washing, the use of gloves and mask by the care provider, and using an antimicrobial rinse with alcohol for cleaning toothbrushes and interdental brushes are critical (Sloane et al., 2013).

Innovative approach to improving oral health care Given the importance of good oral health care to overall health outcomes and quality of life, and the high level of unmet need, researchers have developed some promising practices to improve the oral health care of nursing home residents. Interventions have included developing comprehensive oral health training programs for CNAs and other nursing home staff members, and the identification of a staff member as the oral health specialist (VanArsdall and Aalboe, 2016).

One evidence-based, person-centered care approach, Mouth Care Without a Battle (MCWB), trains nursing home staff to provide oral health care to residents with dementia who typically resist assistance with oral health care. Nursing homes that participated in a MCWB staff training program reduced the incidence of pneumonia in their facilities by 26 to 31 percent during the first year of the program, though that effect faded in the second year of the intervention. Sustaining the benefits of this approach may require the support of dedicated oral care aides to ensure that the nursing home staff continues to follow best practices (Zimmerman et al., 2020).

Among the interventions to improve oral health care in nursing home settings are efforts to enable effective mouth care in nursing home residents with dementia. Residents with dementia tend to exhibit care-resistant behaviors (CRBs) that put them at risk for inadequate mouth care and potential illnesses. Managing Oral Hygiene Using Threat Reduction, a nonpharmacologic, relationship-based intervention, has been shown to be effective in managing CRB during mouth care, resulting in higher rates of completing oral care activities for residents with dementia in a randomized study with a control group (Jablonski et al., 2018).

Hearing and Vision Care

Hearing and vision impairments, common among nursing home residents, can diminish the quality of life for nursing home residents and are associated with falls, social isolation, depression, problems with memory, and cognitive impairment (McCreedy et al., 2018; Williams et al., 2020;

Yurkofsky and Ouslander, 2021). These impairments can also hinder a resident's ability to communicate effectively, particularly if staff members do not face a resident when they are speaking to them or block facial cues by covering their face with their hands or a mask (Andrusjak et al., 2020; McCreedy et al., 2018).

Some hearing and vision impairments can be reversed through cataract surgery, the use of hearing aids or glasses, or regularly checking for impacted earwax (Yurkofsky and Ouslander, 2021). Research has shown that these relatively simple corrective measures improve quality of life and reduce depression and psychological distress among nursing home residents (Owsley et al., 2007a,b). However, most nursing home residents' sensory impairments go undetected for a variety of reasons, including the limited availability of evidence-based guidance or training for staff members, staff members' inability to both identify and manage residents' impairments, and the assumption that hearing and vision loss is a normal part of aging. Moreover, staff or family may mistake sensory loss as evidence of cognitive decline among residents with dementia. A lack of partnership with external hearing and vision services and inadequate insurance coverage can be additional barriers to providing hearing and visual care (Andrusjak et al., 2020).

Estimates suggest that between 67 and 86 percent of adults who could benefit from hearing aids are not using them (Bainbridge and Ramachandran, 2014; Chien and Lin, 2012; NASEM, 2016). The high cost of hearing aids—typically $2,000 per ear—is a significant barrier (McCreedy et al., 2018; Strom, 2014). Medicare covers 80 percent of the cost of a hearing evaluation but does not provide coverage for hearing aids, while Medicaid pays for some of the cost of hearing aids but only in 31 states. Even then, reimbursement rates are typically low (McCreedy et al., 2018; NASEM, 2016; Weber, 2021; Yurkofsky and Ouslander, 2021).

The 2017 Over-the-Counter (OTC) Hearing Aid Act[24] created a class of wearable hearing devices for people with mild to moderate hearing loss. The Food and Drug Administration (FDA) will regulate these hearing aids as medical devices and is expected to issue guidelines for this new category by mid-2022. As an alternative to hearing aids available from audiologists or other hearing specialists, OTC hearing aids will be available for purchase in stores and online (NIDCD, 2021). While the availability of a new class of hearing aids may make such aids more affordable, it may also create additional barriers to accessibility. For example, by separating assessments for hearing aids from health care encounters, people who are unable to afford services may struggle to access care or use their hearing aids without counseling for proper fit and adjustments (Willink et al., 2019).

---

[24] Over-the-Counter Hearing Aid Act of 2017, S. 670, 115th Cong., 1st Sess., Congressional Record, no. 163 (March 21, 2017).

Even if a nursing home identifies a resident as having a hearing or vision impairment, additional barriers exist to managing these impairments. Residents may have limited dexterity or some other limitation that makes it difficult to manage their own hearing aids or glasses, they may feel that the assistive devices would be of no use to them, or they may be put off by the discomfort of wearing an assistive device that has not been properly fitted. Residents can lose or misplace their hearing aids and glasses, batteries for hearing aids may die without being noticed, and residents may refrain from using them because of perceived stigma. Moreover, residents with dementia may be unable to advocate effectively for help with hearing or vision problems (Andrusjak et al., 2020). Finally, the nursing home environment itself can play a large role, given that nursing homes can be noisy, poorly insulated, or poorly lit, creating additional challenges for residents with sensory impairments (McCreedy et al., 2018).

Current Challenges in Physiological Care Quality

Ensuring that nursing home residents' basic physiological care needs are met is critically important to providing person-centered care and to maintaining or improving a resident's quality of life. Resident needs such as toileting, repositioning, mobility, and feeding assistance "represent a care activity that is both time-consuming and required multiple times per day for a substantial proportion of LTC residents" (Simmons et al., 2013, p. 152). Inadequate attention to residents' basic care needs can endanger their health and well-being and can lead to residents' feelings of distress, helplessness, and dissatisfaction as well as family members' concerns about further physical decline of the resident (see Box 4-5 for a family member's note to

---

BOX 4-5
Family Member Perspective

"Further, while the [nursing home] company website and PR touted their commitment to person-centered care and treating residents like their own family, the facility was never able to provide even the most basic, routine services—such as removing and cleaning partial dentures, repositioning wheelchair-bound individuals every two hours, serving nutritional lactose-free and non-pork foods per medical/religious requirements—uniformly and consistently."

— **Anonymous, St. Louis, Missouri**

This quote was collected from the committee's online call for resident, family, and nursing home staff perspectives.

the committee on their initial expectations of physiological care in nursing homes). For example, insufficient attention paid to granting residents preferred food choices might lead to undernutrition and weight loss. Similarly, providing residents with insufficient liquids might lead to dehydration, bladder infections, and potential hospitalization (Basinska et al., 2021).

However, it is important to recognize that meeting one physiological need can create tensions with another. For example, helping nursing home residents remain mobile is important, as is keeping them safe from harm. Given that older adults tend to have health problems that affect their balance, increasing mobility can raise the risk of falls. Thus it is imperative that nursing homes ensure smooth and unobstructed walkways and proper lighting and also consider the impact of medications and health conditions that can influence an individual's balance as discussed further in Chapter 6 (Alzheimer's Association, 2009; Pioneer Network, 2016).

CMS regulations require nursing homes to monitor processes and outcomes of care.[25] The quality of nursing home care is a central focus of the survey process and of public reporting. Quality measurement and quality assurance programs in nursing homes are discussed in greater detail in Chapters 3 and 8 of this report. Despite regulatory oversight, significant gaps remain in the quality of physiological care delivered in the nursing home setting (see Box 4-6). Such shortcomings in care delivery exist due to a variety of factors, including inadequately prepared staff (Stone and Harahan, 2010), hierarchical structures that impede cohesive team building and functioning (Forbes-Thompson et al., 2006), and inadequate staffing and high staff and leadership turnover (Castle and Lin, 2010; Castle et al., 2007; Collier and Harrington, 2008), all of which impair the strong staff–resident relationships that are critical to providing quality care (see Chapter 5 for a complete discussion on workforce issues).

Other factors associated with poorer quality care include care that is not aligned with evidence-based best practices (Ersek and Jablonski, 2014); poor care coordination resulting from inadequate health information technology support (Alexander and Madsen, 2021; Alexander et al., 2020a; Vest et al., 2019) (see Chapter 9 for more detailed discussion of health information technology); infrequent visits and limited involvement of medical directors and primary care providers; regulations that incentivize certain types of care (e.g., rehabilitation) that are not aligned with residents' goals and preferences (Carpenter, 2020; Flint et al., 2019); and insufficient resources to provide ready access to ancillary services such as laboratory tests and intravenous therapy (Cantor et al., 2020). Moreover, low-quality communication between nursing homes and hospitals such as missing, incomplete,

---

[25] CMS Requirements for Long-Term Care Facilities—Quality assurance and performance improvement, 42 CFR § 483.75 (2016).

> **BOX 4-6**
> **Family Member Perspectives**
>
> "I would love to see patient-centered care be a requirement in all nursing homes."
>
> — Frustrated Family Member
>
> "My loved ones have had their rights, dignity taken away. They are mistreated — mostly treated like throw away objects. There is too much to note on what to change . . ."
>
> — Essential Caregiver
>
> "There is no quality of care/quality of life/ . . . and worse, person-centered care is next to impossible. Aides and nurses do not want to be short/quick, but residents are now just a box on the check-list to be done. More is being added to do and resentment builds. We all know shortcuts happen often, staff are frustrated with residents when [they] need something, keep dementia residents to last for [care] because can't speak up or won't be believed if [they] do, and alert and oriented residents are left waiting and seeing the future for themselves."
>
> — K.S.
>
> "[I] try to make a positive impact so that the system becomes more responsive and residents are not just kept alive but are enabled to thrive"
>
> — Anonymous, St. Louis, Missouri
>
> These quotes were collected from the committee's online call for resident, family, and nursing home staff perspectives.

and inaccurate information has been identified as a significant risk factor for negative patient outcomes related to care transitions (Gillespie et al., 2010; King et al., 2013; Scott et al., 2017; Terrell and Miller, 2006).

Behavioral Health Care

Moving beyond the physiological needs discussed in the previous section, the next category in Maslow's hierarchy is psychological needs. These include needs ranging from companionship and relationships, a sense of inclusion, and support of an individual's cognitive needs. In terms of the life of a nursing home resident, this also includes dignity, autonomy, the ability to engage in meaningful activities, and attention to behavioral health needs.

Two different but overlapping elements of behavioral health are important to the optimal mental health and well-being of nursing home residents (Keyes, 2002). The first element reflects the objective presence of mental disorders, which for nursing home residents can be existing diagnoses, undiagnosed conditions, or conditions that emerge during a resident's stay. The second element reflects the subjective state of social well-being, which for nursing home residents includes the resident's ability to cope and their level of functioning (Keyes, 2002).

Environment and services each play a key role in achieving optimal mental health since available resources, environmental demands, and supports can all affect mental well-being (Niclasen et al., 2019). Limited research suggests that the regular presence of behavioral health staff (either on staff or contracted) and the use of interdisciplinary teams enable effective behavioral health care by addressing medical, psychosocial, and environmental issues together (Bartels et al., 2002). However, there is limited evidence in this area, and further research is needed to identify effective service arrangements and the best composition of staff to provide adequate behavioral health care in nursing homes.

Behavioral health or mental health services are traditionally provided within the nursing home facility by physicians, nursing staff, social workers, and activities personnel (Jester et al., 2020). Alternatively, nursing homes may arrange for contracted behavioral health specialists to either provide care in the facility or in the community. The latter would involve transporting residents to and from appointments in the community (Bartels et al., 2002). The primary models of contracted mental health services include psychiatrist-centered, nurse-centered, and multidisciplinary team models.

Regulatory Requirements

The Behavioral Health Services section[26] of the Code of Federal Regulations stipulates that each nursing home resident receive and be provided behavioral health care and services in order that the resident be able to attain and maintain the highest practicable physical, mental, and psychosocial well-being. As outlined in the regulations, behavioral health care starts with a comprehensive resident assessment, which forms the basis for the development of a treatment plan that addresses identified mental health needs. Nursing home facilities are expected to have sufficient staff to enable the provision of direct services while attending to the optimal well-being of residents. The regulations further stipulate that nursing homes must provide residents with mental and psychosocial disorders with the appropriate care to attain the highest well-being possible, emphasizing that using nonpharmacological interventions is a preferred approach. Treatment is to include rehabilitation services and medically related social services. These services can be

---

[26] CMS Requirements for Long-Term Care Facilities—Behavioral health services, 42 CFR § 483.40 (2016).

provided through internal sources using nursing home staff and consultants or through qualified, Medicaid- and Medicare-approved external providers.

OBRA 87 enacted requirements for nursing homes to perform preadmission screening and annual resident reviews (PASRRs) in order to both identify and assess persons with mental illness and developmental disabilities, to ensure that mentally ill persons are not inappropriately admitted to nursing homes, and to make sure that the nursing home setting is the best placement option for the resident.[27] Through the PASRR process, residents with mental illnesses placed in nursing homes are expected to receive appropriate mental health services for their diagnoses.[28] Persons with developmental disabilities are expected to receive appropriate habilitation services to promote optimal functioning.[29]

OBRA 87 also emphasized the importance of a person-centered care approach to providing behavioral health services to nursing home residents (CMS, 2017). Toward that end, the regulations introduced new F-tags[30] that focus on mental health supports and services, specifically in the areas of services that nursing homes made available and offered to the resident, sufficient and competent staff, and behavioral health training for staff. The deficiency categories most closely associated with behavioral health are resident behavior and facility practices, quality of life, and quality of care. In addition, OBRA 87 requires nursing homes to identify the resources needed to care for residents with behavioral health issues, to conduct competency assessments to identify staff ability to provide behavioral health services, and to provide training to increase staff competency.[31]

---

[27] Omnibus Budget Reconciliation Act of 1987, Public Law 100-203; 42 USC 1396r, §1919, 100th Cong., 1st Sess., (December 22, 1987).

[28] Omnibus Budget Reconciliation Act of 1987, Public Law 100-203; 42 USC 1396r, §1919 – subparagraph B, 100th Cong., 1st Sess., (December 22, 1987).

[29] Omnibus Budget Reconciliation Act of 1987, Public Law 100-203; 42 USC 1395i-3, §1919, 100th Cong., 1st Sess., (December 22, 1987).

[30] F-tags are cited when there is noncompliance that is not actual harm but results in minimal discomfort to the resident or has the potential to cause harm. These are very common citations in nursing home surveys. See https://www.cms.gov/Medicare/Provider-Enrollment-and-Certification/GuidanceforLawsAndRegulations/Downloads/List-of-Revised-FTags.pdf (accessed October 21, 2021).

[31] The Social Security Act prohibits federal Medicaid payments to institutions for mental diseases (IMD), defined as "hospital, nursing facility, or other institution of more than 16 beds that is primarily engaged in providing diagnosis, treatment, or care of persons with mental diseases, including medical attention, nursing care, and related services" (MACPAC, 2019, p. xii). Because of the broad definition, it is difficult to determine which facility in a state qualifies as an IMD, leading to great variation and resource allocation by state (MACPAC, 2019, 2020, 2022). This lack of definitional specificity may also serve as a significant barrier to nursing home residents obtaining necessary behavioral health services.

Current State of Behavioral Health Services in Nursing Homes

The widespread closing and downsizing of inpatient psychiatric hospitals, which began in the 1950s and continued for decades in various phases (Koyanagi, 2007; Pan, 2013), combined with inadequate community resources for mental health services, resulted in nursing homes becoming a main setting to care for persons with persistent serious mental illness (SMI). CMS uses a broad definition of SMI to include a diagnosis of schizophrenia, schizoaffective disorder, schizophrenium disorder, delusional disorder, psychotic mood disorders, and anxiety disorders but not a primary diagnosis of depression or Alzheimer's disease and related dementias (ADRD).[32]

Approximately 4 out of 10 long-stay nursing home residents that are Medicaid beneficiaries under the age of 65 have an SMI diagnosis; for those 65 or older, the prevalence is 2 out of 10 (Nelson and Bowblis, 2017). The share of residents diagnosed with schizophrenia or bipolar disorder nearly doubled, from 6.5 percent in 2000 to 12.4 percent in 2017 (Laws et al., 2021). The prevalence of schizophrenia in people aged 65 and over in the general population is 0.1 to 0.5 percent (Rosenberg et al., 2009). Concerns have been raised about nursing home residents with dementia being diagnosed inappropriately with schizophrenia (discussed below and in Chapter 6).

Studies estimate that a disproportionately large share (60 to 90 percent) of nursing home residents have any mental health diagnosis (Brennan and Soohoo, 2019; Burns and Taube, Fullerton et al., 2009; Grabowski et al., 2009, 2010; Orth et al., 2019; Rahman et al., 2013; Smyer et al., 1994; Tariot et al., 1993). Trend analyses indicate that the proportion of residents admitted with mental illness is higher than the proportion with dementia (Aschbrenner et al., 2010; Fullerton et al., 2009; Grabowski et al., 2010). Among individuals with mental illness, individuals diagnosed with schizophrenia or bipolar disorder are more likely to be admitted to a nursing home during the 3-year period following their diagnosis, and older persons with depression are also at an increased risk of being placed in a nursing home (Fullerton et al., 2009). These individuals have a range of complex care needs that present significant challenges for nursing homes (Laws et al., 2021).

Much of the data related to behavioral health conditions of nursing home residents date back more than a decade. More up-to-date prevalence data would likely be higher, reflecting an increase in resident acuity and the proportion of nursing home admissions of residents with mental health conditions (Temkin-Greener et al., 2018a).

---

[32] See https://www.govinfo.gov/content/pkg/CFR-2009-title42-vol5/pdf/CFR-2009-title42-vol5-sec483-100.pdf (accessed February 14, 2022).

Current Challenges

Nursing home use of PASRRs, which was designed to improve access to behavioral health care, has had mixed results, with some conditions, such as schizophrenia, identified more successfully than other conditions, such as depression (Crick et al., 2020). The number of residents with mental health needs in nursing homes is increasing (Temkin-Greener et al., 2018a), and many residents are not having their needs met (Rivera et al., 2020). These unmet needs[33] occur more acutely in certain subpopulations of nursing home residents. For example, nursing homes often overlook the mental health needs of racial and ethnic minorities, who are less likely to receive treatment after an SMI diagnosis (Bailey et al., 2009). Research points to a lack of culturally sensitive assessments and treatment practices as factors contributing to the disparities in care and unmet needs minority populations in nursing homes experience (Fashaw-Walters et al., 2021; Li et al., 2019).

Historically, nursing home care and staffing have primarily focused on the physical health care needs of residents, managing their chronic conditions and maintaining their functional ability. While OBRA 87 was enacted to provide protections for nursing home residents with mental illnesses and developmental disabilities, the treatment of psychiatric conditions and behavioral health conditions in nursing home settings still requires significant improvement (Li, 2010). One of the many aims of the nursing home reforms contained in OBRA 87 was to decrease inappropriate use of medications. In some cases, however, medication use has increased, with little effort made to provide nonpharmacologic approaches to care (Crick et al., 2020). Research has identified numerous barriers to providing nonpharmacologic approaches, including insufficient reimbursement to support care from specialized mental health care teams, inadequate staffing levels and staff training, time pressures, and lack of leadership, among other factors (Crick et al., 2020).

Current funding structures serve as barriers to mental health assessment follow-ups and nonpharmacologic approaches to care (Crick et al., 2020), as these approaches can be resource intensive. Providing high-quality care to residents with SMI requires more direct-care hours, specialized staff training, and services from mental health providers external to nursing home facilities (McGarry et al., 2019), but public payments for residents with SMI do not adequately cover the costs of treating those residents (Rahman et al., 2013). Nursing homes report difficulties in accessing mental health specialists willing to provide services in the nursing home, while

---

[33] Unmet needs are defined here as neglect of care necessary for ADLs. Negative consequences of unmet needs include the resident missing meals, not having appropriate toileting care which results in wetting or soiling clothes, medication error, or not receiving needed assistance in order to walk around (Rivera et al., 2020; Xiang et al., 2017).

the costs to transport residents to external treatment sources may exceed Medicaid coverage in some states (Crick et al., 2020).

Attempts to improve the quality of behavioral health care through regulations have, in many cases, proved to be unsuccessful (Crick et al., 2020), and lower reimbursement rates for SMI care do not encourage quality care (Rahman et al., 2013). In fact, facilities with higher populations of residents requiring SMI care are associated with lower nursing home quality (Rahman et al., 2013) and lower care quality (McGarry et al., 2019). For example, one study of over 14,000 nursing home facilities found that those with greater proportions of residents with SMI also had lower direct-care staffing hours, more residents who were Medicaid beneficiaries, and lower scores on Nursing Home Compare star ratings (Jester et al., 2020) and were more likely to be for-profit facilities.

Eligibility for Medicaid coverage is based on income status as well as disability (including psychiatric disability). There is an increased prevalence of mental illness in high-Medicaid facilities. Moreover, nursing homes with a majority of Medicaid residents are associated with higher rates of psychiatric hospitalization (Becker et al., 2009) and greater rates of antipsychotic medication prescription (Hughes et al., 2000).

Research on access to behavioral health services suggests that there are disparities in access to high-quality nursing homes (Temkin-Greener et al., 2018a). These disparities may be a result of social stigma, nursing home reluctance to accept patients who require medications (which may lower facility quality scores), nursing homes' concerns about their ability to deal with behavioral problems, and the geographical distribution of five-star nursing homes. Research indicates that inadequate access to behavioral health services occurs in both lower and higher star-rated facilities and in both for-profit and nonprofit nursing homes. Moreover, access to such services is not necessarily affected by for-profit status (Orth et al., 2019). Nursing homes located in urban areas, facilities with higher RN staffing and lower turnover, and facilities with more psychiatrically trained physicians were less likely to report inadequate infrastructure to connect residents to behavioral health services (Orth et al., 2019).

A survey of nursing homes identified a number of key challenges to delivering behavioral health care services, including

- lack of staff training (47 percent),
- inability to adequately meet resident's behavioral health needs (33.3 percent),
- inadequate coordination between the facility and community providers (31.8 percent), and
- lack of adequate infrastructure to make referrals and transport residents to services outside the facility (26.2 percent) (Orth et al., 2019).

Of those facilities surveyed, 40 percent viewed PASRRs as hindering admission screening and causing admission delays, and more than 60 percent expressed concerns about the perceived difficulty in accessing psychiatric support after nursing home admission (Orth et al., 2019).

Several studies have identified the challenges of training staff in behavioral health and providing quality care as key challenges for nursing homes (Orth et al., 2019; Roberts et al., 2020). Staff behavioral health education was less problematic in facilities that had dedicated Alzheimer's units, lower turnover of registered nurses, and more psychiatrically trained registered nurses and social workers. Facilities with lower registered nurse turnover and more psychiatrically trained registered nurses were less likely to report inadequate coordination with community providers and being unable to meet resident needs (Orth et al., 2019). Facilities with lower registered nurse turnover, higher registered nurse staffing, and more psychiatrically trained physicians were less likely to report inadequate facility infrastructure (Orth et al., 2019). In a secondary analysis of national data, facilities with social service departments staffed by individuals with higher professional qualifications were associated with improved care through reducing residents' behavioral health symptoms and avoiding the use of antipsychotics (Roberts et al., 2020).

Promising Practices/Innovative Models to Address Behavioral Health Needs

A number of interventions have been found to be effective in treating behavioral health conditions such as depression in the nursing home environment. One systematic review identified cognitive behavioral therapies, reminiscence activities, interventions aimed at reducing social isolation, and exercise-based interventions as having some impact on decreasing depression in cognitively intact nursing home residents (Simning and Simons, 2017). Another study found decreases in depression and increases in quality of life among residents who participated in a 10-week physical activity program (Lok et al., 2017).

Interventions to reduce loneliness linked to depression have also produced positive results in long-term care settings (NASEM, 2020). One systematic review suggests that the interventions that are more successful at reducing loneliness are the ones that do not require high amounts of physical activity and mobility (Quan et al., 2020). Those interventions for which the strongest results have been reported include reminiscence therapy, laughter, and horticultural therapy[34] (Quan et al., 2020).

---

[34] Horticultural therapy refers to the use of flowers, plants, and horticultural activities for treatment. Such therapy has been shown to help individuals learn new skills, adjust to functional loss, and experience hopeful and nurturing feelings, with positive impacts on physical, psychosocial, and cognitive functions such as improving body coordination, encouraging social activity, and improving mood (Chen and Ji, 2015).

Videoconferencing interventions, PARO robot[35] interaction, logotherapy,[36] and pet therapy produced more modest results (Quan et al., 2020).

Other studies have reported success at improving the cognitive functioning of nursing home residents. A systematic review of multimodal, nonpharmacologic interventions for cognitive function in older people with dementia concluded that sessions combining exercise, cognitive training, ADL practice, and activity interventions improved global function, executive function, and memory in persons with dementia when the sessions were at least 30 minutes long and done at least three times a week for at least 8 weeks (Yorozuya et al., 2019). One randomized controlled trial using animal-assisted activities reduced depressive symptomatology and increased the quality of life for persons with cognitive impairment (Olsen et al., 2016).

Research on well-being provides some guidance for developing optimal environments for supporting mental health care. For example, one systematic review of the well-being of long-term care residents with chronic mental illness provided broad recommendations for care, including the development of environments that provide nonstigmatizing specialized care that is accepting and supportive (van der Wolf et al., 2019). Given the lack of evidence of effective treatment approaches, the authors concluded that additional research should be conducted in this area, with attention paid to the well-being of residents.

Use of telehealth for behavioral health care As discussed elsewhere in this report, the COVID-19 pandemic had a particularly deleterious impact in the nursing home setting. This was true not only in terms of morbidity and mortality, but also in terms of residents' mental and behavioral health. In an effort to protect nursing home residents and staff from contracting the coronavirus, nursing homes quickly restricted access to their facilities and curtailed resident activities. While these measures were put in place to provide for the health and safety of residents and staff, the unintended consequence was a significant increase in social isolation and loneliness, depression, and anxiety among residents (also discussed in Chapter 9 of this report) (Mo and Shi, 2020; Rodney et al., 2021). Typically, all residents facing behavioral health challenges rely on visits with family members and personal contact and interaction with other residents and members of the community for various reasons including socialization,

---

[35] A PARO robot is a baby harp seal robot used in nursing homes, which has a calming effect on and elicits emotional responses in patients.

[36] Logotherapy, from the Greek word *logos*, or "meaning," is a form of therapy oriented around helping individuals find meaning in their future.

support, and personal care (Gaugler, 2005). The absence of such coping mechanisms increased the complexity of residents' behavioral health challenges (Nash et al., 2021). Given nursing homes' extremely limited resources such as psychologists that specialize in geriatric populations, behavioral telehealth offers one way to expand access to such necessary, but limited, expertise (Friedrich, 2021). The use of health information technology (HIT) including telehealth in nursing homes is discussed further in Chapter 9.

Remote monitoring and robotics Remote monitoring technology is another innovation that has the potential to improve care delivery and outcomes for nursing home residents. This technology includes devices that can connect remotely to the Internet, which, in the case of mobile devices, makes it possible for the devices to move around independently and collect data about residents. For example, robots can move independently and transmit real-time images to nursing home staff and also open a voice connection between the resident and the remote caregivers to improve communication (Bäck et al., 2012).

In one study, researchers examined the use of assistive robots for the care of nursing home residents with dementia experiencing depression and agitation. In particular, the intervention included a robot device described as being the size of a baby harp seal with a swiveling head, moving legs and tail, and microphones that make authentic sounds like a harp seal; the robot intervention resulted in improved depression and less agitation over time (Jøranson et al., 2015).

It is critical to understand that however useful these and other future innovations might be, the developers and implementers of remote monitoring tools need to always consider the impact of these innovations on resident satisfaction as well as on clinician workflow, burden, and satisfaction (Alexander et al., 2020b).

Research indicates that residents with behavioral health disorders (e.g., schizophrenia, psychosis, bipolar, depression/anxiety, personality disorder, and substance use) are less likely to be admitted to high-quality nursing home facilities than residents without those disorders (Temkin-Greener et al., 2018a). Lower-quality facilities typically have fewer resources available to staff and residents, such as HIT, to help support care delivery during times when in-person access is extremely limited, such as during the pandemic (Alexander et al., 2017). The use of HIT, such as certified electronic health record technology, has been shown to improve communication and clinical integration among behavioral health and all other providers (MACPAC, 2021). The myriad issues related to HIT adoption, implementation, and use in nursing home settings are discussed in Chapter 9.

Care for People with Alzheimer's Disease and Related Dementias

An estimated 48 percent of nursing home residents—59 percent of long-stay and 37 percent of short-stay (post-acute) residents—have a diagnosis of dementia (Harris-Kojetin et al., 2019). These figures for dementia diagnosis are likely underestimates, as studies have demonstrated that when specialists such as neurologists, psychiatrists, and neuropsychologists conduct assessments in long-term care settings, they identify many undiagnosed cases of dementia (Magaziner et al., 2000; Zimmerman et al., 2007).

Alzheimer's disease, the most common dementia, begins subtly, passes through mild cognitive impairment, and progresses to mild, moderate, and finally severe dementia, with the course generally lasting a decade or more. Often, the later stages of the disease, which require 24-hour supervision and assistance with most or all ADLs, result in nursing home placement. A variety of other progressive dementias exist, such as frontotemporal dementia, Lewy body dementia, vascular dementia, and dementia associated with Parkinson's disease. These conditions vary in their presentation, rate of progression, and care needs but share many of Alzheimer's disease's effects on cognitive function (Alzheimer's Association, 2021a,b).

Available research indicates that the key element of dementia care practice should be a focus on the individual's condition, needs, and desires. That focus should be based on knowing the person; recognizing and accepting the person's reality; identifying and supporting opportunities for meaningful engagement; building and nurturing authentic caring relationships; creating and maintaining a supportive community for individuals, family, and staff; and evaluating care practices regularly, using evaluation data to guide appropriate changes in care and policy (Fazio et al., 2018).

Most of the principles of quality care for nursing home residents apply equally to persons with cognitive impairment and to those without. However, providing care for persons with cognitive impairment, including persons with ADRD, raises a number of specific issues. For example, managing Alzheimer's disease and related cognitive disorders largely involves addressing behavioral symptoms such as wandering, resistance to care, repetitive mannerisms, repetitive vocalization, and aggression. Studies show that these behavioral symptoms are often expressions of unmet needs, such as loneliness, boredom, discomfort, anxiety, or pain (Cohen-Mansfield et al., 2015). In this context, a key goal of care should be to identify and meet these needs using individualized approaches and, as first-line methods, nonpharmacological tools and methods (Gaugler et al., 2014). A study found that a diagnosis of cognitive dysfunction upon admission to a nursing home is a stronger predictor of outcome than a diagnosis of dementia. This highlights the need to individualize decisions regarding the risks and benefits of nursing home care for those individuals with cognitive impairment (Burke et al., 2021).

It is also important to recognize that for a person with advanced dementia, the sensory experiences of the present are very important, since awareness of the meaning or future implications of such activities as waiting for a meal, positioning in a bed or chair, or receipt of hygiene care are often not understood. Furthermore, the inexorable progression of virtually all ADRD diagnoses places more importance on the experiences of today, something that is also true of many other nursing residents. These factors combine to make addressing unmet needs, creating pleasant events, and attending to day-to-day quality of life critical outcomes of interest in the care of persons with ADRD (Gaugler et al., 2014; Kitwood, 1997; Logsdon et al., 2002). It is important to note that measuring day-to-day quality of life is challenging and that this key outcome is vastly underrepresented in CMS "quality indicators," which focus largely on medical outcomes (Burke and Werner, 2019).

In addition, persons with dementia underreport new symptoms or needs and therefore tend to receive less attention, have more undetected symptoms (e.g., constipation), and receive fewer treatments (e.g., medication for pain) than other residents. Decision making is also difficult, which creates challenges for the current model of shared decision making, particularly if family members are relatively uninvolved or are unaware of the relevant values and preferences of the person with dementia (Miller et al., 2016b). As ADRD progresses, cognitive impairment advances, limiting the person's ability to participate in decision making. Consequently, formal procedures to facilitate early discussion with family and health care professionals about care goals and advance care planning (see Box 4-8 below) are important, as studies have demonstrated that such planning improves end-of-life outcomes (Wendrich-van Dael et al., 2020).

Antipsychotic medications have been used to treat nursing home residents with behavioral and psychological symptoms of dementia, but FDA warnings about the danger of such medications for people with dementia have led to increased efforts to limit their use (also discussed in Chapter 6). CMS launched the National Partnership to Improve Dementia Care in 2012[37] to reduce potentially inappropriate use of antipsychotics by reorienting nursing homes toward nonpharmacologic person-centered care, including music and exercise programs (Lucas and Bowblis, 2017). Through the initiative, CMS, in partnership with federal and state agencies, nursing homes, advocacy groups and caregivers, working in concert with state-based coalitions, aims to advance best practices to promote person-centered care and improve the quality of life for residents with dementia (Fashaw-Walters et al., 2021; Lucas and Bowblis, 2017).

---

[37] See https://www.cms.gov/Medicare/Provider-Enrollment-and-Certification/Survey CertificationGenInfo/National-Partnership-to-Improve-Dementia-Care-in-Nursing-Homes (accessed February 9, 2022).

Although the rates of antipsychotic medication use for dementia care in nursing homes declined overall between 2012 and 2019, significant variation exists across states (Rosenthal et al., 2022). Recent research has revealed unintended consequences of the National Partnership's efforts. For example, an initial examination has shown that rates of schizophrenia, as documented in residents' MDS assessments, increased after implementation of the Partnership and are higher for Black residents with ADRD than non-Black residents. Such disparities in diagnoses raise concerns that nursing homes are reporting schizophrenia diagnoses in an effort to bypass the Partnership's goal of reducing antipsychotic medication use. Disparities in schizophrenia diagnoses could be due to a number of factors, including differences in quality of care for Black residents compared to non-Black residents, perceptions of nursing home staff regarding the management of challenging behaviors, or structural racism (Fashaw-Walters et al., 2021).

The U.S. Alzheimer's Association published a comprehensive set of dementia care practice recommendations and a series of supporting papers (Fazio et al., 2018), which can help inform a greater focus on dementia care in nursing home practice, training, and regulation (Alzheimer's Association, 2018).[38] Additional research has identified shortcomings in the current evidence base on initiatives designed to improve care for people with ADRD in nursing homes, including an overrepresentation of short-term studies with small sample sizes, making it challenging to determine which interventions are effective. Further research is needed on interventions at the community level (care protocols, dementia villages), policy level (paid family leave policies, payment policies, and transportation policies), and societal level (public awareness campaigns). A balance of short-term and long-term studies is needed, as well as including assessments of interventions in real-world settings where people receive care, including the home and long-term care facilities (NASEM, 2021).

Psychosocial Care

The committee's conceptual model of quality care in nursing homes considers meeting residents' psychological and social needs—situated in the mid-range of Maslow's hierarchy—as a critical component of comprehensive person-centered care. The psychosocial needs of older adults incorporate physical, psychological, intellectual, and social dimensions of care. Nursing homes organize these care services to enhance their residents' mental, social, and emotional well-being; improve outcomes related to their quality of life and quality of care and to resident rights; and support the

---

[38] For the full recommendations, see https://www.alz.org/media/documents/alzheimers-dementia-care-practice-recommendations.pdf (accessed October 21, 2021).

residents' family members and other loved ones. Social services, activities, and nursing departments within the nursing home typically deliver these services, which are augmented by consultants and contractual services that require specialized training or expertise, such as psychiatric services and music and art programs. Research has shown that an interdisciplinary team perspective produces better outcomes (Simons et al., 2012a,b), as the team is trained to address psychological, social, and environmental factors that affect care and quality of life (Simons et al., 2012a).

Providing effective individualized care requires a knowledge of residents' psychosocial preferences (Carpenter et al., 2000). According to one systematic review, nursing home residents identified nine factors important to them that influenced their idea of quality care: staffing levels, staff attitudes, continuity of care, daily routine, environment, decision making/choice, dignity, activities, and attention to culture and spirituality (Gilbert et al., 2021; see also Travers et al., 2021). Research on older adults living in the community has identified preferences for care, trade-offs between freedom and safety, family/friend involvement, privacy issues, avoiding pain, participation in events, and daily routine as areas in which preferences correlate with a better quality of life (Degenholtz et al., 1997). Other studies emphasize preferences in the areas of social contact, growth and leisure activities, personal choice/control, the use of assistive devices, and care and caregivers as being important to an enhanced quality of life (Carpenter et al., 2000). Honoring the choices of nursing home residents is associated with an improved quality of life. Processes such as the initial and ongoing assessment of psychosocial preferences of residents as well as the documentation and communication of these preferences with the interdisciplinary team are central to meeting the needs of residents for optimal delivery of person-centered care.

Regulatory Requirements

The Code of Federal Regulations section on behavioral health services[39] mandates that a nursing home provide psychosocial care as detailed in its comprehensive assessment and plan of care. Including the resident, significant others, and members of the interdisciplinary team responsible for psychosocial care is key to developing and reviewing the assessment and plan-of-care document. The regulations also outline a process through which the care plan should address psychosocial care needs and specify that nursing homes must employ qualified staff to provide the services that meet these needs.

As discussed earlier, regulations require Medicare- and Medicaid-certified nursing homes to conduct patient care surveys as part of the

---

[39] CMS Requirements for Long-Term Care Facilities—Behavioral health services, 42 CFR § 483.40 (2016).

certification process.[40] Two areas of assessment pertinent to psychosocial needs are (1) activities and social participation and (2) medical, nursing, and rehabilitative care. A nursing home that fails to meet one or more federal requirements is cited for a deficiency by surveyors. The deficiency categories most closely associated with psychosocial care needs include resident rights; admission, transfer, and discharge rights; resident behavior and facility practices; and quality of life and quality of care.

Although psychosocial care needs are part of the federal requirements, the regulations place a greater emphasis on medical indicators of high-quality care. While physical health indicators are clearly an important area of focus for quality improvement, psychosocial indicators such as enhancing social engagement, supporting self-worth and resident dignity, and addressing the psychological and spiritual needs of the residents are important elements of nursing home care and should be an integral component of the survey process and quality improvement initiatives (Bowen and Zimmerman, 2009).

Current Status

A growing body of evidence suggests that it is important to provide a variety of services and activities to address the psychosocial care needs of nursing home residents, including attending to spiritual needs, counseling, and other psychosocial support services (Johnston and Narayanasamy, 2016; Koenig, 2012; Lok et al., 2017; Olsen et al., 2016; Zhang et al., 2020). However, despite the importance of these services to person-centered care and resident quality of life, the current emphasis on nursing home care in the United States aligns with a medical model of care, with a limited focus on social care.

Research supports the role of a stronger emphasis on psychosocial care in order to ensure a more person-centered approach to nursing home care. As noted above, nursing home residents cite factors related to dignity, activities, and attention to culture and spirituality as being critical to quality care (Gilbert et al., 2021). An emphasis on improving the performance and outcomes of these factors may strengthen the responsiveness of nursing homes to resident concerns.

Wellness, physical activities, and art activities are vital for health, functional mobility, and performing ADLs. Research suggests that physical activity can protect against and lessen ADL disability, improve cognition and quality of life for residents and those with dementia, and improve mental health (de Souto Barreto et al., 2016). One intervention, Function-Focused Care, engages residents with moderate to severe cognitive impairment in physical activities and functional tasks using motivational and individualized techniques. It has the potential to improve older adults' psychosocial

---

[40] CMS Requirements for Long-Term Care Facilities—Survey frequency, 42 CFR §488.308 (a) and (b) (2016).

and physical well-being, increase physical activity, and reduce risk of hospitalization and falls (Galik et al., 2013, 2015; Resnick et al., 2016).

There is also evidence that wellness interventions such as tai chi and yoga in nursing homes can improve the quality of life among residents (Saravanakumar et al., 2018), and some evidence suggests that ADL training combined with physical exercise can improve well-being in nursing home residents with moderately severe dementia (Henskens et al., 2018). Studies have also shown that art interventions in nursing homes can improve the quality of life for dementia patients (Schneider, 2018), promote person-centered care among nursing home residents (Vaartio-Rajalin et al., 2021), reduce depression and improve the self-esteem of residents (Ching-Teng et al., 2019), and promote overall resident well-being (Curtis et al., 2018).

Research has identified a number of other areas that require improvement, including an emphasis on stronger staffing requirements to deliver psychosocial care (Bern-Klug et al., 2010; Simons et al., 2012a,b), acquiring outcome data that link care provision with improved quality of care (Bowen and Zimmerman, 2008), and better definition of the processes of psychosocial care in nursing homes (Simons et al., 2012b). Factors associated with the quality of psychosocial care include staffing and payer source; in particular, it has been shown that increases in qualified social service staffing produce higher-quality psychosocial care (Zhang et al., 2008; Zimmerman et al., 2005).

Current Challenges

The Agency for Healthcare Research and Quality conducted an environmental scan of nursing homes and found evidence of omissions in psychosocial care which led to severe adverse events such as avoidable hospitalizations, cognitive decline, death (all-cause and suicide), loneliness, and poor resident-centered care (Ogletree et al., 2020). In addition, several studies have documented omissions in psychosocial care, particularly in the areas of addressing emotional and mental health needs, listening to the resident, and honoring care preferences (Hirst, 2002; Poghosyan et al., 2017; Recio-Saucedo et al., 2018). Other studies have reported serious omissions in psychosocial care leading to loss of dignity, abuse, and neglect of the resident (Hirst, 2002; Malmedal et al., 2009; Nåden et al., 2013). One study reported that nursing home staff limit social care more than ADL care (Zúñiga et al., 2016). An earlier report by the HHS OIG on psychosocial services provided to nursing home residents found that only slightly more than half of Medicare beneficiaries received all the psychosocial services identified in their care plans during their nursing home stay, while 41 percent received some, but not all of the psychosocial services identified in their care plans. Five percent of beneficiaries did not receive any of the psychosocial services identified in their care plans (OIG, 2003).

Promising Practices

While psychosocial care in nursing homes has improved over the years (IOM, 2001), it is still evolving. Notable changes and new models of care strongly support implementing a person-centered care approach. For example, the meaningful activity movement requires nursing homes to employ the elements of active participation, activity content related to past roles and interests of the participants, and activities that meet the needs of identity and belonging for all activity offerings (Genoe and Dupuis, 2012). Promising programs such as MemPics, designed to promote meaningful activity for people with mild to moderate dementia using cognitive stimulation (Mansbach et al., 2017), have been tested in the nursing home setting with positive results. The Preference Match Tracker is a tool to identify activity preferences which can be used to document and track individual recreation preferences and activities. Such preferences can be incorporated in the assessment and care planning process to improve the quality of care and quality of life for residents (Van Haitsma et al., 2016).

Videoconferencing for remote health care provision, counseling, and the delivery of specialized activities such as music therapy (Groom et al., 2021; Newbould et al., 2017) and for counseling family and significant others (Gaugler et al., 2020) is proving to be a promising approach for improving psychosocial care. Several studies have established the feasibility of using such methods for assessment, health care management, clinical support, and diagnosis (Alexander et al., 2020a; Groom et al., 2021; Hale et al., 2018; LeadingAge CAST, 2013). Delivering care through videoconferencing may increase access to specialized services and increase access to care for those living in rural areas. Both staff members and residents report satisfaction with providing services though videoconferencing.

Using care preference tools, such as The Conversation Project, in nursing home settings is one approach to honoring resident choices in care (Galambos et al., 2021). New methods for care planning, such as the adoption of a person-directed care planning process (Lepore et al., 2018), can provide a structure for honoring resident choices. When nursing homes use these tools along with other preference assessment instruments, broadly and consistently, they will strengthen a person-centered approach to providing care for their residents.

Another way for nursing homes to improve the psychosocial well-being of their residents and staff is through the establishment of resident and family councils. Every nursing home resident has the right to form or participate in a resident and family council, and the nursing home must provide space for the group to meet and must listen to the complaints and recommendations provided by the council.[41] These councils are described in Box 4-7.

---

[41] For more information from CMS, see https://downloads.cms.gov/medicare/your_resident_rights_and_protections_section.pdf (accessed November 16, 2021).

> **BOX 4-7**
> **Resident and Family Councils**
>
> The Omnibus Budget and Reconciliation Act of 1987 (OBRA 87) mandated resident and family councils in nursing homes as mechanisms to ensure family and resident participation in nursing homes' operations and quality improvement activities. The 2016 CMS revised nursing facility regulations reiterated these rights (National Consumer Voice, 2021).
>
> Resident councils are organized groups of nursing home residents that meet regularly to raise issues of concern, discuss what is working well, and offer suggestions for change or provide suggestions for resolving differences. Activities personnel, social service departments, and, in some cases, administrators facilitate resident council meetings. Resident councils serve to empower the residents of nursing homes and can promote life-long citizenship within the nursing home facility (Freeman, 1997). The committee structure of resident councils allows residents to raise concerns without identifying any one person or family with the concern, enhancing resident empowerment and resident-centered advocacy.
>
> Limited research exists on the effectiveness of resident councils. One study, published 40 years ago, found that while resident councils facilitate communication, they are not effective in changing policy or providing power to residents, and they do not ensure resident participation in council matters (Devitt and Checkoway, 1982). Clearly, more research is needed on best practices for resident councils in nursing homes.
>
> Just as resident councils empower residents, family councils provide a forum for empowering families. Regulations require nursing homes to provide a private meeting place, listen and respond to issues identified by the family council, and designate a staff person to address and provide assistance to the family council as needed (Curry et al., 2007). The revised 2016 CMS regulations mandate that residents have the right to ask family members to participate in a family council, thus providing residents a mechanism for selecting specific family members they want involved in their care.[a]
>
> Generally, when a family council exists, nursing home social services staff or activities personnel assume the responsibility of council liaison. While family councils are an important means to empower families and keep them integrally connected to the facility, estimates suggest that fewer than half of all long-term care facilities have a family council (Curry et al., 2007). Recognizing that family councils are an important means for families to advocate for their resident family members, advocates have called for nursing homes to adopt alternative ways for family councils to meet, communicate, and receive information about facility operations through the use of e-mails, virtual meetings, or phone trees (Hado and Friss Feinberg, 2020).
>
> ---
>
> [a] CMS Medicare and Medicaid Programs; Reform of Requirements for Long-Term Care Facilities, 42 CFR § 405, 431, 447, 482, 483, 485, 488, and 489 (2016).

Palliative Care and End-of-Life Care

Palliative care focuses on persons with serious, life-limiting illnesses and is characterized by openly discussing illness trajectories and identifying, documenting, and honoring patient- and family-directed goals that guide health care; aggressively preventing, promptly identifying, and effectively treating illness-related symptoms; and identifying psycho-spiritual needs and therapeutic approaches to mitigate suffering (National Consensus Project for Quality Palliative Care, 2018). Palliative care is appropriate for patients throughout the illness trajectory, including, but not solely, at the end of life, and individuals can receive palliative care alongside disease-focused treatments. Despite the need for palliative care services, access to this type of care often is limited in the nursing home setting.

Hospice care is palliative by nature, but it focuses specifically on individuals with terminal illness—usually those with the prognosis of 6 months or less. For these individuals, the goals of care focus on comfort (NHPCO, 2019).

Palliative and end-of-life care are critical components of high-quality nursing home care (Ersek et al., 2014), given that the majority of nursing home residents have multiple chronic illnesses which result in distressing symptoms and marked impairments in ADLs (Boscart et al., 2020; CMS, 2015). Indeed, older adults receiving end-of-life care in nursing homes have high symptom burdens and other needs that make them eligible for palliative care or hospice services (Esteban-Burgos et al., 2021; Stephens et al., 2018). Most hospice care in the United States is funded by Medicare under a specific benefit (NHPCO, 2020).

Nursing homes are the venue of death for approximately 25 percent of Medicare beneficiaries and an estimated 43.5 percent of fee-for-service beneficiaries. In addition, 33.2 percent of Medicare Advantage enrollees had a nursing home stay in the last 90 days of life (Teno et al., 2018). The share of Medicare beneficiaries who die in hospice care increased from 22 percent in 2000 to more than 50 percent in 2019 (MedPAC, 2021; Sheingold et al., 2015). Medicare's hospice benefit paid for services provided to more than 1.6 million beneficiaries in 2019 (MedPAC, 2021).

Nursing homes rely on one of three common models for delivering palliative care in their facilities: hospice, external palliative care consultation, or internal, facility-based services (Ersek et al., 2014).

Hospice care Hospice is the most common and well-established approach for delivering palliative care in U.S. nursing homes. CMS extended the Medicare hospice benefit to nursing homes in 1989, and by 2004, 78 percent of nursing homes reported a contract with a hospice agency (Miller and Han, 2008). Approximately one-quarter of deaths among Medicare beneficiaries occurs in a nursing home (Teno et al., 2018).

In order to be eligible, nursing home residents must meet standard hospice admission criteria, including a period of life expectancy of 6 months or less should the terminal illness run its usual course accompanied by a decision that aggressive "curative" treatments would not be pursued (CMS, 2020c). In nursing homes, the Medicare hospice benefit covers the costs of the hospice agency to oversee the individual's care plan, as well as the costs of all medical supplies and medications related to the individual's terminal condition. The benefit also covers supplemental support, as needed, from hospice interdisciplinary team members, including chaplains, social workers, and home health aides, as well as bereavement services for up to 1 year following the patient's death. While providing hospice care, the facility continues to deliver 24-hour nursing care and supportive services for the resident. The Medicare hospice benefit does not provide the resident's payment for room and board, leaving other sources such as Medicaid or out-of-pocket payments to cover those expenses (CMS, 2020a).

Research comparing end-of-life care for residents with and without hospice has shown that hospice care is associated with better psychosocial support, bereavement care, and pain management (Miller et al., 2002; Stevenson and Bramson, 2009). Hospice enrollment is also associated with fewer hospitalizations and lower health care costs for nursing home residents at the end of life (Gozalo and Miller, 2007; Miller et al., 2012; Stevenson and Bramson, 2009).

Despite the strengths of the hospice model, it has its limitations. For example, many nursing home residents have a life-limiting illness with an uncertain trajectory, which can make it difficult to determine hospice eligibility. Some nursing home administrators believe that hospice involvement does not improve end-of-life care for residents and may complicate the coordination of care (Hanson et al., 2005; Rice et al., 2004). In that vein, successful collaboration between hospice agencies and nursing homes requires a commitment to ensuring excellent communication, including soliciting input from and sharing information with nursing home staff and responding to concerns voiced by nursing home staff and administrators (Ersek et al., 2022; Miller, 2010).

Perverse financial incentives are a major barrier to nursing home hospice enrollment, at least among individuals entering the facility from the hospital and who are eligible for the Medicare skilled nursing facility benefit. Only in rare instances can patients access the Medicare skilled nursing facility and Medicare hospice benefit concurrently (e.g., in circumstances where there are unrelated diagnoses for each benefit). Reimbursement to nursing homes for the Medicare hospice benefit is much lower than for the skilled nursing facility benefit, meaning that facilities prioritize skilled nursing facility care over hospice stays, even when individuals' care needs are more palliative than rehabilitative (Hanson and Ersek, 2010). Similarly, these same financial incentives lead families to choose the skilled nursing facility benefit because the skilled nursing facility payment covers all costs in the facility including room and board, unlike the Medicare hospice benefit (Flint et al., 2019). Hospice interdisciplinary team members can supplement the nursing home workforce, which can improve care (Gage et al., 2016; Hwang et al., 2014). Issues related to the inappropriate use of hospice and poor-quality care, particularly for nursing home residents, have increased over the past decade (Chiedi, 2018; MedPAC, 2020; OIG, 2018). Policy makers have paid particular attention to the increase in hospice use in nursing homes, expressing concern that for-profit hospice agencies were aggressively targeting more profitable, long-stay patients (Chiedi, 2018). An investigation by HHS OIG found that hospices do not always provide the services that residents need, such as for pain management, and that in many cases poor-quality care was provided. OIG also cited communication and information gaps that prevented residents and their families and caregivers from making informed decisions about their care. Furthermore, the investigation identified cases of inappropriate billing for higher levels of care than needed and a number of fraud schemes. The current payment system for hospice care creates incentives for hospices to seek out beneficiaries who do not have complex care needs. Hospice is paid on a per diem basis for each day an individual is in hospice, regardless of the quantity or quality of services provided (Chiedi, 2018).

Another trend that raises questions is the growing proportion of nursing homes and hospice agencies that are owned by the same company, coupled with the increasing proportion of nursing home residents receiving hospice services from these providers (Canavan et al., 2013; Stevenson et al., 2020). Co-ownership represents a potential conflict of interest in that residents may be referred to hospice inappropriately to bolster revenue for the hospice agency that is co-owned by the nursing home (usually a for-profit corporation). In addition, co-ownership may limit consumer choice if the nursing home or hospice does not inform residents and family decision makers that they can choose which hospice they want to receive care from. There may also be pressure from the corporate entity for nursing homes to limit contracts with outside hospice agencies (Ersek et al., 2022; Stevenson and Bramson, 2009; Stevenson et al., 2020).

Palliative care consultants In the second model of end-of-life care, nursing homes contract with external palliative care consultation teams to provide specialized, onsite palliative care services. Consultation teams can be an extension of existing hospital-based teams, outpatient or hospice teams, or independent practitioners. Depending on the team and its resources, consultations focus on symptom management, advance care planning (Box 4-8), or assisting with prognostication or hospice entry. Staff or leadership identify the need for a consultation, which the resident's primary care provider then requests. The consultant bills under Medicare Part B, and thus the nursing home does not incur any costs for these services.

A nationally representative study found that 34 percent of nursing homes reported having an arrangement with external specialty palliative care consultants (Schwartz et al., 2019). Nursing homes that had these arrangements were 40 percent more likely to perform above the median on an end-of-life culture change index compared with those without any external or internal palliative care services. Other studies have found that external palliative care consultation is associated with better end-of-life outcomes, such as fewer emergency department visits and hospitalizations in the last months of life and lower likelihood of late admission to hospice (i.e., less than 3 days before death) (Miller et al., 2016a, 2017).

One challenge with this model is the need for consulting practitioners to understand the nursing home environment and to recognize that certain interventions used in other settings may not be used in nursing home settings. Certain palliative care medications, for instance, are not included in nursing home formularies. Moreover, there may be significant limitations in nursing home settings in terms of the ability to administer and titrate pain medication such as intravenous opioids. Another challenge is that implementing consultants' recommendations depends on the primary care provider's and nursing home staff's willingness to accept and implement palliative care recommendations (CAPC, 2008). More broadly, some have pointed to the relatively low reimbursement of these Part B services as a major barrier to their broader use (IOM, 2015).

Facility-based palliative care programs The third model for palliative care delivery in nursing homes is through facility-based programs (Ersek and Wilson, 2003). This model, sometimes referred to as primary palliative care, is promising in that it does not solely rely on access to specialists, it eliminates the challenges of joint management among multiple organizations, and it provides flexibility in how individual facilities implement such teams (Carlson et al., 2011). Furthermore, this model places the expertise and authority with the nursing home itself, which is responsible and held accountable for residents' quality of care (Huskamp et al., 2010a). In a 2004 survey, 27 percent of nursing homes reported having a special program or specially trained staff for hospice or palliative/end-of-life care (Miller and Han, 2008). In a 2016 survey, some 40 percent of nursing homes' directors of nursing reported having a palliative care program; however, the study sample was small and not representative of all U.S. nursing homes (Lester et al., 2016).

Although growing numbers of facilities indicate that they have implemented internal palliative care services, the composition, scope, and

> **BOX 4-8**
> **Advance Care Planning**
>
> Advance care planning (ACP) involves discussing and documenting a patient's values, goals of care, and preferences for future treatment in light of those values and goals, as well as identifying a proxy decision maker. In doing so, advance care planning honors patients' rights, aligns with person-directed care, and increases the likelihood that care received is concordant with care preferences (Hickman et al., 2011, 2020; Miller et al., 2020; Tark et al., 2020a).
>
> Documenting patient preferences take several forms, the most common of which are advance directives, which include naming a surrogate decision maker through a durable power of attorney for health care, and a living will, which identifies choices around specific treatments such as cardiopulmonary resuscitation, mechanical ventilation or antibiotic therapy, or general approaches to care (e.g., comfort-focused versus aggressive, life-prolonging therapies). Treatment preferences for seriously ill patients also can be expressed via a do not resuscitate (DNR) order or a state-authorized portable order, e.g., physicians order for life-sustaining treatment (POLST). These orders differ from advance directives in that they are medical orders that are immediately actionable. In contrast, preferences documented in a living will must be interpreted in light of the patient's current clinical context and translated into medical orders and formal plans of care (NIA, 2018).
>
> As with other health care organizations, nursing homes must notify individuals entering their facility of their right to execute an advance directive (CMS, 2012). The prevalence of advance care planning conversations and documentation in nursing homes is unclear, as there is no standardized measure or required reporting across nursing facilities (the Advance Directive item on the MDS 2.0 was eliminated in the currently mandated MDS 3.0). However, research suggests that approximately 58 to 65 percent of nursing home residents have at least one advance directive on record (Jones et al., 2011; Tjia et al., 2018). Other evidence suggests that the most common advance directives in nursing homes are durable powers of attorney for health care and DNR orders were the most common documented treatment preference (Galambos et al., 2016). In Maryland, where a state

activities of these programs are not well characterized. Generally, they encompass one or more of the following features:

- Implementing specific policies related to palliative care (e.g., the identification of residents who might benefit from this approach);
- Regular, robust advance care planning;
- Standardized symptom assessment and management;
- Training the staff to increase their palliative care knowledge and skills; or
- Creating interdisciplinary palliative care teams and establishing specialty palliative care units (Carpenter et al., 2020; Ersek et al., 2014).

> order completion is required upon admission to a nursing home, investigators found that 84 percent of residents had an order in the medical record (Tarzian and Cheevers, 2017). It should be noted, however, that requiring an order be completed runs counter to the POLST paradigm, which asserts that completion of an advance directive must always be voluntary (Hickman and Critser, 2018).
>
> Despite the benefits of ACP for persons receiving care in nursing homes, there are concerns. First, the quality of advance care planning in nursing homes is largely unstudied, but existing evidence suggests that there is great variability. Particular concerns include problems with providers communicating insufficient or inaccurate information about prognosis, treatment options, and legal requirements for ACP documents and failing to engage in robust shared decision-making approaches. (Goossens et al., 2020; Hickman et al., 2017; Kim et al., 2019). There also is evidence that goals of care conversations often are limited to discussions about CPR (Hickman et al., 2021). Second, many nursing home residents, particularly those with cognitive impairment, are excluded from advance care planning conversations despite their desire to be engaged and ability to voice treatment preferences (Miller et al., 2016b). Third, non-White and Hispanic patients are less likely to have complete advance directives and documented care preferences (Frahm et al., 2012; Jones et al., 2011). Fourth, there is evidence of mismatches between documented preferences and care received, particularly for "do not hospitalize" orders (Nemiroff et al., 2019). Finally, a recent study conducted in nursing homes was unable to show a robust association between ACP and goal-concordant care or quality of life (Mitchell et al., 2020).
>
> The SARS-CoV-2 pandemic underscored the urgency of ACP while also exacerbating barriers to conducting goals of care conversations and documenting treatment preferences. The high COVID-19 mortality rates among nursing home residents have led to calls for increased ACP discussions, regular review of existing documentation of preferences, and the use of COVID-specific ACP approaches and documents (Bender et al., 2021; Gaur et al., 2020; Ye et al., 2021). Because of ongoing restrictions in family visitation and in-person provider interactions with residents, there have also been calls for expansion of telehealth options for ACP (Bender et al., 2021).

However, there is great variability between programs and no assurances that the care provided by a particular nursing home meets commonly accepted palliative care standards. Moreover, there are no nationally recognized and agreed-upon standards and quality measures for nursing home–based palliative care services, although some efforts have been made to identify such guidelines (Temkin-Greener et al., 2015).

Several studies have examined the benefits of nursing home–based palliative care services. One study found a decrease in the use of unnecessary medications following admission of residents to a nursing home–based palliative care unit (Suhrie et al., 2009). Research has shown that specialized dementia "comfort care" units are associated with higher staff satisfaction, less observed resident discomfort, and lower costs than standard nursing home care (Kovach et al., 1996). A systematic review of facility-based palliative care programs (Carpenter et al., 2020) found that overall, study quality was generally low and that the results of the different studies were mixed, with some evidence that facility-based palliative care teams can decrease rehospitalizations of patients at skilled nursing facilities (Berkowitz et al., 2011), reduce emergency department visits (Comart et al., 2013), decrease agitation and pain (Chapman and Toseland, 2007), and demonstrate cost savings (Teo et al., 2014). Evidence for enhanced symptom assessment, documentation, and management and engagement in advance care planning was weak (Strumpf et al., 2004). Given the weakness of the evidence, the study's authors concluded that further research is needed to determine the effectiveness of facility-based palliative care programs (Carpenter et al., 2020).

A major barrier to developing internal nursing home palliative care services is the required financial and human resources. The need to train staff and the additional time necessary to deliver high-quality palliative care are other barriers. High turnover among staff and leadership at nursing homes also threaten the long-term viability of facility-based palliative care teams and programs (Meier et al., 2010). As noted, the evidence base for this model is particularly weak, and little is known about the most effective components and approaches for implementing and sustaining facility-based palliative care and hospice services. Moreover, there are limited financial incentives to provide high-quality palliative care, since the highest reimbursement rates are for post-acute, skilled care (Carlson et al., 2011; Ersek and Carpenter, 2013; Ersek et al., 2014; National Consensus Project for Quality Palliative Care, 2018). Specific measures added to Care Compare would support improved monitoring of the quality of palliative care services provided in nursing home settings (see Chapter 3).

Challenges to Providing Quality, Equitable End-of-Life Care to Nursing Home Residents

There is a wide variation in palliative care services provided by nursing homes (Tark et al., 2020b). In addition to the barriers and limiting factors outlined above, an overarching challenge to providing quality end-of-life care in nursing homes is the pervasive disparities in care. A systematic review (Estrada et al., 2021) revealed that racial and ethnic minority residents had lower rates of completion of advance directives, were more likely to be hospitalized at the end of life, and reported higher levels of pain and less use of hospice care at the end of life than White residents (Araw et al., 2014; Cai et al., 2016; Frahm et al., 2012, 2015; Huskamp et al., 2010b; Lage et al., 2020; Lepore et al., 2011; Monroe and Carter, 2010; Tjia et al., 2018; Zheng et al., 2011).

The review pointed out that the majority of the studies relied on data that were more than 10 years old and thus do not accurately reflect the current diversity of nursing home populations. The review also concluded that more culturally competent research is needed to explore not only the experiences of racial and ethnic minorities at the end of life, but also to characterize the specific barriers to high-quality end-of-life care in nursing homes faced by racial and ethnic minority residents (Estrada et al., 2021). The disproportionate impact of the COVID-19 pandemic on nursing home residents in general, and on racial and ethnic minorities in particular, calls for palliative care interventions. As Rosa and colleagues (2021) explain:

> Palliative care health equity frameworks promote assessment of the social and moral determinants of health as well as systemic injustices to tailor services to the individual, context, and culture at hand.

This is also relevant for other minority populations in nursing homes, such as LGBTQ+ residents who could benefit from "inclusive palliative care practices that foster trust, transparency and value-concordant care delivery" (Rosa et al., 2021).

MODELS OF CARE DELIVERY

This chapter has provided an overview of the wide-ranging needs of nursing home residents and the associated complexity of the care challenges faced by nursing homes in addressing those needs. Research on best practices related to clinical, behavioral, and psychosocial care delivery in nursing homes is relatively scarce, however (Andrusjak et al., 2020; Carpenter et al., 2020; Ersek and Jablonski, 2014; NASEM, 2021; van der Wolf et al., 2019). A robust evidence base on specific models of care delivery that could serve as the most effective approach to providing high-quality person-centered care to all nursing home residents, while ensuring equitable care, has yet to be developed.

Moreover, nursing homes are often not well connected to the communities in which they are located, nor to the broader health care system (Lane and McGrady, 2016; Orth et al., 2019). Research that examines models of care that strengthen ties to the broader community and all sectors of the broader health care system is needed to improve these connections. Finally, research on care delivery needs to focus on the specific factors that affect care directly, such as optimal staffing, physical environment, financing and payment, technology, leadership, and organizational policy. Once research has successfully identified the most effective care models, that research should be translated into practice by launching demonstration projects, designed with an eye toward sustainability, to test specific models in nursing home settings.

KEY FINDINGS AND CONCLUSIONS

- The intensity of care needs is as varied as each individual nursing home resident and requires a broad range of resources and staffing.
- The care plan is critical to the identification of residents' needs, goals, and care preferences and documenting and communicating these preferences with the interdisciplinary team are central to person-centered care.
- Despite their key role, many nursing homes are not meeting care plan requirements.
- Nursing homes are required by law to provide a range of services including medical, nursing, mental and behavioral health, psychosocial care, oral health, among other services, but many residents are not receiving adequate care.
- Despite regulatory oversight and industry reforms, the care for nursing home residents often falls short due to several factors:
    - Delivery of care by inadequately trained staff,
    - Hierarchical structures that impede cohesive team building and functioning,
    - Inadequate staffing and high staff and leadership turnover,
    - Providing care that is not aligned with evidence-based best practices,
    - Need to provide care to meet the complex and evolving needs of residents,
    - The lack of health information technology support for care coordination,
    - Infrequent visits and limited involvement of medical directors and primary care providers, and
    - Regulations that incentivize care that is not aligned with the residents' goals and preferences.
- The lack of culturally sensitive assessments and treatment practices contribute to disparities in care and unmet needs experienced by minority populations.
- Psychosocial needs are highly ranked in most studies of unmet needs among nursing home residents.
- The number of residents with mental health needs is increasing, and the mental health needs of many residents remain unmet.
- Further research is needed to identify effective service arrangements and the requisite composition of staff to provide adequate behavioral health care in nursing homes.

- Inadequate access to behavioral health services occurs in both lower- and higher-rated facilities. Moreover, access to such services is not necessarily affected by for-profit status or the size of the facility. Some of the most commonly cited reasons for inadequate access include a lack of staff education, inadequate staffing, and inadequate infrastructure.
- Additional research needs to be conducted on the development of environments that provide nonstigmatizing specialized care that is accepting and supportive of individuals with behavioral health needs, with special attention paid to the well-being of residents.
- Dementia care practice needs to focus on the individual's condition, needs, and desires, based on knowing the person, recognizing and accepting the person's reality, identifying and supporting opportunities for meaningful engagement, building and nurturing authentic caring relationships, and creating and maintaining a supportive community for individuals, family, and staff.
- There is great variability among palliative care programs in nursing homes.
- There are no nationally recognized and agreed-upon standards and quality measures for nursing home–based palliative care services.
- Barriers to the development and viability of facility-based palliative care include
  - Lack of financial and human resources,
  - The need for staff training,
  - Additional time needed to deliver such care, and
  - High turnover of staff and leadership.
- The evidence base for best practices for behavioral and psychosocial care and palliative care delivery in nursing home settings is particularly weak, and little is known about the most effective components and approaches for implementing and sustaining facility-based services.
- Research is needed to identify specific models of high-quality nursing home care, which would then inform demonstration projects to test the effectiveness of care models in nursing homes.

REFERENCES

Abraham, S. 2011. Fall prevention conceptual framework. *Health Care Manager* 30(2):179–184.

Achterberg, W., S. Lautenbacher, B. Husebo, A. Erdal, and K. Herr. 2019. Pain in dementia. *Pain Reports* 5(1):e803.

Adams-Wendling, L., U. Piamjariyakul, M. Bott, and R. L. Taunton. 2008. Strategies for translating the resident care plan into daily practice. *Journal of Gerontological Nursing* 34(8):50–56.

Agarwal, K. 2021. *Failure to thrive in older adults: Management.* https://www.uptodate.com/contents/failure-to-thrive-in-older-adults-management (accessed January 20, 2022).

Ahmed, T., and N. Haboubi. 2010. Assessment and management of nutrition in older people and its importance to health. *Clinical Interventions in Aging* 5:207–216.

Al Shamsi, H., A. G. Almutairi, S. Al Mashrafi, and T. Al Kalbani. 2020. Implications of language barriers for healthcare: A systematic review. *Oman Medical Hournal* 35(2):e122.

Alexander, G. L., and R. W. Madsen. 2021. A report of information technology and health deficiencies in U.S. nursing homes. *Journal of Patient Safety* 17(6):e483–e489.

Alexander, G. L., R. W. Madsen, E. L. Miller, D. S. Wakefield, K. K. Wise, and R. L. Alexander. 2017. The state of nursing home information technology sophistication in rural and nonrural U.S. markets. *Journal of Rural Health* 33(3):266–274.

Alexander, G. L., K. R. Powell, and C. B. Deroche. 2020a. An evaluation of telehealth expansion in U.S. nursing homes. *Journal of the American Medical Informatics Association* 28(2):342–348.

Alexander, G. L., C. Deroche, K. Powell, A. S. M. Mosa, L. Popejoy, and R. Koopman. 2020b. Forecasting content and stage in a nursing home information technology maturity instrument using a Delphi method. *Journal of Medical Systems* 44(3):60.

Allen, R. S., G. M. Harris, L. D. Burgio, C. B. Azuero, L. A. Miller, H. J. Shin, M. K. Eichorst, E. L. Csikai, J. DeCoster, L. L. Dunn, E. Kvale, and P. Parmelee. 2014. Can senior volunteers deliver reminiscence and creative activity interventions? Results of the Legacy Intervention Family Enactment randomized controlled trial. *Journal of Pain and Symptom Management* 48(4):590–601.

Alzheimer's Association. 2009. *Dementia care practice recommendations for assisted living residences and nursing homes.* Chicago, IL: Alzheimer's Association.

Alzheimer's Association. 2018. *Dementia care practice recommendations.* https://www.alz.org/professionals/professional-providers/dementia_care_practice_recommendations (accessed October 21, 2021).

Alzheimer's Association. 2021a. *2021 Alzheimer's disease facts and figures: Special report—Race, ethnicity and Alzheimer's in America.* Chicago, IL: Alzheimer's Association.

Alzheimer's Association. 2021b. *Types of dementia.* https://www.alz.org/alzheimers-dementia/what-is-dementia/types-of-dementia (accessed November 4, 2021).

Andersson, S., K. Årestedt, O. Lindqvist, C.-J. Fürst, and M. Brännström. 2018. Factors associated with symptom relief in end-of-life care in residential care homes: A national register-based study. *Journal of Pain and Symptom Management* 55(5):1304–1312.

Andrusjak, W., A. Barbosa, and G. Mountain. 2020. Identifying and managing hearing and vision loss in older people in care homes: A scoping review of the evidence. *The Gerontologist* 60(3):e155–e168.

Araw, A. C., A. M. Araw, R. Pekmezaris, C. N. Nouryan, C. Sison, B. Tommasulo, and G. P. Wolf-Klein. 2014. Medical orders for life-sustaining treatment: Is it time yet? *Palliative & Supportive Care* 12(2):101–105.

Aschbrenner, K., D. C. Grabowski, S. Cai, S. J. Bartels, and V. Mor. 2011. Nursing home admissions and long-stay conversions among persons with and without serious mental illness. *Journal of Aging & Social Policy* 23(3):286–304.

Avila Institute of Gerontology. 2017. *Palliative care: Implementation guide book.* https://static1.squarespace.com/static/59dd966ee45a7c496fd4d1be/t/5db20e165e4b5f0984b5efd3/1571950106099/Palliative-Care-Implementation-Guide-0917-1.pdf (accessed August 23, 2021).

Bäck, I., J. Kallio, S. Perälä, and K. Mäkelä. 2012. Remote monitoring of nursing home residents using a humanoid robot. *Journal of Telemedicine and Telecare* 18(6):357–361.

Bailey, R. K., H. L. Blackmon, and F. L. Stevens. 2009. Major depressive disorder in the African American population: Meeting the challenges of stigma, misdiagnosis, and treatment disparities. *JAMA* 101(11):1084–1089.

Bainbridge, K. E., and V. Ramachandran. 2014. Hearing aid use among older U.S. adults; the National Health and Nutrition Examination Survey, 2005–2006 and 2009–2010. *Ear and Hearing* 35(3):289–294.

Bartels, S. J., G. S. Moak, and A. R. Dums. 2002. Mental health services in nursing homes: Models of mental health services in nursing homes: A review of the literature. *Psychiatric Services* 53(11):1390–1396.

Basinska, K., P. Kunzler-Heule, R. A. Guerbaai, F. Zuniga, M. Simon, N. I. H. Wellens, C. Serdaly, and D. Nicca. 2021. Residents' and relatives' experiences of acute situations: A qualitative study to inform a care model. *The Gerontologist* 61(7):1041–1052.

Batchelor-Murphy, M., S. M. Kennerly, S. D. Horn, R. Barrett, N. Bergstrom, L. Boss, and T. L. Yap. 2019. Impact of cognition and handfeeding assistance on nutritional intake for nursing home residents. *Journal of Nutrition in Gerontology and Geriatrics* 38(3):262–276.

Bayoumi, M. 2012. Identification of the needs of haemodialysis patients using the concept of Maslow's hierarchy of needs. *Journal of Renal Care* 38(1):43–49.

Beck, C., K. J. Gately, S. Lubin, P. Moody, and C. Beverly. 2014. Building a state coalition for nursing home excellence. *The Gerontologist* 54(Suppl 1):S87–S97.

Becker, M., R. Andel, T. Boaz, and T. Howell. 2009. The association of individual and facility characteristics with psychiatric hospitalization among nursing home residents. *International Journal of Geriatric Psychiatry* 24(3):261–268.

Behrens, L., K. Van Haitsma, J. Brush, M. Boltz, D. Volpe, and A. M. Kolanowski. 2018. Negotiating risky preferences in nursing homes: A case study of the Rothschild person-centered care planning approach. *Journal of Gerontological Nursing* 44(8):11–17.

Bekkema, N., A. Niemeijer, B. Frederiks, and C. de Schipper. 2021. Exploring restrictive measures using action research: A participative observational study by nursing staff in nursing homes. *Journal of Advanced Nursing* 77(6):2785–2795.

Bender, M., K. N. Huang, and J. Raetz. 2021. Advance care planning during the COVID-19 pandemic. *Journal of the American Board of Family Medicine* 34(Suppl):S16–S20.

Bennett, C. 1980. *Nursing home life: What it is and what it could be*, 1st ed. New York: Tiresias Press, Inc.

Berkowitz, R. E., R. N. Jones, R. Rieder, M. Bryan, R. Schreiber, S. Verney, and M. K. Paasche-Orlow. 2011. Improving disposition outcomes for patients in a geriatric skilled nursing facility. *Journal of the American Geriatrics Society* 59(6):1130–1136.

Bern-Klug, M., K. W. Kramer, P. Sharr, and I. Cruz. 2010. Nursing home social services directors' opinions about the number of residents they can serve. *Journal of Aging and Social Policy* 22(1):33–52.

Berridge, C., and V. Mor. 2018. Disparities in the prevalence of unmet needs and their consequences among black and white older adults. *Journal of Aging and Health* 30(9):1427–1449.

Bhattacharya, S., and R. K. Mishra. 2015. Pressure ulcers: Current understanding and newer modalities of treatment. *Indian Journal of Plastic Surgery: Official Publication of the Association of Plastic Surgeons of India* 48(1):4–16.

Bhattacharyya, K. K., V. Molinari, and K. Hyer. 2021. Self-reported satisfaction of older adult residents in nursing homes: Development of a conceptual framework. *The Gerontologist*. https://doi.org/10.1093/geront/gnab061.

Boscart, V., L. E. Crutchlow, L. Sheiban Taucar, K. Johnson, M. Heyer, M. Davey, A. P. Costa, and G. Heckman. 2020. Chronic disease management models in nursing homes: A scoping review. *BMJ Open* 10(2):e032316.

Bowen, S. E., and S. Zimmerman. 2008. Understanding and improving psychosocial services in long-term care. *Health Care Financing Review* 30(2):1–4.

Brauner, D., R. M. Werner, T. P. Shippee, J. Cursio, H. Sharma, and R. T. Konetzka. 2018. Does Nursing Home Compare reflect patient safety in nursing homes? *Health Affairs (Project Hope)* 37(11):1770–1778.

Brennan, P. L., and S. SooHoo. 2019. Effects of mental health disorders on nursing home residents' nine-month pain trajectories. *Pain Medicine* 21(3):488–500.

Burke, R. E., and R. M. Werner. 2019. Quality measurement and nursing homes: Measuring what matters. *BMJ Quality & Safety* 28(7):520–523.

Burke, R. E., Y. Xu, and A. Z. Ritter. 2021. Outcomes of post-acute care in skilled nursing facilities in Medicare beneficiaries with and without a diagnosis of dementia. *Journal of the American Geriatrics Society* 69(10):2899–2907.

Burns, B. J., and C. A. Taube. 1990. Mental health services in general medical care and in nursing homes. In B. S. Fogel, A. Furino, and G. L. Gottlieb (eds.), *Mental health policy for older Americans: Protecting minds at risk*. Arlington, VA: American Psychiatric Association. Pp. 63–84.

Cai, S., S. C. Miller, and D. B. Mukamel. 2016. Racial differences in hospitalizations of dying Medicare–Medicaid dually eligible nursing home residents. *Journal of the American Geriatrics Society* 64(9):1798–1805.

Calkins, M., and J. Brush. 2016. Honoring individual choice in long-term residential communities when it involves risk: A person-centered approach. *Journal of Gerontological Nursing* 42(8):12–17.

Canavan, M. E., M. D. Aldridge Carlson, H. L. Sipsma, and E. H. Bradley. 2013. Hospice for nursing home residents: Does ownership type matter? *Journal of Palliative Medicine* 16(10):1221–1226.

Cantor, M., C. Liu, M. Wong, J. Chiang, D. Polakoff, and J. Dave. 2020. *Reducing COVID-19 deaths in nursing homes: Call to action*. https://www.healthaffairs.org/do/10.1377/hblog20200522.474405/full (accessed February 25, 2021).

CAPC (Center to Advance Palliative Care). 2008. *Improving palliative care in nursing homes*. New York: CAPC. https://www.capc.org (accessed April 26, 2021).

Carlson, M. D. A., B. Lim, and D. E. Meier. 2011. Strategies and innovative models for delivering palliative care in nursing homes. *Journal of the American Medical Directors Association* 12(2):91–98.

Carpenter, B. D., K. Van Haitsma, K. Ruckdeschel, and M. P. Lawton. 2000. The psychosocial preferences of older adults: A pilot examination of content and structure. *The Gerontologist* 40(3):335–348.

Carpenter, J. G. 2020. Forced to choose: When Medicare policy disrupts end-of-life care. *Journal of Aging and Social Policy* 1–8.

Carpenter, J. G., K. Lam, A. Z. Ritter, and M. Ersek. 2020. A systematic review of nursing home palliative care interventions: Characteristics and outcomes. *Journal of the American Medical Directors Association* 21(5):583–596.e2.

Castle, N. G., and R. A. Anderson. 2011. Caregiver staffing in nursing homes and their influence on quality of care: Using dynamic panel estimation methods. *Medical Care* 49(6):545–552.

Castle, N. G., and J. Engberg. 2007. The influence of staffing characteristics on quality of care in nursing homes. *Health Services Research* 42(5):1822–1847.

Castle, N. G., and M. Lin. 2010. Top management turnover and quality in nursing homes. *Health Care Management Review* 35(2):161–174.

Castle, N. G., J. Engberg, and A. Men. 2007. Nursing home staff turnover: Impact on nursing home compare quality measures. *The Gerontologist* 47(5):650–661.

Chapman, D. G., and R. W. Toseland. 2007. Effectiveness of advanced illness care teams for nursing home residents with dementia. *Social Work* 52(4):321–329.

Chen, J., C. D. Mullins, P. Novak, and S. B. Thomas. 2016. Personalized strategies to activate and empower patients in health care and reduce health disparities. *Health Education & Behavior* 43(1):25–34.

Chen, Y.-M., and J.-Y. Ji. 2015. Effects of horticultural therapy on psychosocial health in older nursing home residents: A preliminary study. *Journal of Nursing Research* 23(3):167–171.

Chiedi, J. M. 2018. *Vulnerabilities in the Medicare hospice program affect quality care and program integrity: An OIG portfolio.* https://oig.hhs.gov/oei/reports/oei-02-16-00570.asp (accessed February 25, 2021).

Chien, W., and F. R. Lin. 2012. Prevalence of hearing aid use among older adults in the United States. *Archives of Internal Medicine* 172(3):292–293.

Ching-Teng, Y., Y. Ya-Ping, and C. Yu-Chia. 2019. Positive effects of art therapy on depression and self-esteem of older adults in nursing homes. *Social Work in Health Care* 58(3):324–338.

Chisholm, L., N. J. Zhang, K. Hyer, R. Pradhan, L. Unruh, and F.-C. Lin. 2018. Culture change in nursing homes: What is the role of nursing home resources? *Inquiry* 55:46958018787043.

CMS (Centers for Medicare & Medicaid Services). 2012. *Memorandum: F tag 155—Advance directives—Advance copy.* https://www.cms.gov/medicare/provider-enrollment-and-certification/surveycertificationgeninfo/downloads/survey-and-cert-letter-12-47.pdf (accessed February 25, 2021).

CMS. 2015. *Nursing home data compendium.* Baltimore, MD: Centers for Medicare & Medicaid Services.

CMS. 2017. *State operations manual appendix PP—Guidance to surveyors for long term care facilities.* https://www.cms.gov/Medicare/Provider-Enrollment-and-Certification/GuidanceforLawsAndRegulations/Downloads/Appendix-PP-State-Operations-Manual.pdf (accessed March 26, 2021).

CMS. 2019a. *Medicare coverage of skilled nursing facility care.* https://www.medicare.gov/Pubs/pdf/10153-Medicare-Skilled-Nursing-Facility-Care.pdf (accessed April 29, 2021).

CMS. 2019b. *Jimmo settlement.* https://www.cms.gov/Center/Special-Topic/Jimmo-Center (accessed April 26, 2021).

CMS. 2020a. *Medicare benefit policy manual, chapter 9—Coverage of hospice services under hospital insurance.* https://www.cms.gov/Regulations-and-guidance/Guidance/Manuals/Downloads/bp102c09.pdf (accessed January 7, 2021).

CMS. 2020b. *Minimum Data Set (MDS) 3.0 for nursing homes and swing bed providers.* https://www.cms.gov/Medicare/Quality-Initiatives-Patient-Assessment-Instruments/NursingHomeQualityInits/NHQIMDS30 (accessed January 23, 2021).

CMS. 2020c. *Medicare hospice benefits.* https://www.medicare.gov/Pubs/pdf/02154-medicare-hospice-benefits.pdf (accessed September 21, 2021).

CMS. 2021a. *COVID-19 emergency declaration blanket waivers for health care providers.* https://www.cms.gov/files/document/covid-19-emergency-declaration-waivers.pdf (accessed January 12, 2022).

CMS. 2021b. *MDS 3.0 frequency report.* https://www.cms.gov/Research-Statistics-Data-and-Systems/Computer-Data-and-Systems/Minimum-Data-Set-3-0-Public-Reports/Minimum-Data-Set-3-0-Frequency-Report (accessed February 15, 2022).

CMS. 2021c. *Frequently asked questions (FAQS) regarding Jimmo settlement agreement.* https://www.cms.gov/Center/Special-Topic/Jimmo-Settlement/FAQs (accessed January 24, 2022).

Cohen-Mansfield, J., M. Dakheel-Ali, M. S. Marx, K. Thein, and N. G. Regier. 2015. Which unmet needs contribute to behavior problems in persons with advanced dementia? *Psychiatry Research* 228(1):59–64.

Coleman, P., and N. M. Watson. 2006. Oral care provided by certified nursing assistants in nursing homes. *Journal of the American Geriatrics Society* 54(1):138–143.

Collier, E., and C. Harrington. 2008. Staffing characteristics, turnover rates, and quality of resident care in nursing facilities. *Research in Gerontological Nursing* 1(3):157–170.

Comart, J., A. Mahler, R. Schreiber, C. Rockett, R. N. Jones, and J. N. Morris. 2013. Palliative care for long-term care residents: Effect on clinical outcomes. *The Gerontologist* 53(5):874–880.

Cooper, C., P. Rapaport, S. Robertson, L. Marston, J. Barber, M. Manela, and G. Livingston. 2018. Relationship between speaking English as a second language and agitation in people with dementia living in care homes: Results from the MARQUE (Managing Agitation and Raising Quality of Life) English national care home survey. *International Journal of Geriatric Psychiatry* 33(3):504–509.

Corbett, A., B. Husebo, M. Malcangio, A. Staniland, J. Cohen-Mansfield, D. Aarsland, and C. Ballard. 2012. Assessment and treatment of pain in people with dementia. *Nature Reviews Neurology* 8(5):264–274.

Crick, M., R. Devey-Burry, J. Hu, D. E. Angus, and C. Backman. 2020. The role of regulation in the care of older people with depression living in long-term care: A systematic scoping review. *BMC Geriatrics* 20(1):273.

Cuevas, P. E., P. Davidson, J. Mejilla, and T. Rodney. 2021. Dignity therapy for end-of-life care patients: A literature review. *Journal of Patient Experience* 8:2374373521996951.

Curry, L. C., C. Walker, M. O. Hogstel, and M. B. Walker. 2007. A study of family councils in nursing homes. *Geriatric Nursing* 28(4):245–253.

Curtis, A., L. Gibson, M. O'Brien, and B. Roe. 2018. Systematic review of the impact of arts for health activities on health, wellbeing and quality of life of older people living in care homes. *Dementia* 17(6):645–669.

Cutler, L. J., and R. A. Kane. 2006. As great as all outdoors. *Journal of Housing for the Elderly* 19(3–4):29–48.

Davila, H., T. P. Shippee, Y. S. Park, D. Brauner, R. M. Werner, and R. T. Konetzka. 2021. Inside the black box of improving on nursing home quality measures. *Medical Care Research and Review* 78(6):758–770.

de Souto Barreto, P., J. E. Morley, W. Chodzko-Zajko, H. P. K, E. Weening-Djiksterhuis, L. Rodriguez-Mañas, M. Barbagallo, E. Rosendahl, A. Sinclair, F. Landi, M. Izquierdo, B. Vellas, and Y. Rolland. 2016. Recommendations on physical activity and exercise for older adults living in long-term care facilities: A taskforce report. *Journal of the American Medical Directors Association* 17(5):381–392.

Degenholtz, H., R. A. Kane, and H. Q. Kivnick. 1997. Care-related preferences and values of elderly community-based LTC consumers: Can case managers learn what's important to clients? *The Gerontologist* 37(6):767–776.

Dellefield, M. E. 2006. Interdisciplinary care planning and the written care plan in nursing homes: A critical review. *The Gerontologist* 46(1):128–133.

Dellefield, M., N. Castle, K. McGilton, and K. Spilsbury. 2015. The relationship between registered nurses and nursing home quality: An integrative review (2008–2014). *Nursing Economics* 33(2):95–108.

Devitt, M., and B. Checkoway. 1982. Participation in nursing home resident councils: Promise and practice. *The Gerontologist* 22(1):49–53.

Doll, G. A., L. J. Cornelison, H. Rath, and M. L. Syme. 2017. Actualizing culture change: The Promoting Excellent Alternatives in Kansas nursing homes (PEAK 2.0) program. *Psychological Services* 14(3):307–315.

Duan, Y., T. P. Shippee, W. Ng, O. Akosionu, M. Woodhouse, H. Chu, J. S. Ahluwalia, J. E. Gaugler, B. A. Virnig, and J. R. Bowblis. 2020. Unmet and unimportant preferences among nursing home residents: What are key resident and facility factors? *Journal of the American Medical Directors Association* 21(11):1712–1717.

Dubeau, C. E., S. E. Simon, and J. N. Morris. 2006. The effect of urinary incontinence on quality of life in older nursing home residents. *Journal of the American Geriatrics Society* 54(9):1325–1333.

Edelman, L. S., J. Drost, R. P. Moone, K. Owens, G. L. Towsley, G. Tucker-Roghi, and J. E. Morley. 2021. Editorial: Applying the age-friendly health system framework to long-term care settings. *Journal of Nutrition, Health, and Aging* 25(2):141–145.

Edemekong, P. F., D. L. Bomgaars, S. Sukumaran, and S. B. Levy. 2021. Activities of daily living. In *StatPearls*. Treasure Island, FL: StatPearls Publishing.

Ersek, M., and J. G. Carpenter. 2013. Geriatric palliative care in long-term care settings with a focus on nursing homes. *Journal of Palliative Medicine* 16(10):1180–1187.

Ersek, M., and A. Jablonski. 2014. A mixed-methods approach to investigating the adoption of evidence-based pain practices in nursing homes. *Journal of Gerontological Nursing* 40(7):52–60.

Ersek, M., and S. A. Wilson. 2003. The challenges and opportunities in providing end-of-life care in nursing homes. *Journal of Palliative Medicine* 6(1):45–57.

Ersek, M., J. Sefcik, and D. Stevenson. 2014. Palliative care in nursing homes. In A. S. Kelley and D. E. Meier (eds.), *Meeting the needs of older adults with serious illness: Clinical, public health, and policy perspectives*. New York: Humana Press. Pp. 73–90.

Ersek, M., K. T. Unroe, J. G. Carpenter, J. G. Cagle, C. E. Stephens, and D. G. Stevenson. 2022. High-quality nursing home and palliative care—one and the same. *Journal of the American Medical Directors Association* 23(2):247–252.

Esteban-Burgos, A. A., M. J. Lozano-Terrón, D. Puente-Fernandez, C. Hueso-Montoro, R. Montoya-Juárez, and M. P. García-Caro. 2021. A new approach to the identification of palliative care needs and advanced chronic patients among nursing home residents. *International Journal of Environmental Research and Public Health* 18(6):3171.

Estrada, L. V., M. Agarwal, and P. W. Stone. 2021. Racial/ethnic disparities in nursing home end-of-life care: A systematic review. *Journal of the American Medical Directors Association* 22(2):279–290.e271.

Fashaw, S. A., K. S. Thomas, E. McCreedy, and V. Mor. 2020. Thirty-year trends in nursing home composition and quality since the passage of the Omnibus Reconciliation Act. *Journal of the American Medical Directors Association* 21(2):233–239.

Fashaw-Walters, S. A., E. McCreedy, J. P. W. Bynum, K. S. Thomas, and T. I. Shireman. 2021. Disproportionate increases in schizophrenia diagnoses among black nursing home residents with ADRD. *Journal of the American Geriatrics Society* 69(12):3623–3630.

Fazio, S., D. Pace, K. Maslow, S. Zimmerman, and B. Kallmyer. 2018. Alzheimer's Association dementia care practice recommendations. *The Gerontologist* 58(Suppl 1):S1–S9.

Flint, L. A., D. J. David, and A. K. Smith. 2019. Rehabbed to death. *New England Journal of Medicine* 380(5):408–409.

Forbes-Thompson, S., B. Gajewski, J. Scott-Cawiezell, and N. Dunton. 2006. An exploration of nursing home organizational processes. *Western Journal of Nursing Research* 28(8):935–954.

Forsgren, E., C. Skott, L. Hartelius, and C. Saldert. 2016. Communicative barriers and resources in nursing homes from the enrolled nurses' perspective: A qualitative interview study. *International Journal of Nursing Studies* 54:112–121.

Frahm, K. A., L. M. Brown, and K. Hyer. 2012. Racial disparities in end-of-life planning and services for deceased nursing home residents. *Journal of the American Medical Directors Association* 13(9):819.e7–819.e11.

Frahm, K. A., L. M. Brown, and K. Hyer. 2015. Racial disparities in receipt of hospice services among nursing home residents. *American Journal of Hospice and Palliative Medicine* 32(2):233–237.

Freedman, V. A., and B. C. Spillman. 2014. The residential continuum from home to nursing home: Size, characteristics and unmet needs of older adults. *Journals of Gerontology, Series B: Psycholocial Sciences* 69(Suppl 1):S42–S50.

Freeman, I. C. 1997. Nursing home politics at the state level and implications for quality: The Minnesota example. *Generations* 21(4):44–48.

Friedrich, S. L. 2021. *Behavioral telemedicine can improve geriatric mental health.* https://www.mcknights.com/marketplace/marketplace-experts/behavioral-telemedicine-can-improve-geriatric-mental-health (accessed October 26, 2021).

Fullerton, C. A., T. G. McGuire, Z. Feng, V. Mor, and D. C. Grabowski. 2009. Trends in mental health admissions to nursing homes, 1999–2005. *Psychiatric Services* 60(7):965–971.

Gage, L. A., K. Washington, D. P. Oliver, R. Kruse, A. Lewis, and G. Demiris. 2016. Family members' experience with hospice in nursing homes. *American Journal of Hospice & Palliative Care* 33(4):354–362.

Galambos, C., J. Starr, M. J. Rantz, and G. F. Petroski. 2016. Analysis of advance directive documentation to support palliative care activities in nursing homes. *Health & Social Work* 41(4):228–234.

Galambos, C., M. Rantz, L. Popejoy, B. Ge, and G. Petroski. 2021. Advance directives in the nursing home setting: An initiative to increase completion and reduce potentially avoidable hospitalizations. *Journal of Social Work in End-of-Life & Palliative Care* 17(1):19–34.

Galik, E., B. Resnick, M. Hammersla, and J. Brightwater. 2013. Optimizing function and physical activity among nursing home residents with dementia: Testing the impact of function-focused care. *The Gerontologist* 54(6):930–943.

Galik, E., B. Resnick, N. Lerner, M. Hammersla, and A. L. Gruber-Baldini. 2015. Function focused care for assisted living residents with dementia. *The Gerontologist* 55(Suppl 1):S13–S26.

Gaugler, J. E. 2005. Family involvement in residential long-term care: A synthesis and critical review. *Aging & Mental Health* 9(2):105–118.

Gaugler, J. E., F. Yu, H. W. Davila, and T. Shippee. 2014. Alzheimer's disease and nursing homes. *Health Affairs (Millwood)* 33(4):650–657.

Gaugler, J. E., T. L. Statz, R. W. Birkeland, K. W. Louwagie, C. M. Peterson, R. Zmora, A. Emery, H. R. McCarron, K. Hepburn, C. J. Whitlatch, M. S. Mittelman, and D. L. Roth. 2020. The residential care transition module: A single-blinded randomized controlled evaluation of a telehealth support intervention for family caregivers of persons with dementia living in residential long-term care. *BMC Geriatrics* 20(1):133.

Gaur, S., N. Pandya, G. Dumyati, D. A. Nace, K. Pandya, and R. L. P. Jump. 2020. A structured tool for communication and care planning in the era of the COVID-19 pandemic. *Journal of the American Medical Directors Association* 21(7):943–947.

Genoe, M. R., and S. L. Dupuis. 2014. The role of leisure within the dementia context. *Dementia* 13(1):33–58.

Gilbert, A. S., S. M. Garratt, L. Kosowicz, J. Ostaszkiewicz, and B. Dow. 2021. Aged care residents' perspectives on quality of care in care homes: A systematic review of qualitative evidence. *Research on Aging* 43(7–8):294–310.

Gillespie, S. M., L. J. Gleason, J. Karuza, and M. N. Shah. 2010. Health care providers' opinions on communication between nursing homes and emergency departments. *Journal of the American Medical Directors Association* 11(3):204–210.

Goddard, C., P. Speck, P. Martin, and S. Hall. 2013. Dignity therapy for older people in care homes: A qualitative study of the views of residents and recipients of "generativity" documents. *Journal of Advanced Nursing* 69(1):122–132.

Goossens, B., A. Sevenants, A. Declercq, and C. Van Audenhove. 2020. Shared decision-making in advance care planning for persons with dementia in nursing homes: A cross-sectional study. *BMC Geriatrics* 20(1):381.

Gozalo, P. L., and S. C. Miller. 2007. Hospice enrollment and evaluation of its causal effect on hospitalization of dying nursing home patients. *Health Services Research* 42(2):587–610.

Grabowski, D. C., K. A. Aschbrenner, Z. Feng, and V. Mor. 2009. Mental illness in nursing homes: Variations across states. *Health Affairs (Millwood)* 28(3):689–700.

Grabowski, D. C., K. A. Aschbrenner, V. F. Rome, and S. J. Bartels. 2010. Quality of mental health care for nursing home residents: A literature review. *Medical Care Research and Review* 67(6):627–656.

Grabowski, D. C., A. Elliot, B. Leitzell, L. W. Cohen, and S. Zimmerman. 2014a. Who are the innovators? Nursing homes implementing culture change. *The Gerontologist* 54(Suppl 1): S65–S75.

Grabowski, D. C., A. J. O'Malley, C. C. Afendulis, D. J. Caudry, A. Elliot, and S. Zimmerman. 2014b. Culture change and nursing home quality of care. *The Gerontologist* 54(Suppl 1): S35–S45.

Graham, J. 2019. *How to find and use new federal ratings for rehab services at nursing homes.* https://khn.org/news/how-to-find-and-use-new-federal-ratings-for-rehab-services-at-nursing-homes (accessed April 26, 2021).

Greene, C., J. Wilson, A. Tingle, and H. Loveday. 2019. Practical solutions for optimising hydration in care home residents. *Nursing Times* 115(9):30–33.

Groom, L. L., M. M. McCarthy, A. W. Stimpfel, and A. A. Brody. 2021. Telemedicine and telehealth in nursing homes: An integrative review. *Journal of the American Medical Directors Association* 22(9):1784–1801.

Hado, E., and L. Friss Feinberg. 2020. Amid the COVID-19 pandemic, meaningful communication between family caregivers and residents of long-term care facilities is imperative. *Journal of Aging and Social Policy* 32(4–5):410–415.

Hale, A., L. M. Haverhals, C. Manheim, and C. Levy. 2018. Vet Connect: A quality improvement program to provide telehealth subspecialty care for veterans residing in VA-contracted community nursing homes. *Geriatrics* 3(3):57.

Hall, S., C. Goddard, P. Speck, and I. J. Higginson. 2013. "It makes me feel that I'm still relevant": A qualitative study of the views of nursing home residents on dignity therapy and taking part in a phase II randomised controlled trial of a palliative care psychotherapy. *Palliative Medicine* 27(4):358–366.

Hanson, L. C., and M. Ersek. 2010. Meeting palliative care needs in post-acute care settings: "To help them live until they die." In S. J. McPhee, M. A. Winker, M. W. Rabow, S. Z. Pantilat, and A. J. Markowitz (eds.), *Care at the close of life: Evidence and experience.* New York: McGraw-Hill. Pp. 513–521.

Hanson, L. C., S. Sengupta, and M. Slubicki. 2005. Access to nursing home hospice: Perspectives of nursing home and hospice administrators. *Journal of Palliative Medicine* 8(6):1207–1213.

Harrington, C., H. Carrillo, R. Garfield, and E. Squires. 2018. *Nursing facilities, staffing, residents and facility deficiencies, 2009 through 2016.* https://www.kff.org/medicaid/report/nursing-facilities-staffing-residents-and-facility-deficiencies-2009-through-2016 (accessed October 22, 2020).

Harris-Kojetin, L., M. Sengupta, J. P. Lendon, V. Rome, R. Valverde, and C. Caffrey. 2019. *Long-term care providers and services users in the United States, 2015–2016.* https://www.cdc.gov/nchs/data/series/sr_03/sr03_43-508.pdf (accessed April 26, 2021).

Henskens, M., I. M. Nauta, M. C. A. van Eekeren, and E. J. A. Scherder. 2018. Effects of physical activity in nursing home residents with dementia: A randomized controlled trial. *Dementia and Geriatric Cognitive Disorders* 46(1–2):60–80.

Herr, M., J.-J. Arvieu, P. Aegerter, J.-M. Robine, and J. Ankri. 2014. Unmet health care needs of older people: Prevalence and predictors in a French cross-sectional survey. *European Journal of Public Health* 24(5):808–813.

Hickman, S. E., and R. Critser. 2018. National standards and state variation in physician orders for life-sustaining treatment forms. *Journal of Palliative Medicine* 21(7):978–986.

Hickman, S. E., C. A. Nelson, A. H. Moss, S. W. Tolle, N. A. Perrin, and B. J. Hammes. 2011. The consistency between treatments provided to nursing facility residents and orders on the physician orders for life-sustaining treatment form. *Journal of the American Geriatrics Society* 59(11):2091–2099.

Hickman, S. E., B. J. Hammes, A. M. Torke, R. L. Sudore, and G. A. Sachs. 2017. The quality of physician orders for life-sustaining treatment decisions: A pilot study. *Journal of Palliative Medicine* 20(2):155–162.

Hickman, S. E., A. M. Torke, G. A. Sachs, R. L. Sudore, Q. Tang, G. Bakoyannis, N. H. Smith, A. L. Myers, and B. J. Hammes. 2020. Do life-sustaining treatment orders match patient and surrogate preferences? The role of POLST. *Journal of General Internal Medicine* 36(2):413–421.

Hickman, S. E., K. Steinberg, J. Carney, and H. D. Lum. 2021. POLST is more than a code status order form: Suggestions for appropriate POLST use in long-term care. *Journal of the American Medical Directors Association* 22(8):1672–1677.

Hirst, S. P. 2002. Defining resident abuse within the culture of long-term care institutions. *Clinical Nursing Research* 11(3):267–284.

Hoben, M., H. Hu, T. Xiong, A. Kent, N. Kobagi, and M. N. Yoon. 2016. Barriers and facilitators in providing oral health care to nursing home residents, from the perspective of care aides—A systematic review protocol. *Systematic Reviews* 5:53.

Horn, S. D., S. A. Bender, M. L. Ferguson, R. J. Smout, N. Bergstrom, G. Taler, A. S. Cook, S. S. Sharkey, and A. C. Voss. 2004. The national pressure ulcer long-term care study: Pressure ulcer development in long-term care residents. *Journal of the American Geriatrics Society* 52(3):359–367.

Horn, S. D., P. Buerhaus, N. Bergstrom, and R. J. Smout. 2005. RN staffing time and outcomes of long-stay nursing home residents: Pressure ulcers and other adverse outcomes are less likely as RNs spend more time on direct patient care. *American Journal of Nursing* 105(11):58–70; quiz 71.

Horn, S. D., S. S. Sharkey, S. Hudak, R. J. Smout, C. C. Quinn, B. Yody, and I. Fleshner. 2010. Beyond CMS quality measure adjustments: Identifying key resident and nursing home facility factors associated with quality measures. *Journal of the American Medical Directors Association* 11(7):500–505.

Hughes, C. M., K. L. Lapane, and V. Mor. 2000. Influence of facility characteristics on use of antipsychotic medications in nursing homes. *Medical Care* 38(12):1164–1173.

Hunnicutt, J. N., J. Tjia, and K. L. Lapane. 2017a. Hospice use and pain management in elderly nursing home residents with cancer. *Journal of Pain and Symptom Management* 53(3):561–570.

Hunnicutt, J. N., C. M. Ulbricht, J. Tjia, and K. L. Lapane. 2017b. Pain and pharmacologic pain management in long-stay nursing home residents. *Pain* 158(6):1091–1099.

Huskamp, H. A., D. G. Stevenson, M. E. Chernew, and J. P. Newhouse. 2010a. A new Medicare end-of-life benefit for nursing home residents. *Health Affairs* 29(1):130–135.

Huskamp, H. A., D. G. Stevenson, D. C. Grabowski, E. Brennan, and N. L. Keating. 2010b. Long and short hospice stays among nursing home residents at the end of life. *Journal of Palliative Medicine* 13(8):957–964.

Hwang, D., J. M. Teno, M. Clark, R. Shield, C. Williams, D. Casarett, and C. Spence. 2014. Family perceptions of quality of hospice care in the nursing home. *Journal of Pain and Symptom Management* 48(6):1100–1107.

IOM (Institute of Medicine). 1986. *Improving the quality of care in nursing homes.* Washington, DC: National Academy Press.

IOM. 2001. *Improving the quality of long-term care.* Washington, DC: National Academy Press.

IOM. 2015. *Dying in America: Improving quality and honoring individual preferences near the end of life.* Washington, DC: The National Academies Press.

Jablonski, R. A., A. M. Kolanowski, A. Azuero, V. Winstead, C. Jones-Townsend, and M. L. Geisinger. 2018. Randomised clinical trial: Efficacy of strategies to provide oral hygiene activities to nursing home residents with dementia who resist mouth care. *Gerodontology* 35(4):365–375.

Jackson, J. C., M. J. Santoro, T. M. Ely, L. Boehm, A. L. Kiehl, L. S. Anderson, and E. W. Ely. 2014. Improving patient care through the prism of psychology: Application of Maslow's hierarchy to sedation, delirium, and early mobility in the intensive care unit. *Journal of Critical Care* 29(3):438–444.

Jester, D. J., K. Hyer, and J. R. Bowblis. 2020. Quality concerns in nursing homes that serve large proportions of residents with serious mental illness. *The Gerontologist* 60(7):1312–1321.

Johnston, B., and M. Narayanasamy. 2016. Exploring psychosocial interventions for people with dementia that enhance personhood and relate to legacy—An integrative review. *BMC Geriatrics* 16(1):77.

Jones, A. L., A. J. Moss, and L. D. Harris-Kojetin. 2011. Use of advance directives in long-term care populations. *NCHS Data Brief* (54):1–8.

Jøranson, N., I. Pedersen, A. M. M. Rokstad, and C. Ihlebæk. 2015. Effects on symptoms of agitation and depression in persons with dementia participating in robot-assisted activity: A cluster-randomized controlled trial. *Journal of the American Medical Directors Association* 16(10):867–873.

Kalánková, D., M. Stolt, P. A. Scott, E. Papastavrou, and R. Suhonen. 2020. Unmet care needs of older people: A scoping review. *Nursing Ethics* 28(2):149–178.

Katz, P. R., K. Ryskina, D. Saliba, A. Costa, H. Y. Jung, L. M. Wagner, M. A. Unruh, B. J. Smith, A. Moser, J. Spetz, S. Feldman, and J. Karuza. 2021. Medical care delivery in U.S. nursing homes: Current and future practice. *The Gerontologist* 61(4):595–604.

Kemp, C. L. 2021. #MoreThanAVisitor: Families as "essential" care partners during COVID-19. *The Gerontologist* 61(2):145–151.

Keser, I., S. Cvijetić, A. Ilić, I. Colić Barić, D. Boschiero, and J. Z. Ilich. 2021. Assessment of body composition and dietary intake in nursing-home residents: Could lessons learned from the COVID-19 pandemic be used to prevent future casualties in older individuals? *Nutrients* 13(5):1510.

Keyes, C. L. M. 2002. The mental health continuum: From languishing to flourishing in life. *Journal of Health and Social Behavior* 43(2):207–222.

Kilgore, C. 2014. An all-hands-on-deck approach to mealtime. *Caring for the Ages* 15(11):12.

Kim, H., C. Bradway, S. E. Hickman, and M. Ersek. 2019. Exploring provider-surrogate communication during POLST discussions for individuals with advanced dementia. *Aging & Mental Health* 23(6):781–791.

King, B. J., A. L. Gilmore-Bykovskyi, R. A. Roiland, B. E. Polnaszek, B. J. Bowers, and A. J. Kind. 2013. The consequences of poor communication during transitions from hospital-to skilled nursing facility: A qualitative study. *Journal of the American Geriatrics Society* 61(7):1095–1102.

Kitwood, T. M. 1997. *Dementia reconsidered: The person comes first.* Philadelphia: Open University Press.

Koenig, H. G. 2012. Religion, spirituality, and health: The research and clinical implications. *ISRN Psychiatry* 2012:278730.

Koren, M. J. 2010. Person-centered care for nursing home residents: The culture change movement. *Health Affairs (Millwood)* 29(2):312–317.

Kovach, C. R., S. A. Wilson, and P. E. Noonan. 1996. The effects of hospice interventions on behaviors, discomfort, and physical complications of end stage dementia nursing home residents. *American Journal of Alzheimer's Disease* 11(4):7–15.

Koyanagi, C. 2007. *Learning from history: Deinstitutionalization of people with mental illness as precursor to long-term care reform.* https://www.kff.org/wp-content/uploads/2013/01/7684.pdf (accessed November 18, 2021).

Lage, D. E., C. DuMontier, Y. Lee, R. D. Nipp, S. L. Mitchell, J. S. Temel, A. El-Jawahri, and S. D. Berry. 2020. Potentially burdensome end-of-life transitions among nursing home residents with poor-prognosis cancer. *Cancer* 126(6):1322–1329.

Lane, S. J., and E. McGrady. 2016. Nursing home self-assessment of implementation of emergency preparedness standards. *Prehospital and Disaster Medicine* 31(4):422–431.

Laws, M. B., A. Beeman, S. Haigh, I. B. Wilson, and R. R. Shield. 2021. Prevalence of serious mental illness and under 65 population in nursing homes continues to grow. *Journal of the American Medical Directors Association* S1525-8610(21):00941-00945. Online ahead of print. https://doi.org/10.1016/j.jamda.2021.10.020.

LeadingAge CAST (Center for Aging Services Technologies). 2013. *Telehealth and remote patient monitoring for long-term and post-acute care: A primer and provider selection guide.* https://mtelehealth.com/pdf/studies/Telehealth_and_Remote_Patient_Monitoring_(RPM)_for_Long-Term_and_Post-Acute_Care_-_A_Primer_and_Provider_Selection_Guide_2013.pdf (accessed April 26, 2021).

Lepore, M. J., S. C. Miller, and P. Gozalo. 2011. Hospice use among urban black and white U.S. nursing home decedents in 2006. *The Gerontologist* 51(2):251–260.

Lepore, M., K. Scales, R. A. Anderson, K. Porter, T. Thach, E. McConnell, and K. Corazzini. 2018. Person-directed care planning in nursing homes: A scoping review. *International Journal of Older People Nursing* 13(4):e12212.

Lester, P. E., R. G. Stefanacci, and M. Feuerman. 2016. Prevalence and description of palliative care in U.S. nursing homes: A descriptive study. *American Journal of Hospice and Palliative Medicine* 33(2):171–177.

Leung, F. W., and J. F. Schnelle. 2008. Urinary and fecal incontinence in nursing home residents. *Gastroenterology Clinics of North America* 37(3):697-707, x. doi:10.1016/j.gtc.2008.06.005.

Li, Y. 2010. Provision of mental health services in U.S. nursing homes, 1995–2004. *Psychiatric Services* 61(4):349–355.

Li, Y., X. Cai, C. Harrington, M. Hasselberg, Y. Conwell, X. Cen, and H. Temkin-Greener. 2019. Racial and ethnic differences in the prevalence of depressive symptoms among U.S. nursing home residents. *Journal of Aging & Social Policy* 31(1):30–48.

Liu, W., J. Cheon, and S. A. Thomas. 2014. Interventions on mealtime difficulties in older adults with dementia: A systematic review. *International Journal of Nursing Studies* 51(1):14–27.

Logsdon, R. G., L. E. Gibbons, S. M. McCurry, and L. Teri. 2002. Assessing quality of life in older adults with cognitive impairment. *Psychosomatic Medicine* 64(3):510–519.

Lok, N., S. Lok, and M. Canbaz. 2017. The effect of physical activity on depressive symptoms and quality of life among elderly nursing home residents: Randomized controlled trial. *Archives of Gerontology and Geriatrics* 70:92–98.

Lucas, J. A., and J. R. Bowblis. 2017. CMS strategies to reduce antipsychotic drug use in nursing home patients with dementia show some progress. *Health Affairs* 36(7):1299–1308.

Lyons, S. S. 2010. How do people make continence care happen? An analysis of organizational culture in two nursing homes. *The Gerontologist* 50(3):327–339.

MACPAC (Medicaid and CHIP Payment and Access Commission). 2019. *Report to Congress on oversight of institutions for mental diseases.* Washington, DC: Medicaid and CHIP Payment and Access Commission.

MACPAC. 2020. *MACPAC releases report to Congress on oversight of institutions for mental diseases.* https://www.macpac.gov/wp-content/uploads/2020/01/MACPAC-Releases-Report-to-Congress-on-Oversight-of-Institutions-for-Mental-Diseases.pdf (accessed February 3, 2022).

MACPAC. 2021. Integrating clinical care through greater use of electronic health records for behavioral health. Chapter 4 in *June 2021 report to Congress on Medicaid and CHIP*. Washington, DC: Medicaid and CHIP Payment and Access Commission.

MACPAC. 2022. *Payment for services in institutions for mental diseases (IMDs)*. https://www.macpac.gov/subtopic/payment-for-services-in-institutions-for-mental-diseases-imds/ (accessed February 3, 2022, 2022).

Magaziner, J., P. German, S. I. Zimmerman, J. R. Hebel, L. Burton, A. L. Gruber-Baldini, C. May, and S. Kittner. 2000. The prevalence of dementia in a statewide sample of new nursing home admissions aged 65 and older: Diagnosis by expert panel. Epidemiology of dementia in nursing homes research group. *The Gerontologist* 40(6):663–672.

Mäki-Turja-Rostedt, S., M. Stolt, H. Leino-Kilpi, and E. Haavisto. 2018. Preventive interventions for pressure ulcers in long-term older people care facilities: A systematic review. *Journal of Clinical Nursing* 28(13–14):2420–2442.

Malmedal, W., R. Hammervold, and B. I. Saveman. 2009. To report or not report? Attitudes held by Norwegian nursing home staff on reporting inadequate care carried out by colleagues. *Scandinavian Journal of Public Health* 37(7):744–750.

Mansbach, W. E., R. A. Mace, K. M. Clark, and I. M. Firth. 2017. Meaningful activity for long-term care residents with dementia: A comparison of activities and raters. *The Gerontologist* 57(3):461–468.

Maramaldi, P., T. Cadet, S. L. Burke, M. LeCloux, E. White, E. Kalenderian, and T. Kinnunen. 2018. Oral health and cancer screening in long-term care nursing facilities: Motivation and opportunity as intervention targets. *Gerodontology* 35(4):407–416.

Maslow, A. H. 1943. A theory of human motivation. *Psychological Review* 50(4):370–396.

Maslow, A. H. 1954. *Motivation and personality*. New York: Harper and Row.

McArthur, C., J. Gibbs, A. Papaioannou, J. Hirdes, J. Milligan, K. Berg, and L. Giangregorio. 2015. Scoping review of physical rehabilitation interventions in long-term care: Protocol for tools, models of delivery, outcomes and quality indicators. *BMJ Open* 5(6):e007528.

McCabe, M., J. Byers, L. Busija, D. Mellor, M. Bennett, and E. Beattie. 2021. How important are choice, autonomy, and relationships in predicting the quality of life of nursing home residents? *Journal of Applied Gerontology* 40(12):1743–1750.

McCreedy, E. M., B. E. Weinstein, J. Chodosh, and J. Blustein. 2018. Hearing loss: Why does it matter for nursing homes? *Journal of the American Medical Directors Association* 19(4):323–327.

McGarry, B. E., N. R. Joyce, T. G. McGuire, S. L. Mitchell, S. J. Bartels, and D. C. Grabowski. 2019. Association between high proportions of seriously mentally ill nursing home residents and the quality of resident care. *Journal of the American Geriatrics Society* 67(11):2346–2352.

McGarry, B. E., E. M. White, L. J. Resnik, M. Rahman, and D. C. Grabowski. 2021. Medicare's new patient driven payment model resulted in reductions in therapy staffing in skilled nursing facilities. *Health Affairs* 40(3):392–399.

Mead, R. 2013. *The sense of an ending*. https://www.newyorker.com/magazine/2013/05/20/the-sense-of-an-ending-2 (accessed April 26, 2021).

MedPAC (Medicare Payment Advisory Commission). 2020. *March 2020 report to the Congress: Medicare payment policy*. Washington, DC: Medicare Payment Advisory Commission. Original edition, Chapter 12.

MedPAC. 2021. *March 2021 report to the Congress: Medicare payment policy*. Washington, DC: Medicare Payment Advisory Commission.

Meier, D. E., B. Lim, and M. D. Carlson. 2010. Raising the standard: Palliative care in nursing homes. *Health Affairs (Millwood)* 29(1):136–140.

Miller, L. M., C. J. Whitlatch, and K. S. Lyons. 2016b. Shared decision making in dementia: A review of patient and family carer involvement. *Dementia* 15(5):1141–1157.

Miller, S. C. 2010. A model for successful nursing home–hospice partnerships. *Journal of Palliative Medicine* 13(5):525–533.

Miller, S. C., and B. Han. 2008. End-of-life care in U.S. nursing homes: Nursing homes with special programs and trained staff for hospice or palliative/end-of-life care. *Journal of Palliative Medicine* 11:866–877.

Miller, S. C., V. Mor, N. Wu, P. Gozalo, and K. Lapane. 2002. Does receipt of hospice care in nursing homes improve the management of pain at the end of life? *Journal of the American Geriatrics Society* 50(3):507–515.

Miller, S. C., J. C. Lima, J. Looze, and S. L. Mitchell. 2012. Dying in U.S. nursing homes with advanced dementia: How does health care use differ for residents with, versus without, end-of-life Medicare skilled nursing facility care? *Journal of Palliative Medicine* 15(1):43–50.

Miller, S. C., N. Cohen, J. C. Lima, and V. Mor. 2014. Medicaid capital reimbursement policy and environmental artifacts of nursing home culture change. *Gerontologist* 54(Suppl 1):S76–S86.

Miller, S. C., J. C. Lima, O. Intrator, E. Martin, J. Bull, and L. C. Hanson. 2016a. Palliative care consultations in nursing homes and reductions in acute care use and potentially burdensome end-of-life transitions. *Journal of the American Geriatrics Society* 64(11):2280–2287.

Miller, S. C., J. C. Lima, O. Intrator, E. Martin, J. Bull, and L. C. Hanson. 2017. Specialty palliative care consultations for nursing home residents with dementia. *Journal of Pain and Symptom Management* 54(1):9–16.e15.

Miller, S. C., W. J. Scott, M. Ersek, C. Levy, R. Hogikyan, V. S. Periyakoil, J. G. Carpenter, J. Cohen, and M. B. Foglia. 2020. Honoring veterans' preferences: The association between comfort care goals and care received at the end of life. *Journal of Pain and Symptom Management* 61(4):743-754.e1.

Mitchell, S. L., A. E. Volandes, R. Gutman, P. L. Gozalo, J. A. Ogarek, L. Loomer, E. M. McCreedy, R. Zhai, and V. Mor. 2020. Advance care planning video intervention among long-stay nursing home residents: A pragmatic cluster randomized clinical trial. *JAMA Internal Medicine* 180(8):1070–1078.

Mitty, E. L. 2005. *Culture change in nursing homes: An ethical perspective.* https://www.hmpgloballearningnetwork.com/site/altc/article/3870 (accessed September 30, 2021).

Mo, S., and J. Shi. 2020. The psychological consequences of the COVID-19 on residents and staff in nursing homes. *Work, Aging and Retirement* 6(4):254–259.

Moilanen, T., M. Kangasniemi, O. Papinaho, M. Mynttinen, H. Siipi, S. Suominen, and R. Suhonen. 2021. Older people's perceived autonomy in residential care: An integrative review. *Nursing Ethics* 28(3):414–434.

Monroe, T. B., and M. A. Carter. 2010. A retrospective pilot study of African-American and Caucasian nursing home residents with dementia who died from cancer. *Journal of Pain and Symptom Management* 40(4):e1.

Mor, V., J. Zinn, J. Angelelli, J. M. Teno, and S. C. Miller. 2004. Driven to tiers: Socioeconomic and racial disparities in the quality of nursing home care. *The Milbank Quarterly* 82(2):227–256.

Morgan, C., N. Endozoa, C. Paradiso, M. McNamara, and M. McGuire. 2008. Enhanced toileting program decreases incontinence in long term care. *Joint Commission Journal on Quality Patient Safety* 34(4):206–208.

Morley, J. E., and A. M. Sanford. 2014. The god card: Spirituality in the nursing home. *Journal of the American Medical Directors Association* 15(8):533–535.

Morris, J. N., C. Hawes, B. E. Fries, C. D. Phillips, V. Mor, S. Katz, K. Murphy, M. L. Drugovich, and A. S. Friedlob. 1990. Designing the national Resident Assessment Instrument for nursing homes. *The Gerontologist* 30(3):293–307.

Morrison, R., B. Jesdale, C. Dube, S. Forrester, A. Nunes, C. Bova, and K. L. Lapane. 2021. Racial/ethnic differences in staff-assessed pain behaviors among newly admitted nursing home residents. *Journal of Pain and Symptom Management* 61(3):438-448.e3.

Munshi, M. N., H. Florez, E. S. Huang, R. R. Kalyani, M. Mupanomunda, N. Pandya, C. S. Swift, T. H. Taveira, and L. B. Haas. 2016. Management of diabetes in long-term care and skilled nursing facilities: A position statement of the American Diabetes Association. *Diabetes Care* 39(2):308-318.

Nåden, D., A. Rehnsfeldt, M.-B. Råholm, L. Lindwall, S. Caspari, T. Aasgaard, Å. Slettebø, B. Sæteren, B. Høy, B. Lillestø, A. K. T. Heggestad, and V. Lohne. 2013. Aspects of indignity in nursing home residences as experienced by family caregivers. *Nursing Ethics* 20(7):748-761.

Nakashima, T., Y. Young, and W.-H. Hsu. 2019. Do nursing home residents with dementia receive pain interventions? *American Journal of Alzheimer's Disease & Other Dementias* 34(3):193-198.

NASEM (National Academies of Sciences, Engineering, and Medicine). 2016. *Hearing health care for adults: Priorities for improving access and affordability.* Washington, DC: The National Academies Press.

NASEM. 2020. *Social isolation and loneliness in older adults: Opportunities for the health care system.* Washington, DC: The National Academies Press.

NASEM. 2021. *Meeting the challenge of caring for persons living with dementia and their care partners and caregivers: A way forward.* Washington, DC: The National Academies Press.

Nash, W. A., L. M. Harris, K. E. Heller, and B. D. Mitchell. 2021. "We are saving their bodies and destroying their souls": Family caregivers' experiences of formal care setting visitation restrictions during the COVID-19 pandemic. *Journal of Aging & Social Policy* 33(4-5):398-413.

National Consensus Project for Quality Palliative Care. 2018. *Clinical practice guidelines for quality palliative care.* 4th ed. Richmond, VA: National Coalition for Hospice and Palliative Care.

National Consumer Voice. 2021. *Resident council center.* https://theconsumervoice.org/issues/recipients/nursing-home-residents/resident-council-center#resident_council_rights (accessed May 17, 2021).

Nelson, M., and J. R. Bowblis. 2017. *A new group of long-stay Medicaid nursing home residents: The unexpected trend of those under age 65 using nursing homes in Ohio.* https://sc.lib.miamioh.edu/bitstream/handle/2374.MIA/6176/Nelson-A-New-Group-Medicaid-10-09-2017.pdf (accessed February 15, 2022).

Nemiroff, L., E. G. Marshall, J. L. Jensen, B. Clarke, and M. K. Andrew. 2019. Adherence to "No transfer to hospital" advance directives among nursing home residents. *Journal of the American Medical Directors Association* 20(11):1373-1381.

Newbould, L., G. Mountain, M. S. Hawley, and S. Ariss. 2017. Videoconferencing for health care provision for older adults in care homes: A review of the research evidence. *International Journal of Telemedicine and Applications* 2017:5785613.

NHPCO (National Hospice and Palliative Care Organization). 2019. *Palliative care or hospice?* https://www.nhpco.org/wp-content/uploads/2019/04/PalliativeCare_VS_Hospice.pdf (accessed December 28, 2020).

NHPCO. 2020. *Hospice facts & figures.* https://www.nhpco.org/hospice-care-overview/hospice-facts-figures (accessed September 21, 2021).

NIA (National Institute on Aging). 2018. *Advance care planning: Health care directives.* https://www.nia.nih.gov/health/advance-care-planning-health-care-directives (accessed October 26, 2021).

Niclasen, J., L. Lund, C. Obel, and L. Larsen. 2019. Mental health interventions among older adults: A systematic review. *Scandinavian Journal of Public Health* 47(2):240-250.

NIDCD (National Institute on Deafness and Other Communication Disorders). 2021. *Over-the-counter hearing aids*. https://www.nidcd.nih.gov/health/over-counter-hearing-aids (accessed November 3, 2021).

Northridge, M. E., A. Kumar, and R. Kaur. 2020. Disparities in access to oral health care. *Annual Review of Public Health* 41:513–535.

Nydén, K., M. Petersson, and M. Nyström. 2003. Unsatisfied basic needs of older patients in emergency care environments—Obstacles to an active role in decision making. *Journal of Clinical Nursing* 12(2):268–274.

Ogletree, A. M., R. Mangrum, Y. Harris, D. R. Gifford, R. Barry, L. Bergofsky, and D. Perfetto. 2020. Omissions of care in nursing home settings: A narrative review. *Journal of the American Medical Directors Association* 21(5):604–614.

OIG (Office of the Inspector General). 2003. *Psychosocial services in skilled nursing facilities*. Washington, DC: HHS Office of the Inspector General.

OIG. 2013. *Skilled nursing facilities often fail to meet care planning and discharge planning requirements*. Washington, DC: HHS Office of the Inspector General.

OIG. 2018. *Vulnerabilities in the Medicare hospice program affect quality care and program integrity: An OIG portfolio*. Washington, DC: HHS Office of the Inspector General.

OIG. 2019. *Trends in deficiencies at nursing homes show that improvements are needed to ensure the health and safety of residents*. Washington, DC: HHS Office of the Inspector General.

Olsen, C., I. Pedersen, A. Bergland, M. J. Enders-Slegers, G. Patil, and C. Ihlebaek. 2016. Effect of animal-assisted interventions on depression, agitation and quality of life in nursing home residents suffering from cognitive impairment or dementia: A cluster randomized controlled trial. *International Journal of Geriatric Psychiatry* 31(12):1312–1321.

Orth, J., Y. Li, A. Simning, and H. Temkin-Greener. 2019. Providing behavioral health services in nursing homes is difficult: Findings from a national survey. *Journal of the American Geriatrics Society* 67(8):1713–1717.

Ostaszkiewicz, J., V. Dickson-Swift, A. Hutchinson, and A. Wagg. 2020. A concept analysis of dignity-protective continence care for care dependent older people in long-term care settings. *BMC Geriatrics* 20(1):266.

Owsley, C., G. McGwin, Jr., K. Scilley, G. C. Meek, D. Seker, and A. Dyer. 2007a. Effect of refractive error correction on health-related quality of life and depression in older nursing home residents. *Archives of Ophthalmology* 125(11):1471–1477.

Owsley, C., G. McGwin, Jr., K. Scilley, G. C. Meek, D. Seker, and A. Dyer. 2007b. Impact of cataract surgery on health-related quality of life in nursing home residents. *British Journal of Ophthalmology* 91(10):1359–1363.

Palese, A., V. Bressan, T. Kasa, M. Meri, M. Hayter, and R. Watson. 2018. Interventions maintaining eating independence in nursing home residents: A multicentre qualitative study. *BMC Geriatrics* 18(1):292.

Pan, D. 2013. *Timeline: Deinstitutionalization and its consequences*. https://www.motherjones.com/politics/2013/04/timeline-mental-health-america (accessed November 18, 2021).

Pilgrim, A. L., S. M. Robinson, A. A. Sayer, and H. C. Roberts. 2015. An overview of appetite decline in older people. *Nursing Older People* 27(5):29–35.

Pioneer Network. 2016. *Lighting: Partner in quality care environments*. https://www.pioneernetwork.net/wp-content/uploads/2016/10/Lighting-A-Partner-in-Quality-Care-Environments-Symposium-Paper-3.pdf (accessed October 26, 2021).

Pioneer Network. 2021. *Artifacts of culture change 2.0: Nursing homes*. https://www.pioneernetwork.net/wp-content/uploads/2021/02/Artifacts_2.0_NH_Form_030521.pdf (accessed June 7, 2021).

Poghosyan, L., A. A. Norful, E. Fleck, J. M. Bruzzese, A. Talsma, and A. Nannini. 2017. Primary care providers' perspectives on errors of omission. *Journal of the American Board of Family Medicine* 30(6):733–742.

Porter, J., A. Ntouva, A. Read, M. Murdoch, D. Ola, and G. Tsakos. 2015. The impact of oral health on the quality of life of nursing home residents. *Health and Quality of Life Outcomes* 13:102.

Quan, N. G., M. C. Lohman, N. V. Resciniti, and D. B. Friedman. 2020. A systematic review of interventions for loneliness among older adults living in long-term care facilities. *Aging & Mental Health* 24(12):1945–1955.

Rahman, M., D. C. Grabowski, O. Intrator, S. Cai, and V. Mor. 2013. Serious mental illness and nursing home quality of care. *Health Services Research* 48(4):1279–1298.

Rantz, M. J., L. Hicks, V. Grando, G. F. Petroski, R. W. Madsen, D. R. Mehr, V. Conn, M. Zwygart-Staffacher, J. Scott, M. Flesner, J. Bostick, R. Porter, and M. Maas. 2004. Nursing home quality, cost, staffing, and staff mix. *The Gerontologist* 44(1):24–38.

Recio-Saucedo, A., C. Dall'Ora, A. Maruotti, J. Ball, J. Briggs, P. Meredith, O. C. Redfern, C. Kovacs, D. Prytherch, G. B. Smith, and P. Griffiths. 2018. What impact does nursing care left undone have on patient outcomes? Review of the literature. *Journal of Clinical Nursing* 27(11–12):2248–2259.

Reitman, N. C. 2010. Care at home of the patient with advanced multiple sclerosis: Part 2. *Home Healthcare Now* 28(5):270–275.

Resnick, B., E. Galik, E. Vigne, and A. P. Carew. 2016. Dissemination and implementation of function focused care for assisted living. *Health Education & Behavior* 43(3):296–304.

Rice, K. N., E. A. Coleman, R. Fish, C. Levy, and J. S. Kutner. 2004. Factors influencing models of end-of-life care in nursing homes: Results of a survey of nursing home administrators. *Journal of Palliative Medicine* 7(5):668–675.

Rivera, E., K. B. Hirschman, and M. D. Naylor. 2020. Reported needs and depressive symptoms among older adults entering long-term services and supports. *Innovation in Aging* 4(3):igaa021.

Roberts, A. R., A. C. Smith, and J. R. Bowblis. 2020. Nursing home social services and post-acute care: Does more qualified staff improve behavioral symptoms and reduce antipsychotic drug use? *Journal of the American Medical Directors Association* 21(3):388–394.

Rodney, T., N. Josiah, and D.-L. Baptiste. 2021. Loneliness in the time of COVID-19: Impact on older adults. *Journal of Advanced Nursing* 77(9):e24–e26.

Roelofs, T. S., K. G. Luijkx, and P. J. Embregts. 2015. Intimacy and sexuality of nursing home residents with dementia: A systematic review. *International Psychogeriatrics* 27(3):367–384.

Rosa, W. E., B. R. Ferrell, and D. J. Mason. 2021. Integration of palliative care into all serious illness care as a human right. *JAMA Health Forum* 2(4):e211099.

Rosenberg, I., D. Woo, and D. Roane. 2009. *The aging patient with chronic schizophrenia.* https://www.hmpgloballearningnetwork.com/site/altc/articles/aging-patient-chronic-schizophrenia (accessed February 15, 2022).

Rosenthal, M., J. Poling, A. Wec, E. Connolly, B. Angell, and S. Crystal. 2022. "Medication is just one piece of the whole puzzle": How nursing homes change their use of antipsychotic medications. *Journal of Applied Gerontology* 41(1):62–72.

Ruopp, M. D. 2020. Overcoming the challenge of family separation from nursing home residents during COVID-19. *Journal of the American Medical Directors Association* 21(7):984–985.

Saliba, D., D. L. Weimer, Y. Shi, and D. B. Mukamel. 2018. Examination of the new short-stay nursing home quality measures: Rehospitalizations, emergency department visits, and successful returns to the community. *INQUIRY: The Journal of Health Care Organization, Provision, and Financing* 55:0046958018786816.

Saravanakumar, P., I. J. Higgins, P. J. Van Der Riet, and D. Sibbritt. 2018. Tai chi and yoga in residential aged care: Perspectives of participants: A qualitative study. *Journal of Clinical Nursing* 27(23–24):4390–4399.

Scales, K., M. Lepore, R. A. Anderson, E. S. McConnell, Y. Song, B. Kang, K. Porter, T. Thach, and K. N. Corazzini. 2019. Person-directed care planning in nursing homes: Resident, family, and staff perspectives. *Journal of Applied Gerontology* 38(2):183–206.

Schneider, J. 2018. The arts as a medium for care and self-care in dementia: Arguments and evidence. *International Journal of Environmental Research and Public Health* 15(6):1151.

Schwartz, M. L., J. C. Lima, M. A. Clark, and S. C. Miller. 2019. End-of-life culture change practices in U.S. nursing homes in 2016/2017. *Journal of Pain and Symptom Management* 57(3):525–534.

Scott, A. M., J. Li, S. Oyewole-Eletu, H. Q. Nguyen, B. Gass, K. B. Hirschman, S. Mitchell, S. M. Hudson, and M. V. Williams. 2017. Understanding facilitators and barriers to care transitions: Insights from project achieve site visits. *Joint Commission Journal on Quality and Patient Safety* 43(9):433–447.

Sheingold, S., S. Bogasky, and S. Stearns. 2015. *Medicare's hospice benefit: Revising the payment system to better reflect visit intensity.* Washington, DC: HHS Office of the Assistant Secretary for Planning and Evaluation.

Sherwin, S., and M. Winsby. 2011. A relational perspective on autonomy for older adults residing in nursing homes. *Health Expectations* 14(2):182–190.

Shield, R. R., J. Looze, D. Tyler, M. Lepore, and S. C. Miller. 2014. Why and how do nursing homes implement culture change practices? Insights from qualitative interviews in a mixed methods study. *Journal of Applied Gerontology* 33(6):737–763.

Sifuentes, A. M. F., and K. L. Lapane. 2020. Oral health in nursing homes: What we know and what we need to know. *Journal of Nursing Home Research* 6:1–5.

Simard, J., and L. Volicer. 2020. Loneliness and isolation in long-term care and the COVID-19 pandemic. *Journal of the American Medical Directors Association* 21(7):966–967.

Simmons, S. F., and R. M. Bertrand. 2010. *Enhancing the quality of nursing home dining assistance: New regulations and practice implications.* Paper presented at Creating Home in the Nursing Home II Symposium.

Simmons, S. F., and J. F. Schnelle. 2004. Individualized feeding assistance care for nursing home residents: Staffing requirements to implement two interventions. *Journals of Gerontology: Series A* 59(9):M966–M973.

Simmons, S. F., and J. F. Schnelle. 2006. Feeding assistance needs of long-stay nursing home residents and staff time to provide care. *Journal of the American Geriatrics Society* 54(6):919–924.

Simmons, S. F., E. Keeler, X. Zhuo, K. A. Hickey, H.-W. Sato, and J. F. Schnelle. 2008. Prevention of unintentional weight loss in nursing home residents: A controlled trial of feeding assistance. *Journal of the American Geriatrics Society* 56(8):1466–1473.

Simmons, S. F., D. W. Durkin, A. N. Rahman, L. Choi, L. Beuscher, and J. F. Schnelle. 2013. Resident characteristics related to the lack of morning care provision in long-term care. *The Gerontologist* 53(1):151–161.

Simning, A., and K. V. Simons. 2017. Treatment of depression in nursing home residents without significant cognitive impairment: A systematic review. *International Psychogeriatrics* 29(2):209–226.

Simons, K., R. P. Connolly, R. Bonifas, P. D. Allen, K. Bailey, D. Downes, and C. Galambos. 2012a. Psychosocial assessment of nursing home residents via MDS 3.0: Recommendations for social service training, staffing, and roles in interdisciplinary care. *Journal of the American Medical Directors Association* 13(2):190.e9-190.e15.

Simons, K., M. Bern-Klug, and S. An. 2012b. Envisioning quality psychosocial care in nursing homes: The role of social work. *Journal of the American Medical Directors Association* 13(9):800–805.

Sloane, P. D., J. Ivey, M. Helton, A. L. Barrick, and A. Cerna. 2008. Nutritional issues in long-term care. *Journal of the American Medical Directors Association* 9(7):476–485.

Sloane, P. D., S. Zimmerman, X. Chen, A. L. Barrick, P. Poole, D. Reed, M. Mitchell, and L. W. Cohen. 2013. Effect of a person-centered mouth care intervention on care processes and outcomes in three nursing homes. *Journal of the American Geriatrics Society* 61(7):1158–1163.

Smyer, M. A., D. G. Shea, and A. Streit. 1994. The provision and use of mental health services in nursing homes: Results from the National Medical Expenditure Survey. *American Journal of Public Health* 84(2):284–287.

Stephens, C. E., L. J. Hunt, N. Bui, E. Halifax, C. S. Ritchie, and S. J. Lee. 2018. Palliative care eligibility, symptom burden, and quality of life ratings in nursing home residents. *JAMA Internal Medicine* 178(1):141–142.

Stevenson, D. G., and J. S. Bramson. 2009. Hospice care in the nursing home setting: A review of the literature. *Journal of Pain and Symptom Management* 38(3):440–451.

Stevenson, D. G., N. Sinclair, S. Zhang, L. M. Meneades, and H. A. Huskamp. 2020. Trends in contracting and common ownership between hospice agencies and nursing homes. *Medical Care* 58(4):329–335.

Stone, R., and M. F. Harahan. 2010. Improving the long-term care workforce serving older adults. *Health Affairs (Millwood)* 29(1):109–115.

Strom, K. E. 2014. *HR 2013 hearing aid dispenser survey: Dispensing in the age of internet and big box retailers.* https://www.hearingreview.com/hearing-products/hearing-aids/ite/hr-2013-hearing-aid-dispenser-survey-dispensing-age-internet-big-box-retailers-comparison-present-past-key-business-indicators-dispensing-offices (accessed October 26, 2021).

Strumpf, N. E., H. Tuch, D. Stillman, P. Parrish, and N. Morrison. 2004. Implementing palliative care in the nursing home. *Annals of Long-Term Care* 12:35–41.

Suhrie, E. M., J. T. Hanlon, E. J. Jaffe, M. A. Sevick, C. M. Ruby, and S. L. Aspinall. 2009. Impact of a geriatric nursing home palliative care service on unnecessary medication prescribing. *American Journal of Geriatric Pharmacotherapy* 7(1):20–25.

Sullivan, D. H., L. E. Johnson, M. M. Bopp, and P. K. Roberson. 2004. Prognostic significance of monthly weight fluctuations among older nursing home residents. *Journals of Gerontology: Series A* 59(6):M633–M639.

Talley, K. M., J. F. Wyman, K. Savik, R. L. Kane, C. Mueller, and H. Zhao. 2015. Restorative care's effect on activities of daily living dependency in long-stay nursing home residents. *The Gerontologist* 55(Suppl 1):S88–S98.

Tariot, P. N., C. A. Podgorski, L. Blazina, and A. Leibovici. 1993. Mental disorders in the nursing home: Another perspective. *American Journal of Psychiatry* 150(7):1063–1069.

Tark, A., J. Song, J. Parajuli, S. Chae, and P. W. Stone. 2020a. Are we getting what we really want? A systematic review of concordance between physician orders for life-sustaining treatment (POLST) documentation and subsequent care delivered at end-of-life. *American Journal of Hospice and Palliative Care* 38(9):1142–1158.

Tark, A., L. V. Estrada, M. E. Tresgallo, D. D. Quigley, P. W. Stone, and M. Agarwal. 2020b. Palliative care and infection management at end of life in nursing homes: A descriptive survey. *Palliative Medicine* 34(5):580–588.

Tarzian, A. J., and N. B. Cheevers. 2017. Maryland's medical orders for life-sustaining treatment form use: Reports of a statewide survey. *Journal of Palliative Medicine* 20(9):939–945.

Temkin-Greener, H., S. Ladwig, T. Caprio, S. Norton, T. Quill, T. Olsan, X. Cai, and D. B. Mukamel. 2015. Developing palliative care practice guidelines and standards for nursing home-based palliative care teams: A Delphi study. *Journal of the American Medical Directors Association* 16(1):86.e1–86.e867.

Temkin-Greener, H., L. Campbell, X. Cai, M. J. Hasselberg, and Y. Li. 2018. Are post-acute patients with behavioral health disorders admitted to lower-quality nursing homes? *American Journal of Geriatric Psychiatry* 26(6):643–654.

Teno, J. M., P. Gozalo, A. N. Trivedi, J. Bunker, J. Lima, J. Ogarek, and V. Mor. 2018. Site of death, place of care, and health care transitions among U.S. Medicare beneficiaries, 2000–2015. *JAMA* 320(3):264–271.

Teo, W. S., A. G. Raj, W. S. Tan, C. W. Ng, B. H. Heng, and I. Y. Leong. 2014. Economic impact analysis of an end-of-life programme for nursing home residents. *Palliative Medicine* 28(5):430–437.

Terrell, K. M., and D. K. Miller. 2006. Challenges in transitional care between nursing homes and emergency departments. *Journal of the American Medical Directors Association* 7(8):499–505.

Tjia, J., M. Dharmawardene, and J. L. Givens. 2018. Advance directives among nursing home residents with mild, moderate, and advanced dementia. *Journal of Palliative Medicine* 21(1):16–21.

Tobis, S., K. Wieczorowska-Tobis, D. Talarska, M. Pawlaczyk, and A. Suwalska. 2018. Needs of older adults living in long-term care institutions: An observational study using Camberwell assessment of need for the elderly. *Clinical Interventions in Aging* 13:2389–2395.

Travers, J. L., K. B. Hirschman, and M. D. Naylor. 2022. Older adults' goals and expectations when using long-term services and supports. *Journal of Applied Gerontology* 41(3):709–717.

Vaartio-Rajalin, H., R. Santamäki-Fischer, P. Jokisalo, and L. Fagerström. 2021. Art making and expressive art therapy in adult health and nursing care: A scoping review. *International Journal of Nursing Sciences* 8(1):102–119.

VanArsdall, P. S., and J. Aalboe. 2016. *Improving the oral health of long term care facility residents.* https://decisionsindentistry.com/article/improving-oral-health-long-term-care-facility-residents/ (accessed February 1, 2022).

Van Den Bos, J., K. Rustagi, T. Gray, M. Halford, E. Ziemkiewicz, and J. Shreve. 2011. The $17.1 billion problem: The annual cost of measurable medical errors. *Health Affairs* 30(4):596–603.

van den Brink, A. M. A., D. L. Gerritsen, M. M. H. de Valk, A. T. Mulder, R. C. Oude Voshaar, and R. Koopmans. 2018. What do nursing home residents with mental–physical multimorbidity need and who actually knows this? A cross-sectional cohort study. *International Journal of Nursing Studies* 81:89–97.

van der Wolf, E., S. A. H. van Hooren, W. Waterink, and L. Lechner. 2019. Well-being in elderly long-term care residents with chronic mental disorder: A systematic review. *Aging and Mental Health* 23(3):287–296.

Van Haitsma, K., K. M. Abbott, A. R. Heid, A. Spector, K. Eshraghi, C. Duntzee, S. Humes, V. Crumbie, S. D. Crespy, and M. Van Valkenburgh-Schultz. 2016. Honoring nursing home resident preferences for recreational activities to advance person-centered care. *Annals of Long-Term Care* 24(2):25–33.

Vest, J. R., H. Y. Jung, K. Wiley, Jr., H. Kooreman, L. Pettit, and M. A. Unruh. 2019. Adoption of health information technology among U.S. nursing facilities. *Journal of the American Medical Directors Association* 20(8):995–1000.

Weber, P. C. 2021. *Hearing amplification in adults.* https://www.uptodate.com/contents/hearing-amplification-in-adults (accessed October 26, 2021).

Wells, J. L., and A. C. Dumbrell. 2006. Nutrition and aging: Assessment and treatment of compromised nutritional status in frail elderly patients. *Clinical Interventions in Aging* 1(1):67–79.

Wendrich-van Dael, A., F. Bunn, J. Lynch, L. Pivodic, L. Van den Block, and C. Goodman. 2020. Advance care planning for people living with dementia: An umbrella review of effectiveness and experiences. *International Journal of Nursing Studies* 107:103576.

White-Chu, E. F., W. J. Graves, S. M. Godfrey, A. Bonner, and P. Sloane. 2009. Beyond the medical model: The culture change revolution in long-term care. *Journal of the American Medical Directors Association* 10(6):370–378.

Williams, N., N. A. Phillips, W. Wittich, J. L. Campos, P. Mick, J. B. Orange, M. K. Pichora-Fuller, M. Y. Savundranayagam, and D. M. Guthrie. 2020. Hearing and cognitive impairments increase the risk of long-term care admissions. *Innovation in Aging* 4(2):igz053.

Willink, A., N. S. Reed, and F. R. Lin. 2019. Access to hearing care services among older Medicare beneficiaries using hearing aids. *Health Affairs* 38(1):124–131.

Woods, B., L. O'Philbin, E. M. Farrell, A. E. Spector, and M. Orrell. 2018. Reminiscence therapy for dementia. *Cochrane Database of Systematic Reviews* 3(3):CD001120.

Xiang, X., R. An, and A. Heinemann. 2017. Depression and unmet needs for assistance with daily activities among community-dwelling older adults. *The Gerontologist* 58(3):428–437.

Xu, D., and R. L. Kane. 2013. Effect of urinary incontinence on older nursing home residents' self-reported quality of life. *Journal of the American Geriatrics Society* 61(9):1473–1481.

Ye, P., L. Fry, and J. D. Champion. 2021. Changes in advance care planning for nursing home residents during the COVID-19 pandemic. *Journal of the American Medical Directors Association* 22(1):209–214.

Yorozuya, K., Y. Kubo, N. Tomiyama, S. Yamane, and H. Hanaoka. 2019. A systematic review of multimodal non-pharmacological interventions for cognitive function in older people with dementia in nursing homes. *Dementia and Geriatric Cognitive Disorders* 48(1–2):1–16.

Yurkofsky, M., and J. G. Ouslander. 2021. *Medical care in skilled nursing facilities (SNFs) in the United States.* https://www.uptodate.com/contents/medical-care-in-skilled-nursing-facilities-snfs-in-the-united-states (accessed July 16, 2021).

Zalenski, R. J., and R. Raspa. 2006. Maslow's hierarchy of needs: A framework for achieving human potential in hospice. *Journal of Palliative Medicine* 9(5):1120–1127.

Zhang, N. J., D. Gammonley, S. C. Paek, and K. Frahm. 2008. Facility service environments, staffing, and psychosocial care in nursing homes. *Health Care Financing Review* 30(2):5–17.

Zhang, Y., H. Xiao, and B. Yong. 2020. Interventions for improving psychosocial adjustment in nursing home residents: A network meta-analysis. *Innovation in Aging* 4(Suppl 1):279.

Zheng, N. T., D. B. Mukamel, T. Caprio, S. Cai, and H. Temkin-Greener. 2011. Racial disparities in in-hospital death and hospice use among nursing home residents at the end-of-life. *Medical Care* 49(11):992.

Zimmerman, S., P. D. Sloane, C. S. Williams, P. S. Reed, J. S. Preisser, J. K. Eckert, M. Boustani, and D. Dobbs. 2005. Dementia care and quality of life in assisted living and nursing homes. *The Gerontologist* 45(1):133–146.

Zimmerman, S., P. D. Sloane, C. S. Williams, D. Dobbs, R. Ellajosyula, A. Braaten, M. F. Rupnow, and D. I. Kaufer. 2007. Residential care/assisted living staff may detect undiagnosed dementia using the Minimum Data Set cognition scale. *Journal of the American Geriatrics Society* 55(9):1349–1355.

Zimmerman, S., S. Austin, L. Cohen, D. Reed, P. Poole, K. Ward, and P. D. Sloane. 2017. Readily identifiable risk factors of nursing home residents' oral hygiene: Dementia, hospice, and length of stay. *Journal of the American Geriatrics Society* 65(11):2516–2521.

Zimmerman, S., P. D. Sloane, K. Ward, C. J. Wretman, S. C. Stearns, P. Poole, and J. S. Preisser. 2020. Effectiveness of a mouth care program provided by nursing home staff vs. standard care on reducing pneumonia incidence: A cluster randomized trial. *JAMA Network Open* 3(6):e204321.

Zúñiga, F., M. Schubert, J. P. H. Hamers, M. Simon, R. Schwendimann, S. Engberg, and D. Ausserhofer. 2016. Evidence on the validity and reliability of the German, French and Italian nursing home version of the Basel extent of rationing of nursing care instrument. *Journal of Advanced Nursing* 72(8):1948–1963.

Zweig, S. C., L. L. Popejoy, D. Parker-Oliver, and S. E. Meadows. 2011. The physician's role in patients' nursing home care: "She's a very courageous and lovely woman. I enjoy caring for her." *JAMA* 306(13):1468–1478.

The Nursing Home Workforce

Nursing homes rely on 1.2 million health care and support workers in a wide range of occupations to help residents achieve their goals through the provision of medical, nursing, and social care to both treat illness and meet basic human needs. Nursing home workers also attend to infection prevention and control, therapeutic and recreational activities, housekeeping, and other needs of the residents. One challenge is that the heterogeneity and complexity of care needs has increased dramatically over the last 20 years, while average direct-care staffing has changed very little (MedPAC, 2016; Tyler et al., 2013). Federal guidelines dictate that facilities must "have sufficient staff to assure the safety of residents and attain or maintain the highest feasible level of physical, mental, and psychosocial well-being of each resident."[1] However, adequate staffing in nursing homes has been difficult to achieve for multiple reasons, including a negative perception of nursing homes, unsupportive working conditions, and poor pay and benefits. In his remarks to this committee, Donald Berwick, a president emeritus and senior fellow at the Institute for Healthcare Improvement, said

> You can't get patient and family experience as a central point in a demoralized workforce or undersupported workforce. And I'm thoroughly convinced that the conditions of work in the American nursing home are unsupportable if we want improvement.

This chapter provides an overview of the nursing home workforce, including their education and training, turnover rates, necessary competencies,

---

[1] CMS Requirements for Long-Term Care Facilities—Administration, 42 CFR § 483.70(e) (2016).

challenges with recruitment and retention, and connection to quality of care. Chapter 4 discusses the range of services provided by different members of the nursing home workforce.

THE OVERALL NURSING HOME WORKFORCE

The number and types of staff members in a nursing home vary depending on the number of residents, the complexity of their needs, and the scope of services provided. While nursing homes employ many workers directly, they may also provide care through referrals to consultants or by contracting workers rather than hiring them as employees. Additionally, family members and volunteers provide various needed services for the care of nursing home residents. Given the scope of care needed, interdisciplinary teams involving multiple staff members with distinct skills and responsibilities are critical to providing high-quality care to nursing home residents. While there are specific regulations for reporting nurse staffing data and steps to ensure the accuracy of those data, much less information is available about the wide range of other providers, and the information that is provided on public sites may not be accurate (OIG, 2021).

Nursing Home Employees

People employed by nursing homes represent a wide variety of occupations from 19 different major groups of the North American Industry Classification System for business establishments in the United States (BLS, 2020a). As Figure 5-1 shows, the bulk of workers are in health care support occupations (41 percent) and health care practitioners and technical occupations (27 percent). As these data only represent individuals employed directly by nursing homes, they may not be fully reflective of the entire workforce that helps to support nursing home residents. Examples from each of the reported categories are presented in Table 5-1. While not all of these occupations will be discussed at length in this chapter, these examples show the breadth of the nursing home workforce.

Temporary Agency Staff and Consultants

Nursing homes may employ temporary staff to fill in during staff absences and shortages. These temporary staff, usually referred to as "contract" or "agency" staff (because they are typically obtained through contracts with staffing agencies), can cost the facility (because of additional agency fees) up to twice as much as a permanent employee (Hale and Hale, 2019; Seavey, 2004). Many nursing homes increased their use

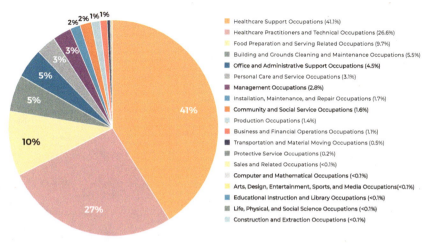

FIGURE 5-1 U.S. employment in nursing homes, May 2020.
SOURCE: BLS, 2020a.

of agency staff to fill gaps during the COVID-19 pandemic (Peck, 2021; Stulick, 2021). Contract staff accounted for about 5.8 percent of all nursing staff hours in the second quarter of 2021 (LTCCC, 2022).

Nursing home residents may also receive care in the nursing home setting from consultant health care professionals who are not employed directly by nursing homes. Instead, these providers bill insurers directly for the care they provide and do not require supervision from nursing home staff. Examples include care provided by podiatrists, optometrists, and dental professionals (CMS, 2021a; Hill, 2017; Lee et al., 2001; NHLC, 2021). Consultant care may also be provided by transferring residents to health care professionals in private offices for care that cannot be provided within the nursing home setting.

Family Caregivers and Volunteers

Family caregivers (including both family and other care partners) and volunteers from the community (who are neither friends nor family members of residents) also play an important role in the care of nursing home residents. Family caregivers, described as "an invisible workforce in nursing homes," are an essential component of the workforce, providing care even

TABLE 5-1 Occupation Classifications and Examples of Roles in U.S. Nursing Homes

NAICS Occupations	Examples of Roles
Health Care Support (41 percent)	Nursing assistants; orderlies; occupational therapy, physical therapy, and recreational therapy assistants and aides; and medical assistants
Health Care Practitioners and Technical (27 percent)	Dietitians; occupational, physical, respiratory, recreational and speech-language therapists; licensed nurses (e.g., registered nurses, advanced practice registered nurses); physicians; physician assistants; pharmacists; dentists and dental hygienists; clinical laboratory and radiologic technologists and technicians; medical records specialists; and health information technologists
Food Preparation/Serving-related (10 percent)	Food preparation and serving workers, cooks, cafeteria attendants, and dishwashers, and supervisors
Building and Grounds Cleaning and Maintenance (5 percent)	Housekeeping and janitorial workers, landscaping and groundskeeper workers, and supervisors
Office and Administrative Support (5 percent)	Financial clerks, information and record clerks, office clerks, secretaries, and receptionists
Personal Care and Service (3 percent)	Entertainment workers and hairdressers
Management Occupations (3 percent)	Chief executives, general and operations managers, marketing and sales managers, financial managers, human resources managers, food service managers, and medical and health services managers
Installation, Maintenance, and Repair (2 percent)	General maintenance and repair workers and their supervisors
Community and Social Service (2 percent)	Social workers, social and human service assistants, substance abuse and mental health counselors, community health workers, and clergy
Production Occupations (1 percent)	Laundry workers
Business and Financial Operations (1 percent)	Human resources workers, marketing and management analysts, and financial specialists
Transportation and Material Moving (0.5 percent)	Drivers, parking attendants, and stockers and order fillers, and supervisors
Protective Services (0.2 percent)	Security guards
Sales and Related (<0.1 percent)	Sales and marketing representatives
Computer and Mathematical (<0.1 percent)	Computer network support specialists, computer user support specialists, and network and computer systems administrators
Arts, Design, Entertainment, Sports, and Media (<0.1 percent)	Public relations specialists and interpreters and translators

continued

TABLE 5-1 Continued

NAICS Occupations	Examples of Roles
Educational Instruction and Library (<0.1 percent)	Special education teachers
Life, Physical, and Social Science (<0.1 percent)	Occupational health and safety specialists and technicians
Construction and Extraction (<0.1 percent)	Carpenters and painters

SOURCE: BLS, 2020a,b.
NOTE: NAICS = North American Industry Classification System.

after their loved ones have entered the nursing home (Coe and Werner, 2021, p. 110; also see Davies and Nolan, 2006; Gaugler, 2005; Reid and Chappell, 2017). Indeed, care provided by family caregivers is even more critical today than in the past, given the nationwide shortage of direct-care workers and high turnover (Antwi and Bowblis, 2018; Gandhi et al., 2021). Furthermore, the COVID-19 pandemic revealed the impact of family caregivers in several ways. Notably, policies that prohibited family and friends from entering nursing homes may have exacerbated staffing shortages because these family members and friends were not able to contribute to the care of their loved ones (Werner and Coe, 2021). Additionally, family caregivers often provided needed social connections, and COVID-related visitation policies contributed to social isolation and loneliness for residents (Abbasi, 2020a; Bethell et al., 2021; Veiga-Seijo et al., 2021).

While volunteers from the community may also assist with the care of nursing home residents, very limited research exists on this segment of the nursing home workforce, including on their training and on its impact on the quality of care. (See later in this chapter for more on family caregivers and volunteers.)

Interdisciplinary Team Care in the Nursing Home

Meeting the physical, psychosocial, mental, emotional, and spiritual needs of persons in nursing homes requires an interdisciplinary approach. "Interdisciplinary team work is a complex process in which different types of staff work together to share expertise, knowledge, and skills to impact on patient care" (Nancarrow et al., 2013). Consistent features of successful interdisciplinary interventions include formal team-based care, communication, coordination, and leadership (Nazir et al., 2013). The 2001 Institute of Medicine (IOM) report *Crossing the Quality Chasm* identified interdisciplinary teams as an essential component of high-quality care delivery and improved patient safety (IOM, 2001a). In long-term care settings, interdisciplinary teams result in improved resident outcomes for a variety of reasons. For example, interdisciplinary teams are better able to adapt to complex systems of care through improved cooperation, collaboration, and communication that ensures that care is continuous and reliable (IOM, 2003). They are also better equipped to meet residents' needs, keep pace with the demands of new technology, respond to the demands of payers, and deliver care across settings (IOM, 2003). In addition, there is also evidence that an interdisciplinary approach for assessing and planning care is related to the psychological well-being of residents, earlier intervention of residents' medical conditions, lower costs, reduced staff turnover, and increased staff satisfaction (IOM, 1996; Mukamel et al., 2009; Temkin-Greener et al., 2009; Zimmerman et al., 2016).

Federal nursing home regulations refer repeatedly to the interdisciplinary team in areas such as care and discharge planning, using physical and chemical restraints, preventing falls, treating incontinence and pressure injuries, managing pain, addressing behavioral health needs, accounting for significant change in health status, and preparing advance directives. Most nursing homes today have some form of an interdisciplinary team in order to comply with the Resident Assessment Instrument/Minimum Data Set process and accreditation requirements[2] (Dellefield, 2006; Temkin-Greener et al., 2009). (See Box 4-3 in Chapter 4 for a description of the requirements for the interdisciplinary care team.) According to the Centers for Medicare & Medicaid Services (CMS) Resident Assessment Instrument manual, the interdisciplinary team, along with the resident and resident's family, engages in developing a person-centered care plan that includes assessment, decision making, identification of outcomes, care planning, implementation of the care plan, and evaluation of care (CMS, 2019a). In its 2016 revised regulations for nursing homes, CMS required that certified nursing assistants (CNAs) be part of the interdisciplinary team and involved in care planning (CMS, 2016). Some have argued that to meet this requirement, nursing homes need to specifically delineate CNAs' responsibilities on the interdisciplinary team and to provide training in order for CNAs to participate effectively in care planning (Travers et al., 2021). (See Chapter 4 for more on care planning and the role of the interdisciplinary care team.)

NURSING HOME ADMINISTRATION AND LEADERSHIP

A variety of personnel provide high-level leadership in nursing homes. The national median for turnover of "top level executives" at nursing

---

[2] The Resident Assessment Instrument collects data to guide care planning and monitoring for long-term care residents.

homes is 20.46 percent (HHCS, 2020). In his testimony to this committee, Michael Wasserman, California Association of Long Term Care Medicine, noted:

> Effectively providing care for a complex group of individuals requires competencies at every level of the organizational chart. Aside from having an appropriate level of staffing, nursing homes require properly prepared highly skilled leadership teams that can balance the financial, operational, and clinical aspects of this incredibly complex business.

Administrator

A nursing home administrator has oversight and operational responsibilities, including ensuring regulatory compliance, supporting the rights of residents, and maintaining financial accountability. The domains of practice that provide the framework for the national examination of nursing home administrators include (1) customer care, supports, and services; (2) human resources; (3) finance; (4) environment; and (5) management and leadership (NAB, 2017). In 2020, the median salary for a nursing home administrator was $113,000 (HHCS, 2020).

Education and Training

Federal regulations for nursing homes require that the administrator of a nursing home is licensed by the state. However, state requirements for the licensure of nursing home administrators vary in terms of minimum education requirements, training hours, examination requirements, and continuing education requirements (NAB, 2021). Thirty-three of the 50 states and the District of Columbia require a minimum of a bachelor's degree to be a nursing home administrator, while eight states require only an associate's degree, and six states require only a high school degree (NAB, 2021). Four states (i.e., Delaware, Indiana, New York, and Wisconsin) do not indicate a minimum degree requirement.

Additionally, 47 of the states and the District of Columbia specify continuing education requirements for nursing home administrators on either an annual or biennial basis (NAB, 2021). However, there is much variation among states regarding these requirements. Eleven states require an average of 24 to 30 hours annually, 26 states and the District of Columbia require an average of 20 hours annually, and 9 states require an average of 12 to 18 hours annually. Four states (i.e., Alaska, Colorado, Hawaii, and New York) do not require continuing education for nursing home administrators.

Characteristics, Tenure, and Turnover

Few studies provide insight on the characteristics of nursing home administrators, and most of the studies that are available are quite old. While these studies may not fully reflect the characteristics of nursing home administrators today, they do provide some insight.

A 2007 study conducted in just two states found the average age of nursing home administrators to be 54 years, with an average tenure of 3.5 years, and with 96 percent holding a baccalaureate or higher degree (Castle et al., 2007). This is important since higher quality of care has been associated with nursing home administrators with higher levels of education and more experience (Castle et al., 2015; Lerner et al., 2014). Older studies of nursing home administrators found annual turnover rates of over 40 percent (Castle, 2001; Castle et al., 2007) and evidence of high instability of tenure within the first 3 years (Singh and Schwab, 2000); they also found that nursing home administrators with lower job satisfaction were more likely to leave within 1 year than administrators with higher job satisfaction. Lower job satisfaction was attributed to several factors, including the administrators' perceptions of high work demands and inadequate work skills (Castle et al., 2007). The sources of stress for nursing home administrators include challenges with regulations, difficulty with families, limited funds and resources, challenges with staffing, meeting the needs of residents, and corporate issues (Myers et al., 2018).

High turnover among the top management at nursing homes has been associated with a higher turnover of nursing assistants and licensed nursing staff (Castle, 2005), a lower quality of care (e.g., presence of pressure ulcers, use of psychoactive drugs, use of restraints) (Castle, 2001), and a number of inspection deficiencies (Geletta and Sparks, 2013). For a family member perspective on nursing home management, see Box 5-1.

BOX 5-1
Family Member Perspective

"Management is removed from the trenches. They are concerned with business and money aspect and forget the human person centered care. The staff once get courage will speak up for concerns of staff and residents. Sadly they are not listened to, are retaliated against or fired."

— K.S.

This quote was collected from the committee's online call for resident, family, and nursing home staff perspectives.

Medical Director

Federal regulations mandate that all certified nursing homes have a medical director who is a physician licensed in the state where the facility is located.[3] Requirements of the role include

(1) Coordinating medical care and providing clinical guidance;
(2) Overseeing the implementation of resident care policies;
(3) Ensuring policies and procedures align with current standards of practice; and
(4) Identifying and addressing issues with resident care or quality of life (CMS, 2005).

The medical director's role has been described to include the promotion of high-quality clinical care, assistance in reviewing the quality of care, advising on infection prevention and control issues, promoting employee health and safety, and being active in facility-related education and communication (AMDA, 2005). In fact, the 2020 CMS Coronavirus Commission on Safety and Quality in Nursing Homes report reinforced "the importance of medical director engagement in nursing home emergency management planning and execution" (MITRE, 2020, p. 41). Regulations also note that the role of the medical director is separate and independent of that of the attending physician. While most medical directors are also attending physicians in the facility, they do not need to be (CMS, 2005). Regulations require nursing home surveyors to evaluate whether medical directors are licensed, serving, and collaborating with the facility to implement policies. Given the expansive role of medical directors, some facilities have identified a need for an assistant or associate medical director who can be a physician, advanced practice registered nurse (APRN), or physician assistant (Medical Direction and Medical Care Work Group, 2011).

Characteristics

Medical directors are paid for their time and expertise. Compensation arrangements generally allow payment for providing clinical care and referring patients; however, medical directors cannot receive direct payment for future referrals to the facility or other businesses of the facility (Turner, 2015). Data on the compensation, recruitment, retention, and turnover of nursing home medical directors are extremely limited. CMS does not keep any record of the characteristics of nursing home medical directors (e.g., age, medical specialty, certification status, geriatric or medical director

---

[3] CMS Requirements for Long-Term Care Facilities—Administration, 42 CFR § 483.70 (h) (2016).

training, number of patients served, time spent in the nursing homes) in its databases, which makes research in this area challenging.

Education, Training, and Certification

To carry out their duties, medical directors need specialized knowledge, including high-level knowledge about geriatric syndromes, palliative care principles, dementia care, nursing home regulation and structure, care transitions, infection prevention and control, and quality improvement. However, except for the requirement of a license to practice medicine in the state, there are no additional specific education and training requirements for medical directors. The American Board of Post-Acute and Long-Term Care Medicine offers certification for medical directors in post-acute and long-term care medicine (ABPLM, 2022a). The board requires applicants for this training to meet specific criteria, including previous clinical and management experience in post-acute and long-term care settings (ABPLM, 2022b). Applicants must also complete the Core Curriculum on Medical Direction in Post-Acute and Long-Term Care, a course provided by the Society for Post-Acute and Long-Term Care Medicine (AMDA) (AMDA, 2022). The course focuses on the role and responsibilities of the medical director; the long-term care environment; organizational dynamics; communication skills, leadership skills, and team building skills; and resident care responsibilities (e.g., emergency care, quality management, family systems, and ethics) (AMDA, 2022). In 2021, California enacted a requirement for the certification of all medical directors in nursing homes (CALTCM, 2021).

In his testimony to this committee, Michael Wasserman, California Association of Long Term Care Medicine, noted:

> There are far too many medical directors who lack even basic knowledge of geriatric medicine concepts and who have little expertise or even interest in the complex regulatory framework of nursing homes. [Additionally,] residents and their families have a right to know the identity of the medical director, who, under federal regulations, is responsible for resident care policies and coordination of care.

Relationship to Quality of Care

Limited evidence links medical director certification and activities to the quality of care in nursing homes. One 2009 study found that the 547 nursing homes with a certified medical director performed up to 15 percent better on standardized quality scores than the other 15,230 nursing homes in the CMS Online Survey Certification and Reporting database (Rowland et al., 2009).

Director of Nursing

The director of nursing is the nursing home's chief nurse executive and is pivotal in influencing organizational and clinical outcomes (Rao and Evans, 2015; Siegel et al., 2010). A survey of directors of nursing in Florida nursing homes found that two-thirds or more held additional roles such as infection prevention and control (68 percent), quality management (79.2 percent), staff education (64 percent), and risk management (57.3 percent) (Sherman and Touhy, 2017).

Each nursing home is required to have a full-time director of nursing who is a registered nurse (RN), although there are waivers to this requirement. Directors of nursing have an average tenure of 6.8 years in their current position and 16.2 years of experience in long-term care, although 42 percent of directors of nursing have been in their current position less than 1 year (Lerner et al., 2014). A 2005 survey found a 36 percent annual turnover rate for directors of nursing (Castle, 2005). The average reported salary for directors of nursing is $92,756 with variation based on size and geographic location of the facility and the experience and education of the director of nursing (AADNS, 2019). Directors of nursing in for-profit nursing homes earn about $10,000 more annually than directors of nursing in nonprofit facilities (HHCS, 2020).

In many nursing homes, the director of nursing may be one of a few registered nurses (RNs) or even the only RN. Therefore, in addition to his or her administrative responsibilities, the director of nursing is often called upon to address the clinical needs of residents. Two-thirds of directors of nursing report they are often needed to provide direct care to residents ("pulled to the floor"), and 42 percent report this occurring daily or weekly (AADNS, 2019).

Competencies

The director of nursing needs to have knowledge and competencies in geriatric nursing as well as in administrative areas such as human resource management, staffing, budgeting and cost management, compliance and regulatory standards, and quality improvement. The director of nursing also needs effective leadership and supervision skills. Directors of nursing report spending half of their time in four areas: (1) management meetings, (2) addressing incidents and accidents, (3) staff scheduling, and (4) medication management (AADNS, 2019). Staffing and staff turnover are most consistently noted by directors of nursing as the greatest challenge and as taking most of their time (AADNS, 2019; Sherman and Touhy, 2017; Siegel et al., 2010).

The American Association of Directors of Nursing Services provides certification for directors of nursing based on seven competency domains, and the American Organization for Nursing Leadership has identified

TABLE 5-2 Director of Nursing Competencies

AADNS Director of Nursing Competencies	AONL Director of Nursing Competencies
Leadership	Communication and relationship building
Management and supervision	Knowledge of the health care environment
Organizational oversight and management	Leadership
Business acumen	Professionalism
Quality improvement	Business skills
Regulatory compliance	
Professional development	

SOURCES: AADNS, 2021; AONE/AONL, 2015.
NOTE: AADNS = American Association of Directors of Nursing Services; AONL = American Organization for Nursing Leadership.

five competency areas for the post-acute care nurse executive (see Table 5-2). More broadly, the American Nurses Association outlines the competencies needed by nurses holding administrative positions in any health care organization (ANA, 2016).

Education and Training

The majority of directors of nursing have an associate degree or diploma in nursing (Holle et al., 2019; Olson and Zwygart-Stauffacher, 2008; Sherman and Touhy, 2017; Trinkoff et al., 2015). However, associate degree nursing programs provide no educational preparation to function in an administrative nursing role and limited training in geriatric nursing. Several reports on competencies for directors of nursing have recommended a requirement for a bachelor's degree in nursing, with a preference for a master's degree (ANA, 2016; Lodge, 1985). At least one analysis suggests that they should have a master's degree in nursing administration (Siegel et al., 2010), and 22 experts in gerontological nursing joined to recommend that all directors of nursing attain certification in core geriatric nursing and leadership competencies (Kolanowski et al., 2021). Fewer than half of directors of nursing (42.5 percent) hold any national certification (Trinkoff et al., 2015).

While effective leadership from a director of nursing has been associated with high-quality care (Castle and Decker, 2011; McKinney et al., 2016), no federal or state requirements specify minimum education requirements, continuing education requirements, or additional training requirements for directors of nursing. Previous IOM reports on nursing home quality pointed to the lack of educational preparation for directors of nursing to serve as the top-level nurse leader and administrator of the organization in the context of the complexity of the environment and role (IOM, 1996, 2001b);

concern persists about the lack of administrative and leadership preparation of directors of nursing and its impact on the quality of care (Harvath et al., 2008; Olson and Zwygart-Stauffacher, 2008; Siegel et al., 2010).

Nursing home member organizations, universities, and director-of-nursing organizations have developed continuing education and certification programs to compensate for the lack of preparation that directors of nursing have for the role (LeadingAge Minnesota, 2021; Vogelsmeier et al., 2010). For example, American Association of Directors of Nursing Services and the National Association of Directors of Nursing in Long-Term Care offer the opportunity to attain national certification as a director of nursing (AAPACN, 2021).[4]

Director of Social Services

The director of social services oversees all social service programs and supervises social workers and social service designees within the facility. Occasionally, the director of social services assists with the implementation of some resident activities, such as the resident council, and assists in the facilitation of admissions tasks. Other leadership positions related to social care focus on activities and the spiritual health of residents, and may include a director of health and wellness, fitness coordinator, activities director/coordinator, and director of pastoral services/spiritual director.

In 2003, the National Association of Social Workers (NASW) developed a consensus statement for professional standards for social work directors in long-term care settings, stating

> It is preferable that the social work director be a graduate of a master's degree program from an accredited school of program of social work, have a minimum of 2 years postgraduate experience in long-term care or related programs, and meet equivalent state requirements for social work practice or, in jurisdictions not having such legal regulation, is a member of the Academy of Certified Social Workers (NASW, 2003, p. 8).

One recent analysis found that while most nursing homes employ social services staff, only 37 percent of nursing homes have a degreed and licensed social worker at the helm of social services, and 42 percent of social services directors do not have a degree in social work (Bern-Klug et al., 2021a). (See later in this chapter for more on the federal requirements of social workers in nursing homes.) Larger not-for-profit nursing homes and nursing homes that are not part of a chain are the most likely to hire a degreed and licensed social worker as a social services director. In 2020, the median salary for a director

---

[4] For more information on the certification exam, see https://www.nadona.org/product/cert-director-of-nursing-cdon (accessed November 3, 2021).

of social services was $55,188 (HHCS, 2020). Evidence on the characteristics, education and training, job satisfaction, and turnover of social services directors is limited or nonexistent. The few studies that exist are dated and examine very narrow topics (Bell et al., 2010; Bern-Klug and Sabri, 2012; Liu and Bern-Klug, 2013). See the discussion of psychosocial care providers later in this chapter for more about social work staff in nursing homes.

PRIMARY CARE PROVIDERS

Primary care providers actively authorize and supervise the care of residents and review the resident's total program of care (e.g., medications, treatments) and status (e.g., current condition; progress; and problems maintaining physical, mental, and psychosocial well-being). Regulations mandate that all nursing home residents must have 24-hour access to health care provided by a physician or other qualified practitioner such as APRNs (e.g., nurse practitioner, clinical nurse specialist) and physician assistants. State laws and regulations govern care provided by clinicians other than physicians in terms of physician supervision or collaboration.

Federal nursing home regulations require an initial visit by a physician within the first 30 days of a nursing home resident's admission, although other required visits may alternate between a physician and other qualified practitioners.[5] For initial visits at nursing homes that are not specifically designated as skilled nursing facilities, clinicians not employed by the facility may do the initial visit and documentation.[6] Primary care providers are also responsible for writing and signing progress notes for each medical care visit and signing and dating all medical orders. The American Medical Directors Association outlines the comprehensive role of the attending primary care provider in the nursing home (AMDA, 2003).

Only limited and dated evidence exists regarding primary care providers for nursing home residents, particularly for physicians and physician assistants. A national survey of medical directors in nursing homes found that the majority were also the practicing physician in the nursing home and often served as medical directors in two nursing homes (Levy et al., 2007). The survey found that "nearly 80 percent of medical directors served as attending physicians and, on average, were the attending physician to 44 percent of the patients in their facilities" (p. 562). Only 12.5 percent of physicians who bill Medicare have claims for nursing home visits (Jung et al., 2021). Barriers to attracting physicians to nursing home care include the

---

[5] CMS Requirements for Long-Term Care Facilities—Physician Services, 42 CFR § 483.30 (c)(1) (2016).

[6] CMS Requirements for Long-Term Care Facilities—Physician Services, 42 CFR § 483.30 (c) (2016).

minimal geriatrics training that most physicians receive in medical school, low reimbursement, nonreimbursable activities associated with providing medical care in nursing homes, burden of regulations on the physician's practice and time, and malpractice risk (Kane, 1993; Levy et al., 2007).

At least one recent analysis concluded that research is needed on the practice quality of medical providers and the impact of provider quality on resident outcomes as well as concluding that practice-based quality measures are needed (Katz et al., 2021). Recently, investigators identified a set of quality indicators for the practice of post-acute and long-term care by primary care providers (Mays et al., 2018).

Skilled Nursing Facility Specialists

Care models with physicians, APRNs, and physician assistants serving as skilled nursing facility specialists (SNFists) are increasing. SNFists (akin to hospitalists) are full-time providers to nursing home residents (Teno et al., 2018). For example, one study reported that between 2007 and 2014, the proportion of billing by SNFists increased from 22 to 31.5 percent (Teno et al., 2017). From 2012 to 2015, the mean number of nursing home specialists increased by nearly 34 percent, particularly for practitioners other than physicians (Ryskina et al., 2017). While the numbers of SNFists are growing, particularly among APRNs, there is extreme variation; many nursing homes have almost no full-time primary care providers while in others, almost all residents have a full-time provider (Goodwin et al., 2021). While most SNFists who are physicians have training in primary care (e.g., internal medicine, family medicine), only 6.5 percent specialized in geriatrics (Jung et al., 2021).

One study found that nursing home residents receiving care from SNFists have lower avoidable hospitalizations, are more likely to be discharged to the community, and have more provider visits (Katz et al., 2021). However, another study suggested that nursing home residents may experience a small increased benefit when they are cared for by the same physicians and advanced practice clinicians in both the hospital and nursing home (White et al., 2020a).

The nursing home specialist model often involves a collaborative practice between physicians and APRNs. An AMDA ad hoc workgroup with representation from the Gerontological Advanced Practice Nurses Association provides an in-depth description of collaborative practice between a medical doctor and an APRN and outlines the core medical competencies, roles, and responsibilities of the APRN in long-term care (AMDA, 2011). In an older national survey, 63 percent of medical directors reported APRN involvement in care of nursing home residents—with two APRNs per responding facility, on average (Rosenfeld et al., 2004). These APRNs were most frequently part of a physician group practice (60 percent) or part of an organization practice (38 percent). Only 19 percent of APRNs were employed directly by nursing homes (Rosenfeld et al., 2004). The proportion of nursing homes employing APRN and physician assistant providers increased from 20.4 percent in 2000 to 35.0 percent in 2010 (up from less than 10 percent in the early 1990s), although there was significant variability across states (Intrator et al., 2005, 2015).

Physician Assistants

Limited and dated evidence suggests that care provided by physician assistants can improve the quality of care for nursing home residents as well as provide cost savings (Ackermann and Kemle, 1998). Many studies of the nursing home workforce consider physician assistants and APRNs together and do not distinguish the specific impact of the physician assistant (Caprio, 2006; Gupta et al., 2014). A 2017 report suggested that physician assistants may represent an underused segment of the workforce available to support nursing home residents (Himmerick et al., 2017).

Advanced Practice Registered Nurses

The APRN role in providing care in nursing homes emerged in the early 1980s and grew in popularity after the 1986 IOM report *Improving the Quality of Care in Nursing Homes* (IOM, 1986). A 2008 review identified the roles APRNs were playing, including as primary-care (and acute-care) providers for both long-stay and post-acute residents; educators of residents, family, and staff; and consultants on improving system-wide and facility-wide care resident care issues (Bakerjian, 2008). Medical directors have previously reported high effectiveness of and high satisfaction with nurse practitioners (Rosenfeld et al., 2004). Family and resident satisfaction has been also associated positively with APRN-provided care in nursing homes (Bakerjian, 2008; Liu et al., 2011; Mileski et al., 2020), and APRNs are effective at building relationships with families and residents for more informed care decision making (Mileski et al., 2020).

Numerous reviews have identified key outcomes resulting from APRN-provided care in nursing homes, including improved management of chronic illnesses, improved functional and health status, improved quality of life, reduced or equivalent mortality and hospital admissions, improved self-care, reduced emergency department use and transfers, lower costs, increased time spent with residents, and increased resident, family, and staff satisfaction (Bakerjian, 2008; Christian and Baker, 2009; Donald et al., 2013; Liu et al., 2011; Mileski et al., 2020; Morilla-Herrera et al., 2016; Popejoy et al., 2017; Rantz et al., 2017; Xing et al., 2013).

Strategies to decrease hospitalizations have included APRN-led advanced care planning, medication reconciliation interventions, and employing APRNs full time at nursing homes (Mileski et al., 2020; Popejoy et al., 2017). However, one literature review identified the most frequently mentioned barrier for increasing the role of APRNs in nursing homes is their restricted scope of practice due to Medicare regulations and state regulatory constraints (Mileski et al., 2020). Nursing homes are unable to employ APRNs to bill Medicare for direct-care services (Popejoy et al., 2019; Rantz et al., 2017). In 2011, the IOM report *The Future of Nursing* recommended that the U.S. Congress "expand the Medicare program to include coverage of [APRN] services that are within the scope of practice under applicable state law, just as physician services are now covered" (IOM, 2011, p. 9). The report further recommended that the Medicare program be amended to authorize APRNs to perform assessments for admission to nursing homes.

A core component of the Missouri Quality Initiative demonstration project to reduce avoidable hospitalizations of nursing home residents is the use of APRNs working full time in a nursing home with an interdisciplinary team (Rantz et al., 2017, 2018a). The APRNs focus primarily on the geriatric clinical management of the residents and work with the staff to embed changes in their daily care delivery in areas such as hydration, fall prevention and management, and continence management. This model successfully reduced all-cause hospitalizations, avoidable hospitalizations, all-cause emergency department visits, avoidable emergency department visits, use of antipsychotic medications, and improved composite quality measure scores (Flesner et al., 2019; Rantz et al., 2018a,b; RTI International, 2017; Vogelsmeier et al., 2018, 2020). Additionally, significant cost savings were realized, including a reduction in total Medicare expenditures (Rantz et al., 2018b). (See Chapter 3 for more on the Missouri Quality Initiative.)

LICENSED NURSES

Two types of licensed nurses work in nursing homes: licensed practical/vocational nurses (LPNs/LVNs) and RNs. An LPN/LVN has completed training through a technical education program and then taken a national licensing examination. Each respective state board of nursing determines the LPN/LVN scope of practice, and in all cases, these nurses work under the supervision of an RN. Several types of education programs prepare an individual to take the national examination for licensure as an RN, including associate degree programs, hospital-based diploma programs, baccalaureate programs (bachelor of science in nursing), or post-baccalaureate programs (master of science in nursing).

Nursing homes and extended care settings in the United States employ 4.4 percent of the country's RNs, compared with 27.5 percent of the country's LPN/LVNs (down from 31.7 percent in 2017) (NCSBN, 2017; Smiley et al., 2021). On average, RNs make up 12 percent of the licensed nurses in nursing homes, whereas in hospitals the majority of, if not all, licensed nurses are RNs (Denny-Brown et al., 2020; Harris-Kojetin et al., 2019). While 64 percent of RNs in the United States have a bachelor's or master's degree in nursing (HRSA, 2019), the percentage of nurses with a bachelor's degree or higher working in nursing homes is unknown. In 2020, RNs at the median earned $31.00 per hour while LPNs earned $23.64 per hour (HHCS, 2020).

Roles and Responsibilities

Traditionally, nursing homes have focused on the roles of licensed nurses in general (e.g., medication administration, treatments, carrying out physician orders) and have failed to differentiate the responsibilities of RNs and LPN/LVNs. Consequently, RNs and LPN/LVNs have been used interchangeably in nursing homes at the expense of the residents' unmet professional nursing needs (Mueller et al., 2018), and LPN/LVNs often work outside their scope of practice (Corazzini et al., 2015; Mueller et al., 2012). For example, in a survey of LPN/LVNs in two states, LPN/LVNs were actively engaged in nursing assessments and developing and evaluating care plans; the unavailability of RNs was reported as the most common reason that LPN/LVNs found themselves engaged in activities that were outside their scope of practice (Mueller et al., 2012). Corazzini and colleagues (2013) examined how RNs and LPN/LVNs in nursing homes enacted core components of their scopes of practice (i.e., assessment, care planning, delegation and supervision). Three factors influenced the effectiveness of the collaboration between RNs and LPN/LVNs and their ability to function within their scopes of practice: (1) quality of connections, (2) degree of interchangeability between RNs and LPN/LVNs, and (3) staffing ratios.

RNs also fill other roles in nursing homes aside from direct clinical care. Federal regulations require that an RN conducts or coordinates required assessments using the Resident Assessment Instrument with the appropriate participation of other health professionals.[7] Additional roles that RNs may have in nursing homes include quality improvement, infection prevention and control, staff development, management, and supervision. LPN/LVNs may fulfill those roles in some nursing homes.

---

[7] CMS Requirements for Long-Term Care Facilities—Resident Assessment, 42 CFR § 483.20 (b)(1)(xviii), (g), and (h) (2016).

Education and Training

RNs are accountable for a wide range of resident care needs, including assessment, diagnosis, outcomes identification, planning, implementation, and evaluation (ANA, 2015). Furthermore, an RN is prepared to provide ongoing assessment of the residents' clinical condition and to use critical thinking approaches to prevent or mitigate negative outcomes such as infections, exacerbation of chronic conditions, adverse medication events, pressure injuries, falls that can lead to hospitalizations, emergency admissions, and even death (Clarke and Donaldson, 2008; Horn et al., 2005; Mileski et al., 2020).

From 2007 to 2010, the Geriatric Nursing Education Consortium carried out a national effort to provide faculty in schools of nursing with "the necessary skills, knowledge, and competency to implement sustainable curricular innovations in care of older adults" (Gray-Miceli et al., 2014, p. 447). Faculty from over 400 baccalaureate nursing programs participated in this program and subsequently incorporated geriatric content into their curricula. However, no long-term data demonstrate whether geriatric nursing content and clinical experiences have been sustained in nursing curricula. Without faculty who have expertise in geriatric nursing, the focus on the nursing care of older adults is at high risk of being minimized in nursing curricula. The 2008 IOM report *Retooling for an Aging America: Building the Health Care Workforce* called for requiring health care workers to demonstrate competencies in basic geriatric care in order to receive and maintain their licenses and certifications and recommended that all health professional schools and health care training programs expand coursework and training in the treatment of older adults (IOM, 2008). The CMS Coronavirus Commission on Safety and Quality in Nursing Homes also called for training of RNs, LPNs, and CNAs in long-term care settings (MITRE, 2020).

The annual mean turnover rate of RNs in nursing homes is estimated at 140.7 percent, with the median rate being 102.9 percent (Gandhi et al., 2021). Recruiting and retaining RNs in nursing homes is challenging because nursing homes generally offer nurses lower wages than they would earn in other health care settings; the annual mean wage for RNs in nursing homes ($72,090) is approximately $10,000 (roughly 12 percent) less than RNs employed in acute-care hospitals ($81,680) and approximately $17,000 (nearly 20 percent) less than RNs employed in outpatient care settings ($89,300), for example (BLS, 2020c). Furthermore, the nursing home environment is often not conducive to supporting the professional practice and development of RNs. Supportive environments include the implementation of evidence-based practices; shared decision making regarding resident care, staffing, and work environment; involvement and leadership in quality improvement initiatives; and support for professional development

(Lyons et al., 2008; Rondeau and Wagar, 2006). Supportive work environments for RNs in nursing homes lead to better resident outcomes, lower nurse burnout, and higher nurse satisfaction (White et al., 2020b).

NURSE STAFFING, REGULATION, AND QUALITY OF CARE

Increasing RN staffing and overall nurse staffing has been a consistent recommendation for improving the quality of care in nursing homes (Harrington et al., 2016, 2020). While inadequate staffing is a widespread concern, it is also cited relatively infrequently by surveyors (CMA, 2014; Harrington et al., 2008, 2020). The following sections give an overview of the evidence base for the relationship between nurse staffing and the quality of care for nursing home residents, the regulations for nurse staffing levels, the success (or failure) of meeting these standards, and other challenges.

Quality of Care

Decades of evidence support the association between inadequate nurse staffing and poor quality of care in nursing homes, particularly in the case of RNs (Aiken, 1981; Eagle, 1968; Harrington et al., 2021; IOM, 1996; Spilsbury et al., 2011; Wells, 2004). Five systematic literature reviews conducted between 2006 and 2015 examined the relationship between nurse staffing and quality of care in nursing homes (Backhaus et al., 2014; Bostick et al., 2006; Castle, 2008; Dellefield et al., 2015; Spilsbury et al., 2011). Four of the reviews concluded that there were positive and significant relationships between nurse staffing and quality, while one review found the relationship to be inconsistent. The results were mixed in regard to the relationship between quality and LPN/LVN staffing or nursing assistant staffing. (See later in this chapter for more on CNAs.) The reviews consistently noted study limitations and called for better staffing data sources, longitudinal study designs, accounting for case mix, and strengthening ways to measure quality. For example, most studies relied on self-reported staffing data collected at the time of a nursing home's state survey (Castle, 2008; Dellefield et al., 2015; Spilsbury et al., 2011).

Studies of nurse staffing typically examine nurse staffing levels as determined by the number of nursing hours per resident; a higher staffing level indicates that there are more nursing hours per resident day (discussed in the next section on regulations). Individual studies have demonstrated associations between higher nursing assistant staffing levels and fewer numbers of deficiencies found in inspections (Harrington, 2000; Hyer et al., 2011; Lerner, 2013) and between higher RN staffing levels and the number and severity of deficiencies (Lerner, 2013). Higher RN staffing levels have also been associated with lower rates of rehospitalizations, hospitalizations, and emergency department use (Min and Hong, 2019; Spector et al., 2013; Yang et al., 2021a).

However, fully understanding the relationship between nurse staffing and quality of care requires more than an examination of the numbers of staff or hours per resident day. Rather, the connection between staffing and quality likely also depends on the skills of the staff, the complexity of resident care needs, and the organizational context of care delivery (e.g., allocation of work assignments, supervision, teamwork, use of care-related technologies, and physical layout of the nursing home) (Arling and Mueller, 2014; Arling et al., 2007). That is to say that some well-run facilities may be able to achieve high quality with fewer staff as compared to facilities in which care delivery is poorly organized.

Regulations for Nurse Staffing

In 2001, CMS conducted a large-scale study to identify appropriate nurse staffing ratios in nursing homes (Feuerberg, 2001; Harrington et al., 2020). The resulting report concluded that a "range of serious problems including malnutrition, dehydration, pressure sores, abuse and neglect . . . have pointed to nurse staffing as a potential root cause" (Feuerberg, 2001, p. 1). In addition to the numbers of staff in nursing homes being insufficient to meet the needs of residents, the CMS report identified several other staffing-related issues that contributed to poor quality in nursing homes, including high staff turnover and low retention, inadequate expenditures on nurse staffing, needs related to staff training/competencies, and ineffective or inadequate management and supervision (Feuerberg, 2001). The report also identified staffing thresholds below which residents were at risk for serious quality-of-care issues (Table 5-3).

Since 2016, CMS has required nursing homes to electronically submit direct-care staffing data on a daily basis through their Payroll-Based Journal (CMS, 2021b). However, the 2001 proposed CMS minimum staffing standards have not been addressed in any subsequent regulatory rules, so that

TABLE 5-3 Proposed Minimum Nurse Staffing Standards for U.S. Nursing Homes in 2001

	Short-stay	Long-stay
RN Hours per Resident Day	.55	.75
LPN/LVN Hours per Resident Day	1.15	1.3
Nursing Assistant Hours per Resident Day	2.4	2.8
Total Nursing Hours per Resident Day	4.1	4.1

SOURCE: Feuerberg, 2001.

there is no minimum federal standard for RN hours per resident day and great variation in state standards (Harrington et al., 2016). Instead, current regulations include a vague nurse staffing requirement that nursing homes must provide "sufficient nursing staff to attain or maintain the highest practicable . . . well-being of each resident."[8] (See later in this chapter for more on CNA staffing levels.) In the second quarter of 2021, the average number of staff hours per resident day was 0.66 for RNs (excluding administrative RNs and directors of nursing), 0.82 for LPNs (excluding administrative LPNs), 2.04 for CNAs, and 3.75 for total nursing hours—well below the recommended thresholds for most nursing home residents (LTCCC, 2022).

The 1996 IOM report *Nursing Staff in Hospitals and Nursing Homes* further recommended a requirement for 24-hour RN coverage in nursing homes by the year 2000 (IOM, 1996). The recommendation was endorsed by a subsequent IOM study in 2001, and then recommended again in the 2004 IOM report *Keeping Patients Safe* (IOM, 2001b, 2004). Yet today the requirement is a 24-hour daily presence of *licensed* nurse coverage (i.e., RN or LPN/LVN) with an RN fulfilling at least 8 of those hours.[9] The CMS Coronavirus Commission on Safety and Quality in Nursing Homes noted the importance of 24-hour daily presence of RNs for nursing homes with positive COVID-19 cases (MITRE, 2020). The Build Back Better Act, introduced in 2021, called for 24-hour daily presence of RNs in all nursing homes and for the U.S. Department of Health and Human Services to study what minimum nursing staff requirements would best help meet resident needs.[10]

An analysis of 2019 data by the U.S. Government Accountability Office (GAO) found that while virtually all nursing homes met the federal requirement of the 8-hour presence of an RN, only about one-quarter of nursing homes met the proposed staffing minimums for RN and total nurse staffing (see Table 5-3) (GAO, 2021). The GAO recommended that CMS should report on nursing homes' minimum staffing standards below which residents are at increased risk of quality problems (such as those proposed in 2001) on Care Compare.

States may also have specific nurse staffing standards for nursing homes (Harrington, 2010). For example, in June 2021, New York State passed a law requiring minimum clinical staffing levels in nursing homes (Brown, 2021). These standards include 3.5 hours per day of clinical staffing, of which at least 2.2 hours are provided by a CNA or nurse aide and at least 1.1 hours are provided by a licensed nurse. States that regulate the level of nursing home staff have higher levels of nurse staffing (Mueller et al., 2006;

---

[8] CMS Requirements for Long-Term Care Facilities—Nursing Services, 42 CFR § 483.35 (2016).
[9] Ibid.
[10] Build Back Better Act, HR 5376, 117th Cong., 1st sess., Congressional Record 167, no. 200, daily ed. (November 17, 2021).

Paek et al., 2016), with one study finding that nursing homes that meet their state's nurse staffing standards had fewer total deficiencies and fewer quality-of-care deficiencies than nursing homes that did not meet the staffing standards (Kim et al., 2009). However, in 2021, the Consumer Voice noted that "twenty years after the CMS study found that at least 4.1 [hours per resident day] of direct care nursing staff time are needed just to prevent poor outcomes, state staffing requirements, with a few exceptions, are nowhere near that recommended level" (Consumer Voice, 2021, p. 8). For family member perspectives on staffing standards and understaffing, see Box 5-2.

BOX 5-2
Family Member Perspectives

"State and federal governments need to enact minimum staffing requirement. It is ridiculous how little staff they have at my husband's facility. Sometimes one aide is responsible for 30+ patients. My husband is a Type 1 diabetic, is blind, and can't walk. There's been several instances of his blood sugar going low, and when he calls for help it can take an hour or more for someone to respond. I have to provide him food to eat when he goes low because I can't rely on staff to help him. As his mental acuity diminishes, I fear that it could become a life-or-death situation."

— K.R.

"Insufficient staffing!!!! For forty residents there is usually one nurse and 3 or 4 (sometimes 5) aides. It's hard enough when things are running fairly smooth but when there is an emergency, everything falls apart and residents suffer because of it."

— 87-year-old wife of an 89-year-old resident

"There are so many types of facilities I have been in and no matter what, staffing is what makes or breaks it. Over the years, it has been clear the staffing ratio is outdated for higher levels of care for living in any long term care setting. Concerns with staffing ratios not allowing staff time to take with residents needed, staff overworked, stressed and shows in how they care/don't care for dependent residents. Sure on paper, numbers look good, but, real-life scenarios are not taken into account."

— K.S.

"Unfortunately, my family member and I swam in a sea of nightmares most of the time because of severe understaffing that affected multiple departments (e.g., nursing, food service, occupational therapy, physical therapy, recreational therapy). My family member's speech therapist acknowledged the problem of understaffing and uneven feeding skills; the therapist told me they could not complain, for fear of losing their job."

— M.K.

These quotes were collected from the committee's online call for resident, family, and nursing home staff perspectives.

Additionally, staffing level patterns show a drop in nurse staffing (i.e., RNs, LPN/LVNs, and nurse aides) during the weekends (GAO, 2021; Harrington et al., 2020). The GAO found that RN staffing hours decrease by around 40 percent on the weekends (see Figure 5-2) (GAO, 2021). GAO noted that this was an important detail for the informed decision making of consumers and recommended that CMS report weekend RN and total nursing staffing levels on Care Compare. Data collected by CMS are helpful to the state survey process. For example, CMS shares weekend staffing data with state survey agencies so that they may target weekend inspections to nursing homes that report lower weekend staffing levels (OIG, 2021). The Office of the Inspector General recommended that CMS report more types of staffing data to state survey agencies, such as nursing homes with frequent reports of lower staffing levels (including specific dates) and nursing homes at risk of having insufficient staffing (OIG, 2021).

Current staffing requirements are not adjusted by resident case mix (CMS, 2016, 2019b). A large proportion of nursing homes have staffing levels below CMS's case-mix adjusted expected staffing levels (GAO, 2021; Geng et al., 2019). For RNs, including both the directors of nursing and RNs with administrative responsibilities, 91 percent of the facilities met the expected level less than 60 percent of the time (Geng et al., 2019). An Office of the Inspector General (OIG) report also noted that by not taking resident

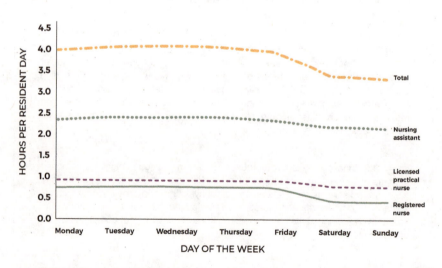

FIGURE 5-2 Average adjusted nursing home staffing by nurse type and day of week.
SOURCE: GAO, 2021.

acuity into account, CMS's assessments of nursing homes with the lowest weekend staffing levels likely miss up to one-quarter of facilities that have a greater level of staffing need (OIG, 2021). For family member perspectives on staffing standards and resident acuity, see Box 5-3.

Meeting specific minimum staffing standards while also moving toward smaller, more home-like models of care may add challenges to achieving these standards. However, innovative approaches to meeting these standards will ensure that all nursing homes have the necessary expertise to achieve high-quality care.

INFECTION PREVENTION AND CONTROL LEADERSHIP

In 2016, CMS issued a final rule revising the requirements that nursing homes (and other long-term care facilities) must meet to participate in Medicare and Medicaid programs. (See Chapter 8 for more on quality assurance.) As part of the rule, nursing homes were required to designate at least one part-time or full-time staff member as the infection prevention and control specialist (also known as an infection preventionist). The role of the

---

BOX 5-3
Family Member Perspectives

"Aides needing to spend more time with dementia resident depending on what needs are at that time and the behaviors can determine need for slower pace and more time, some examples that are not taken into account for staffing levels. It is a domino effect, the staff taking longer with one resident, in turn, puts a longer wait for other residents. Especially when more residents are 2 person assists and Hoyer lifts. Oh yes, they are over minimum staffing ratio, but, in reality it does not present that way."

— K.S.

"My family member was a resident of a 500+-bed, five star-rated facility from May 2015 to May 2019. My family member resided in the facility's rehab wing from March 2015 to May 2015; resided in a blended wing from June 2015 to Sept. 2016; and resided in a memory care wing from Sept. 2016 to May 2019. All three types of wings had the same staff-to-resident ratio, meaning that the memory care wing, where nearly every resident was memory impaired, elderly, and frail, had the same staff-to-resident ratio (one CNA to eight residents, with a census of roughly 39) as the blended wing where higher functioning residents were in the majority."

— M.K.

These quotes were collected from the committee's online call for resident, family, and nursing home staff perspectives.

infection prevention and control specialist includes assessing, implementing, and managing the facility's infection prevention and control plan and participating in the facility's quality assessment and assurance committees. The final rule suggested that an RN would assume the role of the infection prevention and control specialist in most facilities and that the individual would need to spend around 15 percent of his or her time on this role.[11] The CMS Coronavirus Commission on Safety and Quality in Nursing Homes noted the position of infection prevention and control specialist is "traditionally assigned to a supervisor, nursing manager, or provider as an added (rather than a core) responsibility" (MITRE, 2020, p. 41). However, the commission noted that "there are no national standards for training and licensure requirements of infection preventionists that nursing homes are mandated to employ" and subsequently recommended higher qualifications and training (MITRE, 2020, p. 48).

A 2015 survey by the Association for Professionals in Infection Control and Epidemiology found that only 15 percent of infection prevention and control specialists in non–acute care settings (including nursing homes) were certified in infection control (Pogorzelska-Maziarz and Kalp, 2017). Before the 2016 rule, staffing levels for infection prevention and control specialists in nursing homes varied widely across nursing homes (Stone et al., 2020). Between 2014 and 2018, staffing levels were higher in large for-profit nursing homes than in large nonprofit nursing homes (Stone et al., 2020). Furthermore, studies have found a lack of training among the personnel responsible for infection prevention and control in nursing homes (Stone et al., 2018; Trautner et al., 2017). CDC TRAIN offers the Nursing Home Infection Preventionist Training Course; the course is free, qualifies for various continuing education credits, and covers a variety of topics such as infection surveillance, hand hygiene, injection safety, water and linen management, antibiotic stewardship, and preventing respiratory infections (CDC TRAIN, 2021).

The 2020 CMS Coronavirus Commission on Safety and Quality in Nursing Homes noted that the current regulations on infection prevention and control specialists in nursing homes yielded an "insufficient response to the demands" of the [COVID-19] pandemic (MITRE, 2020, p. 41). The commission made several recommendations related to the role of the infection preventionist, including

- Employ infection preventionists with educator capabilities and document their training of the nursing homes staff;
- Assess infection prevention and control competency among all nursing home staff;

---

[11] CMS Requirements for Long-Term Care Facilities—Infection Control, 42 CFR § 483.80 (2016).

THE NURSING HOME WORKFORCE

- Establish a full-time-equivalent-to-bed ratio for an infection preventionist educator for every nursing home (with consideration for health professional shortage areas); and
- Develop and provide a training curriculum and certification for infection preventionists in nursing homes.

See later in this chapter for more on infection prevention and control during the COVID-19 pandemic, particularly the role of strike teams.

PSYCHOSOCIAL AND SPIRITUAL CARE PROVIDERS

A variety of workers are engaged in the psychosocial care of nursing home residents. These include social workers, chaplains, and staff involved with activities, art, and wellness. (See Chapter 4 for more on psychosocial care needs.)

Social Workers

Social workers' roles in nursing homes support person-centered care and include identifying and assessing residents' psychosocial needs; working as part of the interdisciplinary care team; communicating and assisting residents and their families with care needs (e.g., behavioral health and psychosocial care) (see Chapter 4); eliciting and honoring resident care preferences; advocating for at-risk populations (e.g., residents belonging to racial and ethnic minorities, LGBTQ+ residents); and providing transitional care, counseling, and conflict management to residents, families, and staff (Bern-Klug and Kramer, 2013; Kusmaul et al., 2017; Miller et al., 2021; NASW, 2003, 2016). In addition, social services directors are often involved in discharge planning, transitions of care, psychosocial care planning, and interactions with family members (Bern-Klug et al., 2021a). Box 5-4 outlines the major tasks involved in providing medically related social services.

Qualifications

Professionally trained social workers with a bachelor's degree in social work (B.S.W.) or master's degree in social work (M.S.W.) hold a professional degree that includes training to develop clinical, organizational, and community engagement skills. Social work programs provide competency-based education to practitioners who agree to abide by a standard code of ethics and conduct, complete fieldwork, and demonstrate professional behavior and skills (CSWE, 2015). The Council on Social Work Education (CSWE)[12] accredits baccalaureate-level (generalist social work practice)

---

[12] For more information, see www.cswe.org (accessed November 3, 2021).

> **BOX 5-4**
> **Medically Related Social Services: Major Tasks**
>
> - Assist with resident rights and serve as resident advocate in the facility
> - Manage grievance processes including assisting residents with making grievances and obtaining a resolution
> - Refer and obtain outside services and supports
> - Arrange for transitional care (e.g., community placement options and supports)
> - Provide or arrange for mental and psychosocial health counseling services
> - Assist with advance care planning, including facilitating discussions with resident and families and completion of advance directives
> - Identify and promote person-centered, nonpharmacologic interventions for behavioral health care
> - Assist with financial and legal matters
> - Educate residents and family members about care options
> - Ensure that residents' needs are met through initial and ongoing assessment and care planning
> - Provide support and services when a resident is in distress, during times of suspected abuse, and when there is a lack of family support
>
> SOURCE: Content adapted from Simons et al., 2012.

and master's level (specialty practice) social work programs. CSWE defines social work competence as the ability to integrate and apply social work knowledge and values to provide professional services promoting human and community well-being (CSWE, 2015, 2021). Students who graduate from a CSWE-accredited social work program demonstrated competence, both in the classroom and through fieldwork, served under the supervision of a professional social worker (Bern-Klug et al., 2016).

Regulatory Requirements

Currently, federal regulations[13] require nursing homes with 120 or more beds to hire a qualified social worker on a full-time basis, although this "qualified social worker" need not have a social work degree (Bern-Klug et al., 2021a). Specifically, the "qualified social worker" is defined as an individual with a minimum of a B.S.W. or a bachelor's degree in a human services field including, but not limited to, sociology, gerontology, special education, rehabilitation counseling, or psychology and who has 1 year of

---

[13] CMS Requirements for Long-Term Care Facilities—Administration, 42 CFR § 483.70 (2016).

supervised social work experience in a health care setting working directly with individuals.[14] Because this requirement applies only to nursing homes with 120 or more beds, some two-thirds of nursing homes do not have to employ a social services staff member (Bern-Klug et al., 2021b). Social work is the only profession affected by the "120-bed rule" (Bern-Klug et al., 2018). However, Roberts and Bowblis (2017) concluded that the 120-bed rule "does not account for the level of psychosocial need among residents in smaller nursing homes, nor does it consider the caseload of practitioners."

Many individual states have their own regulations regarding social work services in nursing homes, and while most do not require nursing homes with 120 or fewer beds to employ social workers, Connecticut, Maine, and Oklahoma do require that nursing home residents have access to social work services regardless of the size of the nursing home. However, 10 states do not require a "qualified social worker" to have either a social work license or a social work degree, though some require either completing a state-approved course or having some direct supervision and minimum years of experience (Bern-Klug, 2008; Bern-Klug et al., 2018).

Both state and federal guidelines provide unrealistic recommendations for social service staffing patterns. In a recent study of social service directors, 66 percent of social service directors stated that one full-time social service staff member could handle 60 residents at most, with 75 percent of social service directors recommending fewer than 30 short-term (skilled/rehab/post/sub-acute care) nursing home residents per full-time social worker (Bern-Klug et al., 2021b). One older study found that social workers serving older adults face challenges including lower pay and higher caseloads (especially in nursing facilities), which affect job satisfaction (Whitaker et al., 2006).

In 2003, the NASW developed a consensus statement for professional standards for social workers in long-term care settings. It stated:

> A social worker has, at a minimum, a bachelor's degree from an accredited school or program of social work; has 2 years of postgraduate experience in long-term care or related programs; and meets equivalent state requirements for social work practice, or, in jurisdictions not having such legal regulation, holds certification or credentialing from the National Association of Social Workers. In no instance shall a social worker have less than a baccalaureate from an accredited school or program of social work. (NASW, 2003, p. 7)

Regulatory requirements are inadequate to address the complexities of psychosocial and behavioral health care with qualified staffing, and there is a long history of advocacy for increased standards in this area

---

[14] CMS Conditions of Participation Organization Environment—Personnel Qualifications, 42 CFR § 418.114 (2016).

(Li, 2010; Orth et al., 2019; Streim et al., 2002). Two recent developments are contributing to this push. First, CMS's adoption of the Minimum Data Set 3.0 as the updated resident assessment instrument places more emphasis on resident-centered care, quality of life, and enhanced psychosocial and behavioral health care. In addition, in response to the industry's move to encourage resident and family participation in care choices and the movement toward more holistic care, recommendations emerged to increase the presence of bachelor's and master's prepared social workers and to increase the training of all staff on behavioral health and quality-of-life issues (Simons et al., 2012).

During the required comment period prior to the updating of CMS's 2016 rule for nursing home requirements, members of the National Nursing Home Social Work Network recommended that nursing home facilities hire graduates of accredited social work programs to fulfill the social work role in nursing homes (Bern-Klug et al., 2016). These same organizations asked that all nursing homes, regardless of size, employ a full-time social worker. In spite of these recommendations, the final rule did not require social workers as core members of the team developing a resident's comprehensive care plan. Furthermore, the rule added an undergraduate degree in gerontology as an acceptable degree for a "qualified social worker." The reduction in standards for qualified social workers in nursing homes occurred at the same time that these updated regulations increased requirements for psychosocial care, person-centered care, and behavioral health care (CMS, 2016).

Evidence of Social Work Contributions to Nursing Home Care

Social workers' contributions to resident care often involve tasks that are complex and clinically challenging. The results of a national survey of social service directors indicated strong involvement in care transitions, with more than 55 percent of the respondents reporting that they spent over 50 percent of their time with short-term residents (Galambos et al., 2021). Almost 62 percent of social service directors and their staff were consistently involved in disaster planning and response activities at the nursing home facility (Kusmaul et al., 2021). Studies also point to the positive outcomes that social workers achieve in complex care situations (Sussman and Dupuis, 2014). Research has shown, for example, that social service staff with higher qualifications are integral to improving behavioral symptoms and reducing antipsychotic medications (Roberts et al., 2020), that social workers routinely intervene in resident-to-resident aggression (Bonifas, 2015), and that social workers increase advance directive completion, contributing to a reduction in potentially avoidable hospitalizations (Galambos et al., 2021).

A systematic review that examined the impact of social work interventions in aging and quality of life found that 71 percent of the studies reported significant quality-of-life outcomes, and 15 of these studies documented cost savings achieved through social work interventions, with these cost outcomes achieved through care coordination, palliative care, and end-of-life care (Rizzo and Rowe, 2016). Furthermore, a study on social integration and mental and functional health outcomes for nursing home residents found that nursing homes with degreed social workers have the capacity to provide better psychosocial care (Leedahl et al., 2015).

Given the evidence of social workers' contributions to nursing home care, inclusion of social workers on interdisciplinary care teams can help ensure resident care preferences are met. See later in this chapter for more on the role of social workers during the COVID-19 pandemic.

Chaplains

As Chapter 4 discusses, attending to the spiritual needs of nursing home residents is a critical part of their quality of life and well-being (Gilbert et al., 2021; Koenig, 2012; Morley and Sanford, 2014). Chaplains provide residents, their families, and even staff with spiritual support. In addition, they provide human connection for residents, listening to their stories; leading prayers, religious services and rituals, and group meetings; supporting family and friends; and providing grief and bereavement support (Seidman, 2021). Their role is especially critical in the area of palliative care. Unfortunately, nursing homes employ too few chaplains to meet the needs of seriously ill patients, and those chaplains that are available have limited time to support staff (Ferrell et al., 2020). One analysis found that most post-acute and long-term care facilities do not have a budget for a chaplain or a full-time spiritual counselor and instead designate an already overworked social worker to get additional education or find a volunteer chaplain (McKnight, 2016). The COVID-19 pandemic has shed light on the urgent need to include chaplains in care teams and for chaplains to provide consistent spiritual care services (Ferrell et al., 2020).

Activities Staff

As noted in Chapter 4, wellness activities, physical activities, and art activities are vital for health, functional mobility, and the performance of everyday activities. Federal regulations require facilities to provide an ongoing activities program that is "designed to meet the interests of and support the physical, mental, and psychosocial well-being of each resident, encouraging both independence and interaction in the community." They also require that the program be directed by a qualified professional who is either "a qualified therapeutic recreation specialist or an activities professional," meaning they are licensed or registered by the state, are a qualified occupational therapist or assistant, and have completed a training course by the state.[15] However, data on whether nursing homes are complying with this regulation are scarce.

OTHER CLINICAL STAFF

In addition to the professionals discussed above, a variety of other health care practitioners, specialists, and staff also help support residents in nursing homes. However, evidence on these individuals specifically in nursing homes is extremely limited.

Dental Health Care Workforce

As Chapter 4 describes, "oral disease impacts physical, psychological, and social well-being through pain, diminished function, and reduced quality of life" (Dunbar, 2019; Sifuentes and Lapane, 2020). However, most nursing homes do not contract with dentists or dental hygienists, so residents tend to only receive emergency and acute care rather than routine and preventative dental care (Dunbar, 2019; Maramaldi et al., 2018). Assistance with daily oral health care for nursing home residents is typically the responsibility of the CNAs (Dunbar, 2019; Sifuentes and Lapane, 2020), who not only lack the training to provide such care, but typically face significant competing demands for their time. Other challenges include staff perceptions that oral health care is not a priority, staff hesitancy or unwillingness to perform the tasks, and residents' resistance to staff assistance (Patterson Norrie et al., 2019; Porter et al., 2015). In addition, the dental health care workforce is often not well prepared to address the specific oral health needs of older adults. Surveys of dental students indicate that many find the geriatric dentistry training curriculum to be inadequate, and geriatric dentistry is not among the 12 specialty areas recognized by the American Dental Association (ADA, 2021).[16]

---

[15] CMS Requirements for Long-Term Care Facilities—Quality of Life, 42 CFR § 483.24 (2016).

[16] For a full list of the specialty areas, see https://www.ada.org/en/ncrdscb/dental-specialties/specialty-definitions (accessed November 3, 2021).
Moreover, a 2011 IOM study, *Improving Access to Oral Health Care for Vulnerable and Underserved Populations,* found that the American Board of General Dentistry did not explicitly require questions on geriatric dental care for board certification and that of the more than 500 residencies recognized by the American Dental Education Association, none were specifically devoted to the care of elderly patients (IOM, 2011).

Pharmacists

Nursing home residents tend to require a large number of prescriptions to help manage their health. The use of a large number of medications by a single person, including potentially inappropriate medications or duplication, is a significant concern among nursing home residents, as it can lead to adverse drug events, disability, hospitalization, and death (Hoel et al., 2021; Lee et al., 2019). Federal regulations require a nursing home contract with a consultant pharmacist to review each resident's drug regimen monthly and to report irregularities, which the attending physician must review and respond to in the medical record.[17] Problems identified by consultant pharmacists typically include missing information, an unnecessary drug, and excessive duration or dose of a drug (Lapane and Hughes, 2006). Concerns have been raised that consultant pharmacists may have conflicts of interest when their services are provided by the dispensing pharmacy of the nursing home (Barlas, 2012; Sullivan, 2018). In fact, two large nursing home pharmacies agreed to pay settlements in response to claims of kickbacks under whistleblower provisions of the False Claims Act (DOJ, 2015; McCrystal et al., 2010). These claims included that a dispensing pharmacy provided the services of consultant pharmacists at a reduced rate in order to secure pharmacy contracts, and that a dispensing pharmacy accepted incentives from a drug company in exchange for the consultant pharmacist recommending that physicians prescribe specific drugs.

Recently, the role of pharmacists has evolved from being product centered to being more person centered, with a greater emphasis on their role in ensuring quality care (Lee et al., 2019). A systematic review by Lee and colleagues (2019) found that the presence of pharmacy services in a nursing home led to an improvement in the quality of prescribing, positive trends in de-prescribing and reducing the number of medications used per resident, an improvement of nursing home staff knowledge on medication use, and a reduction in the number of resident falls. However, the study found more mixed results in terms of mortality, hospitalization, and resident admission rates. The role of consultant pharmacists in antibiotic stewardship programs has also been considered to help improve overall antibiotic use (Ashraf and Bergman, 2021).

Registered Clinical Dieticians and Feeding Assistants

Registered clinical dietitians assess, evaluate, and recommend appropriate nutrition interventions based on residents' preferences and their health status (e.g., malnutrition, diabetes, obesity), but not all residents have access to a registered clinical dietician (Dorner and Friedrich, 2018). Federal regulation only mandates that CMS-certified facilities must have a

---

[17] CMS Requirements for Long-Term Care Facilities—Pharmacy Services, 42 CFR § 483.45 (2022).

"qualified dietitian or other clinically qualified nutrition professional either full-time, part-time, or on a consultant basis."[18] Despite the regulations, nursing home staff may not have the resources to fully address the nutritional needs of residents (Simmons and Schnelle, 2004, 2006; Simmons et al., 2008). For example, there may be too few CNAs to assist with feeding, especially in the evenings, and too few RNs and dietitians to oversee the dining experience in nursing homes (IOM, 2000). To fill the gap in nutrition and feeding assistance, some nursing facilities employ or contract with a registered dietitian nutritionist or nutrition and dietetics technicians (Dorner and Friedrich, 2018), but it is often not enough.

In 2003, CMS allowed nursing homes to use paid feeding assistants "to provide more residents with help in eating and drinking and reduce the incidence of unplanned weight loss and dehydration" (CMS, 2007, p. 1). Paid feeding assistants are required to complete an approved state-based training program (with a minimum of 8 hours of training) and must be supervised by RNs or LPNs. Furthermore, the paid feeding assistant may only help residents who do not have complicated feeding problems (e.g., difficulty swallowing, tube feedings). Current nursing home staff may be used as paid feeding assistants as long as they have completed the required training. A small evaluation of paid feeding assistants found the quality of their care to be comparable to CNAs (Simmons et al., 2007).

The 2000 IOM report *The Role of Nutrition in Maintaining Health in the Nation's Elderly* recommended that "licensing agencies need to develop more effective oversight with respect to feeding, supervision of staff, and other nutrition-related issues" (IOM, 2000, p. 235).

Therapists

A variety of types of therapists, assistants, and aides are among the extended nursing home workforce. Nursing homes are required to provide or consult for specialized rehabilitative services for a mental disorder and intellectual disability (e.g., physical therapy, speech–language pathology, occupational therapy, respiratory therapy) for nursing home residents as required by their care plans.[19]

Occupational Therapists and Assistants

In nursing homes, occupational therapists "address training in self-care skills; training in the use of adaptive equipment, compensatory techniques,

---

[18] CMS Requirements for Long-Term Care Facilities—Food and Nutrition Services, 42 CFR § 483.60 (2016).

[19] CMS Requirements for Long-Term Care Facilities—Specialized Rehabilitative Services, 42 CFR § 483.65 (2016).

and environmental modifications; and behavioral and mental health issues" (AOTA, 2015). Occupational therapists help residents increase physical activity, engage in self-care, reduce pain, and maintain independence (Livingstone et al., 2019, 2021). Studies have found a positive relationship between occupational therapy staffing levels and the quality of life and care for nursing home residents (Jette et al., 2005; Livingstone et al., 2019). As outlined in Chapter 4, occupational therapists can also help reduce length of stay by helping residents make the gains in function needed to be able to be discharged from the nursing home (Yurkofsky and Ouslander, 2021). However, when Medicare significantly altered the way nursing homes are paid through its patient-driven payment model (PDPM), staffing levels fell by almost 6 percent for occupational therapists and by about 10 percent for occupational therapist assistants. These cuts were also almost entirely among contracted staff (McGarry et al., 2021a).

Physical Therapists, Assistants, and Aides

Physical therapy providers in nursing homes work with residents to "reduce impairment, rehabilitate from an injury or illness, improve functioning and cognition, and prevent adverse effects or onset of disease" (Livingstone et al., 2021). This includes strength and endurance training, balance improvement exercises, and mobility training. Therapists and assistants tend to work together, rather than using assistants as an alternative to therapists. As was the case with occupational therapists, the 2019 introduction of Medicare's PDPM resulted in a reduction of physical therapy staff. Specifically, staffing levels in nursing homes fell by about 6 percent for physical therapists and 10 percent for physical therapy assistants (McGarry et al., 2021a). Contract staffing again accounted for most of the decrease in staffing levels (McGarry et al., 2021a). One analysis suggested that some facilities may start using assistants and aides as lower-cost substitutes for therapists (Livingstone et al., 2021). A 2021 report by the OIG stated that "CMS does not audit the physical-therapist staffing information reported by nursing homes and included on Care Compare. Because CMS does not use any accuracy checks on these data, we cannot determine whether the data reported on Care Compare are accurate" (OIG, 2021, p. 15).

Respiratory Therapists

Respiratory therapists work with residents who are suffering from breathing issues resulting from illnesses such as chronic obstructive pulmonary disease, asthma, surgery, or injury or who are recovering from an illness. The full array of respiratory therapy services can include oxygen therapy, inhalation medication management, pulmonary rehabilitation, and ventilator management (AARC, 2016). Respiratory therapists are educated and trained in all aspects of pulmonary medicine and can help residents manage all respiratory diseases and conditions. Under current regulations, respiratory therapy is considered a nontherapy ancillary service (AARC, 2017).

Speech–Language Pathologists and Speech Therapists

Speech–language pathologists help evaluate and treat a range of conditions that lead to communication, cognition, memory, problem-solving, language expression, or swallowing disorders in long-term care residents (Casper, 2013). Approximately 5 percent of all speech–language pathologists work in nursing and residential care facilities (BLS, 2021a). Among speech–language pathologists working in nursing homes, 83.4 percent are employed full time, and 82.8 percent are paid on an hourly basis; 61.7 percent work for one employer, 24.7 percent work for two employers, and 9.4 percent work for three or more employers (ASHA, 2021). More than one in five nursing homes have funded, unfilled positions (ASHA, 2021).

DIRECT-CARE WORKERS

Direct-care workers—nursing assistants (also called nurse aides), personal care aides, and home health aides—provide the majority of hands-on care to residents in nursing homes (Campbell et al., 2021). Direct-care workers provide care that includes everyday tasks such as assistance with eating, bathing, toileting, and dressing, as well as more advanced tasks such as infection control and taking care of cognitively impaired residents (BLS, 2021b; McMullen et al., 2015; PHI, 2021). Taken together, these tasks are critical to maintaining the function, well-being, and quality of life of the resident. CNAs—nursing assistants who have met specific federal and state educational and training requirements—make up the largest proportion of direct-care workers in nursing homes.

Demographics

More than 527,000 nursing assistants were employed or contracted by nursing homes across the United States in 2020 (12 percent of the total direct-care workforce) (BLS, 2021c). Among these workers, the median age was 38, and 91 percent were women; 58 percent were people of color (38 percent Black/African American, 13 percent Hispanic/Latino, 5 percent Asian or Pacific Islanders, 2 percent other), and 21 percent were born outside of the United States (PHI, 2021). More than 90 percent had completed at least high school, and 13 percent had an associate's degree or higher (PHI, 2021).

As the demand for direct-care workers increases, nursing homes in the United States will need to fill approximately 561,800 nursing assistant jobs between 2019 and 2029 (Campbell et al., 2021; PHI, 2021). This effort will not come without challenges which have plagued the ability for nursing homes to recruit and retain an adequate supply of direct-care workers for decades, however. Many of these challenges are rooted in structural and systemic factors that play out in the form of low wages, minimal training requirements, and a lack of respect and recognition, which, to a significant degree, represent the legacy of long-standing institutional racism, sexism, and ageism (Drake, 2020; Ryosho, 2011; Sloane et al., 2021; Squillace et al., 2009; Travers et al., 2020; Truitt and Snyder, 2020). Because of the crucial role of this position in nursing homes, significantly improving the quality of care requires investment in quality jobs for direct-care workers.

Immigrant workers, both documented and undocumented, fill critical gaps in the direct-care workforce, especially in nursing homes that serve a high share of Black and Latinx residents (Lee et al., 2020; Zallman et al., 2019). As such, this group may be a primary target for recruitment efforts. However, when entering the workforce, immigrant workers face additional barriers, such as barriers in language, health literacy, and uninsured rates, compared with native-born individuals (Campbell, 2018; Lee et al., 2020). One strategy to support immigrant workers and attract them to direct-care worker positions includes a pathway to citizenship (Katz, 2019; White House, 2021).

Wages

The mean hourly wage in 2020 for nursing assistants in nursing homes was $15.41, and the mean annual wage was $32,050 (BLS, 2021c). The bottom quartile of nursing assistants earn less than $26,650 annually, and the bottom 10 percent earn less than $22,750 (BLS, 2021c). The level of pay for direct-care workers in nursing homes has drawn stark attention to comparable wages for other types of work that might be considered more desirable. For example, while nursing assistants provide increasingly complex care and face persistent challenges with inadequate training and risk of on-the-job injury, they may earn little more than cashiers ($25,020 per year), food service workers ($24,130 per year), or retail sales workers ($27,320 per year) (BLS, 2021d,e,f). A 2021 story found that many nursing home workers were leaving for jobs at Amazon:

> The average starting pay for an entry-level position at Amazon warehouses and cargo hubs is more than $18 an hour, with the possibility of as much as $22.50 an hour and a $3,000 signing bonus, depending on location and shift. Full-time jobs with the company come with health benefits, 401(k)s and parental leave (Varney, 2021).

Direct-care workers often have to work multiple jobs, forgo important necessities such as health insurance and retirement benefits because of an inability to afford premiums, and live in congregate housing (Morris, 2009). Because of their low wages, 34 percent of direct-care workers require some form of public assistance, and many live in poverty; direct-care workers who are also women of color are more likely than White women and men to require public assistance, live in poverty, or live in low-income households (PHI, 2019, 2021). This could in part be a result of the fact that Black female direct-care workers make 20 cents per hour less than White female direct-care workers and 70 cents per hour less than White male direct-care workers (Scales et al., 2020). For family member perspectives on the compensation of nursing home workers, particularly CNAs, see Box 5-5.

BOX 5-5
Family Member Perspectives

"I would improve the wages and benefits for nursing home staff so they would be fairly compensated for their work and so the best and brightest worker would be attracted to the profession."

— Family Member, Schenectady, New York

"I believe the greatest improvement to care would be addressing nurse aide issues comprehensively; pay a living wage of at least $15 per hour, support fixing employability barriers like adequate childcare and public transportation availability. The reality is that the staff is underpaid, overworked, under supported, and insufficiently trained to care for residents."

— Family Member, Wilmington, North Carolina

"Staff on front lines are not paid well, are not trained well regarding person-centered care, do not have skills to succeed."

— K.S.

"Staff are incredibly caring people who need to be paid a living wage."

— Family Member, Berkeley, California

"If they paid workers more, maybe there would be more and better care and at the prices being charged per month, I don't see why they can't."

— Wendy

"I wonder if the pay should be higher for people in the trenches and not corporate level."

— Family Member, Sioux Falls, South Dakota

These quotes were collected from the committee's online call for resident, family, and nursing home staff perspectives.

Education and Training

CNAs are required[20] to have a minimum of 75 hours of training plus at least 12 hours of continuing education annually, including 16 hours of "supervised practical training," that covers basic nursing services, personal care services, basic restorative services, mental health and social services, care of cognitively impaired residents, residents' rights, and other topics (Hernández-Medina et al., 2006). The minimum number of hours and topics covered by CNA trainings have been a cause for concern as these requirements have not changed since the passing of the Nursing Home Reform Act, part of the Omnibus Budget Reconciliation Act of 1987. Given the marked increase in nursing home resident acuity, complexity, and care needs, current requirements are inadequate (Hernández-Medina et al., 2006). For example, one small study found that CNAs in nursing homes had inadequate knowledge related to aging, cognition, and mental health (Kusmaul, 2016). Some states and facilities have implemented more robust training efforts, with many states requiring additional hours and topics of training beyond federal minimum requirements. CNAs themselves have expressed interest in including education on dementia and infection control (Lerner et al., 2010).

Additional training of CNAs has been associated with improved nursing home quality indicators (Hernández-Medina et al., 2006; PHI, 2011; Trinkoff et al., 2013; Zheng and Temkin-Greener, 2010). As a result, various bodies have suggested that the number of required hours for training be increased to between 100 and 120 hours, with 50 to 60 of those hours going toward clinical training (Hernández-Medina et al., 2006). Specifically, the 2008 IOM report *Retooling for an Aging America* recommended that "Federal requirements for the minimum training of [CNAs] and home health aides should be raised to at least 120 hours and should include demonstration of competence in the care of older adults as a criterion for certification" (IOM, 2008, p. 218). While many states have increased their requirements since 2007, only the District of Columbia and 13 states (up from 12 states in 2007) require at least 120 hours (IOM, 2008; PHI, 2020).

CNAs reporting high-quality training are more likely to work in states requiring additional initial training hours and were more satisfied with their jobs than those with low-quality training (Han et al., 2014). Training that focused specifically on work-life skills, such as problem solving, task organization, and working with others, helped to increase satisfaction (Han et al., 2014). Additionally, the implementation of orientation programs for newly hired staff in all states and facilities is needed (IOM, 2004).

---

[20] CMS Requirements for Long-Term Care Facilities—Requirements for Approval of a Nurse Aide Training and Competency Evaluation Program, 42 CFR § 483.152 (2016).

Because the care needs of the resident are complex, dynamic, and growing, CNAs need ongoing professional development to adapt to the changing needs of the resident population. The current federal requirement for professional development is that CNAs must receive 12 hours of in-service or continuing education each year.[21] The inclusion of topics such as infection control, care of the cognitively impaired, behavioral health, resident rights, skin care, communication techniques, safety and disaster training, and resident confidentiality may help ensure the competency of CNAs in carrying out their responsibilities. The National Institute of CNA Excellence, a project seeking to recruit and train CNAs, is expected to launch in 2022 (NICE, 2021). Created by the National Association of Health Care Assistants, the project provides virtual training that goes beyond traditional training in clinical skills to include topics like team building, leadership skills, conflict resolution, resident advocacy, and communication. The project further plans to support the CNA candidate through certification and job placement. For family member perspectives on the training of nursing home staff, particularly CNAs, see Box 5-6.

BOX 5-6
Family Member Perspectives

On behalf of my mother, there is inadequate amount of properly trained staff. They barely know the rudimentary basics of personal care. There is no medical, transfer, aging, or infection control training.

— **Concerned Citizen**

Improvements to care include mandating staffing ratios for aides and increasing competency with more skill lab time during initial training, and require annual skill demonstration.

— **Family Member, Wilmington, North Carolina**

Need to provide much better training in areas including feeding of memory care residents, infection control, communicating with memory care residents, interacting with residents from cultures/ethnicities different from their own, and treating residents with dignity, compassion, and respect.

— **M.K.**

These quotes were collected from the committee's online call for resident, family, and nursing home staff perspectives.

---

[21] CMS Requirements for Long-Term Care Facilities—Training Requirements, 42 CFR § 483.95(g) (2016).

Job Requirements and Characteristics

Unlike licensed personnel such as RNs, direct-care workers do not have an official scope of practice. Instead, nine authorized duties are listed by the Code of Federal Regulations to be allowable by each state: (1) personal care, (2) safety/emergency procedures, (3) basic nursing, (4) infection control, (5) communication and interpersonal activities, (6) care of cognitively impaired residents, (7) basic restorative care, (8) mental health and social service activities, and (9) residents' rights (McMullen et al., 2015). While these are duties that direct-care workers are authorized to perform, depending on the state, they may or may not be tasked to do so. Moreover, there are a number of additional duties that direct-care workers have been permitted to carry out, such as medication management, wound care, catheter care tasks, and the management of medical information, because they benefit residents and alleviate pressure from other members of the workforce (McMullen et al., 2015).

Medication aides are most often CNAs who have received training to administer medications in some capacity based on the regulations provided by the state. There are variations in the requirements of the medication aides related to supervision, hours of training, continuing education, and length of time working as a CNA and in the facility. For example, in Iowa, medication aides can only administer medications under the supervision of an RN (ANA Enterprise, 2015). As of March 2020, certified medication technicians (as defined in the 2020–2021 Nursing Home Salary and Benefits Report by the Hospital and Healthcare Compensation Service and the American Health Care Association) had a median hourly wage of $15.66 in nursing homes (HHCS, 2020).

Staffing Levels

As noted earlier in this chapter, a 2001 study by CMS proposed that minimum staffing standards for nursing assistants (thresholds below which residents were at risk for serious quality-of-care issues) should be 2.4 hours per resident day for short-stay residents and 2.8 hours per resident day for long-stay residents (Feuerberg, 2001). However, these levels are rarely achieved in all nursing homes. Furthermore, these minimum staffing standards may not reflect the acuity of the residents' needs, and lead to excessive workloads or the inability of CNAs to provide high-quality care. For example, one simulation estimated that nurse aides needed between 2.8 and 3.6 hours per resident per day in order to meet resident needs for assistance with activities of daily living (depending on resident acuity); however, reported staffing levels averaged only between 2.3 and 2.5 hours per resident per day (Schnelle et al., 2016). On average, 1 nursing assistant supports 12 residents per shift, and 1 in 10 nursing assistants supports 16 or more residents (PHI, 2019).

Turnover and Burnout

Adequate staffing in nursing homes has been difficult to achieve because of high turnover, stigmatized perception of the CNA role, and poor working conditions (Manchha et al., 2021). One recent analysis using data from the Payroll-Based Journal found the average turnover rate among CNAs to be 129.1 percent; in comparison, turnover rates were 140.7 percent for RNs and 114.1 percent for LPNs, with some individual facilities found to have nursing staff turnover rates over 300 percent (Gandhi et al., 2021). High turnover is expensive for nursing homes and negatively affects the quality of the services delivered and the quality of life in nursing homes (Feuerberg, 2001; IOM, 2004; Seavey, 2004). Contributors to these high turnover rates among direct-care workers in nursing homes include characteristics related to the nature of the job itself and the working environment found in nursing homes, including factors that result in injury. One analysis, for example, found that more than half of CNAs had incurred at least one work-related injury within the past year and almost one-quarter of CNAs were unable to work for at least 1 day as a result of being injured (Squillace et al., 2009).

The top reasons for direct-care workers leaving their jobs include lack of respect, low salary, staff shortages, personal health concerns, lack of appreciation by the facility, lack of teamwork among the staff, lack of trusting relationships with residents and families, lack of tools to do the job, lack of good relationships with supervisors, and not being informed of changes before they are made (Bryant, 2017; Mickus et al., 2004; U.S. Congress, 2001; Zhang et al., 2016). For example, one study of nearly 400 nursing homes in Iowa found that higher wages were associated with lower CNA turnover (Sharma and Xu, 2022). Moreover, CNAs are also often undervalued for their skills, mistreated and disrespected, and experience workplace violence in the form of physical and verbal abuse (Tak et al., 2010). While the work of the direct-care workforce has commonly been referred to as physically demanding, in 2020 during the midst of the COVID-19 pandemic, nursing home workers saw one of the highest death rates among all occupations (Lewis, 2021). The direct-care workforce is likely to experience even higher rates of burnout, though most of the literature on the topic focuses on the rate of burnout among licensed nurses and physicians (Cooper et al., 2016). For a family member perspective on staff burnout, see Box 5-7.

Greater retention of CNAs has been found to be associated with improved functional status and fewer pressure ulcers, electrolyte imbalances, and urinary tract infections among nursing home residents (Kimmey and

> **BOX 5-7**
> **Family Member Perspective**
>
> "Unfortunately, many well intended staff end up frustrated, burnt-out, and numbed by lacking support of management."
>
> — K.S.
>
> *This quote was collected from the committee's online call for resident, family, and nursing home staff perspectives.*

Stearns, 2015; Trinkoff et al., 2017). Many approaches to support the retention of this direct-care workforce have been proposed, including

- Pay a wage reflective of the risks and physical demand that direct care workers assume daily.
- Provide a separate payment that can go toward wages, benefits (e.g., sick leave, health insurance), or both, similar to New York's Home Care Worker Parity Law.[22]
- Enhance work relationships by improving communication and supervision so that CNAs feel appreciated, listened to, and treated with respect.
- Improve management systems by increasing and improving staffing and scheduling along with increasing the availability of more robust training and better career ladders.
- Improve work system factors, including helping CNAs with directions, providing resources and supplies, and preventing injury and exposure to hazards or violence (Kemper et al., 2008; Morris, 2009).
- Create formal promotion programs, peer mentoring programs, and tuition reimbursement programs and proactively engage nursing assistants in efforts to enact such programs (Kemper et al., 2008; Stone and Dawson, 2008).

Tailored and ongoing training programs improve job satisfaction and reduce turnover (Ejaz and Noelker, 2006; Han et al., 2014). For example, an approach based on the occupational adaptation framework (Schkade and McClung, 2001) has been found to show greater gains in skills mastery and more cooperative approaches to solving complex problems such as dementia care needs than traditional skills training approaches (McKay et al., 2021).

---

[22] Additional information available at https://dol.ny.gov/home-health-care-aides-and-wage-parity (accessed November 3, 2021).

There is also a need for opportunities for job advancement and upgrading the skill of CNAs (Campbell, 2021; IOM, 2004; PHI, 2016; Wiener et al., 2009). Career advancement opportunities include attaining a specialized skill or expertise area (e.g., medication aide) or advancing to a higher level of licensing (e.g., LPN/LVN, RN). One older study demonstrated that empowering CNAs led to reductions in health deficiency citations, reduced staff turnover, and a decline in urinary incontinence rates among residents (Stone et al., 2002). Strategies specific to empowerment were mostly focused on having CNAs participate in care planning and care plan implementation.

Supervision and Support

The immediate supervision of direct-care workers is carried out by both LPN/LVNs and RNs. These relationships are often challenging as a result of power dynamics arising from the hierarchical structure of most nursing homes, incivility, bullying, and undue time demands (Cooke and Baumbusch, 2021; Lundin et al., 2021). When these groups work together to communicate and support one another, it makes for a better relationship, so decentralization of hierarchical systems can promote better teamwork across disciplines and roles (Kemper et al., 2008), and encourage supervisors to demonstrate supportive behaviors (McGilton et al., 2004). Relationships among personnel can also be improved by implementing leadership training for all levels of supervisors and managers, developing self-managed work teams, improving information sharing between nurses and direct-care staff, enhancing responsibilities for direct-care workers, facilitating team building and peer mentoring, and involving direct-care workers in care management decisions (Eaton, 2000; Eaton et al., 2001; Rantz et al., 2013; Stone and Dawson, 2008). Furthermore, nursing homes need to create a culture of values that fosters respect, trust, collaboration, and interprofessional health care team building (Kemper et al., 2008). Ultimately, nursing home leadership is responsible for creating a desirable working environment in the nursing home. For nursing home workers' perspectives on supervision, support, and the workplace environment, see Box 5-8.

Expanded Roles for CNAs

One notable example of expanding recognition of the role and importance of the CNA is the Green House model for nursing home care (see Chapter 6). Green House nursing homes employ modified staff roles to split work, empower staff, and have staff members work together. Direct-care workers in Green Houses, referred to as "shahbazim" (singular, "shahbaz"), "work in self-managed teams and are responsible for direct resident care, cleaning, laundry, meal preparation, staff scheduling, and activities, and simulating how families might organize work" (Bowers and Nolet, 2014).

> **BOX 5-8**
> **Nursing Home Staff Perspectives**
>
> "There is strong evidence for cross-training staff in other disciplines to increase autonomy, job satisfaction, career path possibilities and career development. Not only does this support the CNA, but it also supports the nursing home resident. There are better clinical outcomes when staff are engaged, a real part of the interdisciplinary team, and can act as resident advocates."
>
> — **Physician and researcher from Amherst, Massachusetts who has worked in long-term care facilities**
>
> "I work in a nursing home chain. I honestly believe that our company genuinely cares about residents and want to give the best care possible. However, it's not perfect by any means. I want to have more nurses making high-impact decisions; want more scrutiny into training requirements of administrators; want advanced practice nurses to lead nursing teams; nursing homes to initiate and lead evidence-based projects to improve quality of life and quality of care instead of having to rely on quality improvement organizations."
>
> — **Nursing Home Worker, Los Angeles, California**
>
> *These quotes were collected from the committee's online call for resident, family, and nursing home staff perspectives.*

The shahbaz provides general oversight, while the nurse provides more clinical direction. One study found that an integrated model (with high interaction and coordination) between shabazim and nurses resulted in the best resident outcomes (Bowers and Nolet, 2014).

FAMILY CAREGIVERS

Family caregivers provide critical supports to nursing home residents, but they do not receive sufficient support, recognition, resources, or inclusion. Family involvement in the care of a nursing home resident is a multidimensional construct that entails visiting the resident, providing hands-on care and assistance with activities of daily living, supervising and monitoring the quality of care of the resident, providing emotional support, representing the resident's perspective and history, and advocating for the resident in terms of safety and security (Bern-Klug and Forbes-Thompson, 2008; Coe and Werner, 2021; Gaugler, 2005; Lopez et al., 2013; NASEM, 2016). Family caregivers also often play a key role as surrogate decision makers for their loved ones, which can be particularly stressful (Givens et al., 2012; NASEM, 2016). For family member perspectives on the role of family in caring for nursing home residents, see Box 5-9.

> **BOX 5-9**
> **Family Member Perspectives**
>
> "My mother was well-cared for, but even in the best of facilities there were clearly not enough staff. Family was heavily depended upon to augment staff for meal supervision, as activity volunteers, and general personal care-related issues such as maintaining the residents' room in an orderly fashion, meeting clothing and toiletry supply needs, etc. The labor-intensive care of dementia patients does not allow for much more than moving the person from his/her room, to living room, to dining room and back again. They need to be taken outdoors into the patio or garden, on rides to enjoy seeing the world, etc. Without family visitors, those activities don't happen . . . . Many times, while in rehab, I had to track people down to help my mother get assistance to go to the bathroom. It was extremely stressful as her daughter, and heartbreaking."
>
> — Daughter and caregiver of two parents with dementia who needed nursing home care
>
> "I like that the majority of staff are nice to both the residents and family members. What I don't like is the lack of staffing and the lack of communication between the staff and the family members."
>
> — J.C.
>
> *These quotes were collected from the committee's online call for resident, family, and nursing home staff perspectives.*

However, upon a loved one's entrance to a nursing home, the role of the family caregiver may become indirect as the family members endeavor to ensure that high-quality care is provided by facility staff. One analysis found that family caregivers feel responsible for maintaining continuity by

- Helping the resident maintain his or her sense of identity through the continuation of loving relationships and helping staff to get to know the resident as an individual;
- Monitoring the care received, providing feedback to staff, and filling gaps; and
- Contributing to community by interacting with other residents, relatives, and staff; taking part in social events; and generally providing a link with the outside world (Davies and Nolan, 2006).

Family caregivers may be especially important for the continuity of care for nursing home residents with dementia, with responsibilities such as ensuring that the resident is being treated with respect and receiving high-quality care (Aneshensel et al., 1995; Duncan and Morgan, 1994; Graneheim et al., 2014; Reid and Chappell, 2017; Ross et al., 2001). Recognition of family caregivers as partners in the care of the person with dementia contributes to the overall quality of care (Graneheim et al., 2014). For example, family members often can help advocate for and help provide support for nonpharmacologic alternatives to help manage residents' behavioral and psychological symptoms of dementia (Tjia et al., 2017). Overall, family involvement is a "strong predictor of perceived resident quality of life" (Roberts and Ishler, 2018).

As such, it is important to include the family members as essential members of the resident interdisciplinary care team. Family caregivers can serve as an extension of the staff and help workers better understand the resident's goals and preferences, so that CNAs, nurses, and other staff can deliver sensitive, nurturing, and person-centered care to the resident (Kellett, 2007). This requires the development and maintenance of effective relationships and communication between family and staff (Bauer et al., 2014; Brown Wilson et al., 2009; Cohen et al., 2014; Henkusens et al., 2014; Maas et al., 2004). Keys to such development are trust in staff (Bauer et al., 2014; Bern-Klug and Forbes-Thompson, 2008; Rosemond et al., 2017) and ongoing monitoring of staff (Bramble et al., 2009). In her presentation to this committee, Beverley Laubert, a long-term care ombudsman for the Ohio Department of Aging, said

> Quality care is relationship-based. For example, a CNA is given education in the basic principles of dementia care, but to truly be equipped to support a resident with memory impairment, that CNA must know something about the resident's family and life story. Only then can the staff know and respond to the unique needs of the resident in their care. Similarly, the housekeeper should know something about the resident to understand that moving the resident's Bible into a drawer could be disruptive.

Among the strategies and interventions that can facilitate collaborative and partnership efforts between family and staff are support groups and family councils (Baumbusch et al., 2022; Hoek et al., 2021). (See Chapters 4 and 8 for more on resident and family councils.) The Partners in Caregiving program developed by Pillemer et al. (2003) was designed to intervene not only on the part of family members (e.g., the formation of councils or support groups), but also to engage staff and administrators to effectively change facility policies focused on integrating family caregivers (CITRA, 2021). The Families Involved in Nursing Home Decision-Making program uses video-conferencing to include family in care plan meetings (Oliver et al., 2021). Family caregivers can also experience high levels of stress and can benefit from improved education and support for themselves.

For example, family caregivers express a desire for better education about disease course, treatment options, and surrogate decision making (e.g., placement of feeding tubes, end-of-life decisions) (Givens et al., 2012).

VOLUNTEERS

Apart from the family and friends of nursing home residents, volunteers from the local community (unrelated to the nursing home resident) may contribute to the care of nursing home residents. The organizational structure of the long-term care facility influences the "amount of volunteers in a nursing home, the types of activities in which volunteers engage and [the] quality of care" (Falkowski, 2013, p. 61). For example, data from the 2004 National Nursing Home Survey show that nonprofit facilities were likely to have more volunteers, more frequent visits by volunteers, and to use volunteers to support staff (e.g., for "clerical duties, helping at mealtime, and providing personal care"), while for-profit facilities tended to use volunteers in socialization activities (e.g., "game playing, conducting religious services, and making social visits") (Falkowski, 2013, p. 4). Both the percentage of Medicare residents and the percentage of Medicaid residents in the nursing home were associated with a lower number of volunteers that visit weekly, and the number of volunteers in a nursing home was associated with the amount of socialization activities for nursing home residents. Finally volunteers need to be properly trained for their duties to support the relationships and trust between volunteers and staff so that staff can focus on more technical work (Falkowski, 2013). However, little is known about the best practices of training for maintaining an effective volunteer workforce.

Several studies provide evidence of the impact that volunteer services can have on the quality of life for nursing home residents (Saunders et al., 2019; van der Ploeg et al., 2012; Zhao et al., 2015), including mitigating the adverse effects of social isolation (Claxton-Oldfield, 2015; Cohen-Mansfield, 2001, 2013; Damianakis et al., 2007; van der Ploeg et al., 2012, 2014). Families also appreciate and benefit from volunteer support (Candy et al., 2015). For example, during the COVID-19 pandemic, the Yale School of Medicine Geriatrics Student Interest Group initiated the Telephone Outreach in the COVID-19 Outbreak Program in which student volunteers connected with older adults in nursing homes via weekly phone calls (van Dyck et al., 2020). In the three nursing homes that implemented the program for 30 residents, initial results have been generally positive, with residents expressing appreciation for the conversations, the student volunteers perceiving personal benefits (e.g., greater sense of purpose, improved well-being), and actionable needs being identified (e.g., obtaining desired books for a resident).

Research also suggests that volunteers are successful in supporting and caring for hospice patients and residents with dementia (Candy et al., 2015; Claxton-Oldfield, 2015; Damianakis et al., 2007). They are able to support residents at the end of life by performing a variety of tasks, including emotional support (e.g., comforting the residents' fears), social support (e.g., engaging with the resident and their family), practical support (e.g., helping the resident with personal care), informational support (e.g., providing education so families and residents know what to expect), and more. In fact, one older study found that satisfaction and emotional well-being were higher in hospice programs that involved more volunteers (Block et al., 2010). Volunteers are also beneficial in caring for residents with dementia by facilitating activities that fill unmet needs (e.g., boredom, need for relaxation, loneliness agitation, etc.) by providing or removing stimuli (Cohen-Mansfield, 2013). However, more education and research is necessary to truly understand and promote the value of volunteer support services (Claxton-Oldfield, 2015; Cohen-Mansfield, 2013). For a family member perspective on volunteers, see Box 5-10.

EQUITY AND THE WORKFORCE

Occupational segregation is defined as overrepresentation or underrepresentation of a particular group (e.g., defined by race, sex, or immigration status) in specific jobs or fields (Bahn and Cumming, 2020). This type of segregation is characterized as a process fueled by a desire for social distance from a marginalized group (Tomaskovic-Devey, 2018), where opportunity or positions with greater authority are reserved for the group with the most social power (i.e., White men) (Bahn and Cumming, 2020). Workplace segregation for women and racial and ethnic minorities leads to

---

BOX 5-10
Family Member Perspective

"I have boundless respect, admiration, and gratitude for two volunteer programs the facility coordinated with. Thanks to these volunteer programs, my family member received extra oversight from bimonthly visits by a very caring nurse supervisor as well as deeply supportive (often weekly) visits from volunteers."

— M.K.

This quote was collected from the committee's online call for resident, family, and nursing home staff perspectives.

these groups holding positions with more routinized and controlled work and less supervisory authority (Tomaskovic-Devey, 2018). The overrepresentation of historically marginalized groups in occupations reduces their wages "irrespective of other measures of productivity such as required skill level" (Bahn and Cumming, 2020).

There are substantial differences in the racial and ethnic diversity among the roles within the nursing home workforce. The percent of racial and ethnic minorities in higher-level positions in the long-term care workforce decreases as the level of educational attainment required for a given position increases (Bates et al., 2018). For example, as shown in Figure 5-3, CNAs themselves are more diverse than the nursing home workforce overall.

Specifically, a higher percentage of CNAs are either Black/African American or Hispanic/Latinx as compared with the nursing home workforce overall, suggesting that higher-level positions within nursing homes are much less diverse. When such workforce disparities exist, they affect how work is organized (e.g., the autonomy and control afforded those jobs) as well the level of compensation and benefits associated with specific job titles, with racial and ethnic minorities and women often at the bottom of the workplace hierarchy (Tomaskovic-Devey, 2018). For example, one recent analysis (Travers et al., 2020) found that racial and ethnic minorities and immigrant direct-care workers—over 90 percent of whom

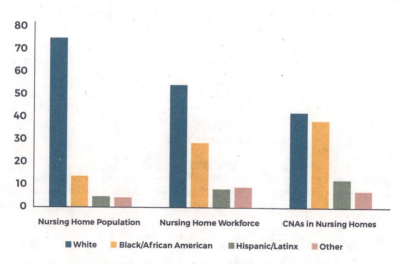

FIGURE 5-3 Racial and ethnic diversity (percentage) among nursing home residents, nursing home staff, and CNAs in nursing homes.
SOURCES: Bates et al., 2018; Harris-Kojetin et al., 2004; PHI, 2021.

are women—performed over 50 percent of the tasks related to helping residents with activities of daily living (Probst et al., 2010; Stacey, 2005).

A root cause for these types of disparities is systemic/structural racism, which is defined as a set of "historically and contextually specific ideological justifications for a society's racialized social system" (Ray, 2019, p. 31). A 2021 review articulated the pathways through which systemic/structural racism has created and sustained disparities in the long-term care system in the United States (Sloane et al., 2021). Specific pathways include institutional factors such as

- Biased hiring, pay, and promotion practices that concentrate racial and ethnic minority and immigrant workers in specific low-resource nursing homes;
- Cultural factors, such as current and historic patterns of microaggressions, discrimination, and racial violence throughout society that influence the nursing home work environment; and
- Interpersonal factors, such as racial bias from residents and other staff members, directed at racial and ethnic minority and immigrant workers.

Therefore, all workers in nursing homes, including leadership, will likely benefit from training in principles of diversity, equity, and inclusion.

Providing Culturally Sensitive Care

In addition to concerns for the power dynamics and hierarchies of the workforce itself, the contrast between the diversity of the nursing home workforce and the residents they serve (see Figure 5-3) may create challenges in the delivery of high-quality care. For example, as noted in the 2008 IOM report *Retooling for an Aging America*, the diversity of the workforce is important because patients may prefer to be treated by health care professionals of the same ethnic background and a provider from a patient's same ethnic background may have a better understanding of culturally appropriate demonstrations of respect or speak the same language (IOM, 2008). While the nursing home population is becoming more diverse, the patterns of diversity still may not match the workforce that cares for them.

FACTORS THAT INFLUENCE THE RELATIONSHIP BETWEEN STAFFING AND QUALITY

Several factors influence the relationship between staffing and quality, including the ownership status of the nursing home and employment patterns.

Ownership Status

As noted in Chapter 8, while there are important nuances related to the case mix of certain nursing homes and nursing home chains, the published literature suggests that in general, for-profit nursing homes consistently demonstrate lower levels of quality and satisfaction with care than not-for-profit nursing homes (Banaszak-Holl et al., 2002; GAO, 2011; Grabowski and Hirth, 2003; Harrington et al., 2001, 2012; Hillmer et al., 2005; Stevenson and Grabowski, 2008; You et al., 2016). In general, inadequate staffing and lower salaries have been long-standing issues in nursing homes as compared with acute-care settings. A 2012 study comparing staffing levels and deficiencies of for-profit nursing homes and five other ownership groups found that the 10 largest for-profit nursing home chains had lower RN and total nurse staffing hours than government facilities when controlling for other factors, and that they received 36 percent higher deficiencies (and 41 percent higher serious deficiencies) than government facilities (Harrington et al., 2012). (See Chapter 8 for more on transparency and ownership issues.)

Use of Temporary and Agency Staff

While many of the studies are old or not specific to nursing homes, considerable research has established that the use of high levels of temporary staff is an indicator of poor quality care and poor outcomes (Castle, 2009; Castle and Engberg, 2008; Senek et al., 2020). One study, for example, found that approximately 60 percent of nursing homes use at least some agency staff and that having agency staff account for 25 percent or more of the workforce was associated with 1 to 2 percent lower scores on quality measures (Castle, 2009). The manner in which nursing homes use agency staff may be the reason for lower quality (Castle, 2009).

Consistent Assignment

The consistent assignment of nursing staff to residents in nursing homes is a critical component of culture change and one that may help achieve quality of care and life for residents (Advancing Excellence, 2021a; Castle, 2013; Roberts et al., 2015). Advancing Excellence in America's Nursing Homes, a campaign to improve the quality of care and life in nursing homes, defines consistent assignment as "a resident receives care from the same nursing assistants 85 percent of the time" (Advancing Excellence, 2021b). However, studies have found that an average of only 68 percent of nursing homes use consistent assignment and only 28 percent of homes achieve the recommended level of 85 percent consistent staffing (Castle, 2011, 2013). Despite limited research on the topic, the available literature suggests that consistent staffing has been associated with lower turnover and absenteeism among staff, fewer quality-of-care deficiency citations, and fewer quality-of-life deficiency citations (Castle, 2011, 2013). In her presentation to this committee, Beverley Laubert, a long-term care ombudsman for the Ohio Department of Aging, said

> Current staff training requirements are insufficient to support residents' quality of living. The best practice that I've seen for such relationship-based care is consistent assignment of staff. We know that consistent assignment matters to both the quality of work life and the residents' living experience. Staff get to know specific residents, learn their preferences, and work proactively and efficiently. It makes the job more fulfilling. Residents and family don't have to repeatedly train staff on their preferences then. But until consistent assignment is required and enforced, not just recommended as a best practice, that it's the minimum practice, we won't see sustained quality care.

For a family member perspective on consistent assignment, see Box 5-11.

COVID-19 AND NURSING HOME STAFFING

The COVID-19 pandemic resulted in disproportionate deaths of residents in nursing homes. The key predictors of nursing home COVID-19 cases and deaths—nursing home size and location—leave little room for immediate and direct intervention by the nursing homes themselves. However, staffing as a contributor to poor outcomes might be more under the control of nursing homes and more amenable to policy changes. The 2020 CMS Coronavirus Commission on Safety and Quality in Nursing Homes made many recommendations related to staff in nursing homes, including

- Mobilization of resources to support the workforce (e.g., increased breaks, identification of surges);
- Provision of safety guidance (e.g., related to testing of staff and residents, quarantine options, workers with multiple employers);

BOX 5-11
Family Member Perspective

"I like consistent caregivers—nursing assistants that work on a regular basis to ensure that routine cares are done according to my family member."

— Anonymous, Minnesota

This quote was collected from the committee's online call for resident, family, and nursing home staff perspectives.

- Provision of guidance and training on the use and reuse of personal protective equipment (PPE);
- Support of 24-hour daily RN staffing in nursing homes with positive cases;
- Use of certified infection prevention and control specialists with educator capabilities; and
- Targeted recruitment of CNAs (MITRE, 2020).

Staffing Patterns and COVID-19 Impact

Multiple studies found that higher nurse staffing ratios mitigated the effect of an outbreak and resulted in fewer deaths once an outbreak occurred (Gorges and Konetzka, 2020; Konetzka et al., 2021; Li et al., 2020). At the same time, higher staffing ratios were not able to prevent the outbreak from starting, given that staff were often the source of bringing COVID-19 into facilities. One study found that while nursing homes with higher staffing ratios (just prior to the pandemic) did not have a reduced probability of an initial outbreak, higher baseline staffing ratios were helpful in stemming an outbreak once it started (Figueroa et al., 2020). Nursing homes with the highest staff hours per resident day experienced fewer cases and deaths than those at the bottom of the distribution. Several other studies demonstrated connections between staffing and impact of the COVID-19 pandemic, including

- Nursing homes with increased RN staffing had fewer confirmed COVID-19 cases and fewer deaths from COVID-19 (Li et al., 2020).
- Nursing homes in California with lower RN staffing had higher COVID-19 infections (Harrington et al., 2020).
- Staff size, including those not involved in direct resident care, was associated with more COVID-19 cases; therefore, "reducing the number of unique staff members without decreasing direct-care hours, such as by relying on full-time rather than part-time staff, could help prevent outbreaks" (McGarry et al., 2021b, p. 1261).
- Nearly half of nursing home COVID cases were attributable to cross-facility staff movement (Chen et al., 2021), contributing to the evidence of the impact of consistent staffing on quality of care.

Nurse practitioners working in nursing homes were found to be essential for containing the spread within the nursing homes and for providing much needed guidance to staff and care to residents during the pandemic (McGilton et al., 2021; Popejoy et al., 2020). Additionally, social workers (along with others) helped residents stay connected to their families (Kusmaul et al., 2020). This was particularly challenging as "access to technology was sporadic, and access to personal protective equipment, even worse" (Kusmaul et al., 2020, p. 651). Additionally, some social workers were prevented from entering facilities or encouraged to work from home. In part, these challenges stemmed from social workers not being recognized as being "frontline workers" but rather as "non-essential."

Staffing Shortages

Several studies and many anecdotal stories documented exacerbation of staffing shortages at various times throughout the COVID-19 pandemic (Abbasi, 2020b; Davidson and Szanton, 2020; Denny-Brown et al., 2020; Fernandez, 2021; Kirkham and Lesser, 2020; McGarry et al., 2020; Murray, 2021; Peck, 2021; Quinton, 2020; Sedensky, 2021; Weber, 2021; Xu et al., 2020). Early in the pandemic, staff shortages were found to be greater in nursing homes with lower quality scores that have a higher Medicaid population and where COVID-19 cases were more prevalent among staff or residents (McGarry et al., 2020; Xu et al., 2020). Many nursing homes increased their use of contract (agency) staff to fill these gaps (Peck, 2021; Stulick, 2021). A cross-sectional time-series study of over 15,000 nursing homes found that while urban nursing homes reported a relatively constant staffing shortage, rural nursing homes saw an increase in staffing shortages until November 2020 (Yang et al., 2021b). In December 2021, on average, 30.1 percent of nursing homes had shortages of nurses or nurse aides (AARP, 2022). However, this varied dramatically by state. For example, 73.5 percent of nursing homes in Wyoming had shortages of nurses or nurse aides, while only 3.6 percent of nursing homes in California had such shortages (AARP, 2022). Eight states had shortages in more than half of the nursing homes in the state.

Many nursing home workers, especially low-wage workers (e.g., CNAs, housekeepers) left their jobs for other positions in part due to working conditions and opportunities for higher-paying jobs (Quinton, 2020; Tan, 2022; Varney, 2021). Dr. David Gifford, chief medical officer for the American Health Care Association and the National Center for Assisted Living (AHCA/NCAL), noted

> Nursing homes are in constant competition for staff. Many providers struggle to recruit and retain caregivers who can often find less demanding jobs in other settings, such as hospitals and industries that can offer better pay. (Romero, 2021)

However, Werner and Coe (2021) found a decline in the average total number of staff hours per day that was accompanied by a decline in the resident census itself, resulting in a slight increase in the number of staff hours per resident day (Werner and Coe, 2021). They suggested that this discrepancy might be explained by the increased use of contractors, the increased intensity of the work (i.e., caring for residents during the pandemic requires more staff time), increased hours among the existing staff, or the loss of the contributions of family caregivers (Werner and Coe, 2021).

CMS Staffing Waivers and Temporary Nurse Aides

Early in the COVID-19 pandemic, CMS provided blanket waivers for a variety of regulations related to nursing home workers. For example, CMS waived certain requirements for in-person visits by physicians and others, allowed physicians to delegate certain tasks to APRNs and physician assistants, and reduced paid feeding assistant training to just one hour (CMS, 2021c). In addition, CMS waived training and certification requirements for new CNAs; these temporary nurse aides only needed to "demonstrate competency in skills and techniques necessary to care for residents' needs" (CMA, 2021, p. 17). Serious concerns were raised about the risks that a lack of training creates for both nursing home residents and the workers themselves (Hauslohner and Sacchetti, 2020; Scales, 2020; Severens, 2020). In response, many states imposed their own training requirements for temporary nurse aides and AHCA/NCAL developed a free 8-hour online training program that many states recognized as satisfying their requirements (either alone or in conjunction with other stipulations) (AHCA/NCAL, 2022; Scales, 2021; Van Houtven et al., 2021). The Nurses Certification and Recognition of Experience (CARE) Act of 2021[23] proposes a pathway for temporary nurse aides to continue in their jobs after the pandemic without fulfilling the full requirements to become a CNA. However, concerns have been raised about the lack of formal training many of these workers have received (less than the current 75 hours of required training, which as discussed earlier in this chapter, has been found to be insufficient) and the provision that allows employers to attest to the competency of these workers (without testing) (CMA, 2021; Scales, 2021; Van Houtven et al., 2021). Currently, there is no systematic tracking of temporary nurse aides (Edelman, 2020; Scales, 2021).

Worker Health and Safety

Nursing home staff commonly suffered from a lack of PPE. McGarry and colleagues (2020) found that early in the pandemic, about one in five nursing homes had shortages of PPE, particularly gowns and N95 respirators. Labor unions representing health care workers advocated for improved access to personal protective equipment and infection control practices. In New York, the presence of a union for health care workers was associated with a 30 percent lower mortality rate from COVID-19 for nursing home residents. Nursing homes with unions also had lower COVID-19

---

[23] Nurses Certification and Recognition of Experience (CARE) Act of 2021, HR 331, 117th Cong., 1st sess. (January 15, 2021).

infection rates as well as a 13.8 percent greater access to N95 respirators and 7.3 percent greater access to eye shields for staff (Dean et al., 2020)

Additionally, COVID-19 affected the health of nursing home workers themselves. Given the vulnerability of the nursing home population, nursing home workers may have increased exposure to COVID-19 as compared to workers in other settings. As of November 2021, there have been 673,591 confirmed cases of COVID-19 among nursing home staff and 2,166 deaths (CMS, 2021d). In fact, one analysis suggests that nursing home workers had one of the highest death rates among all occupations (Lewis, 2021). However, vaccination rates among nursing home workers remain relatively low (AARP, 2021; CMS, 2021d; Gharpure et al., 2021; McGarry et al., 2021c), particularly among CNAs (49.2 percent as of July 2021). Nursing home staff also experienced high rates of stress and burnout due to fears of contracting COVID-19, fear of infecting their families, and increased intensity of the work (Weber, 2021; Werner and Coe, 2021; White et al., 2021). The use of telehealth has been suggested as one modality that could lower stress among staff, enable planning and information sharing between families and staff, and provide "flexible options for staff education and training" (Edelman et al., 2020, p. 1).

Strike Teams

The COVID-19 pandemic offered unique opportunities for collaboration among public health stakeholders; health care providers; local, state, and federal governments; and other organizations. Strike teams, defined as "multidisciplinary teams deployed to support public health emergency response efforts," supported long-term care facilities experiencing outbreaks and resource shortages by providing technical assistance and guidance to "improve infection control practices as a short-term strategy to minimize the impact of the virus" (ASTHO, 2021). Strike teams address a variety of issues, including visitor guidance, vaccine administration, infection prevention and control education, the supply of personal PPE, and more (AMDA, 2021).

Several states implemented strike teams during the COVID-19 pandemic. Massachusetts invested $130 million over 2 months to create a 28-item checklist of infection control practices which were subject to state audits and to deploy infection control teams to 123 facilities that were struggling to pass the audits (Lipsitz et al., 2020). The program also went beyond immediate technical assistance and provided weekly educational webinars, assisted with procurement of resources, and provided payment incentives to nursing homes (Lipsitz et al., 2020). Other states (e.g., Louisiana and Washington) collaborated with the CDC to support PPE distribution, arrange COVID testing and cohorting practices, and develop infection control practices and guidelines (ASTHO, 2021).

In October 2021, the CDC, in partnership with CMS, joined state efforts by allocating $500 million to allow state and other jurisdictional health departments to staff, train, and deploy strike teams to expand clinical surge capacity, address staffing shortages, and strengthen infection control policies and procedures in a variety of health care settings (including nursing homes) (CDC, 2021a,b). Awardees are required to use funds for technical assistance to prevent COVID outbreaks and may optionally use funds to supply resources and other infrastructure support (e.g., environmental assessments of ventilation) (CDC, 2021b).

KEY FINDINGS AND CONCLUSIONS

The Overall Nursing Home Workforce

- A wide variety of workers help to support nursing home residents in achieving their goals and preferences.
- Very little evidence exists about many members of the nursing home workforce, including their impact on the quality of care as well as basic demographic information.
- Family caregivers (including chosen families) provide critical supports to nursing home residents, but they do not receive sufficient support, recognition, resources, or inclusion.
- There is high turnover of many types of nursing home staff, which is associated with lower levels of quality.
- An interdisciplinary care team approach is related to reduced staff turnover and increased staff satisfaction.
- Many health care practitioners are not adequately prepared for their specific role and responsibilities in the nursing home setting.
- Many nursing home workers earn less than their counterparts in other settings of care.
- Systemic and structural racism have created and sustained racial and ethnic disparities in the long-term care system.
- Factors that can influence the relationship between staffing and quality of care include the ownership status of the nursing home, the use of temporary or agency staff, and a lack of consistent assignment.

Nursing Home Administration and Leadership

- Nursing home federal regulations require that the administrator of a nursing home is licensed by the state. However, states vary in their requirements for minimum education, training hours, examinations, and continuing education.

- Except for the requirement of a license to practice medicine in the state, there are no additional specific education and training requirements for medical directors.
- Limited data exist on the characteristics of nursing home administrators, medical directors, and directors of nursing.
- The director of nursing is often called upon to address the clinical needs of residents in addition to his or her administrative responsibilities.
- No federal or state requirements specify minimum education requirements, continuing education requirements, or additional training requirements for directors of nursing.
- Evidence on the characteristics, education and training, job satisfaction, and turnover of social services directors is limited or nonexistent.
- Forty-two percent of social services directors do not have a degree in social work.

Primary Care Providers

- Limited and dated evidence exists focusing on primary care providers for nursing home residents, particularly for physicians and physician assistants.
- APRN-provided care has been associated with improved quality of care for nursing home residents and increased resident, family, and staff satisfaction.
- The most frequently mentioned barrier for increasing the role of APRNs in nursing homes is their restricted scope of practice due to Medicare regulations and state regulatory constraints.

Nurse Staffing

- Nursing staff (including RNs, LPN/LVNs, and CNAs) are key to providing comprehensive nursing home care.
- RNs and LPN/LVNs have been used interchangeably in nursing homes, with LPN/LVNs working outside their scope of practice.
- Decades of evidence support the association between inadequate nurse staffing and poor quality of care in nursing homes, particularly for RNs.
- While several studies have called for 24-hour RN coverage in nursing homes, today the requirement is a 24-hour daily presence of a *licensed* nurse (i.e., RN or LPN/LVN) with an RN fulfilling at least 8 of those hours.
- The 2001 proposed CMS minimum staffing standards have not been addressed in any regulations, and current staffing requirements are not adjusted by resident case mix.

- Most nursing homes do not have sufficient nursing staff to meet the needs of residents and are not adjusting staffing to take resident acuity into account.
- Nursing levels decrease significantly over weekends; GAO recommended reporting these measures on Care Compare.
- CMS can provide staffing data to state survey agencies to help with their approach to timing of inspections.

Psychosocial and Spiritual Care Providers

- Social workers have a positive impact on quality of care.
- Two-thirds of nursing homes are not required to employ a social services staff member.
- According to federal regulations, a "qualified social worker" does not need to have a degree in social work.
- Nursing homes employ too few chaplains to meet the needs of seriously ill patients and may instead designate social workers to get additional education or find a volunteer chaplain.

Certified Nursing Assistants (CNAs)

- CNAs provide the majority of hands-on care to nursing home residents.
- In spite of decades of calls for enhancing the training of CNAs, minimum training standards for CNAs have not changed since 1987.
- The top reasons for direct-care workers leaving their jobs include a lack of respect, low salary, difficulty of the job, staff shortages, personal health concerns, a lack of appreciation by the facility, a lack of teamwork among the staff, a lack of trusting relationships with residents and families, a lack of tools to do the job, a lack of good relationships with supervisors, and not being informed of changes before they are made.

Infection Prevention and Control Leadership and the Impact of COVID-19

- There are no national standards for training and licensure of infection prevention and control specialists, and most of these specialists are not certified in infection control.
- Presence of APRNs, increased RN staffing, and consistent staffing were associated with better COVID-19 outcomes.

REFERENCES

AADNS (American Association of Directors of Nursing Services). 2019. *2019 AADNS work time study and salary report*. Denver, CO: American Association Post-Acute Care Nursing, American Association of Directors of Nursing Services.

AADNS. 2021. *DNS-CT candidate handbook*. Denver, CO: American Association Post-Acute Care Nursing, American Association of Directors of Nursing Services.

AAPACN (American Association of Post-Acute Care Nursing). 2021. *Director of nursing services–certified*. https://www.aapacn.org/education/dns-ct (accessed July 7, 2021).

AARC (American Association for Respiratory Care). 2016. *Position statement: Delivery of respiratory therapy services in skilled nursing facilities providing ventilator and/or high acuity respiratory care*. https://www.aarc.org/wp-content/uploads/2014/10/delivery_of_services_in_snf.pdf (accessed August 18, 2021).

AARC. 2017. *Skilled nursing facilities (SNF)*. https://www.aarc.org/advocacy/federal-policies-affecting-rts/skilled-nursing-facilities-snf (accessed August 18, 2021).

AARP. 2021. *4 in 5 U.S. nursing homes behind on staff vaccination goal, analysis finds*. https://www.aarp.org/caregiving/health/info-2021/nursing-home-staff-vaccine-threshold.html (accessed November 21, 2021).

AARP. 2022. *AARP nursing home COVID-19 dashboard*. https://www.aarp.org/ppi/issues/caregiving/info-2020/nursing-home-covid-dashboard.html (accessed February 16, 2022).

Abbasi, J. 2020a. Social isolation—The other COVID-19 threat in nursing homes. *JAMA* 324(7):619–620.

Abbasi, J. 2020b. "Abandoned" nursing homes continue to face critical supply and staff shortages as COVID-19 toll has mounted. *JAMA* 324(2):123–125.

ABPLM (American Board of Post-Acute and Long-Term Care Medicine, Inc.) 2022a. *Certified medical director (CMD)*. https://www.abplm.org/home (accessed February 8, 2022).

ABPLM. 2022b. *Certified Medical Director (CMD) initial certification application*. https://www.abplm.org/_files/ugd/c389c5_266ac9b1632c4dd992034a235b2bbbad.pdf (accessed February 8, 2022).

Ackermann, R. J., and K. A. Kemle. 1998. The effect of a physician assistant on the hospitalization of nursing home residents. *Journal of the American Geriatrics Society* 46(5):610–614.

ADA (American Dental Association). 2021. *Specialty definitions*. https://www.ada.org/en/ncrdscb/dental-specialties/specialty-definitions (accessed September 30, 2021).

Advancing Excellence (Advancing Excellence in America's Nursing Homes). 2021a. *Implementation guide: Goal 8—Improving consistent assignment of nursing home staff*. https://theconsumervoice.org/uploads/files/long-term-care-recipient/Auld,Rosenthal-3of4-Concurrent(ConsistentAssignment).pdf (accessed September 17, 2021).

Advancing Excellence. 2021b. *Increasing use of consistent assignment*. https://www.leadingageok.org/ConsistentAssignment.pdf (accessed September 17, 2021).

AHCA/NCAL (American Health Care Association and National Center for Assisted Living). 2022. *Temporary nurse aide*. https://educate.ahcancal.org/tna (accessed February 9, 2022).

Aiken, L. H. 1981. Nursing priorities for the 1980's: Hospitals and nursing homes. *American Journal of Nursing* 81(2):324–330.

AMDA (Society for Post-Acute and Long-Term Care Medicine). 2003. *Role of the attending physician in the nursing home*. https://paltc.org/amda-white-papers-and-resolution-position-statements/role-attending-physician-nursing-home (accessed November 9, 2021).

AMDA. 2005. Roles and responsibilities of the medical director in the nursing home: Position statement A03. *Journal of the American Medical Directors Association* 6(6):411–412.

AMDA. 2011. Collaborative and supervisory relationships between attending physicians and advanced practice nurses in long-term care facilities. *Journal of the American Medical Directors Association* 12(1):12–18.

AMDA. 2021. *Policy brief: Implement nursing home strike teams.* https://paltc.org/sites/default/files/Policy%20Brief%20on%20NH%20Strike%20Teams%20final%20v4.pdf (accessed October 22, 2021).

AMDA. 2022. *Core Curriculum: Medical direction in PALTC.* https://apex.paltc.org/page/core-curriculum-on-medical-direction (accessed February 8, 2022).

ANA (American Nurses Association). 2015. *Nursing: Scope and standards of practice.* Silver Spring, MD: American Nurses Association.

ANA. 2016. *Nursing administration: Scope and standards of practice.* 2nd ed. Silver Springs, MD: American Nurses Association.

ANA Enterprise (American Nurses Association Enterprise). 2015. *Medication aide/technician categories by state.* https://www.nursingworld.org/~4af4e6/globalassets/docs/ana/ethics/state-chart-medication-aide-status-09-15.pdf (accessed June 23, 2021).

Aneshensel, C. S., L. I. Pearlin, J. T. Mullan, S. H. Zarit, and C. J. Whitlatch. 1995. *Profiles in caregiving: The unexpected career.* San Diego: Academic Press.

Antwi, Y. A., and J. R. Bowblis. 2018. The impact of nurse turnover on quality of care and mortality in nursing homes: Evidence from the great recession. *American Journal of Health Economics* 4(2):131–163.

AONE/AONL (American Organization of Nurse Executives, American Organization for Nursing Leadership). 2015. *AONL nurse executive competencies: Post-acute care.* Chicago, IL: AONE and AONL.

AOTA (American Occupational Therapy Association). 2015. *Occupational therapy's role with skilled nursing facilities.* https://www.aota.org/~/media/Corporate/Files/AboutOT/Professionals/WhatIsOT/RDP/Facts/FactSheet_SkilledNursingFacilities.pdf (accessed August 18, 2021).

Arling, G., R. L. Kane, C. Mueller, J. Bershadsky, and H. B. Degenholtz. 2007. Nursing effort and quality of care for nursing home residents. *The Gerontologist* 47(5):672–682.

Arling, G., and C. Mueller. 2014. Nurse staffing and quality: The unanswered question. *Journal of the American Medical Directors Association* 15(6):376–378.

ASHA (American Speech–Language–Hearing Association). 2021. *2021 SLP health care survey: Survey summary report: Number and type of responses.* https://www.asha.org/siteassets/surveys/2021-slp-health-care-survey-summary-report.pdf (accessed August 18, 2021).

Ashraf, M. S., and S. Bergman. 2021. The case for consultant pharmacists as key players in nursing home antibiotic stewardship programs. *Journal of the American Medical Directors Association* 22(1):6–8.

ASTHO (Association of State and Territorial Health Officials). 2021. *Partner coordination efforts to strengthen infection prevention and control practices: Lessons from the COVID-19 response.* https://astho.org/ASTHOReports/Partner-Coordination-Efforts-to-Strengthen-Infection-Prevention-and-Control-Practices/04-09-21 (accessed October 22, 2021).

Backhaus, R., H. Verbeek, E. van Rossum, E. Capezuti, and J. P. Hamers. 2014. Nurse staffing impact on quality of care in nursing homes: A systematic review of longitudinal studies. *Journal of the American Medical Directors Association* 15(6):383–393.

Bahn, K., and C. S. Cumming. 2020. *Factsheet: U.S. occupational segregation by race, ethnicity, and gender.* https://equitablegrowth.org/factsheet-u-s-occupational-segregation-by-race-ethnicity-and-gender (accessed July 7, 2021).

Bakerjian, D. 2008. Care of nursing home residents by advanced practice nurses. A review of the literature. *Research in Gerontological Nursing* 1(3):177–185.

Banaszak-Holl, J., W. B. Berta, D. M. Bowman, J. A. Baum, and W. Mitchell. 2002. The rise of human service chains: Antecedents to acquisitions and their effects on the quality of care in U.S. nursing homes. *Managerial and Decision Economics* 23(4–5):261–282.

Barlas, S. 2012. Medicare wants only 'independent' consultant pharmacists in nursing homes. *Pharmacy and Therapeutics* 37(1):6.

Bates, T., G. Amah, and J. Coffman. 2018. *Racial/ethnic diversity in the long-term care workforce.* San Francisco, CA: UCSF Health Workforce Research Center on Long-term Care.

Bauer, M., D. Fetherstonhaugh, L. Tarzia, and C. Chenco. 2014. Staff–family relationships in residential aged care facilities: The views of residents' family members and care staff. *Journal of Applied Gerontology* 33(5):564–585.

Baumbusch, J., I. Sloan Yip, S. Koehn, R. C. Reid, and P. Gandhi. 2022. A survey of the characteristics and administrator perceptions of family councils in a western Canadian province. *Journal of Applied Gerontology* 41(2):363–370.

Bell, S. A., M. Bern-Klug, K. W. O. Kramer, and J. B. Saunders. 2010. Most nursing home social service directors lack training in working with lesbian, gay, and bisexual residents. *Social Work in Health Care* 49(9):814–831.

Bern-Klug, M. 2008. State variations in nursing home social worker qualifications. *Journal of Gerontological Social Work* 51(3–4):379–409.

Bern-Klug, M., and S. Forbes-Thompson. 2008. Family members' responsibilities to nursing home residents: "She is the only mother I got." *Journal of Gerontological Nursing* 34(2):43–52.

Bern-Klug, M., and K. W. O. Kramer. 2013. Core functions of nursing home social services departments in the United States. *Journal of the American Medical Directors Association* 14(1):75.e1–75.e7.

Bern-Klug, M., and B. Sabri. 2012. Nursing home social services directors and elder abuse staff training. *Journal of Gerontological Social Work* 55(1):5–20.

Bern-Klug, M., R. Connolly, D. Downes, C. Galambos, N. Kusmaul, R. Kane, P. Hector, E. Beaulieu, on behalf of the National Nursing Home Social Work Network. 2016. Responding to the 2015 CMS proposed rule changes for LTC facilities: A call to redouble efforts to prepare students and practitioners for nursing homes. *Journal of Gerontological Social Work* 59(2):98–127.

Bern-Klug, M., E. Byram, N. Sabbagh Steinberg, H. Gamez Garcia, and K. C. Burke. 2018. Nursing home residents' legal access to onsite professional psychosocial care: Federal and state regulations do not meet minimum professional social work standards. *The Gerontologist* 58(4):e260–e272.

Bern-Klug, M., K. M. Smith, A. R. Roberts, N. Kusmaul, D. Gammonley, P. Hector, K. Simons, C. Galambos, R. P. Bonifas, C. Herman, D. Downes, J. C. Munn, G. Rudderham, E. A. Cordes, and R. Connolly. 2021a. About a third of nursing home social services directors have earned a social work degree and license. *Journal of Gerontological Social Work* 64(7):699–720.

Bern-Klug, M., K. A. Carter, and Y. Wang. 2021b. More evidence that federal regulations perpetuate unrealistic nursing home social services staffing ratios. *Journal of Gerontological Social Work* 64(7):811–831.

Bethell, J., H. M. O'Rourke, H. Eagleson, D. Gaetano, W. Hykaway, and C. McAiney. 2021. Social connection is essential in long-term care homes: Considerations during COVID-19 and beyond. *Canadian Geriatrics Journal* 24(2):151–153.

Block, E. M., D. J. Casarett, C. Spence, P. Gozalo, S. R. Connor, and J. M. Teno. 2010. Got volunteers? Association of hospice use of volunteers with bereaved family members' overall rating of the quality of end-of-life care. *Journal of Pain and Symptom Management* 39(3):502–506.

BLS (U.S. Bureau of Labor Statistics). 2020a. *May 2020 national industry-specific occupational employment and wage estimates: NAICS 623100—Nursing care facilities (skilled nursing facilities).* https://www.bls.gov/oes/current/naics4_623100.htm (accessed August 12, 2021).

BLS. 2020b. *2018 SOC definitions*. https://www.bls.gov/soc/2018/soc_2018_definitions.pdf (accessed April 15, 2020).

BLS. 2020c. *Occupational employment and wages, May 2020a, 29-1141: Registered nurses*. https://www.bls.gov/oes/current/oes291141.htm#nat (accessed February 10, 2022).

BLS. 2021a. *Occupational outlook handbook: Speech–language pathologists*. https://www.bls.gov/ooh/Healthcare/Speech-language-pathologists.htm (accessed August 18, 2021).

BLS. 2021b. *Occupational outlook handbook: Nursing assistants and orderlies*. https://www.bls.gov/ooh/healthcare/nursing-assistants.htm (accessed November 21, 2021).

BLS. 2021c. *Occupational employment and wages, May 2020: Nursing assistants*. https://www.bls.gov/oes/current/oes311131.htm (accessed November 30, 2021).

BLS. 2021d. *Occupational outlook handbook: Cashiers*. https://www.bls.gov/ooh/sales/cashiers.htm (accessed February 8, 2022).

BLS. 2021e. *Occupational outlook handbook: Food and beverage serving and related workers*. https://www.bls.gov/ooh/food-preparation-and-serving/food-and-beverage-serving-and-related-workers.htm (accessed February 8, 2022).

BLS. 2021f. *Occupational outlook handbook: Retail sales workers*. https://www.bls.gov/ooh/sales/retail-sales-workers.htm (accessed February 8, 2022).

Bonifas, R. P. 2015. Resident-to-resident aggression in nursing homes: Social worker involvement and collaboration with nursing colleagues. *Health & Social Work* 40(3):e101–e109.

Bostick, J. E., M. J. Rantz, M. K. Flesner, and C. J. Riggs. 2006. Systematic review of studies of staffing and quality in nursing homes. *Journal of the American Medical Directors Association* 7(6):366–376.

Bowers, B. J., and K. Nolet. 2014. Developing the Green House nursing care team: Variations on development and implementation. *The Gerontologist* 54(Suppl 1):S53–S64.

Bramble, M., W. Moyle, and M. McAllister. 2009. Seeking connection: Family care experiences following long-term dementia care placement. *Journal of Clinical Nursing* 18(22):3118–3125.

Brown, D. 2021. *New minimum staffing mandates finalized for NY providers*. https://www.mcknights.com/news/new-minimum-staffing-mandates-finalized-for-ny-providers (accessed November 21, 2021).

Brown Wilson, C., S. U. E. Davies, and M. Nolan. 2009. Developing personal relationships in care homes: Realising the contributions of staff, residents and family members. *Ageing and Society* 29(7):1041–1063.

Bryant, O. A. 2017. *Employee turnover in the long-term care industry*. Walden Dissertations and Doctoral Studies 3389. https://scholarworks.waldenu.edu/dissertations/3389 (accessed May 4, 2022).

CALTCM (California Association of Long Term Care Medicine). 2021. *Understanding the California requirement (AB 749) and the process to become, maintain, or reinstate the certified medical director (CMD) credential*. https://www.caltcm.org/certified-medical-director-cmd-information (accessed February 8, 2022).

Campbell, S. 2018. *Racial disparities in the direct care workforce: Spotlight on Black/African American workers*. https://phinational.org/wp-content/uploads/2018/02/Black-Direct-Care-Workers-PHI-2018.pdf (accessed August 13, 2021).

Campbell, S., A. D. R. Drake, R. Espinoza, and K. Scales. 2021. *Caring for the future: The power and potential of America's direct care workforce*. New York: PHI.

Candy, B., R. France, J. Low, and L. Sampson. 2015. Does involving volunteers in the provision of palliative care make a difference to patient and family wellbeing? A systematic review of quantitative and qualitative evidence. *International Journal of Nursing Studies* 52(3):756–768.

Caprio, T. V. 2006. Physician practice in the nursing home: Collaboration with nurse practitioners and physician assistants. *Annals of Internal Medicine* 14(3):17–24.

Casper, M. L. 2013. Speech–language pathology in the long-term care setting: It isn't your grandmother's nursing home anymore. *Seminars in Speech and Language* 34(1):29–36.

Castle, N. G. 2001. Administrator turnover and quality of care in nursing homes. *The Gerontologist* 41(6):757–767.
Castle, N. G. 2005. Turnover begets turnover. *The Gerontologist* 45(2):186–195.
Castle, N. G. 2008. Nursing home caregiver staffing levels and quality of care: A literature review. *Journal of Applied Gerontology* 27(4):375–405.
Castle, N. G. 2009. Use of agency staff in nursing homes. *Research in Gerontological Nursing* 2(3):192–201.
Castle, N. G. 2011. The influence of consistent assignment on nursing home deficiency citations. *The Gerontologist* 51(6):750–760.
Castle, N. G. 2013. Consistent assignment of nurse aides: Association with turnover and absenteeism. *Journal of Aging & Social Policy* 25(1):48–64.
Castle, N. G., and F. H. Decker. 2011. Top management leadership style and quality of care in nursing homes. *The Gerontologist* 51(5):630–642.
Castle, N. G., and J. B. Engberg. 2008. The influence of agency staffing on quality of care in nursing homes. *Journal of Aging & Social Policy* 20(4):437–457.
Castle, N. G., J. Engberg, and R. A. Anderson. 2007. Job satisfaction of nursing home administrators and turnover. *Medical Care Research and Review* 64(2):191–211.
Castle, N. G., J. Furnier, J. C. Ferguson-Rome, D. Olson, and J. Johs-Artisensi. 2015. Quality of care and long-term care administrators' education: Does it make a difference? *Health Care Management Review* 40(1):35–45.
CDC (Centers for Disease Control and Prevention). 2021a. *CDC to invest $2.1 billion to protect patients and healthcare workers from COVID-19 and future infectious diseases.* https://www.cdc.gov/media/releases/2021/p0917-COVID-19-funding.html (accessed October 25, 2021).
CDC. 2021b. *Nursing home & long-term care facility strike team and infrastructure project guidance: Project E—Emerging issues.* Washington, DC: Centers for Disease Control and Prevention.
CDC TRAIN. 2021. *Nursing home infection preventionist training course.* https://www.train.org/cdctrain/training_plan/3814 (accessed April 29, 2021).
Chen, M. K., J. A. Chevalier, and E. F. Long. 2021. Nursing home staff networks and COVID-19. *Proceedings of the National Academy of Sciences of the United States of America* 118(1):e2015455118.
Christian, R., and K. Baker. 2009. Effectiveness of nurse practitioners in nursing homes: A systematic review. *JBI Library of Systematic Reviews* 7(30):1333–1352.
CITRA (Cornell Institute for Translational Research on Aging). 2021. *Partners in Caregiving (PIC).* http://citra-pic.human.cornell.edu (accessed May 26, 2021).
Clarke, S. P., and N. E. Donaldson. 2008. Chapter 25. Nurse staffing and patient care quality and safety. In R. Hughes (ed.), *Patient safety and quality: An evidence-based handbook for nurses.* Rockville, MD: Agency for Healthcare Research and Quality.
Claxton-Oldfield, S. 2015. Got volunteers? The selection, training, roles, and impact of hospice palliative care volunteers in Canada's community-based volunteer programs. *Home Health Care Management & Practice* 27(1):36–40.
CMA (Center for Medicare Advocacy). 2014. *Staffing deficiencies in nursing facilities: Rarely cited, seldom sanctioned.* https://medicareadvocacy.org/staffing-deficiencies-in-nursing-facilities-rarely-cited-seldom-sanctioned (accessed November 9, 2021).
CMA. 2021. *Who provides care for nursing home residents? An update on temporary nurse aides.* https://medicareadvocacy.org/wp-content/uploads/2021/09/SNF-TNA-Report-09-2021.pdf (accessed January 20, 2022).
CMS (Centers for Medicare & Medicaid Services). 2005. *State operations provider certification: Medical director guidance.* CMS Manual System Pub. 100-07. https://www.cms.gov/Regulations-and-Guidance/Guidance/Transmittals/downloads/R15SOMA.pdf (accessed August 20, 2021).

CMS. 2007. *Nursing homes – issuance of new tag F373 (paid feeding assistants) as part of Appendix PP, State Operations Manual, including training materials.* https://www.cms.gov/Medicare/Provider-Enrollment-and-Certification/SurveyCertificationGenInfo/downloads/SCLetter07-30.pdf (accessed February 9, 2022).

CMS. 2016. *Final rule: Medicare and Medicaid programs; reform of requirements for long-term care facilities.* https://s3.amazonaws.com/public-inspection.federalregister.gov/2016-23503.pdf (accessed August 20, 2021).

CMS. 2019a. *Long-term care facility resident assessment instrument 3.0 user's manual.* https://downloads.cms.gov/files/mds-3.0-rai-manual-v1.17.1_october_2019.pdf (accessed August 20, 2021).

CMS. 2019b. *Medicare and Medicaid programs; requirements for long-term care facilities: Regulatory provisions to promote efficiency, and transparency.* https://www.federalregister.gov/documents/2019/07/18/2019-14946/medicare-and-medicaid-programs-requirements-for-long-term-care-facilities-regulatory-provisions-to (accessed October 15, 2021).

CMS. 2021a. *Consultation services rendered by a podiatrist in a skilled nursing facility.* https://www.cms.gov/medicare-coverage-database/view/ncd.aspx?NCDId=170 (accessed November 21, 2021).

CMS. 2021b. *Staffing data submission Payroll Based Journal (PBJ).* https://www.cms.gov/Medicare/Quality-Initiatives-Patient-Assessment-Instruments/NursingHomeQualityInits/Staffing-Data-Submission-PBJ (accessed November 20, 2021).

CMS. 2021c. *COVID-19 emergency declaration blanket waivers for health care providers.* https://www.cms.gov/files/document/covid-19-emergency-declaration-waivers.pdf (accessed January 12, 2022).

CMS, 2021d. *COVID-19 nursing home data.* https://data.cms.gov/covid-19/covid-19-nursing-home-data (accessed November 21, 2021).

Coe, N. B., and R. M. Werner. 2021. Informal caregivers provide considerable front-line support in residential care facilities and nursing homes. *Health Affairs* 41(1):105–111.

Cohen, L. W., S. Zimmerman, D. Reed, P. D. Sloane, A. S. Beeber, T. Washington, J. G. Cagle, and L. P. Gwyther. 2014. Dementia in relation to family caregiver involvement and burden in long-term care. *Journal of Applied Gerontology* 33(5):522–540.

Cohen-Mansfield, J. 2001. Nonpharmacologic interventions for inappropriate behaviors in dementia: A review, summary, and critique. *American Journal of Geriatric Psychiatry* 9(4):361–381.

Cohen-Mansfield, J. 2013. Nonpharmacologic treatment of behavioral disorders in dementia. *Current Treatment Options in Neurology* 15(6):765–785.

Consumer Voice. 2021. *State staffing nursing home standards.* https://theconsumervoice.org/uploads/files/issues/CV_StaffingReport.pdf (accessed February 8, 2022).

Cooke, H. A., and J. Baumbusch. 2021. Not just how many but who is on shift: The impact of workplace incivility and bullying on care delivery in nursing homes. *The Gerontologist* 61(4):563–572.

Cooper, S. L., H. L. Carleton, S. A. Chamberlain, G. G. Cummings, W. Bambrick, and C. A. Estabrooks. 2016. Burnout in the nursing home health care aide: A systematic review. *Burnout Research* 3(3):76–87.

Corazzini, K. N., R. A. Anderson, C. Mueller, S. Hunt-McKinney, L. Day, and K. Porter. 2013. Understanding RN and LPN patterns of practice in nursing homes. *Journal of Nursing Regulation* 4(1):14–18.

Corazzini, K. N., E. S. McConnell, L. Day, R. A. Anderson, C. Mueller, A. Vogelsmeier, S. Kennerly, B. Walker, J. T. Flanagan, and M. Haske-Palomino. 2015. Differentiating scopes of practice in nursing homes: Collaborating for care. *Journal of Nursing Regulation* 6(1):43–49.

CSWE (Council on Social Work Education). 2015. *Educational policy and accreditation standards* https://www.cswe.org/getattachment/Accreditation/Accreditation-Process/2015-EPAS/2015EPAS_Web_FINAL.pdf.aspx (accessed November 20, 2021).

CSWE. 2021. *CSWE's Educational Policy and Accreditation Standards (EPAS) in diversity and justice.* https://www.cswe.org/Centers-Initiatives/Centers/Center-for-Diversity/Curriculum-Resources/EPAS-Curricular-Guide-on-Diversity-and-Social-Ec (accessed November 20, 2021).

Damianakis, T., L. M. Wagner, S. Bernstein, and E. Marziali. 2007. Volunteers' experiences visiting the cognitively impaired in nursing homes: A friendly visiting program. *Canadian Journal on Aging* 26(4):343–356.

Davidson, P. M., and S. L. Szanton. 2020. Nursing homes and COVID-19: We can and should do better. *Journal of Clinical Nursing* 29(15–16):2758–2759.

Davies, S., and M. Nolan. 2006. "Making it better": Self-perceived roles of family caregivers of older people living in care homes: A qualitative study. *International Journal of Nursing Studies* 43(3):281–291.

Dean, A., A. Venkataramani, and S. Kimmel. 2020. Mortality rates from COVID-19 are lower in unionized nursing homes. *Health Affairs* 39(11):1993–2001.

Dellefield, M. E. 2006. Interdisciplinary care planning and the written care plan in nursing homes: A critical review. *The Gerontologist* 46(1):128–133.

Dellefield, M., N. Castle, K. McGilton, and K. Spilsbury. 2015. The relationship between registered nurses and nursing home quality: An integrative review (2008–2014). *Nursing Economics* 33(2):95–108.

Denny-Brown, N., D. Stone, B. Hays, and D. Gallaghe. 2020. *COVID-19 intensifies nursing home workforce challenges.* Washington, DC: Office of the Assistant Secretary for Planning and Evaluation, U.S. Department of Health and Human Services.

DOJ (U.S. Department of Justice). 2015. *Nation's second-largest nursing home pharmacy to pay $9.25 million to settle kickback allegations.* https://www.justice.gov/opa/pr/nations-second-largest-nursing-home-pharmacy-pay-925-million-settle-kickback-allegations (accessed February 8, 2022).

Donald, F., R. Martin-Misener, N. Carter, E. E. Donald, S. Kaasalainen, A. Wickson-Griffiths, M. Lloyd, N. Akhtar-Danesh, and A. DiCenso. 2013. A systematic review of the effectiveness of advanced practice nurses in long-term care. *Journal of Advanced Nursing* 69(10):2148–2161.

Dorner, B., and E. K. Friedrich. 2018. Position of the Academy of Nutrition and Dietetics: Individualized nutrition approaches for older adults: Long-term care, post-acute care, and other settings. *Journal of the Academy of Nutrition and Dietetics* 118(4):724–735.

Drake, A. D. R. 2020. *Direct care work is real work: Elevating the role of the direct care worker.* http://phinational.org/resource/direct-care-work-is-real-work-elevating-the-role-of-the-direct-care-worker (accessed August 20, 2021).

Dunbar, S. 2019. *Geriatric care: Oral hygiene challenges in care facilities.* https://www.todaysrdh.com/geriatric-care-oral-hygiene-challenges-in-care-facilities (accessed August 16, 2021).

Duncan, M. T., and D. L. Morgan. 1994. Sharing the caring: Family caregivers' views of their relationships with nursing home staff. *The Gerontologist* 34(2):235–244.

Eagle, E. 1968. Nursing homes and related facilities. A review of the literature. *Public Health Reports* 83(8):673–684.

Eaton, S. C. 2000. Beyond "unloving care": Linking human resource management and patient care quality in nursing homes. *International Journal of Human Resource Management* 11(3):591–616.

Eaton, S. C., C. Green, R. Wilson, and T. Osypuk. 2001. *Extended Care Career Ladder Initiative (ECCLI): Baseline evaluation report of a Massachusetts nursing home initiative.* https://www.hks.harvard.edu/publications/extended-care-career-ladder-initiative-eccli-baseline-evaluation-report-massachusetts (accessed August 20, 2021).

Edelman, L. S., E. S. McConnell, S. M. Kennerly, J. Alderden, S. D. Horn, and T. L. Yap. 2020. Mitigating the effects of a pandemic: Facilitating improved nursing home care delivery through technology. *JMIR Aging* 3(1):e20110–e20110.

Edelman, T. 2020. *CMS will not track minimally trained aides at nursing facilities.* https://medicareadvocacy.org/cms-will-not-track-minimally-trained-aides-at-nursing-facilities (accessed February 9, 2022).

Ejaz, F., and L. Noelker. 2006. *Tailored and ongoing training improve job retention.* https://phinational.org/wp-content/uploads/legacy/clearinghouse/EjazSummaryFinal.pdf (accessed April 5, 2021).

Falkowski, P. P. 2013. *Volunteer programming impact on long-term care facilities.* Ph.D. dissertation. The Graduate College at the University of Nebraska, Lincoln, Nebraska.

Fernandez, M. 2021. *America's nursing homes fight to find enough caregivers.* https://www.axios.com/americas-nursing-homes-fight-to-find-enough-caregivers-293e5f15-3ff6-462c-b9dd-e09602fdbd94.html (accessed November 21, 2021).

Ferrell, B. R., G. Handzo, T. Picchi, C. Puchalski, and W. E. Rosa. 2020. The urgency of spiritual care: COVID-19 and the critical need for whole-person palliation. *Journal of Pain and Symptom Management* 60(3):e7–e11.

Feuerberg, M. 2001. *Report to Congress: Appropriateness of minimum nurse staffing ratios in nursing homes: Phase II final report.* Washington, DC: Centers for Medicare & Medicaid Services (CMS).

Figueroa, J. F., R. K. Wadhera, I. Papanicolas, K. Riley, J. Zheng, E. J. Orav, and A. K. Jha. 2020. Association of nursing home ratings on health inspections, quality of care, and nurse staffing with COVID-19 cases. *JAMA* 324(11):1103–1105.

Flesner, M., A. Lueckenotte, A. Vogelsmeier, L. Popejoy, K. Canada, D. Minner, C. Galambos, and M. J. Rantz. 2019. Advanced practice registered nurses' quality improvement efforts to reduce antipsychotic use in nursing homes. *Journal of Nursing Care Quality* 34(1):4–8.

Galambos, C., L. Rollin, M. Bern-Klug, M. Oie, and E. Engelbart. 2021. Social services involvement in care transitions and admissions in nursing homes. *Journal of Gerontological Social Work* 64(7):740–757.

Gandhi, A., H. Yu, and D. C. Grabowski. 2021. High nursing staff turnover in nursing homes offers important quality information. *Health Affairs* 40(3):384–391.

GAO (U.S. Government Accountability Office). GAO. 2011. *Nursing homes: Private investment homes sometimes differed from others in deficiencies, staffing, and financial performance.* Washington, DC: U.S. Government Accountability Office.

GAO. 2021. *Additional reporting on key staffing information and stronger payment incentives needed for skilled nursing facilities.* Washington, DC: U.S. Government Accountability Office.

Gaugler, J. E. 2005. Family involvement in residential long-term care: A synthesis and critical review. *Aging & Mental Health* 9(2):105–118.

Geletta, S., and R. J. Sparks. 2013. Administrator turnover and quality of care in nursing homes. *Annals of Long-Term Care: Clinical Care and Aging* 21(4):27–30.

Geng, F., D. G. Stevenson, and D. C. Grabowski. 2019. Daily nursing home staffing levels highly variable, often below CMS expectations. *Health Affairs* 38(7):1095–1100.

Gharpure, R., A. Patel, and R. Link-Gelles. 2021. First-dose COVID-19 vaccination coverage among skilled nursing facility residents and staff. *JAMA* 325(16):1670–1671.

Gilbert, A. S., S. M. Garratt, L. Kosowicz, J. Ostaszkiewicz, and B. Dow. 2021. Aged care residents' perspectives on quality of care in care homes: A systematic review of qualitative evidence. *Research on Aging* 43(7–8):294–310.

Givens, J. L., R. P. Lopez, K. M. Mazor, and S. L. Mitchell. 2012. Sources of stress for family members of nursing home residents with advanced dementia. *Alzheimer Disease and Associated Disorders* 26(3):254–259.

Goodwin, J. S., P. Agrawal, S. Li, M. Raji, and Y. Kuo. 2021. Growth of physicians and nurse practitioners practicing full time in nursing homes. *Journal of the American Medical Directors Association* 22(12):2534–2539.

Gorges, R. J., and R. T. Konetzka. 2020. Staffing levels and COVID-19 cases and outbreaks in U.S. nursing homes. *Journal of the American Geriatrics Society* 68(11):2462–2466.

Grabowski, D. C., and R. A. Hirth. 2003. Competitive spillovers across non-profit and for-profit nursing homes. *Journal of Health Economics* 22(1):1–22.

Graneheim, U. H., A. Johansson, and B. M. Lindgren. 2014. Family caregivers' experiences of relinquishing the care of a person with dementia to a nursing home: Insights from a meta-ethnographic study. *Scandinavian Journal of Caring Sciences* 28(2):215–224.

Gray-Miceli, D., L. D. Wilson, J. Stanley, R. Watman, A. Shire, S. Sofaer, and M. Mezey. 2014. Improving the quality of geriatric nursing care: Enduring outcomes from the Geriatric Nursing Education Consortium. *Journal of Professional Nursing* 30(6):447–455.

Gupta, S., J. P. Epane, N. Patidar, and R. Weech-Maldonado. 2014. Employing nurse practitioners and physician assistants in nursing homes: Role of market factors. *International Journal of Health Sciences* 2(3):11–25.

Hale, J., and T. Hale. 2019. *Nursing homes turn to temporary employees to fill critical vacancies.* https://www.desmoinesregister.com/story/opinion/columnists/2019/10/15/nursing-homes-turn-temporary-employees-fill-critical-vacancies/3987380002 (accessed May 14, 2021).

Han, K., A. M. Trinkoff, C. L. Storr, N. Lerner, M. Johantgen, and K. Gartrell. 2014. Associations between state regulations, training length, perceived quality and job satisfaction among certified nursing assistants: Cross-sectional secondary data analysis. *International Journal of Nursing Studies* 51(8):1135–1141.

Harrington, C. 2000. Nursing home staffing and its relationship to deficiencies. *Journals of Gerontology: Series B* 55(5):S278–S287.

Harrington, C. 2010. *Nursing home staffing standards in state statutes and regulations.* https://theconsumervoice.org/uploads/files/issues/Harrington-state-staffing-table-2010.pdf (accessed August 20, 2021).

Harrington, C., S. Woolhandler, J. Mullan, H. Carrillo, and D. U. Himmelstein. 2001. Does investor ownership of nursing homes compromise the quality of care? *American Journal of Public Health* 91(9):1452–1455.

Harrington, C., T. Tsoukalas, C. Rudder, R. J. Mollot, and H. Carrillo. 2008. Variation in the use of federal and state civil money penalties for nursing homes. *The Gerontologist* 48(5):679–691.

Harrington, C., B. Olney, H. Carrillo, and T. Kang. 2012. Nurse staffing and deficiencies in the largest for-profit nursing home chains and chains owned by private equity companies. *Health Services Research* 47(1 Pt 1):106–128.

Harrington, C., J. F. Schnelle, M. McGregor, and S. F. Simmons. 2016. The need for higher minimum staffing standards in U.S. nursing homes. *Health Services Insights* 9:13–19.

Harrington, C., M. E. Dellefield, E. Halifax, M. L. Fleming, and D. Bakerjian. 2020. Appropriate nurse staffing levels for U.S. nursing homes. *Health Services Insights* 13:1178632920934785.

Harrington, C., S. Chapman, E. Halifax, M. Dellefield, and A. Montgomery. 2021. Time to ensure sufficient nursing home staffing and eliminate inequities in care. *Journal of Gerontology and Geriatric Medicine* 7:099.

Harris-Kojetin, L., D. Lipson, J. Fielding, K. Kiefer, and R. Stone. 2004. *Recent findings on frontline long-term care workers: A research synthesis 1999–2003.* Washington, DC: Institute for the Future of Aging Services.

Harris-Kojetin, L., M. Sengupta, J. P. Lendon, V. Rome, R. Valverde, and C. Caffrey. 2019. *Long-term care providers and services users in the United States, 2015–2016.* https://www.cdc.gov/nchs/data/series/sr_03/sr03_43-508.pdf (accessed April 2, 2021).

Harvath, T. A., K. Swafford, K. Smith, L. L. Miller, M. Volpin, K. Sexson, D. White, and H. A. Young. 2008. Enhancing nursing leadership in long-term care. A review of the literature. *Research in Gerontological Nursing* 1(3):187–196.

Hauslohner, A., and M. Sacchetti. 2020. *Nursing homes turn to quick fix training to meet pandemic staffing needs.* https://www.washingtonpost.com/national/nursing-homes-turn-to-quick-fix-training-to-meet-pandemic-staffing-needs/2020/05/28/418c3802-a020-11ea-9590-1858a893bd59_story.html (accessed January 21, 2022).

Henkusens, C., H. H. Keller, S. Dupuis, and L. Schindel Martin. 2014. Transitions to long-term care: How do families living with dementia experience mealtimes after relocating? *Journal of Applied Gerontology* 33(5):541–563.

Hernández-Medina, E., S. Eaton, D. Hurd, and A. White. 2006. *Training programs for certified nursing assistants.* https://www.aarp.org/home-garden/livable-communities/info-2006/2006_08_cna.html (accessed August 20, 2021).

HHCS (Hospital & Healthcare Compensation Service). 2020. *2020–2021 nursing home salary & benefits report.* Oakland, NJ: Hospital & Healthcare Compensation Service and John R. Zabka Associates.

Hill, J. 2017. *Consider nursing home optometry as practice option.* https://www.optometrytimes.com/view/consider-nursing-home-optometry-practice-option (accessed November 21, 2021).

Hillmer, M. P., W. P. Wodchis, S. S. Gill, G. M. Anderson, and P. A. Rochon. 2005. Nursing home profit status and quality of care: Is there any evidence of an association? *Medical Care Research and Review* 62(2):139–166.

Himmerick, K. A., J. Miller, C. Toretsky, M. Jura, and J. Spetz. 2017. *Employer demand for physician assistants and nurse practitioners to care for older people and people with disabilities.* https://healthworkforce.ucsf.edu/sites/healthworkforce.ucsf.edu/files/REPORT_2017_PA_NP_Demand_in_LTC_Report_FINAL.pdf (accessed November 30, 2021).

Hoek, L. J., J. C. van Haastregt, E. de Vries, R. Backhaus, J. P. Hamers, and H. Verbeek. 2021. Partnerships in nursing homes: How do family caregivers of residents with dementia perceive collaboration with staff? *Dementia* 20(5):1631–1648.

Hoel, R. W., R. M. Giddings Connolly, and P. Y. Takahashi. 2021. Polypharmacy management in older patients. *Mayo Clinic Proceedings* 96(1):242–256.

Holle, C. L., L. J. Sundean, M. E. Dellefield, J. Wong, and R. P. Lopez. 2019. Examining the beliefs of skilled nursing facility directors of nursing regarding BSN completion and the impact of nurse leader education on patient outcomes. *Journal of Nursing Administration* 49(2):57–60.

Horn, S. D., P. Buerhaus, N. Bergstrom, and R. J. Smout. 2005. RN staffing time and outcomes of long-stay nursing home residents: Pressure ulcers and other adverse outcomes are less likely as RNs spend more time on direct patient care. *American Journal of Nursing* 105(11):58–70; quiz 71.

HRSA (Health Resources and Services Administration). 2019. *Brief summary results from the 2018 National Sample Survey of Registered Nurses.* Rockville, MD: U.S. Department of Health and Human Services Health Resources and Services Administration National Center for Health Workforce Analysis.

Hyer, K., K. S. Thomas, L. G. Branch, J. S. Harman, C. E. Johnson, and R. Weech-Maldonado. 2011. The influence of nurse staffing levels on quality of care in nursing homes. *The Gerontologist* 51(5):610–616.

Intrator, O., Z. Feng, V. Mor, D. Gifford, M. Bourbonniere, and J. Zinn. 2005. The employment of nurse practitioners and physician assistants in U.S. nursing homes. *The Gerontologist* 45(4):486–495.

Intrator, O., E. A. Miller, E. Gadbois, J. K. Acquah, R. Makineni, and D. Tyler. 2015. Trends in nurse practitioner and physician assistant practice in nursing homes, 2000–2010. *Health Services Research* 50(6):1772–1786.

IOM (Institute of Medicine). 1986. *Improving the quality of care in nursing homes.* Washington, DC: National Academy Press.

IOM. 1996. *Nursing staff in hospitals and nursing homes: Is it adequate?* Washington, DC: National Academy Press.

IOM. 2000. *The role of nutrition in maintaining health in the nation's elderly: Evaluating coverage of nutrition services for the Medicare population.* Washington, DC: National Academy Press.

IOM. 2001a. *Crossing the quality chasm: A new health system for the 21st century.* Washington, DC: National Academy Press.

IOM. 2001b. *Improving the quality of long-term care.* Washington, DC: National Academy Press.

IOM. 2003. *Health professions education: A bridge to quality.* Washington, DC: The National Academies Press.

IOM. 2004. *Keeping patients safe: Transforming the work environment of nurses.* Washington, DC: The National Academies Press.

IOM. 2008. *Retooling for an aging America: Building the health care workforce.* Washington, DC: The National Academies Press.

IOM. 2011. *Improving access to oral health care for vulnerable and underserved populations.* Washington, DC: The National Academies Press.

Jette, D. U., R. L. Warren, and C. Wirtalla. 2005. The relation between therapy intensity and outcomes of rehabilitation in skilled nursing facilities. *Archives of Physical Medicine and Rehabilitation* 86(3):373–379.

Jung, H., Y. Qian, P. R. Katz, and L. P. Casalino. 2021. The characteristics of physicians who primarily practice in nursing homes. *Journal of the American Medical Directors Association* 22:468–473.

Kane, R. S. 1993. Factors affecting physician participation in nursing home care. *Journal of the American Geriatrics Society* 41(9):1000–1003.

Katz, P. R., K. Ryskina, D. Saliba, A. Costa, H. Y. Jung, L. M. Wagner, M. A. Unruh, B. J. Smith, A. Moser, J. Spetz, S. Feldman, and J. Karuza. 2021. Medical care delivery in U.S. nursing homes: Current and future practice. *The Gerontologist* 61(4):595–604.

Katz, R. 2019. *Workforce shortages: Bold solutions from LeadingAge.* https://leadingage.org/workforce/workforce-shortaLes-bold-solutions-leadingage (accessed August 13, 2021).

Kellett, U. 2007. Seizing possibilities for positive family caregiving in nursing homes. *Journal of Clinical Nursing* 16(8):1479–1487.

Kemper, P., B. Heier, T. Barry, D. Brannon, J. Angelelli, J. Vasey, and M. Anderson-Knott. 2008. What do direct care workers say would improve their jobs? Differences across settings. *The Gerontologist* 48(Suppl 1):17–25.

Kim, H., C. Kovner, C. Harrington, W. Greene, and M. Mezey. 2009. A panel data analysis of the relationships of nursing home staffing levels and standards to regulatory deficiencies. *Journals of Gerontology, Series B: Psychological Sciences and Social Sciences* 64(2):269–278.

Kimmey, L. D., and S. C. Stearns. 2015. Improving nursing home resident outcomes: Time to focus on more than staffing? *Journal of Nursing Home Research* 1:89–95.

Kirkham, C., and B. Lesser. 2020. *Special report: Pandemic exposes systemic staffing problems at U.S. nursing homes.* https://www.reuters.com/article/us-health-coronavirus-nursing-homes-speci/special-report-pandemic-exposes-systemic-staffing-problems-at-u-s-nursing-homes-idUSKBN23H1L9 (accessed November 19, 2021).

Koenig, H. G. 2012. Religion, spirituality, and health: The research and clinical implications. *ISRN Psychiatry* 2012:278730.

Kolanowski, A., T. Coretes, C. Mueller, B. Bowers, M. Boltz, D. Bakerjian, C. Harrington, L. Popejoy, A. Vogelsmeier, M. Wallhage, D. Fick, M. Batchelor, M. Harris, R. Palan-Lopez, M. Dellefield, A. Mayo, D. Woods, A. Horgas, P. Cacchione, D. Carter, P. Tabloski, and L. Gerdner. 2021. A call to the CMS: Mandate adequate professional nurse staffing in nursing homes. *American Journal of Nursing* 121(3):24–27.

Konetzka, R. T., E. M. White, A. Pralea, D. C. Grabowski, and V. Mor. 2021. A systematic review of long-term care facility characteristics associated with COVID-19 outcomes. *Journal of the American Geriatrics Society* 69(10):2766–2777.

Kusmaul, N. 2016. The content of education for direct caregivers. *Educational Gerontology* 42(1):19–24.

Kusmaul, N., M. Bern-Klug, and R. Bonifas. 2017. Ethical issues in long-term care: A human rights perspective. *Journal of Human Rights and Social Work* 2:86–97.

Kusmaul, N., M. Bern-Klug, J. Heston-Mullins, A. R. Roberts, and C. Galambos. 2020. Nursing home social work during COVID-19. *Journal of Gerontological Social Work* 63(6–7):651–653.

Kusmaul, N., S. Beltran, T. Buckley, A. Gibson, and M. Bern-Klug. 2021. Structural characteristics of nursing homes and social service directors that influence their engagement in disaster preparedness processes. *Journal of Gerontological Social Work* 64(7):775–790.

Lapane, K. L., and C. M. Hughes. 2006. Pharmacotherapy interventions undertaken by pharmacists in the Fleetwood phase III study: The role of process control. *Annals of Pharmacotherapy* 40(9):1522–1526.

LeadingAge Minnesota. 2021. *2020–21 nursing leadership certificate program.* https://www.leadingagemn.org/assets/docs/2020-21_NursingLeadershipCertProgram_Brochure_withLO_1.pdf (accessed January 30, 2021).

Lee, C., A. Podury, J. Kaduthodil, and L. Graham. 2020. *Long-term care facilities must prioritize immigrant workers' needs to contain COVID-19.* https://www.healthaffairs.org/do/10.1377/hblog20200914.520181/full (accessed November 19, 2021).

Lee, E. E., C. A. Thomas, and T. Vu. 2001. Mobile and portable dentistry: Alternative treatment services for the elderly. *Special Care in Dentistry* 21(4):153–155.

Lee, S. W. H., V. S. L. Mak, and Y. W. Tang. 2019. Pharmacist services in nursing homes: A systematic review and meta-analysis. *British Journal of Clinical Pharmacology* 85(12):2668–2688.

Leedahl, S. N., R. K. Chapin, and T. D. Little. 2015. Multilevel examination of facility characteristics, social integration, and health for older adults living in nursing homes. *Journals of Gerontology, Series B: Psychological Sciences and Social Sciences* 70(1):111–122.

Lerner, N. B. 2013. The relationship between nursing staff levels, skill mix, and deficiencies in Maryland nursing homes. *Health Care Manager* 32(2):123–128.

Lerner, N. B., B. Resnick, E. Galik, and K. G. Russ. 2010. Advanced nursing assistant education program. *Journal of Continuing Education in Nursing* 41(8):356–362.

Lerner, N. B., A. Trinkoff, C. L. Storr, M. Johantgen, K. Han, and K. Gartrell. 2014. Nursing home leadership tenure and resident care outcomes. *Journal of Nursing Regulation* 5(3):48–52.

Levy, C., S.-I. T. Palat, and A. M. Kramer. 2007. Physician practice patterns in nursing homes. *Journal of the American Medical Directors Association* 8(9):558–567.

Lewis, T. 2021. *Nursing home workers had one of the deadliest jobs of 2020.* https://www.scientificamerican.com/article/nursing-home-workers-had-one-of-the-deadliest-jobs-of-2020 (accessed February 18, 2021).

Li, Y. 2010. Provision of mental health services in U.S. nursing homes, 1995–2004. *Psychiatric Services* 61(4):349–355.

Li, Y., H. Temkin-Greener, G. Shan, and X. Cai. 2020. COVID-19 infections and deaths among Connecticut nursing home residents: Facility correlates. *Journal of the American Geriatrics Society* 68(9):1899–1906.

Lipsitz, L. A., A. M. Lujan, A. Dufour, G. Abrahams, H. Magliozzi, L. Herndon, and M. Dar. 2020. Stemming the tide of COVID-19 infections in Massachusetts nursing homes. *Journal of the American Geriatrics Society* 68(11):2447–2453.

Liu, J., and M. Bern-Klug. 2013. Nursing home social services directors who report thriving at work. *Journal of Gerontological Social Work* 56:127–145.

Liu, L., A. Guarino, and R. Palan-Lopez. 2011. Family satisfaction with care provided by nurse practitioners to nursing home residents with dementia at the end of life. *Clinical Nursing Research* 21:350–367.

Livingstone, I., J. Hefele, P. Nadash, D. Barch, and N. Leland. 2019. The relationship between quality of care, physical therapy, and occupational therapy staffing levels in nursing homes in 4 years' follow-up. *Journal of the American Medical Directors Association* 20(4):462–469.

Livingstone, I., J. Hefele, and N. Leland. 2021. Characteristics of nursing home providers with distinct patterns of physical and occupational therapy staffing. *Journal of Applied Gerontology* 40(4):443–451.

Lodge, M. P. 1985. *Professional education and practice of nurse administrators/directors of nursing in long-term care: Executive summary*. Kansas City, MO: American Nurses' Foundation, Inc.

Lopez, R. P., K. M. Mazor, S. L. Mitchell, and J. L. Givens. 2013. What is family-centered care for nursing home residents with advanced dementia? *American Journal of Alzheimer's Disease & Other Dementias* 28(8):763–768.

LTCCC (Long Term Care Community Coalition). 2022. *Nursing home staffing Q2 2021*. https://nursinghome411.org/data/staffing/staffing-q2-2021 (accessed February 16, 2022).

Lundin, A., P. H. Bülow, and J. Stier. 2021. Assistant nurses' positioned accounts for prioritizations in residential care for older people. *The Gerontologist* 61(4):573–581.

Lyons, S. S., J. P. Specht, S. E. Karlman, and M. L. Maas. 2008. Everyday excellence. A framework for professional nursing practice in long-term care. *Research in Gerontological Nursing* 1(3):217–228.

Maas, M. L., D. Reed, M. Park, J. P. Specht, D. Schutte, L. S. Kelley, E. A. Swanson, T. Trip-Reimer, and K. C. Buckwalte. 2004. Outcomes of family involvement in care intervention for caregivers of individuals with dementia. *Nursing Research* 53(2):76–86.

Manchha, A. V., N. Walker, K. A. Way, D. Dawson, K. Tann, and M. Thai. 2021. Deeply discrediting: A systematic review examining the conceptualizations and consequences of the stigma of working in aged care. *The Gerontologist* 61(4):e129–e146.

Maramaldi, P., T. Cadet, S. L. Burke, M. LeCloux, E. White, E. Kalenderian, and T. Kinnunen. 2018. Oral health and cancer screening in long-term care nursing facilities: Motivation and opportunity as intervention targets. *Gerodontology* 35(4):407–416.

Mays, A. M., D. Saliba, S. Feldman, M. Smalbrugge, C. M. P. M. Hertogh, T. L. Booker, K. A. Fulbright, S. A. Hendriks, and P. R. Katz. 2018. Quality indicators of primary care provider engagement in nursing home care. *Journal of the American Medical Directors Association* 19(10):824–832.

McCrystal, T., M. Burghardt, and S. Ferranti. 2010. *Buyer beware: OIG shines a spotlight on provider relationships with long term care pharmacies and scrutinizes contract pricing structures*. https://www.ropesgray.com/-/media/Files/in-the-news/2010/07/impact-of-omnicare-settlement-for-pharmacy-providers-and-long-term-care-facilities.pdf (accessed January 18, 2022).

McGarry, B. E., D. C. Grabowski, and M. L. Barnett. 2020. Severe staffing and personal protective equipment shortages faced by nursing homes during the COVID-19 pandemic. *Health Affairs* 39(10):1812–1821.

McGarry, B. E., E. M. White, L. J. Resnik, M. Rahman, and D. C. Grabowski. 2021a. Medicare's new patient driven payment model resulted in reductions in therapy staffing in skilled nursing facilities. *Health Affairs* 40(3):392–399.

McGarry, B. E., A. D. C. Grabowski, and M. L. Barnett. 2021b. Larger nursing home staff size linked to higher number of COVID-19 cases in 2020. *Health Affairs* 40(8):1261–1269.

McGarry, B. E., K. Shen, M. L. Barnett, D. C. Grabowski, and A. D. Gandhi. 2021c. Association of nursing home characteristics with staff and resident COVID-19 vaccination coverage. *JAMA Internal Medicine* 181(12):1670–1672.

McGilton, K. S., L. McGillis-Hall, D. Pringle, L. O'Brien-Pallas, and J. Krejci. 2004. *Identifying and testing factors that influence supervisors' abilities to develop supportive relationships with their staff.* https://www.hhr-rhs.ca/index.php?option=com_mtree&task=viewlink&link_id=5287&Itemid=109&lang=en (accessed November 19, 2021).

McGilton, K. S., A. Krassikova, V. Boscart, S. Sidani, A. Iaboni, S. Vellani, and A. Escrig-Pinol. 2021. Nurse practitioners rising to the challenge during the coronavirus disease 2019 pandemic in long-term care homes. *The Gerontologist* 61(4):615–623.

McKay, M. H., N. D. Pickens, A. Medley, D. Cooper, and C. L. Evetts. 2021. Comparing occupational adaptation-based and traditional training programs for dementia care teams: An embedded mixed-methods study. *The Gerontologist* 61(4):582–594.

McKinney, S. H., K. Corazzini, R. A. Anderson, R. Sloane, and N. G. Castle. 2016. Nursing home director of nursing leadership style and director of nursing-sensitive survey deficiencies. *Health Care Management Review* 41(3):224–232.

McKnight, W. 2016. Chaplains play important part in integrated palliative care. *Caring for the Ages* 17(8):6.

McMullen, T. L., B. Resnick, J. Chin-Hansen, J. M. Geiger-Brown, N. Miller, and R. Rubenstein. 2015. Certified nurse aide scope of practice: State-by-state differences in allowable delegated activities. *Journal of the American Medical Directors Association* 16(1):20–24.

Medical Direction and Medical Care Work Group. 2011. *Role of the medical director in the nursing home.* https://www.health.ny.gov/professionals/nursing_home_administrator/docs/11-13_med_dir_role.pdf (accessed August 20, 2021).

MedPAC (Medicare Payment Advisory Commission). 2016. *Report to the Congress: Medicare payment policy.* Washington, DC: Medicare Payment Advisory Commission.

Mickus, M., C. C. Luz, and A. Hogan. 2004. *Voices from the front: Recruitment and retention of direct care workers in long term care across Michigan.* https://phinational.org/wp-content/uploads/legacy/clearinghouse/MI_vocices_from_the_front.pdf (accessed August 20, 2021).

Mileski, M., U. Pannu, B. Payne, E. Sterling, and R. McClay. 2020. The impact of nurse practitioners on hospitalizations and discharges from long-term nursing facilities: A systematic review. *Healthcare* 8(2):114.

Miller, V. J., T. Hamler, S. J. Beltran, and J. Burns. 2021. Nursing home social services: A systematic review of the literature from 2010 to 2020. *Social Work in Health Care* 60(4):387–409.

Min, A., and H. C. Hong. 2019. Effect of nurse staffing on rehospitalizations and emergency department visits among short-stay nursing home residents: A cross-sectional study using the U.S. Nursing Home Compare database. *Geriatric Nursing* 40(2):160–165.

MITRE (The MITRE Corporation). 2020. *Coronavirus Commission for Safety and Quality in Nursing Homes: Commission final report.* https://sites.mitre.org/nhCOVIDcomm/wp-content/uploads/sites/14/2020/09/FINAL-REPORT-of-NH-Commission-Public-Release-Case-20-2378.pdf (accessed August 20, 2021).

Morley, J. E., and A. M. Sanford. 2014. The God card: Spirituality in the nursing home. *Journal of the American Medical Directors Association* 15(8):533–535.

Morilla-Herrera, J. C., S. Garcia-Mayor, F. J. Martín-Santos, S. Kaknani Uttumchandani, Á. Leon Campos, J. Caro Bautista, and J. M. Morales-Asencio. 2016. A systematic review of the effectiveness and roles of advanced practice nursing in older people. *International Journal of Nursing Studies* 53:290–307.

Morris, L. 2009. Quits and job changes among home care workers in Maine: The role of wages, hours, and benefits. *The Gerontologist* 49(5):635–650.

Mukamel, D. B., S. Cai, and H. Temkin-Greener. 2009. Cost implications of organizing nursing home workforce in teams. *Health Services Research* 44(4):1309–1325.

Mueller, C., G. Arling, R. Kane, J. Bershadsky, D. Holland, and A. Joy. 2006. Nursing home staffing standards: Their relationship to nurse staffing levels. *The Gerontologist* 46(1):74–80.

Mueller, C., R. A. Anderson, E. S. McConnell, and K. Corazzini. 2012. Licensed nurse responsibilities in nursing homes: A scope-of-practice issue. *Journal of Nursing Regulation* 3(1):13–20.

Mueller, C., Y. Duan, A. Vogelsmeier, R. Anderson, E. McConnell, and K. Corazzini. 2018. Interchangeability of licensed nurses in nursing homes: Perspectives of directors of nursing. *Nursing Outlook* 66(6):560–569.

Murray, T. 2021. *Nursing home safety during Covid: Staff shortages.* https://uspirg.org/sites/pirg/files/reports/StaffShortages/WEB_USP_Nursing-Home-Safety-During-COVID_Staff-Shortages.pdf (accessed September 24, 2021).

Myers, D. R., R. Rogers, H. H. LeCrone, K. Kelley, and J. H. Scott. 2018. Work life stress and career resilience of licensed nursing facility administrators. *Journal of Applied Gerontology* 37(4):435–463.

NAB (National Association of Long-Term Care Administrator Boards). 2017. *NHA/RCAL/HCBS domains of practice.* https://www.nabweb.org/filebin/pdf/Reference_Documents/NAB_NHA_RCAL_HCBS_Domains_of_Practice_effective_07.05.2017.pdf (accessed March 31, 2021).

NAB. 2021. *State licensure requirements.* https://www.nabweb.org/state-licensure-requirements (accessed April 23, 2021).

Nancarrow, S. A., A. Booth, S. Ariss, T. Smith, P. Enderby, and A. Roots. 2013. Ten principles of good interdisciplinary team work. *Human Resources for Health* 11(1):19.

NASEM (National Academies of Sciences, Engineering, and Medicine). 2016. *Families caring for an aging America.* Edited by R. Schulz and J. Eden. Washington, DC: The National Academies Press.

NASW (National Association of Social Workers). 2003. *NASW standards for social work services in long-term care facilities.* https://www.socialworkers.org/LinkClick.aspx?fileticket=cwW7lzBfYxg%3d&portalid=0 (accessed November 20, 2021).

NASW. 2016. *NASW standards for social work practice in health care settings.* https://www.socialworkers.org/LinkClick.aspx?fileticket=fFnsRHX-4HE%3D&portalid=0 (accessed November 20, 2021).

Nazir, A., K. Unroe, M. Tegeler, B. Khan, J. Azar, and M. Boustani. 2013. Systematic review of interdisciplinary interventions in nursing homes. *Journal of the American Medical Directors Association* 14(7):471–478.

NCSBN (National Council of State Boards of Nursing). 2017. *National nursing workforce study.* https://www.ncsbn.org/workforce.htm (accessed August 20, 2021).

NHLC (Nursing Home Law Center). 2021. *Podiatry care in nursing homes? A necessity for many patients with foot injuries and complications.* https://www.nursinghomelawcenter.org/news/nursing-home-abuse/podiatry-care-in-nursing-homes-a-necessity-for-many-patients-with-foot-injuries-complications (accessed November 21, 2021).

NICE (National Institute of CNA Excellence). 2021. *About NICE!* https://www.nicecna.org/about-nice (accessed November 20, 2021).

OIG (Office of the Inspector General). 2021. *CMS use of data on nursing home staffing: Progress and opportunities to do more.* Washington, DC: Department of Health and Human Services Office of the Inspector General.

Oliver, D. P., A. J. Rolbiecki, K. Washington, R. L. Kruse, L. Popejoy, J. B. Smith, and G. Demiris. 2021. A pilot study of an intervention to increase family member involvement in nursing home care plan meetings. *Journal of Applied Gerontology* 40(9):1080–1086.

Olson, D., and M. Zwygart-Stauffacher. 2008. The organizational quality frontier and essential role of the director of nursing. *Journal of Nursing Care Quality* 23(1):11–13.

Orth, J., Y. Li, A. Simning, and H. Temkin-Greener. 2019. Providing behavioral health services in nursing homes is difficult: Findings from a national survey. *Journal of the American Geriatrics Society* 67(8):1713–1717.

Paek, S. C., N. J. Zhang, T. T. H. Wan, L. Y. Unruh, and N. Meemon. 2016. The impact of state nursing home staffing standards on nurse staffing levels. *Medical Care Research and Review* 73(1):41–61.

Patterson Norrie, T., A. R. Villarosa, A. C. Kong, S. Clark, S. Macdonald, R. Srinivas, J. Anlezark, and A. George. 2019. Oral health in residential aged care: Perceptions of nurses and management staff. *Nursing Open* 7(2):536–546.

Peck, L. 2021. *Executive survey insights: Wave 31: July 12 to August 8, 2021.* https://blog.nic.org/executive-survey-insights-wave-31 (accessed October 15, 2021).

PHI. 2011. *Nurse aide training requirements by state.* http://phinational.org/advocacy/nurse-aide-training-requirements-state-2016 (accessed June 23, 2021).

PHI. 2016. *Raise the floor: Quality nursing home care depends on quality jobs.* https://phinational.org/wp-content/uploads/legacy/research-report/phi-raisethefloor-201604012.pdf (accessed November 18, 2021).

PHI. 2019. *U.S. nursing assistants employed in nursing homes.* https://phinational.org/wp-content/uploads/2019/08/US-Nursing-Assistants-2019-PHI.pdf (accessed February 16, 2022).

PHI. 2020. *Nursing assistant training requirements by state.* http://phinational.org/advocacy/nurse-aide-training-requirements-state-2016 (accessed November 18, 2021).

PHI. 2021. *Direct care workers in the United States: Key facts.* https://phinational.org/resource/direct-care-workers-in-the-united-states-key-facts-2 (accessed September 10, 2021).

Pillemer, K., J. J. Suitor, C. R. Henderson, Jr., R. Meador, L. Schultz, J. Robison, and C. Hegeman. 2003. A cooperative communication intervention for nursing home staff and family members of residents. *The Gerontologist* 43(Spec No 2):96–106.

Pogorzelska-Maziarz, M., and E. L. Kalp. 2017. Infection prevention outside of the acute care setting: Results from the MegaSurvey of infection preventionists. *American Journal of Infection Control* 45(6):597–602.

Popejoy, L., A. Vogelsmeier, C. Galambos, M. Flesner, G. Alexander, A. Lueckenotte, V. Lyons, and M. Rantz. 2017. The APRN role in changing nursing home quality: The Missouri Quality improvement Initiative. *Journal of Nursing Care Quality* 32(3):196–201.

Popejoy, L. L., A. A. Vogelsmeier, G. L. Alexander, C. M. Galambos, C. A. Crecelius, B. Ge, M. Flesner, K. Canada, and M. Rantz. 2019. Analyzing hospital transfers using INTER-ACT acute care transfer tools: Lessons from MOQI. *Journal of the American Geriatrics Society* 67(9):1953–1959.

Popejoy, L., A. Vogelsmeier, W. Boren, N. Martin, S. Kist, K. Canada, S. J. Miller, and M. Rantz. 2020. A coordinated response to the COVID-19 pandemic in Missouri nursing homes. *Journal of Nursing Care Quality* 35(4):287–292.

Porter, J., A. Ntouva, A. Read, M. Murdoch, D. Ola, and G. Tsakos. 2015. The impact of oral health on the quality of life of nursing home residents. *Health and Quality of Life Outcomes* 13:102.

Probst, J. C., J. D. Baek, and S. B. Laditka. 2010. The relationship between workplace environment and job satisfaction among nursing assistants: Findings from a national survey. *Journal of the American Medical Directors Association* 11(4):246–252.

Quinton, S. 2020. *Staffing nursing homes was hard before the pandemic. Now it's even tougher.* https://www.pewtrusts.org/en/research-and-analysis/blogs/stateline/2020/05/18/staffing-nursing-homes-was-hard-before-the-pandemic-now-its-even-tougher (accessed May 26, 2021).

Rantz, M. J., M. Zwygart-Stauffacher, M. Flesner, L. Hicks, D. Mehr, T. Russell, and D. Minner. 2013. The influence of teams to sustain quality improvement in nursing homes that "need improvement." *Journal of the American Medical Directors Association* 14(1):48–52.

Rantz, M. J., L. Popejoy, A. Vogelsmeier, C. Galambos, G. Alexander, M. Flesner, C. Crecelius, B. Ge, and G. Petroski. 2017. Successfully reducing hospitalizations of nursing home residents: Results of the Missouri Quality Initiative. *Journal of the American Medical Directors Association* 18(11):960–966.

Rantz, M. J., L. Popejoy, A. Vogelsmeier, C. Galambos, G. Alexander, M. Flesner, C. Murray, C. Crecelius, B. Ge, and G. Petroski. 2018a. Impact of advanced practice registered nurses on quality measures: The Missouri Quality Initiative experience. *Journal of the American Medical Directors Association* 19(6):541–550.

Rantz, M. J., L. Popejoy, A. Vogelsmeier, C. Galambos, G. Alexander, M. Flesner, C. Murray, and C. Crecelius. 2018b. Reducing avoidable hospitalizations and improving quality in nursing homes with APRNs and interdisciplinary support. *Journal of Nursing Care Quality* 33(1):5–9.

Rao, A. D., and L. K. Evans. 2015. The role of directors of nursing in cultivating nurse empowerment. *Annals of Long-Term Care* 23(4):27–32.

Ray, V. 2019. A theory of racialized organizations. *American Sociological Review* 84(1):26–53.

Reid, R. C., and N. L. Chappell. 2017. Family involvement in nursing homes: Are family caregivers getting what they want? *Journal of Applied Gerontology* 36(8):993–1015.

Rizzo, V. M., and J. M. Rowe. 2016. Cost-effectiveness of social work services in aging: An updated systematic review. *Research on Social Work Practice* 26(6):653–667.

Roberts, A. R., and J. R. Bowblis. 2017. Who hires social workers? Structural and contextual determinants of social service staffing in nursing homes. *Health & Social Work* 42(1):15–23.

Roberts, A. R., and K. J. Ishler. 2018. Family involvement in the nursing home and perceived resident quality of life. *The Gerontologist* 58(6):1033–1043.

Roberts, A. R., A. C. Smith, and J. R. Bowblis. 2020. Nursing home social services and post-acute care: Does more qualified staff improve behavioral symptoms and reduce antipsychotic drug use? *Journal of the American Medical Directors Association* 21(3):388–394.

Roberts, T., K. Nolet, and B. Bowers. 2015. Consistent assignment of nursing staff to residents in nursing homes: A critical review of conceptual and methodological issues. *The Gerontologist* 55(3):434–447.

Romero, L. 2021. *Pandemic, labor shortages have left long-term care facilities competing for staff*. https://abcnews.go.com/US/pandemic-labor-shortages-left-long-term-care-facilities/story?id=79508224 (accessed November 21, 2021).

Rondeau, K. V., and T. H. Wagar. 2006. Nurse and resident satisfaction in magnet long-term care organizations: Do high involvement approaches matter? *Journal of Nursing Management* 14(3):244–250.

Rosemond, C., L. C. Hanson, and S. Zimmerman. 2017. Goals of care or goals of trust? How family members perceive goals for dying nursing home residents. *Journal of Palliative Medicine* 20(4):360–365.

Rosenfeld, P., M. Kobayashi, P. Barber, and M. Mezey. 2004. Utilization of nurse practitioners in long-term care: Findings and implications of a national survey. *Journal of the American Medical Directors Association* 5:9–15.

Ross, M. M., A. Carswell, and W. B. Dalziel. 2001. Family caregiving in long-term care facilities. *Clinical Nursing Research* 10(4):347–363; discussion 364–348.

Rowland, F. N., M. Cowles, C. Dickstein, and P. R. Katz. 2009. Impact of medical director certification on nursing home quality of care. *Journal of the American Medical Directors Association* 10(6):431–435.

RTI International. 2017. *Evaluation of the initiative to reduce avoidable hospitalizations among nursing facility residents: Final report.* Waltham, MA: RTI International.

Ryosho, N. 2011. Experiences of racism by female minority and immigrant nursing assistants. *Affilia: Journal of Women and Social Work* 26(1):59–71.

Ryskina, K. L., D. Polsky, and R. M. Werner. 2017. Physicians and advanced practitioners specializing in nursing home care, 2012–2015. *JAMA* 318(20):2040–2042.

Saunders, R., K. Seaman, R. Graham, and A. Christiansen. 2019. The effect of volunteers' care and support on the health outcomes of older adults in acute care: A systematic scoping review. *Journal of Clinical Nursing* 28(23–24):4236–4249.

Scales, K. 2020. *Nursing assistants have training standards for a reason.* https://phinational.org/nursing-assistants-have-training-standards-for-a-reason (accessed November 19, 2021).

Scales, K. 2021. *Temporary nurse aides need job stability and support.* https://phinational.org/temporary-nurse-aides-need-job-stability-and-support (accessed May 14, 2021).

Scales, K., A. Altman, S. Campbell, A. Cook, A. Del Rio Drake, R. Espinoza, and J. M. Sturgeon. 2020. *It's time to care: A detailed profile of America's direct care workforce.* http://phinational.org/resource/its-time-to-care-a-detailed-profile-of-americas-direct-care-workforce (accessed August 20, 2021).

Schkade, J. K., and M. McClung. 2001. *Occupational adaptation in practice: Concepts and cases.* Thorofare, NJ: Slack.

Schnelle, J. F., L. D. Schroyer, A. A. Saraf, and S. F. Simmons. 2016. Determining nurse aide staffing requirements to provide care based on resident workload: A discrete event simulation model. *Journal of the American Medical Directors Association* 17(11):970–977.

Seavey, D. 2004. *The cost of frontline turnover in long-term care.* https://www.leadingage.org/sites/default/files/Cost_Frontline_Turnover.pdf (accessed July 7, 2021).

Sedensky, M. 2021. *Ghost towns: Nursing home staffing falls amid pandemic.* https://apnews.com/article/coronavirus-pandemic-nursing-homes-d1befe76a3a0680b57defb6d9f1cfb66 (accessed February 16, 2022).

Seidman, H. R. 2021. *The changing role of chaplains at long-term care facilities.* https://www.nextavenue.org/the-changing-role-of-chaplains-during-the-pandemic (accessed August 18, 2021).

Senek, M., S. Robertson, T. Ryan, R. King, E. Wood, and A. Tod. 2020. The association between care left undone and temporary nursing staff ratios in acute settings: A cross-sectional survey of registered nurses. *BMC Health Services Research* 20(1):637.

Severens, M. 2020. *Trump team relaxed training rules for nursing home staff just as pandemic hit.* https://www.politico.com/news/2020/07/15/coronavirus-nursing-homes-361510 (accessed January 21, 2022).

Sharma, H., and L. Xu. 2022. Association between wages and nursing staff turnover in Iowa nursing homes. *Innovation in Aging.* https://doi.org/10.1093/geroni/igac004 (accessed February 14, 2022).

Sherman, R. O., and T. Touhy. 2017. An exploratory descriptive study to evaluate Florida nurse leader challenges and opportunities in nursing homes settings. *SAGE Open Nursing* 3:1–7.

Siegel, E. O., C. Mueller, K. L. Anderson, and M. E. Dellefield. 2010. The pivotal role of the director of nursing in nursing homes. *Nursing Administration Quarterly* 34(2):110–121.

Sifuentes, A. M. F., and K. L. Lapane. 2020. Oral health in nursing homes: What we know and what we need to know. *Journal of Nursing Home Research* 6:1–5.

Simmons, S. F., and J. F. Schnelle. 2004. Individualized feeding assistance care for nursing home residents: Staffing requirements to implement two interventions. *Journals of Gerontology: Series A* 59(9):M966–M973.

Simmons, S. F., and J. F. Schnelle. 2006. Feeding assistance needs of long-stay nursing home residents and staff time to provide care. *Journal of the American Geriatrics Society* 54(6):919–924.

Simmons, S. F., R. Bertrand, V. Shier, R. Sweetland, T. J. Moore, D. T. Hurd, and J. F. Schnelle. 2007. A preliminary evaluation of the paid feeding assistant regulation: Impact on feeding assistance care process quality in nursing homes. *The Gerontologist* 47(2):184–192.

Simmons, S. F., E. Keeler, X. Zhuo, K. A. Hickey, H.-W. Sato, and J. F. Schnelle. 2008. Prevention of unintentional weight loss in nursing home residents: A controlled trial of feeding assistance. *Journal of the American Geriatrics Society* 56(8):1466–1473.

Simons, K., M. Bern-Klug, and S. An. 2012. Envisioning quality psychosocial care in nursing homes: The role of social work. *Journal of the American Medical Directors Association* 13(9):800–805.

Singh, D., and R. Schwab. 2000. Predicting turnover and retention in nursing homes administrators: Management and policy implications. *The Gerontologist* 40(3):310–319.

Sloane, P. D., R. Yearby, R. T. Konetzka, Y. Li, R. Espinoza, and S. Zimmerman. 2021. Addressing systemic racism in nursing homes: A time for action. *Journal of the American Medical Directors Association* 22(4):886–892.

Smiley, R. A., C. Ruttinger, C. M. Oliveira, L. R. Hudson, R. Allgeyer, K. A. Reneau, J. H. Silvestre, and M. Alexander. 2021. The 2020 National Nursing Workforce Survey. *Journal of Nursing Regulation* 12(1):S1–S96.

Spilsbury, K., C. Hewitt, L. Stirk, and C. Bowman. 2011. The relationship between nurse staffing and quality of care in nursing homes: A systematic review. *International Journal of Nursing Studies* 48(6):732–750.

Spector, W. D., R. Limcangco, C. Williams, W. Rhodes, and D. Hurd. 2013. Potentially avoidable hospitalizations for elderly long-stay residents in nursing homes. *Medical Care* 51(8)673–681.

Squillace, M. R., R. E. Remsburg, L. D. Harris-Kojetin, A. Bercovitz, E. Rosenoff, and B. Han. 2009. The National Nursing Assistant Survey: Improving the evidence base for policy initiatives to strengthen the certified nursing assistant workforce. *The Gerontologist* 49(2):185–197.

Stacey, C. L. 2005. Finding dignity in dirty work: The constraints and rewards of low-wage home care labour. *Sociology of Health and Illness* 27(6):831–854.

Stevenson, D. G., and D. C. Grabowski. 2008. Private equity investment and nursing home care: Is it a big deal? *Health Affairs* 27(5):1399–1408.

Stone, P. W., C. T. A. Herzig, M. Agarwal, M. Pogorzelska-Maziarz, and A. W. Dick. 2018. Nursing home infection control program characteristics, CMS citations, and implementation of antibiotic stewardship policies: A national study. *Inquiry* 55:1–7.

Stone, P. W., M. Agarwal, and M. Pogorzelska-Maziarz. 2020. Infection preventionist staffing in nursing homes. *American Journal of Infection Control* 48(3):330–332.

Stone, R. I., and S. L. Dawson. 2008. The origins of Better Jobs Better Care. *The Gerontologist* 48(Spec No 1):5–13.

Stone, R. I., S. C. Reinhard, B. Bowers, D. Zimmerman, C. D. Phillips, C. Hawes, J. A. Fielding, and N. Jacobson. 2002. *Evaluation of the Wellspring model for improving nursing home quality*. New York: Commonwealth Fund.

Streim, J. E., E. W. Beckwith, D. Arapakos, P. Banta, R. Dunn, and T. Hoyer. 2002. Mental health services in nursing homes: Regulatory oversight, payment policy, and quality improvement in mental health care in nursing homes. *Psychiatric Services* 53(11):1414–1418.

Stulick, A. 2021. *Nursing homes use of staffing agencies soars during pandemic as workforce crisis deepens*. https://skillednursingnews.com/2021/06/nursing-homes-use-of-staffing-agencies-soars-during-pandemic-as-workforce-crisis-deepens/?euid=1f8e8685ef&utm_source=snn-newsletter&utm_medium=email&utm_campaign=fd29b0ab54 (accessed November 21, 2021).

Sullivan, T. 2018. *CMS proposed rule: Changes to the conditions of participation for long term care facilities—proposing to ban manufacturer rebates to long term care pharmacies.* https://www.policymed.com/2011/10/cms-proposed-rule-changes-to-the-conditions-of-participation-for-long-term-care-facilities-proposing.html (accessed February 8, 2022).

Sussman, T., and S. Dupuis. 2014. Supporting residents moving into long-term care: Multiple layers shape residents' experiences. *Journal of Gerontological Social Work* 57(5): 438–459.

Tak, S., M. H. Sweeney, T. Alterman, S. Baron, and G. M. Calvert. 2010. Workplace assaults on nursing assistants in U.S. nursing homes: A multilevel analysis. *American Journal of Public Health* 100(10):1938–1945.

Tan, R. 2022. *Low-wage workers prop up the nursing home industry. They're quitting in droves.* https://www.washingtonpost.com/dc-md-va/2022/01/23/nursing-home-dc-staffing-omicron (accessed February 9, 2022).

Temkin-Greener, H., S. Cai, P. Katz, H. Zhao, and D. B. Mukamel. 2009. Daily practice teams in nursing homes: Evidence from New York State. *The Gerontologist* 49(1):68–80.

Teno, J. M., P. L. Gozalo, A. N. Trivedi, S. L. Mitchell, J. N. Bunker, and V. Mor. 2017. Temporal trends in the numbers of skilled nursing facility specialists from 2007 through 2014. *JAMA Internal Medicine* 177(9):1376–1378.

Teno, J. M., A. N. Trivedi, and P. Gozalo. 2018. What exactly is a "SNF-ist?"—Reply. *JAMA Internal Medicine* 178(1):154.

Tjia, J., C. A. Lemay, A. Bonner, C. Compher, K. Paice, T. Field, K. Mazor, J. N. Hunnicutt, K. L. Lapane, and J. Gurwitz. 2017. Informed family member involvement to improve the quality of dementia care in nursing homes. *Journal of the American Geriatrics Society* 65(1):59–65.

Tomaskovic-Devey, D. 2018. Labor process inequality and the sex and racial composition of jobs. In D. Tomaskovic-Devey, *Gender and racial inequality at work*. Ithaca, NY: Cornell University Press.

Trautner, B. W., M. T. Greene, S. L. Krein, H. L. Wald, S. Saint, A. J. Rolle, S. McNamara, B. S. Edson, and L. Mody. 2017. Infection prevention and antimicrobial stewardship knowledge for selected infections among nursing home personnel. *Infection Control and Hospital Epidemiology* 38(1):83–88.

Travers, J. L., A. M. Teitelman, K. A. Jenkins, and N. G. Castle. 2020. Exploring social-based discrimination among nursing home certified nursing assistants. *Nursing Inquiry* 27(1):e12315.

Travers, J. L., B. A. Caceres, D. Vlahov, H. Zaidi, J. S. Dill, R. I. Stone, and P. W. Stone. 2021. Federal requirements for nursing homes to include certified nursing assistants in resident care planning and interdisciplinary teams: A policy analysis. *Nursing Outlook* 69(4):617–625.

Trinkoff, A. M., C. L. Storr, M. Johantgen, N. Lerner, K. Han, and K. McElroy. 2013. State regulatory oversight of certified nursing assistants and resident outcomes. *Journal of Nursing Regulation* 3(4):53–59.

Trinkoff, A. M., N. B. Lerner, C. L. Storr, K. Han, M. E. Johantgen, and K. Gartrell. 2015. Leadership education, certification and resident outcomes in U.S. nursing homes: Cross-sectional secondary data analysis. *International Journal of Nursing Studies* 52(1):334–344.

Trinkoff, A. M., C. L. Storr, N. B. Lerner, B. K. Yang, and K. Han. 2017. CNA training requirements and resident care outcomes in nursing homes. *The Gerontologist* 57(3):501–508.

Truitt, A. R., and C. R. Snyder. 2020. Racialized experiences of Black nursing professionals and certified nursing assistants in long-term care settings. *Journal of Transcultural Nursing* 31(3):312–318.

Turner, S. A. 2015. Medical director and other physician compensation arrangements under scrutiny. *Geriatric Nursing* 36(4):314–315.

Tyler, D. A., Z. Feng, N. E. Leland, P. Gozalo, O. Intrator, and V. Mor. 2013. Trends in post-acute care and staffing in U.S. nursing homes, 2001–2010. *Journal of the American Medical Directors Association* 14(11):817–820.

U.S. Congress (U.S. Congress, Senate, Committee on Health, Education, Labor and Pensions). 2001. *Nursing workforce: Recruitment and retention of nurses and nurse aides is a growing concern.* 107th Cong., May 17 (statement of William J. Scanlon, director health care issues).

van der Ploeg, E. S., T. Mbakile, S. Genovesi, and D. W. O'Connor. 2012. The potential of volunteers to implement non-pharmacological interventions to reduce agitation associated with dementia in nursing home residents. *International Psychogeriatrics* 24(11):1790–1797.

van der Ploeg, E. S., H. Walker, and D. W. O'Connor. 2014. The feasibility of volunteers facilitating personalized activities for nursing home residents with dementia and agitation. *Geriatric Nursing* 35(2):142–146.

van Dyck, L. I., K. M. Wilkins, J. Ouellet, G. M. Ouellet, and M. J. Conroy. 2020. Combating heightened social isolation of nursing home elders: The telephone outreach in the COVID-19 outbreak program. *American Journal of Geriatric Psychiatry* 28(9):989–992.

Van Houtven, C., K. Miller, R. Gorges, H. Campbell, W. Dawson, J. McHugh, B. McGarry, R. Gilmartin, N. Boucher, B. Kaufman, L. Chisholm, S. Beltran, S. Fashaw, X. Wang, O. Reneau, A. Chun, J. Jacobs, K. Abrahamson, K. Unroe, C. Bishop, G. Arling, S. Kelly, R. M. Werner, R. T. Konetzka, and E. C. Norton. 2021. State policy responses to COVID-19 in nursing homes. *Journal of Long-Term Care* 264–282.

Varney, S. 2021. *Nursing homes bleed staff as Amazon lures low-wage workers with prime packages.* https://khn.org/news/article/nursing-homes-staff-shortages-amazon-lures-low-wage-workers (accessed February 8, 2022).

Veiga-Seijo, R., M. d. C. Miranda-Duro, and S. Veiga-Seijo. 2021. Strategies and actions to enable meaningful family connections in nursing homes during the COVID-19: A scoping review. *Clinical Gerontologist* 45(1):20–30.

Vogelsmeier, A. A., S. J. Farrah, A. Roam, and L. Ott. 2010. Evaluation of a leadership development academy for RNs in long-term care. *Nursing Administration Quarterly* 34(2):122–129.

Vogelsmeier, A., L. Popejoy, C. Crecelius, S. Orique, G. Alexander, and M. Rantz. 2018. APRN-conducted medication reviews for long-stay nursing home residents. *Journal of the American Medical Directors Association* 19(1):83–85.

Vogelsmeier, A., L. Popejoy, K. Canada, C. Galambos, G. Petroski, C. Crecelius, G. Alexander, and M. Rantz. 2020. Results of the Missouri Quality Initiative in sustaining changes in nursing home care: Six-year trends of reducing hospitalizations of nursing home residents. *Journal of Nutrition, Health & Aging* 25(1):5–12.

Weber, L. 2021. *Nursing homes keep losing workers.* https://www.wsj.com/articles/nursing-homes-keep-losing-workers-11629898200 (accessed November 21, 2021).

Wells, J. C. 2004. The case for minimum nurse staffing standards in nursing homes: A review of the literature. *Alzheimer's Care Today* 5(1):39–51.

Werner, R. M., and N. B. Coe. 2021. Nursing home staffing levels did not change significantly during COVID-19. *Health Affairs* 40(5):795–801.

Whitaker, T., T. Weismiller, E. Clark, and M. Wilson. 2006. *Assuring the sufficiency of a frontline workforce: A national study of licensed social workers.* Executive summary. Washington, DC: National Association of Social Workers.

White, E. M., C. M. Kosar, M. Rahman, and V. Mor. 2020a. Trends in hospitals and skilled nursing facilities sharing medical providers, 2008–16. *Health Affairs* 39(8):1312–1320.

White, E. M., L. H. Aiken, D. M. Sloane, and M. D. McHugh. 2020b. Nursing home work environment, care quality, registered nurse burnout and job dissatisfaction. *Geriatric Nursing* 41(2):158–164.

White, E. M., T. F. Wetle, A. Reddy, and R. R. Baier. 2021. Front-line nursing home staff experiences during the COVID-19 pandemic. *Journal of the American Medical Directors Association* 22(1):199–203.

White House. 2021. *Fact sheet: President Biden sends immigration bill to Congress as part of his commitment to modernize our immigration system.* https://www.whitehouse.gov/briefing-room/statements-releases/2021/01/20/fact-sheet-president-biden-sends-immigration-bill-to-congress-as-part-of-his-commitment-to-modernize-our-immigration-system (accessed August 13, 2021).

Wiener, J. M., M. R. Squillace, W. L. Anderson, and G. Khatutsky. 2009. Why do they stay? Job tenure among certified nursing assistants in nursing homes. *The Gerontologist* 49(2):198–210.

Xing, J., D. B. Mukamel, and H. Temkin-Greener. 2013. Hospitalizations of nursing home residents in the last year of life: Nursing home characteristics and variation in potentially avoidable hospitalizations. *Journal of the American Geriatrics Society* 61(11):1900–1908.

Xu, H., O. Intrator, and J. R. Bowblis. 2020. Shortages of staff in nursing homes during the COVID-19 pandemic: What are the driving factors? *Journal of the American Medical Directors Association* 21(10):1371–1377.

Yang, B. K., M. W. Carter, A. M. Trinkoff, and H. W. Nelson. 2021a. Nurse staffing and skill mix patterns in relation to resident care outcomes in U.S. nursing homes. *Journal of the American Medical Directors Association* 22(5):1081–1087.e1081.

Yang, B. K., M. Carter, and W. Nelson. 2021b. Trends in COVID-19 cases, related deaths, and staffing shortage in nursing homes by rural and urban status. *Geriatric Nursing* 42(6):1356–1361.

You, K., Y. Li, O. Intrator, D. Stevenson, R. Hirth, D. Grabowski, and J. Banaszak-Holl. 2016. Do nursing home chain size and proprietary status affect experiences with care? *Medical Care* 54(3):229–234.

Yurkofsky, M., and J. G. Ouslander. 2021. *Medical care in skilled nursing facilities (SNFs) in the United States.* https://www.uptodate.com/contents/medical-care-in-skilled-nursing-facilities-snfs-in-the-united-states (accessed July 16, 2021).

Zallman, L., K. E. Finnegan, D. U. Himmelstein, S. Touw, and S. Woolhandler. 2019. Care for America's elderly and disabled people relies on immigrant labor. *Health Affairs* 38(6):919–926.

Zhang, Y., L. Punnett, B. Mawn, and R. Gore. 2016. Working conditions and mental health of nursing staff in nursing homes. *Issues in Mental Health Nursing* 37(7):485–492.

Zhao, L., H. Xie, and R. Dong. 2015. Volunteers as caregivers for elderly with chronic diseases: An assessment of demand and cause of demand. *International Journal of Nursing Sciences* 2(3):268–272.

Zheng, N. T., and H. Temkin-Greener. 2010. End-of-life care in nursing homes: The importance of CAN staff communication. *Journal of the American Medical Directors Association* 11(7):494–499.

Zimmerman, S., B. J. Bowers, L. W. Cohen, D. C. Grabowski, S. D. Horn, P. Kemper, and T. R. Collaborative. 2016. New evidence on the Green House model of nursing home care: Synthesis of findings and implications for policy, practice, and research. *Health Services Research* 51(Suppl 1):475–496.

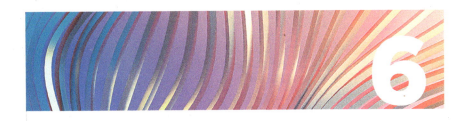

Nursing Home Environment and Resident Safety

Nursing home residents have diverse needs, which can be viewed within the framework of Maslow's hierarchy of needs (as discussed in Chapter 4 and detailed in Table 4-1). This chapter of the report explores two key areas that are critical to residents' quality of care and quality of life: resident safety and the physical environment in which nursing home residents live and receive care and services. These two topics are located within the second level of Maslow's hierarchy—safety and security—as depicted in Figure 4-1.

ENSURING THE SAFETY OF NURSING HOME RESIDENTS

Patient safety is an essential component of high quality care (IOM, 2001). Given the large share of nursing home residents who are frail, vulnerable, and have chronic medical conditions, keeping residents safe from harm is critically important and particularly challenging. As reinforced throughout this report, a nursing home provides care to residents, while also serving as a place to live. Because of this dual function as well as the health characteristics of their residents, nursing homes must balance safety with residents' preferences for autonomy and quality of life (Brauner et al., 2018).

Preventable adverse events constitute more than half of all harms experienced by nursing home residents (OIG, 2014a). The most common of these are falls, infections, and adverse events related to medications. While medical errors, such as providing the wrong medication to a resident, are a common source of patient harm, failure to provide care also results in patient harm (Simmons et al., 2016). Omissions of care, also referred to as missed care, are a key patient safety issue in nursing homes (Ball and

Griffiths, 2018), and have a negative impact on resident outcomes as well as the quality of care in nursing homes (Ogletree et al., 2020).

This chapter discusses some of the more common safety-related areas of focus in nursing homes including improving medication safety, resident falls, preventing elder abuse, improving communication during transitions of care, enhancing infection control, and strengthening emergency planning, preparedness and response.

Improving Medication Safety

All certified nursing homes are required by statute to provide pharmaceutical services to ensure that all drugs needed to meet each resident's needs are dispensed and administered properly.[1] Regulations revised in 2016 require a licensed pharmacist review each resident's drug regimen as well as their medical record on a monthly basis (Barlas, 2016).[2]

Given the prevalence of nursing home residents with multiple chronic conditions, ongoing symptoms (e.g., chronic pain), and acute problems (e.g., infections), polypharmacy—defined as taking five or more medications per day—is common. Research indicates that 91 percent of nursing home residents take more than 5 medications per day, while 65 percent of residents take more than 10 medications per day (Spinewine et al., 2021). Polypharmacy is associated with a high risk of negative clinical outcomes, including cognitive impairments, falls, fractures, adverse drug events (ADEs),[3] and drug interactions (Bernsten et al., 2001; Hoel et al., 2021; NIA, 2021; Wang et al., 2015).

Medication errors, which can occur at any step of the medication use process (prescribing, purchasing, ordering, delivery, storage, preparation, administration, or monitoring), affect between 16 and 27 percent of all nursing home residents (Spinewine et al., 2021). Research shows that approximately 40 percent of medication errors occur at care transitions (Hughes, 2008; Redmond et al., 2018). Poor communication during these transitions can

---

[1] CMS Requirements for Long-Term Care Facilities—Pharmacy Services, 42 CFR § 483.45 (2016).

[2] Concerns over conflict of interest were raised in relation to cases where pharmacists were seen to lack independence from and were thus unduly influenced by pharmaceutical companies (Barlas, 2012). Several cases were filed under the whistleblower provisions of the False Claims Act alleging that nursing home pharmacies accepted kick-backs from drug manufacturers in exchange for prescribing that manufacturers' prescription drugs (CANHR, 2009; DOJ, 2015). Other cases involved a company offering consultant pharmacist services to nursing homes at below market value in exchange for the pharmacist prescribing that drug manufacturer's products (McCrystal et al., 2010). However, the revised rules did not contain any specific requirements to address these concerns (Barlas, 2016).

[3] An adverse drug event (ADE) is an injury resulting from medical intervention related to a drug. This includes medication errors, adverse drug reactions, allergic reactions, and overdoses (ODPHP, 2021).

also lead to adverse drug events (Branch et al., 2021). Thus, ensuring the appropriate use of medications is crucial to ensuring resident safety, preventing unnecessary harm, and improving the quality of care in nursing homes.

Efforts to improve medication safety involve regular, formal pharmacist reviews of medications combined with an enhanced integration of the pharmacist with the interdisciplinary care team. One review found that the introduction of pharmacists into nursing homes contributed positively to reducing the number of drugs taken by nursing home residents (Lee et al., 2019). Earlier studies revealed that interventions by pharmacists in nursing home settings generally reduced inappropriate prescribing and improved the knowledge base of nursing home staff (Verrue et al., 2009).

Another initiative targeting medication safety is deprescribing, which refers to the process of reducing, discontinuing, or withdrawing of medications. Deprescribing has been found to have an impact on improving health outcomes, reducing the number of potentially inappropriate medications, decreasing the number of older people who had falls, and lowering mortality rates (Kua et al., 2019). Approaches to deprescribing medications that are no longer needed or that have more potential for harm than good include, for example, efforts to substitute nonpharmacologic management for psychoactive medications in persons with dementia (O'Mahony et al., 2014; Sloane et al., 2021; Welsh et al., 2020).

Among the quality improvement strategies focused on medication safety are efforts to minimize the adverse effects of potentially inappropriate prescribing, overprescribing, and drug interactions. Approaches to optimize prescribing include the development of and adherence to prescribing guidelines, such as the Beers Criteria[4] for potentially inappropriate medication use in older persons (American Geriatrics Society, 2019). Other approaches include improving communication within the care team and with residents and families about medication issues (e.g., potentially inappropriate antibiotics) and tailoring medication prescribing to resident characteristics and needs (Desai et al., 2011). As one of the four components of age-friendly health systems, effective medication management emphasizes the key role of regular care plan meetings with the interdisciplinary care team (as discussed in Chapter 4) to ensure alignment with "what matters" to the individual nursing home resident and their families (Edelman et al., 2021). For a nursing home resident's perspective on medication safety, see Box 6-1.

Health information technology applications such as electronic medication administration records (eMARs) hold the potential to improve medication safety—particularly in terms of reducing medication errors—in nursing home settings. Such eMARs enable the automatic documentation of medication into the electronic medical record. Nursing home settings have not

---

[4] For more information, see https://dcri.org/beers-criteria-medication-list (accessed November 3, 2021).

> **BOX 6-1**
> **Resident Perspective**
>
> "I decided to read my medical record for the first time only to discover many wrong diagnoses and multiple unnecessary drugs I was getting crushed in applesauce. I had a diagnosis of psychosis for which I was being given Zyprexa and Ativan when my hospital discharge summary said 'No evidence of psychosis.' I supposedly had a sleep disorder for which Trazadone and Ambien for insomnia were prescribed when I'm a night owl who likes to read. I had a diagnosis of pain and was being given Oxycodone when I had no pain. I was on insulin for diabetes when it turned out my case is so mild I had only to eat differently to have a normal A1C."
>
> — 78 year-old nursing home resident, MA
>
> *This quote was collected from the committee's online call for resident, family, and nursing home staff perspectives.*

adopted this technology as broadly as other health care settings, which may be due to a lack of financial support (Spinewine et al., 2021). The integration of eMARs with clinical decision-making would help to improve the safety of medication delivery, the tracking of residents' allergies, and the monitoring of residents' response to medication (Poon et al., 2010; Truitt et al., 2016).

Antipsychotic Medications

A serious patient safety and quality issue in nursing homes is the use of antipsychotic medications. Such medications are used to treat mental health conditions such schizophrenia. The Food and Drug Administration released information about cardiac fatalities in 2005 and issued black box warnings about the association of antipsychotic medications with an increased risk of death when used to treat elderly patients with dementia-related psychosis (Narang et al., 2010).[5] The Office of the Inspector General (OIG) raised concerns about the high use of antipsychotic medications among nursing home residents more than 10 years ago, based on an examination of claims for atypical antipsychotic drugs[6] for nursing home residents. OIG found

---

[5] Drug companies charged with off-label marketing of antipsychotic drugs for nursing home residents paid large penalties in settlements under the False Claims Act. See https://www.justice.gov/opa/pr/johnson-johnson-pay-more-22-billion-resolve-criminal-and-civil-investigations (accessed February 16, 2022).

[6] Atypical antipsychotics—also known as second-generation antipsychotics and serotonin-dopamine antagonists—are a type of psychotropic drug that the Food and Drug Administration has approved to treat medical conditions such as schizophrenia, Tourette's syndrome, Huntington's disease, and bipolar disorder (OIG, 2021).

that nearly 90 percent of claims for atypical antipsychotic drugs were associated with a condition listed in the black box warning (OIG, 2011). In an effort to advance person-centered care and promote the use of nonpharmacologic treatments for nursing home residents with dementia, the Centers for Medicare & Medicaid Services (CMS) launched the National Partnership to Improve Dementia Care in Nursing Homes in 2012 (discussed in Chapter 4). An initial focus of the Partnership was on reducing use of antipsychotic medications for nursing home residents with dementia.

More recently, the OIG conducted an examination of the way in which CMS monitors the use of antipsychotic medication use in nursing homes (OIG, 2021). CMS uses a quality measure to track the number of long-stay nursing home residents who received antipsychotic medication. OIG concluded that CMS's reliance on nursing homes' self-reported data through the Minimum Data Set (MDS) as the only source of information on antipsychotic drug use in nursing homes has resulted in an inaccurate measurement of the full extent of such medication use. The OIG analyzed Medicare claims and found that 5 percent of all Part D beneficiaries who were long-stay residents age 65 and older had a Part D claim in 2018 for an antipsychotic medication, but the MDS did not report those residents as having received an antipsychotic drug in the same quarter in which they had a Part D claim (OIG, 2021). Moreover, the OIG found that nearly one in three of all nursing home residents who had schizophrenia diagnoses documented in the MDS did not have any Medicare service claims for that diagnosis—in other words, there was no documented evidence that the resident received treatment for their schizophrenia diagnosis. Importantly, CMS excludes residents with MDS-reported diagnoses of schizophrenia, Huntington's disease, or Tourette's syndrome from inclusion in its quality measure of antipsychotic drug use. Finally, OIG found that even for the residents whose antipsychotic drug use was captured in the MDS, the MDS does not capture critically important details such as the particular antipsychotic drug prescribed, specific dosage, and duration of use.

Based on its findings, OIG recommended that CMS take steps to improve the accuracy of MDS reports by developing automatic comparisons of Medicare Part D claims and MDS information to identify inconsistencies. OIG also recommended that CMS consider supplementing MDS information with Part D data to facilitate the effective monitoring of medication use in nursing homes (OIG, 2021).

Having an effective electronic health record (EHR) system (discussed in Chapter 9) that is highly integrated with medication prescribing and administration processes, for example, could enable nursing homes to run automated comparisons of MDS survey data and pharmacy data (part of Medicare Part D claims), which may improve oversight and associated prescribing practices for chronic illnesses such as dementia. In the case of nursing home residents with dementia, combining these data sources could improve accuracy of identifying cases of dementia, and reduce errors of omission and commission that might result in inappropriate prescribing and administration practices for the treatment of nursing home residents with dementia (Lin et al., 2010).

Falls Prevention

The prevention of physical injury, including resident harm from falling, is a prominent safety issue in nursing home settings, and preventing falls is a major focus for quality improvement efforts. Approximately half of all nursing home residents fall every year (AHRQ, 2019). Moreover, falls resulting in significant injury represented nearly 1 out of 10 adverse events experienced by Medicare skilled nursing facility residents (OIG, 2014a). Falls are very common occurrences in nursing homes due to the high prevalence of gait, balance, and muscle strength problems among residents (Chang et al., 2010). Systematic reviews have identified a number of factors associated with an elevated risk of falls, including previous falls, whether a resident uses a cane or other assistive walking device, wandering, Parkinson's disease, dizziness, polypharmacy, and the use of sedatives, antipsychotics, or antidepressants (Cameron et al., 2018a; Deandrea et al., 2013; Muir et al., 2012). In addition, residents with cognitive impairment or acute conditions may make errors in judgment that lead to falls (Brauner et al., 2018; Fischer et al., 2014; Meuleners et al., 2016). Thus, falls are associated with a range of issues, including medication management, mobility, and the cognitive state of the resident (Edelman et al., 2021).

The role of medication in falls has been well studied. A number of drugs, aptly referred to as fall-risk increasing drugs, are associated with a significant risk of falls. In particular, the use of psychotropic, cardiac, and analgesic drugs in the older population is associated with higher risk of falls (Leipzig et al., 1999a,b). A 2009 study analyzed nine unique drug classes: antihypertensive agents, diuretics, β blockers, sedatives and hypnotics, neuroleptics and antipsychotics, antidepressants, benzodiazepines, narcotics, and nonsteroidal anti-inflammatory drugs (Woolcott et al., 2009). The authors presented a significant association between falls and the use of sedatives and hypnotics, antidepressants, and benzodiazepines, and noted that the use of antidepressants had the strongest association with falls. Other drug classes have also been associated with an increased fall risk, such as neuroleptics and antipsychotics, and nonsteroidal anti-inflammatory drugs (Woolcott et al., 2009). The most successful fall-prevention strategies are multifactorial, containing elements that address the physical environment, medication prescribing, and physical exercise. Successful efforts also include a focus on education and training, mobility assistance, balance and strength training, reductions in the number of prescribed medications, and increases in staffing levels (Cameron et al., 2018a; Clemson et al., 2012; Leland et al., 2012; Vlaeyen al., 2015). The Agency for Healthcare Research and Quality (AHRQ) developed an interdisciplinary falls management program to reduce falls in nursing homes.[7]

Efficacy trials have demonstrated that multicomponent interventions can reduce the occurrence of falls by as much as one-third. Fall-reduction rates in clinical practice, however, are much lower (Gulka et al., 2020). It is important to recognize that falls in the nursing home setting might be associated with positive changes, such as increased mobility as a result of physical therapy and a resident's ability to get up and walk around rather than being confined to a bed or a chair. This increased resident autonomy, which can be viewed as an improvement in the resident's quality of life, can increase the residents' risk of falling at the same time. Thus, the occurrence of a fall in a nursing home setting may not necessarily be an indicator of poor care, but rather a reflection of the high-risk status of the population, coupled with the importance of promoting independence among residents with the goal of improving quality of life (Cameron et al., 2018b). Certain videogame-based exercises show promise in contributing to reducing the risk of falling in nursing home settings. Such exercises work to enhance older adults' gait, balance, and overall physical performance (Bateni, 2012; Lee et al., 2019; Tay et al., 2018).

Preventing Elder Abuse in the Nursing Home Setting

Despite these protections enshrined in federal legislation, elder abuse in nursing homes continues to represent a serious threat to residents' safety and quality of life. Though a standard or universal definition of elder abuse does not exist (Braaten and Malmedal, 2017), CMS defines abuse as

> the willful infliction of injury, unreasonable confinement, intimidation, or punishment with resulting physical harm, pain or mental anguish. Abuse also includes the deprivation by an individual, including a caretaker, of goods or services that are necessary to attain or maintain physical, mental and psychosocial well-being.[8,9]

---

[7] For access to the AHRQ Fall Program, see https://www.ahrq.gov/patient-safety/settings/long-term-care/resource/injuries/fallspx/man1.html (accessed February 7, 2022).

[8] CMS Survey and Certification of Long-Term Care Facilities—Definitions, 42 CFR § 488.301 (2017).

[9] Other definitions are found in the literature. For example, according to the Centers for Disease Control and Prevention, "Elder abuse is an intentional act or failure to act that causes or creates a risk of harm to an older adult. An older adult is someone age 60 or older. The abuse often occurs at the hands of a caregiver or a person the elder trusts" (CDC, 2021).

Elder abuse can take many forms, including physical, psychological, financial, sexual, and spiritual abuse[10] as well as neglect. In the nursing home setting, abuse of residents can be perpetrated by staff, family members, or other residents (Myhre et al., 2020; NCEA, 2021a).

The Nursing Home Reform Act of 1987, passed as part of the Omnibus Budget Reconciliation Act of 1987 (OBRA 87), established quality-of-life rights for nursing home residents, including freedom from abuse, mistreatment, and neglect and the ability to voice grievances without fear of discrimination or reprisal (Wiener et al., 2007). Physical restraints, the use of which had previously been common in nursing homes, were allowed only under very narrow circumstances, and strict requirements were established limiting the amount of time that residents could be restrained.[11] OBRA 87 also expanded the rights of nursing home residents to communicate with regulators and specified that residents have access to a state long-term care ombudsman.[12]

As emphasized throughout this report, many nursing home residents have physical or mental impairments, and their dependency on others for care amplifies their vulnerability to abuse (Braaten and Malmedal, 2017; Lindbloom et al., 2007). Older adults with Alzheimer's disease and related dementias (ADRD) represent a growing share of the nursing home population and, given their cognitive impairments, are at even greater risk for abuse. Moreover, ADRD can also lead to behavior that may be aggressive and challenging for nursing home staff to manage, which may in turn lead to incidents of abuse of residents by staff (Berridge et al., 2019; Braaten and Malmedal, 2017; IOM and NRC, 2014; Myhre et al., 2020).

Although staff use of physical restraints on residents has significantly declined since OBRA 87, nursing home staff use psychotropic medications to control the symptoms of certain diseases. According to Human Rights Watch, U.S. nursing facilities administer antipsychotic medications to thousands of residents, most of whom have Alzheimer's disease or some other form of dementia with associated symptoms such as agitation, restlessness, and aggression. Not only do these residents not have a diagnosis for which these drugs are approved for use, but antipsychotic drugs are very

---

[10] An element of elder abuse, spiritual abuse refers to efforts to intimidate, pressure, or control a person using religion, faith, or beliefs. Examples include using scripture or beliefs to humiliate a person, and force a person into doing things (e.g., giving money) against their will, or not allowing residents to attend religious ceremonies.

[11] The series of reforms included the requirement that nursing home residents have "the right to be free" from physical and chemical restraints not required to treat their medical symptoms. Viewed as harmful to residents' health and quality of life, the restraints used included physical restraints such as hand mitts, vests that tie residents to chairs or beds, and restrictive chairs that limit mobility as well as chemical restraints such as psychoactive drugs used to affect a resident's mood and behavior (OIG, 2019).

[12] Specifically, OBRA 87 mandated that nursing facility residents have "direct and immediate access to ombudspersons when protection and advocacy services become necessary."

dangerous for older people with dementia, significantly increasing their risk of heart problems, infections, and falls. These drugs are often given to residents without their consent (HRW, 2018). Moreover, research indicates that nursing homes are diagnosing residents as having schizophrenia to justify the use of antipsychotic drugs to render residents more compliant. An investigation of Medicare data by the *New York Times* found that the percentage of nursing home residents diagnosed with schizophrenia has risen 70 percent since 2012. Currently, one in nine nursing home residents have a diagnosis of schizophrenia (Thomas et al., 2021). Thus, there is increasing concern that while physical restraints may no longer be in use in nursing home settings, they have been replaced by chemical restraints and that the use of such medications without the resident's consent constitutes a form of abuse (HRW, 2018).

Other medical conditions common among nursing home residents can cause agitation, confusion, and aggression and thus increase the risk of abuse of residents by staff (Braaten and Malmedal, 2017). Finally, not only is the population aging, but it is becoming increasingly diverse. Little is known, however, about racial or ethnic differences in elder abuse. Available evidence points to a significantly higher prevalence of financial and psychological abuse in African American adults than in White adults (Dong et al., 2014).

Scope of Abuse in Nursing Homes

Abuse in the nursing home setting could take a variety of forms, including physical neglect and depriving residents of their dignity (e.g., not changing their dirty clothes); limiting their choice over daily activities; intentionally providing inadequate care (e.g., neglecting to change their position to avoid pressure sores); and physical, psychological/emotional, sexual, and financial abuse. Research on the prevalence of abuse of residents in nursing home settings is limited, and studies often yield very different prevalence estimates.

Yon et al. conducted a systematic review and meta-analysis of self-reports of abuse by nursing home residents. According to the study's estimates, psychological abuse was the most common, with one-third of respondents reporting incidents of psychological abuse. The next most common forms of abuse were physical abuse (14 percent), financial abuse (14 percent),[13] and neglect (nearly 12 percent) (Yon et al., 2019). The lived experience of one nursing home resident is found in Box 6-2 below.

---

[13] Examples of financial abuse in the nursing home setting include forging a resident's signature, cashing residents' checks without permission, theft or misuse of a resident's funds or possessions, and forcing a resident to sign financial documents (Nursing Home Abuse Guide, 2021).

> **BOX 6-2**
> **Resident Perspective**
>
> "There was one case where a CNA repeatedly and viciously verbally abused me. My administrator did not respond to my requests for assistance in this matter, so I filed a complaint with the MA Disabled Persons Protection Commission and I called the police.
> Now this CNA is not allowed on my unit at all."
>
> — **78-year-old nursing home resident, MA**
>
> *This quote was collected from the committee's online call for resident, family, and nursing home staff perspectives.*

Staff are not the only perpetrators of abuse in nursing homes. One study of more than 2,000 residents in 10 nursing homes revealed that 20 percent of residents experienced at least one incidence of resident-to-resident abuse over the course of one month (Lachs et al., 2016; see also Lachs et al., 2021). Moreover, while the subject has received less attention, research reveals the pervasive nature of resident-to-staff aggression in nursing homes, particularly aggression against certified nursing assistants, who provide most of the direct care to and interact most closely with residents (Brophy et al., 2019; Lachs et al., 2013). A study of nursing home staff found that 15.6 percent of residents had exhibited aggressive behaviors toward staff during a 2-week period. Though verbal abuse (e.g., being screamed at) was the most prevalent, physical abuse of staff was common (Lachs et al., 2013). Resident-to-staff aggression may be due to a number of factors, ranging from resident frustration and aggravation to resident response to aggressive behavior or maltreatment by staff (Lachs et al., 2013). Resident abuse of staff may in turn lead staff to abuse and neglect residents as a reaction to, or out of frustration with, residents' aggressive behavior, thus fueling a dangerous cycle of abuse. Staff who experience abuse may also feel higher levels of burnout, helplessness, self-doubt, and loneliness (Isaksson et al., 2009; Kristiansen et al., 2006) or react by avoiding contact with aggressive residents, which may result in a negative impact on the quality of care they receive (Lachs et al., 2013). One study found significant relationships among abuse and factors such as number of staff, workplace strain, and stress (Gates et al., 2003).

Research indicates that the prevalence of abuse (regardless of perpetrator) in nursing homes is significantly underestimated (Pillemer et al., 2016) and that many incidents of abuse are not reported (Storey, 2020).

Nursing home residents may fear retaliation if they report abuse, may be embarrassed or ashamed to report the incident, or may be unable to report abuse due to physical or cognitive impairments (Baker et al., 2016; Lindbloom et al., 2007). Moreover, conditions typically associated with abuse, such as being withdrawn and uncommunicative, may be easy to conflate with the common symptoms of dementia (Dong et al., 2014). Similarly, staff may not report abuse by residents out of concern about losing their job (Lachs et al., 2013).

Elder abuse is often unnoticed, ignored, and disregarded by nursing home staff. For example, one study of sexual abuse against older nursing home residents involved focus groups with nursing home staff. Interviews revealed that the staff found it difficult to imagine that acts of sexual abuse against nursing home residents could actually take place, which in turn made it very difficult for them to believe that any such abuse had actually happened. Such perceptions by staff make it more challenging to not only discover abuse, but adds to the residents' feeling of vulnerability and heightens their hesitancy to report abuse, based on the fear they will not be believed (Iversen et al., 2015). A 2015 literature review on the state of knowledge of sexual abuse against nursing home residents revealed that both older women and men were victims of sexual abuse, which was perpetrated primarily by nursing home staff and other residents. The study emphasized the need for further research and called for effective reporting systems as one important component of a broader approach to addressing sexual abuse against older persons (Malmedal et al., 2015).

Sexual abuse allegations are not tracked on a national or state level as they are often not categorized apart from other forms of abuse. An analysis of inspection reports by CNN revealed that more than 1,000 nursing homes had been cited for mishandling or failing to prevent sexual assault and sexual abuse cases between 2013 and 2016; many facilities received multiple citations over the time period (Ellis and Hicken, 2017). Ongoing media reports and congressional testimony underscore the urgency of addressing sexual abuse in nursing homes (Fedschun, 2019; U.S. Congress, 2019).

Oversight of Elder Abuse in Nursing Homes

Federal, state, and local agencies as well as individual nursing homes all have a role to play in oversight and investigation of elder abuse in nursing homes. CMS regulations stipulate the specific processes for the reporting and investigation of incidents of abuse. Nursing homes are required to ensure that abuse is reported to state survey agencies; these agencies are in turn required to report incidents to CMS (see Table 6-1). Certain individuals (including nursing home owners, operators, and employees) are required by law to immediately report any incident to the state survey agency as well

TABLE 6-1 Reporting and Investigating Elder Abuse in Nursing Homes

Nursing Homes	State Survey Agency
Reporting Abuse	
Nursing homes must ensure that allegations of elder abuse are reported to the state survey agency immediately. If the allegation involves serious bodily injury, nursing homes must report it no later than **2 hours** after the allegation is made. If the incident does not involve serious bodily injuries, it must be reported within **24 hours**. Federal law requires certain covered individuals at the nursing homes to report incidents immediately to law enforcement in addition to the state survey agency if there is a reasonable suspicion that a crime has occurred. Such covered individuals include nursing home owners, operators, and employees.	State survey agencies must report to the Centers for Medicare & Medicaid Services (CMS) all complaints and certain facility-reported incidents of abuse through a computer-based complaint and incident tracking system. State survey agencies must immediately alert CMS regional offices when an especially significant or sensitive incident occurs that attracts public or broad media attention. State survey agencies are required to enter into CMS's tracking system all complaint information gathered as part of the agency's federal survey and certification responsibilities, as well as all facility-reported incidents that require a federal onsite survey. There is no federal requirement for state survey agencies to notify law enforcement until the state survey agency has substantiated a suspected crime. The U.S. Government Accountability Office (GAO) found that this led to delays in referring suspected crime to law enforcement. In an effort to avoid such delays, GAO recommended that CMS require state survey agencies to refer any suspected crime to law enforcement immediately.
Investigating Abuse	
CMS requires nursing homes to have written policies and procedures for conducting internal investigations of suspected elder abuse. CMS requires nursing homes to submit findings from these investigations to the state survey agency within 5 business days of the incident. Federal law requires nursing homes to establish policies for ensuring that law enforcement is notified of elder abuse that occurs in their facilities.	CMS requires state survey agencies to assess reports of elder abuse in nursing homes and assign a priority investigation status based on the seriousness of the allegations: *Immediate jeopardy* requires the agency to start onsite investigation within 2 business days of receipt. *Non-immediate jeopardy high priority* requires onsite investigation within 10 days of prioritization. *Non-immediate jeopardy medium* requires onsite survey to be scheduled (no time frame specified). *Non-immediate jeopardy low* requires investigation during the next survey. CMS policy requires state survey agencies to notify law enforcement of substantiated findings of elder abuse that occur in nursing homes.

SOURCE: GAO, 2019a.

as to law enforcement if there is a reasonable suspicion that a crime has been committed (GAO, 2019a).[14]

Additionally, other state and local agencies may be involved in investigating abuse in nursing homes. Each state has an adult protective services (APS) program. APS jurisdiction and standards of practice vary from state to state. State and local APS work closely with local law enforcement if criminal abuse is suspected (Ramsey-Klawsnik, 2018). CMS regulations give the nursing home survey agency primary jurisdiction for allegations of abuse of residents by staff, resident-to-resident abuse, and abuse of staff by residents in nursing homes.[15] In contrast, APS has jurisdiction in cases where someone from outside the facility committed abuse against a resident, such as a family member who might commit abuse during a visit (Ramsey-Klawsnik, 2018).

As an indication of increased concern about elder abuse in nursing homes, the U.S. Government Accountability Office (GAO) and OIG at the U.S. Department of Health and Human Services have released a number of investigative reports over the past several years (GAO, 2019a,b,c; OIG, 2019). GAO's investigations revealed that the number of abuse deficiencies in nursing homes cited by state survey agencies more than doubled (from 430 to 875) between 2013 and 2017, with the most common form of abuse being physical and mental or verbal abuse. The increasing number and severity of abuse amplifies concerns about the safety of nursing home residents (GAO, 2019a).

GAO recommended that CMS develop guidance on abuse information that nursing homes should self-report and require state survey agencies to submit data on abuse and perpetrator type (GAO, 2019c). GAO also recommended that actions be taken to refer incidents of abuse to law enforcement in a timely manner; to track abuse referrals; to clarify that evidence exists to support the allegation of abuse; and to share information with law enforcement.

The OIG analyzed high-risk hospital emergency room Medicare claims for treatment and found that one in five claims was due to potential abuse or neglect of nursing home residents (OIG, 2019). OIG's analysis revealed significant failures within each step of the process, showing that nursing homes had failed to report many instances of abuse or neglect to the state survey agencies and that several survey agencies had failed to report abuse to local law enforcement.

---

[14] Mandated reporting laws for elder abuse require individuals such as nursing home staff, doctors, and nurses—referred to as "mandated reporters"—to contact authorities about any concerns related to elder abuse. Laws in eight states require any person who suspects elder abuse to report it to authorities (Nursing Home Abuse Justice, 2021).

[15] CMS Requirements for Long-Term Care Facilities—Resident Rights, 42 CFR § 483.10 (2016).

To address the breakdown of reporting at every level, OIG recommended that CMS work with survey agencies to improve training on how to identify and report incidents of potential abuse and neglect of nursing home residents and to work to enhance existing guidance with examples of incidents of potential abuse and neglect (OIG, 2019). OIG also recommended that CMS require state survey agencies to record and track all incidents of potential abuse and neglect in nursing homes and referrals made to local law enforcement and other agencies. Finally, OIG recommended that CMS monitor the survey agencies' reporting of findings of substantiated abuse to local law enforcement.

CMS' quality reporting system, Care Compare (see Chapter 3), includes an alert icon to help potential residents and their families gain a better understanding of the quality of care provided by specific nursing homes, including citations for resident abuse.[16]

Preventing Elder Abuse

Elder abuse in general, and particularly in the nursing home setting, is not well understood or recognized. Research on elder abuse in nursing homes is still in its early stages, particularly compared with other forms of interpersonal violence (Lindbloom et al., 2007; Myhre et al., 2020; Yon et al., 2019). The nature, origins, and causes of abuse in nursing homes are associated with a complex web of personal, social, and organizational factors (Myhre et al., 2020). Research focused on recognizing and detecting abuse as well as research on strategies to address and prevent abuse of nursing home residents are both limited (Braaten and Malmedal, 2017; Myhre et al., 2020). In particular, research is needed in order to be able to better design intervention strategies and approaches and to clearly establish the linkages between intervention activities and changes in the prevalence of elder abuse (Baker et al., 2016; Kennedy and Will, 2021; Shen et al., 2021).

Nursing homes can be challenging places to work, with staff citing workforce shortages and time pressures as the key sources of stress (Brophy et al., 2019). Research reveals that staff who self-report that they have abused a nursing home resident characterize themselves as "emotionally exhausted" (Yon et al., 2019). Thus, it is important to focus on staffing and staff competence as part of elder abuse prevention strategies. This includes training on identifying abuse and risk factors, effective communication

---

[16] Consumer organizations have been quick to warn consumers that "the absence of an abuse icon on Nursing Home Compare does not necessarily indicate the absence of abuse," noting, "Federal reports over the last few decades have documented that state survey agencies (health inspectors) have missed problems and failed to cite violations. Moreover, violations indicating the existence of abuse or potential abuse may be cited under other federal tags, resulting in their exclusion from this initiative" (CMA, 2019).

and teamwork, creating a work environment that encourages and supports openness and discussion of challenges, and implementation of a person-centered care approach (Braaten and Malmedal, 2017).

Improvement strategies derived from the culture change model for nursing homes (see Chapter 4 and later in this chapter) have been proposed as effective approaches to reduce elder abuse in nursing homes. Characterized by the core elements of staff empowerment, consistent staff assignment, resident-directed care and activities, decentralized decision making, and the creation of home-like living environments, culture change is viewed as an effective approach for promoting the safety of residents (Berridge et al., 2019). The delivery of person-centered care, a hallmark of the model, can ensure that the resident feels seen and recognized by staff as a person (rather than staff focusing on their medical condition or disease state), which can help support stronger bonds between staff and residents (Braaten and Malmedal, 2017).

Successful approaches to intervening in resident abuse incidents, particularly resident-to-resident aggression, include the development of interprofessional protocols with clinical staff in the nursing home for dealing with such situations (Bonifas, 2015). Research has shown that nurse–social work collaborative teams are an effective staffing approach with which to address elder abuse (Bonifas, 2015). Preventive measures to reduce resident-to-resident aggression include preadmission screening for aggressive behaviors, the development of a person-centered approach to providing care based on the screening assessment, and an intentional (in other words, nonrandom) approach to roommate selection (Bonifas, 2015). Other potential approaches to reducing elder abuse include consistent assignment (discussed in Chapter 5), which involves a resident receiving care from the same nursing assistants, who would know the resident well and be more aware of any changes in condition that might be related to potential instances of abuse.

Interventions designed to address residents' aggressive behavior toward staff include training programs such as Bathing Without a Battle, which has been found to be an effective means of improving the bathing experience of residents with dementia in nursing homes (Gozalo et al., 2014). Other interventions include creating awareness on the part of staff as to which residents should not interact during mealtimes or activities; distraction of residents who show escalating aggression; and mediating disagreements among residents to ensure they do not lead to aggressive behavior. Further study is needed to prevent resident abuse of staff and the negative impact on residents and on staff safety, job satisfaction, morale, and turnover (Lachs et al., 2013).

One potential intervention to detect and prevent elder abuse that has become increasingly common is the deployment of surveillance cameras in nursing homes. Seven states have enacted legislation to permit private individuals to use cameras in residents' room in nursing homes, and other states have proposed similar legislation (Levy et al., 2019). The use of cameras carries with it serious ethical concerns and risks to residents as well as nursing home staff members. For residents, concerns include the impact on residents' privacy and dignity, whereas for staff the concerns focus on whether cameras may undermine workers' sense of being responsible for the residents (Levy et al., 2019).

Despite enactment of legislation allowing the use of cameras and the associated ethical and legal concerns (e.g., privacy, dignity), research is limited as to the prevalence, efficacy, or effects of the use of cameras in nursing homes (Berridge et al., 2019). Nursing homes are both places of work and places where people live, and as such they "are a complex space for regulating privacy because they are simultaneously public and private spaces" (Berridge et al., 2019).

Elder abuse prevention strategies need to include efforts on a broad societal level using public awareness campaigns to elevate the importance of understanding and recognizing the dangers of elder abuse. World Elder Abuse Awareness Day, for example, is recognized internationally and serves as a global platform to call attention to the problem (NCEA, 2021b). Another public awareness effort is the National Council on Elder Abuse's Reframing Elder Abuse Project.[17]

It is clear that a constellation of measures will be needed to combat elder abuse. These range from high-quality research to identify the most effective prevention strategies to staff training and education about effective clinical interventions, the implementation of the culture change model for nursing homes, and creating public awareness of the problem of elder abuse more broadly.

Care Transitions

Many nursing home residents have multiple, complex medical conditions and require transitions between the nursing home and the hospital. Poor communication between nursing homes and hospitals is one of the key barriers to safe and effective care transitions (Gillespie et al., 2010). Nine out of 10 nursing home residents arrive in the emergency department (ED) missing critical patient information—such as medication lists and reason for transfer to the ED—necessary to provide safe and efficient care (Terrell and Miller, 2006). Poor-quality communication has also been shown to impact resident care when residents are discharged from the hospital with poor-quality information about ED diagnosis, tests and treatments provided, and

---

[17] For more information, see https://ncea.acl.gov/resources/reframing.aspx (accessed November 3, 2021).

treatment recommendations (Terrell and Miller, 2006). Missing, inaccurate, or conflicting information is a key barrier to effective transitions between nursing homes and hospitals, which contribute to the risk of rehospitalization and inappropriate care for residents (King et al., 2013).

Research highlights the importance of high-quality communication among health care professionals including effective use of EHRs as well as in-person communication to facilitate care transitions (Scott et al., 2017). The use of EHRs in nursing homes is discussed further in Chapter 9 of this report.

Infection Control

A major patient safety concern in nursing homes is infections, with nearly 2 million infections occurring in nursing homes each year (Mody et al., 2015; Montoya et al., 2016; Strausbaugh and Joseph, 2000). Urinary tract infection (UTI) is one of the most common infections among nursing home residents, with many UTIs associated with the use of catheters (Dwyer et al., 2013; Mody et al., 2017). Diagnoses of UTI among nursing home residents present specific challenges as older adults with a UTI may show signs of confusion or agitation rather than pain (Wegerer, 2017). This is particularly problematic for nursing home residents with dementia as signs of confusion and agitation may be interpreted to be related to their dementia or advanced age rather than an indication of a UTI (D'Agata et al., 2013; Hodgson et al., 2011). Moreover, many illnesses present with similar symptoms to UTI and residents with dementia may not be able to verbalize their symptoms. These challenges often lead to diagnostic errors as well as misuse of antimicrobials (D'Agata et al., 2013; Mitchell, 2021).

CMS expanded infection control conditions for nursing homes in its updated 2016 requirements.[18] Existing and updated federal requirements were designed to address a broad range of issues in nursing homes, including strict infection control needs during food preparation, housekeeping, and daily care; influenza prophylaxis, surveillance, and response; norovirus prevention and response; *Clostridioides difficile* detection and response; surveillance for rare but potentially deadly outbreaks such as legionella pneumonia and *Candida auris*; potentially inappropriate overuse of antibiotics for such diagnoses as viral bronchitis and asymptomatic bacteriuria; and the growing prevalence of colonization with and infection by multidrug-resistant organisms (Jump et al., 2018; Montoya and Mody, 2011; Strausbaugh et al., 2003).

---

[18] CMS Requirements for Long Term Care Facilities—Infection Control, 42 CFR § 483.80 (2016).

Lack of Expertise in Infection Control Practices

Infection control has been a long-standing requirement of nursing homes and an area in which many shortcomings were noted by state survey agencies well in advance of the COVID-19 pandemic. Among the new 2016 federal requirements, which were to be implemented over a 2-year period (2017–2019), nursing homes were directed to initiate antibiotic stewardship programs; develop policies and procedures related to identification, reporting, investigation, and control of communicable diseases and infections among residents, staff, and visitors; and employ a staff member who is an infection preventionist. CMS and the Centers for Disease Control and Prevention (CDC) developed a free online training program for infection preventionists in March 2019 to assist nursing homes to prepare for this new staff position (CMS, 2019a). (See Chapter 5 for discussion of the infection preventionist role in nursing homes.)

Given the relatively recent implementation of the new requirements, most nursing homes were unprepared to deal with the wave of infections from the novel coronavirus. Studies found that nearly 75 percent of facilities did not have adequate staffing or infection control measures in place prior to the pandemic (Chapman and Harrington, 2020; Geng et al., 2019). Indeed, GAO found that 82 percent of nursing homes had deficiencies in infection prevention and control between 2013 and 2017; infection prevention and control was the most common reason for deficiencies cited by nursing home surveyors prior to the pandemic. Moreover, approximately two-thirds of nursing homes with infection prevention and control deficiencies had been cited multiple times (GAO, 2020). A 2020 Kaiser Health News analysis found that even among five-star facilities (see Chapter 3 for more on the CMS star rating system), 4 in 10 have been cited for infection control deficiencies (Rau, 2020).

The COVID-19 pandemic was unprecedented in scope and overwhelmed all sectors of the health care system. Nursing homes have increasingly been identified as high-risk settings for the transmission of infectious diseases, and this was confirmed by the devastating impact of the pandemic. The extremely high mortality levels among nursing home residents and staff during the early phases of the public health emergency underscored the extent to which the lack of robust infection prevention and control programs rendered nursing homes extremely vulnerable in the face of a highly transmissible novel pathogen (Andersen et al., 2021). High rates of transmission of the virus were facilitated by the composition of the resident population, which included large numbers of chronically ill, often immunocompromised individuals as well as the physical design of nursing homes: congregate living in multiple-occupancy rooms and with multiple-user bathrooms. Moreover, residents are brought together regularly for congregate indoor meals and activities, and multiple staff have very close contact with residents multiple times a day (Ouslander and Grabowski, 2020).

The pandemic revealed that there was a significant lack of the expertise and experience in infection control practices necessary to limit the introduction and spread of the coronavirus within nursing homes. While nursing homes are required to assign an individual staff member to infection control, this was not typically a full-time position; persons with infection control responsibilities had many other responsibilities as well (Andersen et al., 2021).[19] Efforts to isolate or group those infected or quarantine those exposed were often delayed or inadequate and sometimes nonexistent, resulting in rapid spread of the virus throughout facilities (Blain et al., 2020; Giri et al., 2021).

During the early phases of the pandemic, nursing homes' attempts to contain the spread of the SARS-CoV-2 virus occurred against the backdrop of a lack of prioritization of nursing homes in federal and state responses to the pandemic (Laxton et al., 2020). While CMS, CDC, state departments of health and human services, and provider organizations issued infection-control guidance, the volume and frequently changing nature of the guidance posed significant challenges to nursing home administrators and directors of nursing who struggled to interpret, keep up with, and adapt to the latest guidance. Quality Improvement Organizations have historically lacked both the resources and the expertise to provide assistance to nursing homes to address quality problems, which was made clear during the pandemic (GAO, 2007; Harrington et al., 2017; IOM, 1986; Laxton et al., 2020; Musumeci and Chidambaram, 2020; Spanko, 2020). Assistance often came instead from either local hospital-affiliated health systems or from county or state health departments (Laxton et al., 2020).

The federal government, states, and localities deployed strike teams[20] and, in some cases, the National Guard to provide assistance to nursing homes to handle infection prevention and control (Andersen et al., 2021; CMS, 2021). In addition, the Institute for Healthcare Improvement,[21] PHI,[22] and the Agency for Healthcare Research and Quality's Nursing Home COVID-19 Action Network[23] provided useful resources to bolster nursing homes' responses to the pandemic. CDC published guidance on

---

[19] CMS Requirements for Long Term Care Facilities—Infection Control, 42 CFR § 483.80 (2016).

[20] Federal strike teams deployed nationally to assist nursing homes with significant COVID-19 outbreaks consisted of infection prevention specialists, epidemiologists, Public Health Service officers from CDC, CMS, and the Office of the Assistant Secretary of Health, while local and state public health officials joined when available. In addition, a number of states created state strike teams to provide support to nursing homes (Andersen et al., 2021).

[21] For more information, see http://www.ihi.org/Topics/COVID-19/Pages/default.aspx (accessed November 3, 2021).

[22] For more information, see https://phinational.org/ (accessed November 3, 2021).

[23] For more information, see https://www.ahrq.gov/nursing-home/index.html (accessed November 3, 2021).

antibiotic stewardship (CDC, 2020) and developed a 20-hour training course for infection preventionists (CDC TRAIN, 2020).

Inadequate Supply of PPE

Adequate access to personal protective equipment (PPE)—including masks, gowns, goggles, gloves, and hand sanitizer—did not exist early in the pandemic (McGarry et al., 2020). In addition, nursing home staff were not adequately trained in the appropriate use of PPE. Staff had not been fit-tested for use of N95 respirators or trained in their appropriate use, nor were they trained in the correct donning and doffing of PPE, including gowns, gloves, and respirators or masks, or in which PPE to use in which situations (Denny-Brown et al., 2020; GAO, 2020). One report indicated that as late as August 2020, shortages of PPE, including N95 respirators and medical gowns, had actually intensified rather than diminished. Nearly half of all nursing homes reported that they had less than a week's supply of at least one type of PPE at some point between May and August 2020. A week's supply of PPE is considered the minimum acceptable amount and less than that is considered a "critical shortage"; however, during a major infectious disease outbreak, a nursing home can use up that limited supply in a day or two and should ideally have access to much more (Murray and Friedman, 2020). Another study also found more than one in five nursing homes reported severe PPE shortages of less than a 1-week supply in July 2020 (McGarry et al., 2020). The severe shortages represented "an extremely limited capacity to respond to a COVID-19 outbreak" (McGarry et al., 2020, p. 1813). The CMS Coronavirus Commission on Safety and Quality in Nursing Homes recommended that nursing homes procure and sustain a 3-month supply of PPE, working with federal and state agencies to ensure adequate supply of PPE for nursing homes (MITRE, 2020). One nursing home resident's perspective on the impact of PPE shortages is provided in Box 6-3.

BOX 6-3
Resident Perspective

"During the early phase of the coronavirus pandemic our 11–7 shift staff were unable to get needed PPE to protect themselves because of our administrator's rigid policy that staff had to go to her office to sign for it. Myself and other residents were being neglected, as CNAs were afraid to provide care without PPE."

— **78-year-old nursing home resident, MA**

This quote was collected from the committee's online call for resident, family, and nursing home staff perspectives.

Access to Testing and Timeliness of Results

Early in the pandemic, when availability of testing was very limited, nursing homes depended on symptom screening of staff and residents to protect residents from infection. Unfortunately, symptom screening alone did not identify many of those who were infected and able to transmit the virus. The testing of staff was as important as testing of residents. Staff often were exposed to people infected with the virus in the community, because of their need to use public or shared transportation, because their low wages often led them to work more than one job, and because they and others near them were unable to self-isolate and work from home by the very nature of their jobs (Denny-Brown et al., 2020; Shen, 2020; True et al., 2020).

Another factor that contributed to the rapid transmission of the virus in nursing home settings was the delay in recognizing the importance of asymptomatic infection in disease transmission, with early reports claiming that there was little or no asymptomatic transmission of the virus (CNBC, 2020). It has now been well documented that asymptomatic or presymptomatic infection was often the way the virus was introduced into, and spread within, nursing homes. Overall, inadequate access to testing for COVID-19 to identify those infected, either residents or staff, whether symptomatic or asymptomatic, limited nursing homes' ability to effectively contain the spread of the virus (Ouslander and Grabowski, 2020). The amount of time between COVID-19 testing and results proved to be a significant issue during the pandemic. According to one study, 6 months after the first COVID cases in U.S. nursing homes, less than 15 percent of staff and 10 percent of residents experienced a test turnaround time of less than 1 day (McGarry et al., 2021). Timeliness of receipt of test results is critical to containing the viral spread in both nursing homes and the community (McGarry et al., 2021).

Lockdown of Facilities as Infection Control Response

In an effort to protect residents and staff, in March 2020, CMS directed nursing homes to severely limit or not allow any visitation from family members and loved ones, with a significant impact on residents in the form of social isolation and loneliness (discussed in Chapters 2 and 8). The importance of telehealth and other technologies to help combat social isolation among nursing home residents is discussed in Chapter 9. Moreover, many families of nursing home residents found communication of information concerning COVID-19 infections in the facilities to be inadequate (Hado and Friss Feinberg, 2020; HRW, 2021; National Consumer Voice, 2021). Some states have considered ways to ensure that such isolation does not occur in future public health emergencies (Jaffe, 2021).

One strategy to strengthen infection control in nursing homes in the future would be to address the training requirements and accountability of nursing home infection preventionists as specified in the 2016 updated requirements (Stone et al., 2018). Other potential strategies include encouraging nursing homes to form alliances with hospital-based infectious disease specialists; strengthening infection and antibiotic reporting requirements, including having regular feedback comparing performances of nursing homes with their peers and requiring influenza and coronavirus immunizations for staff (Pugh, 2020); and requiring an increased role for local and state health departments in assisting with nursing home infection control (CMS and CDC, 2020; Laxton et al., 2020).

NURSING HOME EMERGENCY PLANNING, PREPAREDNESS, AND RESPONSE

Another vital safety-related challenge for nursing homes that was revealed in the starkest of terms during the pandemic is planning, preparing, and implementing an effective response to a wide array of public health emergencies to protect residents from harm while also ensuring that residents are cared for during and after an emergency (Powell et al., 2012). The 2016 CMS Medicare and Medicaid requirements for participation (discussed in more detail in Chapter 8) require long-term care facilities to maintain a comprehensive emergency preparedness program, based on a thorough risk assessment, with written policies and procedures in place specific to their population.[24] Additionally, regulations expanded emergency plan requirements to consider items such as sewage disposal, supplies, emergency lighting, and evacuation procedures with a resident/staff tracking system, and more.[25] Beyond having such written plans in place, nursing home staff need to review and audit the plans on a regular basis to ensure that the plans are robust, that nursing home staff can locate supplies, and that there is accurate documentation of participation in emergency management planning discussions and exercises.

Frequent life-threatening events ranging from the COVID-19 pandemic to weather-related disasters such as hurricanes, tornadoes, floods, and wildfires clearly underscore the urgent need for nursing homes to plan and prepare for a broad range of public health emergencies. Weather-related emergencies, with their associated damage resulting from strong winds and flooding, have had a devastating impact on the staff and residents of nursing homes and resulted in higher rates of morbidity, mortality, and

---

[24] CMS Requirements for Long Term Care Facilities—Emergency Preparedness, 42 CFR § 483.73 (2016).
[25] Ibid.

hospitalization than among other members of the community (Lane and McGrady, 2018). Thus it is essential for nursing homes to prepare for serious weather events most likely to occur in the part of the United States in which they are located (i.e., hurricanes on the East Coast, tornadoes in the Midwest and South, severe snowstorms in the West and Midwest, floods in sites near rivers and lakes, and drought-fueled wildfires on the West Coast).

Although evacuation is a significant risk for nursing home residents, who tend to be frail, have multiple medical conditions, and become disoriented in new surroundings, evacuation may still be necessary when disasters pose an immediate risk to a facility and its residents (Brown et al., 2012; Cacchione et al., 2011). Experience during disasters such as hurricanes Katrina, Sandy, and Ida, for example, revealed that nursing home facilities often lacked clear guidance for evacuation procedures, despite calls by experts to develop flexible planning and protocols (IOM, 2012; Powell et al., 2012). Nursing homes house distinct vulnerable populations, such as those with cognitive impairments, vision and hearing impairments, and disabilities, which require specific evacuation planning considerations (Hyer et al., 2010; IOM, 2012).

Research emphasizes the importance of nursing home staff training in psychological first aid (PFA) and general emergency preparedness. Local emergency management's review of nursing home facilities' emergency plans has also been found to be critical. One study indicated that nursing homes may consider including some residents in emergency preparedness staff training efforts (Pierce et al., 2017).

Studies have noted that during disasters and emergencies the emphasis is on physical safety and provision of medical care, and not on nursing home residents' mental health needs. PFA was developed in response to residents' needs immediately following a disaster to reduce distress and promote residents' ability to function. PFA does not require a highly trained licensed mental health provider, and nursing home staff could be trained to provide such care (Brown et al., 2009). The availability of PFA operating manuals for nursing home staff has contributed to the broad application of PFA as an effective tool for disaster intervention (Wang et al., 2021).

Including Nursing Homes in Federal Emergency Preparedness and Response

The Federal Emergency Management Agency (FEMA), an agency of the U.S. Department of Homeland Security, is responsible for the coordination of federal government resources to ensure that communities are prepared for, and capable of effectively responding to, disasters (FEMA, 2021). To facilitate coordination of resources, FEMA created the National Response Framework, which provides an overarching organizational structure for

15 emergency support functions (ESFs) ranging from transportation and communication, firefighting, and search and rescue to public safety and security. The ESFs specify the most critical resources and capabilities needed to respond to a national emergency (FEMA, 2020).

ESF 8 includes specific considerations related to public health and medical services in the context of federal emergency support, and it provides a mechanism for the coordination of federal assistance to support state, tribal, and local officials in response to a disaster, emergency, or incident that may lead to a public health, medical, behavioral, or human service emergency (FEMA, 2016a). ESF 8 outlines the federal government's role in coordinating public health infrastructure and health care delivery to minimize or prevent health emergencies. The Department of Health and Human Services (HHS) coordinates ESF 8 through the Assistant Secretary for Preparedness and Response (ASPR). Core functions that ESF 8 supports include[26]

- Public information and warning (e.g., coordinating public health messaging);
- Critical transportation (e.g., resources to assist the movement of at-risk/medically fragile populations to shelter areas);
- Mass care services (e.g., technical expertise and guidance on the public health issues of the medical needs population, advocacy services, etc.); and
- Public health, health care, and emergency medical services (e.g., health surveillance, triage in the event of a health care surge, assessment of the public health needs of a health care system or facility, technical assistance, etc.) (FEMA, 2016a).

In addition, ESF 15—external affairs—requires government, community organizations, and private-sector authorities to provide accurate, coordinated, timely, and accessible information necessary to develop, coordinate, and deliver messages in the event of an emergency to affected audiences, including the media and local populations. The Department of Homeland Security works closely with HHS as the respective leads for ESF 8 and ESF 15 during a public health emergency (FEMA, 2016b).[27]

The key focus of ESF 8 is on supporting the response to public health and medical disasters. For example, resources for patient care during public health and medical emergencies are directed to "support prehospital triage and treatment, inpatient hospital care, outpatient services,

---

[26] For a complete list of the core capabilities of ESF 8, see FEMA (2016a).
[27] For a complete list of core capabilities of ESF 15, see FEMA (2016b).

behavioral healthcare, medical-needs sheltering, pharmacy services, and dental care to victims with acute injury/illnesses or those who suffer from chronic illnesses/conditions" (FEMA, 2016a). ESF 8, however, does not specify nursing homes among the list of facilities, nor does it designate nursing home residents and staff as a specific vulnerable population. Similarly, ESF 15 also does not specifically include residents of nursing homes in the list of community members (FEMA, 2016b). Clarification of nursing homes in the list of community members is particularly relevant given the inclusion of behavioral health care among the list of services, in light of the prevalence of behavioral health needs among nursing home residents (discussed in Chapter 4) and the importance of providing PFA to nursing home residents in the aftermath of an emergency, as discussed above.

The devastating impact of COVID-19 on nursing home staff and residents described above demonstrates the urgent need to explicitly ensure that long-term care settings such as nursing homes are included in the broad range of emergency planning, preparedness, and response activities for health care settings similar to what is done for acute-care settings. In order to ensure the same level of preparedness and response accorded other health care settings, it is critical to include nursing homes explicitly in federal emergency response protocols, such as ESF 8 and ESF 15.

Partnering with Local and State Emergency Management and Public Health

As discussed above, nursing homes have not been well integrated into federal planning and response efforts. For example, a lack of federal–state integration left individual states responsible for PPE distribution resulting in wide variation in the prioritization and inclusion of nursing homes to receive supplies (Abbasi, 2020; Cohen and Rodgers, 2020; McGarry et al., 2020; Murray and Friedman, 2020). This is also the case for state and local disaster planning and response efforts (Hyer et al., 2010). A federal program, the Hospital Preparedness Program (HPP),[28] directed by ASPR, provides financial support to states, localities, and territories to develop regional coalitions of health care organizations that collaborate on emergency planning, preparedness, and response. Regional coalitions are required to include at least two acute care hospitals, emergency medical services, emergency management, and public health agencies. On average, nearly 90 percent of hospitals belonged to a health care coalition in 2017; in 17

---

[28] See https://www.phe.gov/Preparedness/planning/hpp/Pages/default.aspx (accessed February 4, 2022).

states every hospital was a member of a coalition. An OIG report called on ASPR to encourage those who receive HPP funding to "prioritize exercises for communities and health care coalitions that include hospitals, long-term care facilities, EMS, emergency management, public health, and other essential partners" (OIG, 2014b, p. 22).

Improved coordination with emergency management officials across all levels could enhance the effectiveness of nursing home emergency planning and preparedness (Lane and McGrady, 2016). It is essential that nursing homes be included in state and local emergency planning sessions and drills. Ideally, these state and local agencies would have staff members with expertise, knowledge, and training in long-term care populations and programs. Forging effective partnerships with local emergency management is particularly critical to establishing evacuation standards, plans, sites, and routes as well as ensuring that the nursing home facility is aware of the most up-to-date state and local emergency planning regulations (Andersen et al., 2021; Casey et al., 2020; Lane and McGrady, 2016, 2018; OIG, 2012; U.S. Senate Committee on Finance, 2018).

In addition to coordinating with emergency management for disaster planning, preparedness, and response, nursing home emergency planning efforts should be integrated with those of local public health and local health care facilities for infection control, the need for which was made clear during the COVID-19 pandemic (Andersen et al., 2021; Powell et al., 2012). State and local public health departments, including State Health Department health care–associated infection programs first established in 2009, serve as vital partners for providing technical assistance, education, and training to nursing homes on infection prevention and control (Andersen et al., 2021). Moreover, as discussed above, shortages of essential supplies, such as PPE, for nursing homes during the pandemic underscores the importance of ensuring nursing homes are included in federal and state emergency planning, preparedness, and response measures and initiatives.

Public health plays other key roles during emergencies, providing necessary resources as well as essential expertise concerning food safety, environmental protection, and infection control. Health care facilities will be stressed during emergency events and thus limited in their ability to care for additional patients. Nursing home planning and preparedness efforts therefore need to be closely coordinated with those of public health departments, health and social care organizations, and other health care facilities and emergency services. In this way, an integrated network of care among hospitals, nursing homes, and local and state community services can be established to ensure that nursing home residents' health care needs can be met during emergencies (Harnett et al., 2020).

THE PHYSICAL ENVIRONMENT

The physical environment of the nursing home plays a crucial role in supporting resident health and function, promoting quality of life, enabling staff to provide needed care, and supporting family satisfaction (Wood et al., 2020). Due to the unique dual role of nursing homes as places to live as well as sites in which care is provided, increased attention is being paid to ways to create a nursing home environment that is more like home rather than a health care institution in which people also happen to live (van Hoof et al., 2016a). Indeed, the degree to which residents feel at home may be critical to the success of providing person-centered care and may contribute to the overall quality of care in nursing homes (Edvardsson et al., 2010; van Zadelhoff et al., 2011). Moreover, COVID-19, with its associated disease incidence and visitor/group gathering restrictions, has underlined the importance of the particular design of the nursing home physical environment for resident well-being and quality of life (Anderson et al., 2020).

Key elements of the physical nursing home environment include sensory-related elements such as light, sound, odor, and touch; air flow and temperature control; environmental aspects specifically related to personal care provision and staff function; the building's overall design; room layout and configuration; and indoor and outdoor spaces. These aspects of the physical environment are important to consider in constructing, renovating, and evaluating nursing homes and in planning the nursing home of the future, and are discussed further below.

Sensory-Related Elements of the Physical Environment

It is through the senses of sight, hearing, smell, taste, and touch that one experiences and communicates with the world. Those experiences can be pleasant or unpleasant, depending on how sensory stimulation is provided and regulated. Many nursing home residents have limitations or needs related to one or more senses, and those needs will vary depending on the individual. Therefore, support for positive sensory perception and minimization of unpleasant sensory experiences are critical elements of quality nursing home environments, as summarized in Table 6-2 below.

Building Layout

Many nursing homes were developed using design features adapted from hospitals constructed in the 1960s and 1970s (Eijkelenboom et al., 2017; Schwarz, 1997). These features, which include large units with long corridors, large activity and dining spaces, shared rooms and bathrooms,

TABLE 6-2 Importance of Sensory Perceptions in the Nursing Home Setting

Sense	Key Issues to Consider for Sensory Perceptions in the Nursing Home Setting
Sight	Lighting design issues in nursing homes are complex because common aging changes in the eye cause older persons to need higher light intensities, while at the same time they are also more sensitive to glare and to differences in the consistency of lighting. For this reason, lighting design must take many factors into consideration, including
	The use of indirect rather than direct lighting sources, including overhead illumination and diffusers for skylights.
	The promotion of evenness of lighting within rooms, such as by having daylight sources from more than one side of a room, to achieve a ratio no larger than 3:1 from lightest to darkest areas of a room.
	Adequate illumination in bedroom task areas for reading.
	Design features and policies that reduce glare, for example, from shiny floor surfaces and lighting fixtures.
	Full-spectrum bright light during the day (ideally by exposure to direct or indirect sunlight) to entrain circadian systems, improving sleep and possibly relieving depression.
	Motion-activated systems to provide illumination for nighttime activity, including trips to the bathroom, thereby helping promote safety and prevent falls.
Sound	Most nursing home residents have some degree of hearing loss, including aging-related changes that impair speech discrimination and increase sensitivity to background noise. Noise is common in many nursing homes, due to environmental factors such as poor sound absorbency of surfaces; loud sounds generated by staff communication, meal service, housekeeping, and maintenance; resident vocalization; electronic systems such as televisions, radios, and computers; and alarms. Unwanted noise can reduce sleep and increase agitation, and desired sounds (such as personalized music) can enhance the quality of life.
	Issues to consider in providing optimal sound stimulation include
	Smaller nursing home functional units, such as wards and common areas, as noise increases with the number of residents and staff.
	Private bedrooms, which eliminate distracting sounds of roommates and their care.
	Noise-absorbent materials on walls and ceilings of common rooms and hallways.
	Policies and procedures that limit loud staff communication.
	Use of headphones or other personal communication/listening devices by residents with significant hearing impairment when individualized activities, including resident–staff communication, take place in common areas.
Touch	Many nursing home residents have mobility issues that confine them largely or wholly to beds and chairs, often resulting in them remaining in the same place for hours or longer. In addition, conditions such as advanced dementia, visual impairment, and hearing loss mean that awareness of the immediate environment is mainly by touch. Many residents with significant mobility limitations are unable to reposition themselves when they are uncomfortable, placing them at risk not only for chronic discomfort but also for skin breakdown and pressure ulcers. Among the issues to consider are
	Different individuals can have widely different preferences in terms of ambient temperature; individual room thermostats are an important element of person-centered care.

Continued

TABLE 6-2 Continued

Sense	Key Issues to Consider for Sensory Perceptions in the Nursing Home Setting
	Bed, wheelchair, and other seating surfaces play an important role in a resident's physical comfort. Cushioning designed to provide comfort, facilitate positioning, and prevent pressure ulcers are essential for persons with mobility limitations. Exposure to sunlight, soft blankets, pets (if desired), and other pleasant and stimulating tactile sensations can add to a resident's quality of life.
Smell	The reduction and elimination of noxious odors is an elementary element of nursing home quality. Beyond the absence of negative odors, environmental quality should provide access to pleasantly stimulating odors as well. Examples include
	Cooking-related odors, such as bread baking or brewing coffee.
	Fresh flowers.
	Aromatherapy with scents that have been associated with positive impact on mood, such as lavender in relieving anxiety.

SOURCES: Dichter et al., 2021; Donelli et al., 2019; Figueiro et al., 2014; Forbes et al., 2014; Hickman et al., 2007; Joosse, 2011; Martin and Ancoli-Israel, 2008; Meyer et al., 1992; Riemersma-van der Lek et al., 2008; Schnelle et al., 1999; Sloane et al., 2002, 2007a; Wu et al., 2015.

and lack of ready access to outdoors (Brawley, 2005; Eijkelenboom et al., 2017), are now considered to be detrimental to the residents' quality of life, infection control, and effective staff function in caring for nursing home residents. Newer evidence and experience-based principles of environmental design for older persons have led to the identification of a range of best practices for optimal nursing home design, which are described below.

Air Flow and Filtration

The COVID-19 pandemic has led to building designers giving much greater consideration to the role that air flow and filtration can play in minimizing the cross-contamination of aerosolized droplets that can occur through stagnation in public areas and transmission through ventilation systems. Moreover, there is a greater interest in filtration systems that can capture and eliminate aerosolized viral particles from circulation.

The need to care for residents with active, airborne/droplet infections such as COVID-19 in the nursing home setting has raised the possibility of mandating that nursing homes have some negative pressure rooms, with separate systems to ventilate air outdoors to the facility roof. Lessons learned through the COVID-19 experience underscore the importance of incorporating new air circulation standards in future nursing home design (Lynch and Goring, 2020; Reiling et al., 2008; TROPOS, 2020). Consideration should also be given to the use of air cleaners with upper-room ultraviolet disinfection and air purifiers with high-efficiency particulate absorbing filters as an additional measures, though with the understanding that such purifiers cannot replace the supply of fresh air (TROPOS, 2020; University of Nebraska–Lincoln, 2021).

Facilitation of Staff Activity

The design of a nursing home should also consider issues related to staff convenience and function, such as ensuring ready access to supplies by locating supply closets close to areas where the supplies will be used and by placing personalized resident supplies and, when possible, medications in locked cabinets in resident rooms. In addition, the design layout should include attention to incorporating enhanced infection control practices (e.g., accessible handwashing stations for staff that are integrated with workflow and the use of bacterial resistant surfaces and improved waste disposal). Furthermore, it is important to design bathing areas that facilitate resident transfer and care, prevent infection, keep residents warm, and do not overheat staff (Sloane et al., 1995, 2007b). Moreover, resident monitoring devices, such as motion sensors in bedrooms, are important possibilities to consider as a way to facilitate staff activity (Woodbridge et al., 2018).

Access to Outdoors

Ready access to safe, stimulating outdoor space is important to residents' health and quality of life, but most nursing homes do not provide this amenity (Cutler and Kane, 2006). The average nursing home resident spends little if any time outdoors, even in good weather, despite evidence that exposure to sunlight can raise vitamin D levels, promote better sleep, and improve one's mood (van den Berg et al., 2019). Well-designed outdoor spaces provide opportunity for activities that promote dignity and important personal expression for many older persons (Connell et al., 2007; Martin and Ancoli-Israel, 2008; Sandvoll et al., 2020). Barriers to the use of outdoor space include the nontherapeutic design of many outdoor spaces, difficult access to the outdoors, the need for most residents to have staff or family assistance when they are outdoors, and the need for staff to plan and conduct or monitor activities outdoors. For nursing homes located in areas where the weather presents a barrier to outdoor activities, interior designs should include windows, not only to ensure a sufficient amount of natural light, but also to enable residents to experience the outdoors visually.

Given the important association between access to the outdoors and residents' health, the thoughtful design of outdoor space is an important element of nursing home planning, construction, and use (van den Berg et al., 2019).

Important elements of outdoor space design for nursing homes to consider include

- One outdoor area for each functional unit of the nursing home, both for infection control and to facilitate the oversight of residents;
- Ready access to outdoor space on the ground level, without locks or thresholds, and with easy doorway visibility for residents and ability of staff to monitor the activity of residents from common areas;
- Security by way of a safe, visually appealing barrier at the limits of the area;
- Circular paths to facilitate movement;
- Plantings that are visually pleasant, provide visual and olfactory stimulation, and are nonpoisonous;
- Areas that provide sun and areas that provide shade, with seating availability in each; and
- Opportunities for visual stimulation and activity, such as raised and ground-level gardens, bird feeders, whirligigs, and space for outdoor games (van den Berg et al., 2019; Wrublowsky, 2018).

Private Rooms and Bathrooms

Having one's own private bedroom and bathroom is important for addressing nursing home residents' needs such as privacy, dignity, relationship considerations (e.g., family visitation), and sensory control (e.g., temperature and television noise). It also provides private space for personal expression (e.g., a resident's own furniture and mementos or intimate interactions) (Calkins and Cassella, 2007; Nygaard et al., 2020; van Hoof et al., 2016b). A large body of research has demonstrated the benefits of single occupancy rooms in terms of patient safety, effectiveness and quality of care, and promotion of person-centered care. Private rooms have been shown to reduce the risk of acquiring and spreading infections in hospital settings (Chaudhury et al., 2004; Cohen et al., 2017; Munier-Marion et al., 2016; Stiller et al., 2016; Zhu et al., 2022). Research also shows that single rooms are associated with improved sleep patterns and reduced agitation in people with dementia, fewer medication errors, and fewer adverse outcomes in hospitals (Silow-Carroll et al., 2021). Moreover, research has revealed higher resident satisfaction and family preference for single occupancy rooms (Nakrem et al., 2013; Nguyen Thi et al., 2002; Reid et al., 2015). Overall, the benefits of private rooms include shorter hospital stays, greater privacy for the patient, reduced noise levels and traffic in and out of patient's rooms, contributing to reduced stress on the part of patients, and space for family members to visit and support the individual's healing process (Chaudhury et al., 2004). A family member's perspective is captured in Box 6-4 below.

BOX 6-4
Family Member Perspective

". . . my mother was in a private nursing home for three months recuperating from a broken hip. This home had no private rooms. Her roommate was an obese woman who lived in her bed, lifted by hoist to be moved for bathing and hygiene. The roommate had no visitors and therefore had the television on every waking moment. My mother didn't watch television."

— Daughter and caregiver of two parents who suffered from dementia and needed nursing home care.

This quote was collected from the committee's online call for resident, family and nursing home staff perspectives.

Moreover, it is clear from the COVID-19 experience and from research on colonization of multidrug-resistant bacteria that private rooms and bathrooms promote infection control (Brown et al., 2021; Mody et al., 2021; Siegel et al., 2017). On the other hand, a limited number of nursing home residents will prefer to share a bedroom, for example, with a spouse, partner, or close friend. Therefore, while it is better for the residents if most nursing home rooms and bathrooms are private, reserving a small number of double-occupancy rooms for those who prefer to share a room is important. For a family member's perspective on the importance of having a private room, see Box 6-5.

BOX 6-5
Resident and Family Perspective

"Everyone should be able to have the choice of a private room, not just residents who might qualify for Medicare coverage of their stay or people who are paying privately. *We should all put ourselves in the place of residents and imagine what it would be like to live in half of a room with a stranger in the other half.* Last evening I was talking with a friend who's searching for the right college for her son. That 17 year-old gets more choice in who he lives with and the availability of preferred meals and access to enriching activity than an 80-year old grandmother gets in a nursing home."

— Beverley Laubert

This quote was collected from the committee's public webinar on January 26, 2021.

Impact of the COVID-19 Pandemic and Physical Design of Nursing Homes

The devastating impact of the COVID-19 pandemic on nursing homes, combined with the specific ways in which the physical design of nursing homes facilitated the spread of the virus, has renewed interest in alternative nursing home designs (Sabatino and Harrington, 2021). Many of the recommended features of updated physical environments take into account the factors discussed in the preceding sections of this chapter, including expanded resident living spaces with private rooms and bathrooms, improved ventilation and air circulation, and outdoor areas and room to exercise, along with other physical, environmental, and safety features to improve quality of life for residents (Anderson et al., 2020).

Indeed, the lessons learned during the COVID-19 pandemic, particularly the key factors that contributed to the spread of the virus in nursing home settings, are critical to anyone reimagining nursing homes for the future (see Box 6-6). Central among these factors was the size of the nursing home facility. In 2019, the median capacity of a nursing home facility was 100 beds, although average facility size varied significantly by geographic location as well as by ownership type (MedPAC, 2021; Sabatino and Harrington, 2021). Research has shown nursing home size to be a major predictor of infection rates (Abrams et al., 2020; Figueroa et al., 2020; Harrington et al., 2020; Stall et al., 2020).

Another key factor related to density in facilities is room sharing; most nursing home residents live multi-occupancy rooms, with two to four beds per room and shared bathrooms. Multi-occupancy rooms are standard in nursing homes, as Medicare and Medicaid will only pay for semi-private rooms; residents who want a single room must pay private rates (CMS, 2019b).[29] Reducing the density of all resident spaces with spacious living areas and more single-occupancy rooms (even without reducing total capacity and size) has been shown to reduce transmission of infectious diseases, such as COVID-19 (Zhu et al., 2022).

Innovative Physical Design of Nursing Homes

This chapter has discussed key safety and environmental aspects that influence nursing home quality of care and which have a direct impact on residents' quality of life. The culture in nursing homes has long mirrored an acute-care model in terms of its esthetics, restrictions, and medical focus. Many residents, however, prefer a model that is less institutional and more

---

[29] CMS Requirements for Long-Term Care Facilities—Admission, Transfer, and Discharge Rights, 42 CFR § 483.15 (2016).

> **BOX 6-6**
> **COVID-19 Pandemic and the Nursing Home Environment**
>
> A number of factors related to the typical nursing home design and layout contributed to the widespread devastating impact of COVID-19 on nursing home residents, including
>
> - The closed nursing home environment (Figueroa et al., 2020; Yurkofsky and Ouslander, 2021),
> - The communal nature of nursing home life, including shared dining and common areas (Figueroa et al., 2020; Yurkofsky and Ouslander, 2021),
> - Shared resident rooms (Brown et al., 2021),
> - The intimate nature of nursing home care, which prevents social distancing (Thompson et al., 2020),
> - The number of low-wage staff, especially nursing assistants, who work in more than one facility (Chen et al., 2021),
> - Challenges with residents, such as those with dementia, who have difficulty adhering to social distancing and universal masking policies (Thompson et al., 2020; Yurkofsky and Ouslander, 2021), and
> - Older nursing home layouts, which severely limited options to safely isolate residents who were either infected or suspected of having been in contact with an infected person or to quarantine newly admitted residents in dedicated areas separate from other residents (Andersen et al., 2021).
>
> The 2020 CMS Coronavirus Commission on Safety and Quality in Nursing Homes included a number of recommendations related to the nursing home physical environment (MITRE, 2020).
>
> - Identify short-term facility designs to address immediate risks (e.g., changes in heating, ventilation, and air conditioning systems and single room occupancy)
> - Establish a national forum to share best practices on how to best use physical space
> - Establish a commission to identify long-term priorities and funding to redesign nursing homes (separate wings for cohorting, separate entrances and exits, separate bathrooms and break areas, etc.).

reflective of the homes in which they once lived, which commonly includes private rooms and bathrooms (Roubein, 2021; Waters, 2021). Small-scale[30] nursing home environments eliminate disorienting long corridors and large public spaces, reduce unpleasant noise, create a more "home-like" feel, and can promote staff cohesion (Abrams et al., 2020; Kane et al., 2007; Passini

---

[30] Though there is no formal definition of what constitutes a small nursing home, a common limit is 20 or fewer residents (Sabatino and Harrington, 2021).

et al., 2000; Waters, 2021). Key features in the small household model of nursing home care are depicted in Figure 6-1.

Interest in reconfiguring large, institution-like traditional nursing homes as smaller, more home-like settings is not new; innovative approaches such as the Eden Alternative[31] and the Green House Project[32] have been around for more than 25 years in this country. As discussed in Chapter 4, creating a more home-like atmosphere is a key element of the culture change movement in nursing homes. For one family member's perspective on a more home-like atmosphere for nursing homes, see Box 6-7.

Small-scale home-like environments have been developed in other nations, such as the Netherlands, Denmark, and Norway (de Boer et al., 2018; Kane et al., 2007; Rabig et al. 2006; Regnier, 2018; Verbeek et al., 2009; Waters, 2021), as well as "clustered neighborhood designs" where groups of 8–12 residents have their own rooms yet share living and dining space (Eijkelenboom et al., 2017). Other innovative approaches include nursing home models in the Netherlands that serve to bring together both ends of the age spectrum through a combination of child care and long-term care (Werner et al., 2020).

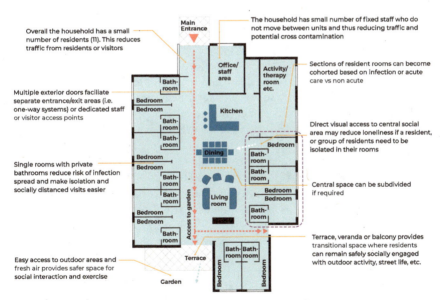

FIGURE 6-1 Generic floor plan of a household model nursing home with 11 single bedrooms.
SOURCE: Anderson et al., 2020.

---

[31] For more information, see https://www.edenalt.org (accessed December 2, 2021).
[32] For more information, see https://thegreenhouseproject.org (accessed December 2, 2021).

> **BOX 6-7**
> **Family Perspective**
>
> "When my widowed mother needed to transfer to a nursing home, I knew enough to make sure it was a non-profit facility. We were fortunate to find one, owned and operated by a coalition of churches, and in my opinion, as good as it gets for those needing to live in a nursing home. They applied the Eden Alternative philosophy, had many design features that made for a home-like atmosphere."
>
> — Daughter and caregiver of two parents with dementia who needed nursing home care
>
> *This quote was collected from the committee's online call for resident, family, and nursing home staff perspectives.*

Another example of an alternate approach to traditional nursing home care that has been in place for nearly 20 years is TigerPlace. Launched in 2004[33] as a state demonstration project, TigerPlace was designed to maximize older adults' independence and function throughout the end of life (Lane et al., 2019; Rantz et al., 2008, 2014a).[34] Though the main service provided is housing (meals, housekeeping, and maintenance are also included), interdisciplinary professional health care team members (e.g., full-time registered nurses, social workers, licensed practical nurses, certified nursing assistants, and consulting advanced practice registered nurse faculty) provide services to residents. TigerPlace was designed as a "living laboratory" for research and development of a wide range of interdisciplinary innovations, such as evaluation of aging in place and of the effectiveness of care coordination (Rantz et al., 2014b, 2015); the development of technology to enhance aging independently (Mishra et al., 2020; Rantz et al., 2005); environmental sensors to detect early illness, automated fall risk, and fall detection (Skubic et al., 2015; Stone et al., 2015; Su et al., 2018); electronic health record data mining (Mishra et al., 2020; Popejoy et al.,

---

[33] The passage of state legislation in 1999 and 2001 enabled a facility with apartments to be built to nursing home standards, licensed as an intermediate care facility (facilitating the use of long-term care insurances by residents). TigerPlace operates as independent housing through waivers granted to enable its innovative approach to providing services to older adults.

[34] A public–private partnership was formed with Americare Systems, Inc., which built, owns, and operates the housing component, with the care delivery provided by a home health agency of the Sinclair School of Nursing, University of Missouri. For more information, see https://agingmo.com/tiger-place-institute (accessed December 3, 2021).

2015), longitudinal functional health and cost-of-care measurement (Rantz et al., 2011, 2014a); and social engagement or other research activities of interest to older adults, faculty, and students (Demiris et al., 2008, 2009; Galambos et al., 2013, 2019). Evaluations of TigerPlace have consistently shown that residents and families prefer TigerPlace's innovative approach. Financial analyses reveal that the total cost of care (beginning at the point when residents would qualify for nursing home placement through the end of life) is less than traditional care (Rantz et al., 2011, 2014a).

Redesigning Nursing Home Environments to Support Quality Care

As noted above, a number of innovative models reflect the preference for less institutional, more home-like settings, including Green House homes. Launched in 2003 with initial funding from the Robert Wood Johnson Foundation (RWJF),[35] a total of approximately 300 independently owned Green House homes operate in 32 states and serve approximately 3,200 older adults. The large majority of Green House homes—more than 80 percent—are owned by nonprofit companies (Waters, 2021).

Research has identified the benefits of the Green House model as including higher quality of life, lower Medicare spending, and reduced staff turnover as compared with traditional nursing homes (Green House Project, 2012; Waters, 2021). Studies have found that, compared with traditional nursing home residents, those living in Green House homes had lower rates of hospitalization, and were 45 percent less likely to need catheters, 38 percent less likely to have pressure ulcers, and 16 percent less likely to be bedridden (Zimmerman et al., 2016). Earlier studies demonstrated that residents and families were more satisfied with Green House homes than traditional nursing homes (Kane et al., 2007; Lum et al., 2008).

Despite the positive impact they have on a range of resident health outcome measures and the enhanced quality of life they provide, Green Houses represent less than 2 percent of all nursing homes and provide care to less than 1 percent of all nursing home residents. A significant limiting factor is their relatively high costs of construction and operation compared with traditional nursing homes. Although costs vary by location, daily rates in Green Houses range from approximately $250 to $500 per day. Medicaid reimbursement rates for nursing home care vary by state (discussed in Chapter 7), but overall, given the higher costs of Green Houses relative to other nursing home settings, residents tend to be primarily White, middle- or upper-income private paying individuals. This raises equity concerns

---

[35] RWJF awarded the Green House Project a 5-year, $10 million grant to pay for technical assistance, support for architects, and evaluations (Waters, 2021).

about the ability of individuals on Medicaid to access high-quality care such as that provided in Green House settings (Waters, 2021).

The pandemic highlighted another benefit of the Green Home model in that nursing homes using this model had significantly lower rates of coronavirus infection. The infection rates in large traditional nursing homes (with 50 or more residents) were nine times higher than the rates in Green House nursing homes. The median mortality rate in Green Houses was 24 for every 100 COVID-19 cases, as compared with 80 per 100 cases in small traditional homes and 53 per 100 cases in large traditional nursing homes. The lower rates of COVID-19 cases and mortality among Green House residents were likely due to residents having private rooms and to the fact that fewer people live and work in Green Houses than in traditional nursing homes (Zimmerman et al., 2021).

A range of incentives and supports will be needed to facilitate the shift to smaller, more home-like designs for nursing homes with features that would enhance patient safety by lessening the impact of a future public health emergency, while improving resident quality of life. Transition to a new model of care will require significant financial investment by the U.S. Congress, as well as a number of regulatory changes, including allowing Medicare and Medicaid to pay for private rooms for residents; private rooms are currently only paid for by CMS if deemed medically necessary (CMS, 2019b).

Federal agencies such as the U.S. Department of Housing and Urban Development (HUD), the Internal Revenue Service, and CMS could help promote the development of smaller nursing homes with private rooms by providing incentives for new construction of smaller homes or renovations for smaller units within larger homes (Sabatino and Harrington, 2021). An existing source of financing assistance to support rehabilitation or construction of smaller nursing home facilities is HUD's Section 232 program, which guarantees mortgages of nearly 2,400 nursing homes across the country.[36] HUD has been criticized, however, for inadequate oversight of the program and for discontinuing its physical inspections of nursing homes that received HUD-backed mortgages, many of which have received one- or two-star ratings under the CMS Five Star rating system (Goldstein and Gebeloff, 2019). The U.S. Department of Agriculture operates a loan program to provide affordable financing to develop essential community facilities in rural areas of the country. Funding can be used to purchase, build, or improve community facilities, which include nursing homes.[37]

---

[36] See https://www.hud.gov/program_offices/housing/mfh/progdesc/procsec232_223f (accessed February 7, 2022).

[37] See https://www.rd.usda.gov/programs-services/community-facilities/community-facilities-direct-loan-grant-program (accessed February 7, 2022).

Clearly, the COVID-19 pandemic has served as the catalyst underscoring the urgency of transforming the nursing home built environment (Werner et al., 2020). The design of nursing homes going forward will need to take into account all the myriad factors discussed in this chapter in order to ensure the highest quality of life for residents and to answer resident, family, and staff safety concerns—on a daily basis as well as in times of future public health emergencies. Such necessary changes will require a collaborative approach that brings together health care leaders, nursing home architects and builders, state and federal agencies, and local communities (Anderson et al., 2020).

KEY FINDINGS AND CONCLUSIONS

- Resident safety is a key aspect of quality of care in nursing homes. Because of the dual role of nursing homes as care settings as well as places to live, nursing homes must balance resident safety with resident autonomy and quality of life.
- Even before the pandemic, infection control issues were the most common reason for citation deficiencies by nursing home surveyors.
- Nursing homes are not well integrated into federal, state, county, and local emergency management planning, preparedness, and response.
- Nursing home emergency management needs to be conducted in partnership with state and local emergency management departments as well as with local public health and health care facilities.
- The physical environment of the nursing home plays a large and important role in supporting or inhibiting resident function and in promoting or detracting from residents' quality of life. This became particularly evident during the COVID-19 pandemic.
- Features such as large units, long corridors, massive activity and dining spaces, shared rooms and bathrooms, and a lack of ready access to outdoor areas are now considered to be detrimental to resident quality of life, infection control, and effective staff function.
- Small nursing homes had fewer COVID-19 infections and lower mortality compared with nursing homes with 50 or more beds.
- Research demonstrates the positive impact of single occupancy rooms and private bathrooms on resident health, safety, and quality of life. However, CMS does not reimburse for private rooms in nursing homes other than in cases of medical necessity.
- COVID-19 affected high-quality nursing homes as well as low-quality nursing homes. The overwhelming impact of the pandemic on nursing homes shines a light on existing, universal, deep-rooted

problems that require systemic solutions across the nursing home industry.

REFERENCES

Abbasi, J. 2020. "Abandoned" nursing homes continue to face critical supply and staff shortages as COVID-19 toll has mounted. *JAMA* 324(2):123–125.

Abrams, H. R., L. Loomer, A. Gandhi, and D. C. Grabowski. 2020. Characteristics of U.S. nursing homes with COVID-19 cases. *Journal of the American Geriatrics Society* 68(8):1653–1656.

AHRQ (Agency for Healthcare Research and Quality). 2019. *Falls.* https://psnet.ahrq.gov/primer/falls (accessed February 4, 2022).

American Geriatrics Society. 2019. Updated AGS Beers criteria® for potentially inappropriate medication use in older adults. *Journal of the American Geriatrics Society* 67(4):674–694.

Andersen, L. E., L. Tripp, J. F. Perz, N. D. Stone, A. H. Viall, S. M. Ling, and L. A. Fleisher. 2021. Protecting nursing home residents from COVID-19: Federal strike team findings and lessons learned. *NEJM Catalyst: Innovations in Care Delivery* 2(3). https://doi.org/10.1056/CAT.21.0144.

Anderson, D. C., T. Grey, S. Kennelly, and D. O'Neill. 2020. Nursing home design and COVID-19: Balancing infection control, quality of life, and resilience. *Journal of the American Medical Directors Association* 21(11):1519–1524.

Baker, P. R. A., D. P. Francis, N. N. Hairi, S. Othman, and W. Y. Choo. 2016. Interventions for preventing abuse in the elderly. *Cochrane Database of Systematic Reviews* 2016(8):CD010321.

Ball, J., and P. Griffiths. 2018. *Missed nursing care: A key measure for patient safety.* https://psnet.ahrq.gov/perspective/missed-nursing-care-key-measure-patient-safety (accessed February 7, 2022).

Barlas, S. 2012. Medicare wants only 'independent' consultant pharmacists in nursing homes. *Pharmacy and Therapeutics* 37(1):6.

Barlas, S. 2016. Medicare adds new long-term-care pharmacy rules: Agency passes again on pharmacist independence requirements. *Pharmacy and Therapeutics* 41(12):762–764.

Bateni, H. 2012. Changes in balance in older adults based on use of physical therapy vs the Wii Fit gaming system: A preliminary study. *Physiotherapy* 98(3):211–216.

Bernsten, C., I. Björkman, M. Caramona, G. Crealey, B. Frøkjaer, E. Grundberger, T. Gustafsson, M. Henman, H. Herborg, C. Hughes, J. McElnay, M. Magner, F. van Mil, M. Schaeffer, S. Silva, B. Søndergaard, I. Sturgess, D. Tromp, L. Vivero, and A. Winterstein. 2001. Improving the well-being of elderly patients via community pharmacy-based provision of pharmaceutical care: A multicentre study in seven European countries. *Drugs and Aging* 18(1):63–77.

Berridge, C., J. Halpern, and K. Levy. 2019. Cameras on beds: The ethics of surveillance in nursing home rooms. *AJOB Empirical Bioethics* 10(1):55–62.

Blain, H., Y. Rolland, J. M. G. A. Schols, A. Cherubini, S. Miot, D. O'Neill, F. C. Martin, O. Guérin, G. Gavazzi, J. Bousquet, M. Petrovic, A. L. Gordon, and A. Benetos. 2020. August 2020 interim EuGMS guidance to prepare European long-term care facilities for COVID-19. *European Geriatric Medicine* 11(6):899–913.

Bonifas, R. P. 2015. Resident-to-resident aggression in nursing homes: Social worker involvement and collaboration with nursing colleagues. *Health & Social Work* 40(3):e101–e109.

Braaten, K. L., and W. Malmedal. 2017. Preventing physical abuse of nursing home residents— as seen from the nursing staff's perspective. *Nursing Open* 4(4):274–281.

Branch, J., D. Hiner, and V. Jackson. 2021. *The impact of communication on medication errors*. https://psnet.ahrq.gov/web-mm/impact-communication-medication-errors (accessed February 7, 2022).

Brauner, D., R. M. Werner, T. P. Shippee, J. Cursio, H. Sharma, and R. T. Konetzka. 2018. Does Nursing Home Compare reflect patient safety in nursing homes? *Health Affairs (Millwood)* 37(11):1770–1778.

Brawley, E. C. 2005. *Design innovations for aging and Alzheimer's: Creating caring environments*. Hoboken, NJ: John Wiley & Sons.

Brophy, J., M. Keith, and M. Hurley. 2019. Breaking point: Violence against long-term care staff. *New Solutions: A Journal of Environmental and Occupational Health Policy* 29(1):10–35.

Brown, K. A., A. Jones, N. Daneman, A. K. Chan, K. L. Schwartz, G. E. Garber, A. P. Costa, and N. M. Stall. 2021. Association between nursing home crowding and COVID-19 infection and mortality in Ontario, Canada. *JAMA Internal Medicine* 181(2):229–236.

Brown, L. M., M. L. Bruce, K. Hyer, W. L. Mills, E. Vongxaiburana, and L. Polivka-West. 2009. A pilot study evaluating the feasibility of psychological first aid for nursing home residents. *Clinical Gerontologist* 32(3):293–308.

Brown, L. M., D. M. Dosa, K. Thomas, K. Hyer, Z. Feng, and V. Mor. 2012. The effects of evacuation on nursing home residents with dementia. *American Journal of Alzheimer's Disease and Other Dementias* 27(6):406–412.

Cacchione, P. Z., L. M. Willoughby, J. C. Langan, and K. Culp. 2011. Disaster strikes! Long-term care resident outcomes following a natural disaster. *Journal of Gerontological Nursing* 37(9):16–27.

Calkins, M., and C. Cassella. 2007. Exploring the cost and value of private versus shared bedrooms in nursing homes. *The Gerontologist* 47(2):169–183.

Cameron, E. J., S. K. Bowles, E. G. Marshall, and M. K. Andrew. 2018b. Falls and long-term care: A report from the care by design observational cohort study. *BMC Family Practice* 19(1):73.

Cameron, I. D., S. M. Dyer, C. E. Panagoda, G. R. Murray, K. D. Hill, R. G. Cumming, and N. Kerse. 2018a. Interventions for preventing falls in older people in care facilities and hospitals. *Cochrane Database of Systematic Reviews* 9(9):CD005465.

CANHR (California Advocates for Nursing Home Reform). 2009. *Omnicare settles drug kickback cases for $98m (November 3, 2009)*. http://www.canhr.org/newsroom/canhrnewsarchive/2009/DOJ110309.html (accessed January 18, 2022).

Casey, B., G. Peters, and R. Wyden. 2020. *COVID-19 in nursing homes: How the Trump Administration failed residents and workers*. https://www.aging.senate.gov/imo/media/doc/COVID-19%20in%20Nursing%20Homes%20Final%20Report.pdf (accessed September 14, 2021).

CDC (Centers for Disease Control and Prevention). 2020. *Core elements of antibiotic stewardship for nursing homes*. https://www.cdc.gov/longtermcare/prevention/antibiotic-stewardship.html (accessed April 29, 2021).

CDC. 2021. *Preventing elder abuse*. https://www.cdc.gov/violenceprevention/elderabuse/fastfact.html (accessed November 3, 2021).

CDC TRAIN. 2021. *Nursing home infection preventionist training course*. https://www.train.org/cdctrain/training_plan/3814 (accessed April 29, 2021).

Chang, H. J., C. Lynm, and R. M. Glass. 2010. Falls and older adults. *JAMA* 303(3):288.

Chapman, S., and C. Harrington. 2020. Policies matter! Factors contributing to nursing home outbreaks during the COVID-19 pandemic. *Policy, Politics, and Nursing Practice* 21(4):191–192.

Chaudhury, H., A. Mahmood, and M. Valente. 2004. *The use of single patient rooms versus multiple occupancy rooms in acute care environments.* https://www.healthdesign.org/sites/default/files/use_of_single_patient_rooms_v_multiple_occ._rooms-acute_care.pdf (accessed January 18, 2022).

Chen, M. K., J. A. Chevalier, and E. F. Long. 2021. Nursing home staff networks and COVID-19. *Proceedings of the National Academy of Sciences of the United States of America* 118(1):e2015455118.

Clemson, L., M. A. Fiatarone Singh, A. Bundy, R. G. Cumming, K. Manollaras, P. O'Loughlin, and D. Black. 2012. Integration of balance and strength training into daily life activity to reduce rate of falls in older people (the LiFE study): Randomised parallel trial. *BMJ* 345:e4547.

CMA (Center for Medicare Advocacy). 2019. *Nursing Home Compare's abuse icon is now live.* https://medicareadvocacy.org/nursing-home-compares-abuse-icon-is-now-live (accessed November 3, 2021).

CMS (Centers for Medicare & Medicaid Services). 2019a. *Specialized infection prevention and control training for nursing home staff in the long-term care setting is now available.* https://www.cms.gov/Medicare/Provider-Enrollment-and-Certification/SurveyCertificationGenInfo/Downloads/QSO19-10-NH.pdf (accessed February 1, 2022).

CMS. 2019b. *Medicare coverage of skilled nursing facility care.* https://www.medicare.gov/Pubs/pdf/10153-Medicare-Skilled-Nursing-Facility-Care.pdf (accessed April 29, 2021).

CMS. 2021. *Toolkit on state actions to mitigate COVID-19 prevalence in nursing homes.* https://www.cms.gov/files/document/covid-toolkit-states-mitigate-covid-19-nursing-homes.pdf (accessed November 8, 2021).

CMS and CDC (Centers for Medicare & Medicaid Services and Centers for Disease Control and Prevention). 2020. *COVID-19 long-term care facility guidance.* https://www.cms.gov/files/document/4220-covid-19-long-term-care-facility-guidance.pdf (accessed August 25, 2021).

CNBC. 2020. *WHO: Coronavirus patients who don't show symptoms aren't driving the spread of the virus.* https://www.cnbc.com/video/2020/06/08/who-coronavirus-patients-who-dont-show-symptoms-arent-spreading-new-infections.html (accessed April 27, 2021).

Cohen, B., C. C. Cohen, B. Løyland, and E. L. Larson. 2017. Transmission of health care-associated infections from roommates and prior room occupants: A systematic review. *Clinical Epidemiology* 9:297–310.

Cohen, J., and Y. v. d. M. Rodgers. 2020. Contributing factors to personal protective equipment shortages during the COVID-19 pandemic. *Preventive Medicine* 141:106263–106263.

Connell, B. R., J. A. Sanford, and D. Lewis. 2007. Therapeutic effects of an outdoor activity program on nursing home residents with dementia. *Journal of Housing for the Elderly* 21(3–4):194–209.

Cutler, L. J., and R. A. Kane. 2006. As great as all outdoors. *Journal of Housing for the Elderly* 19(3–4):29–48.

D'Agata, E., M. B. Loeb, and S. L. Mitchell. 2013. Challenges in assessing nursing home residents with advanced dementia for suspected urinary tract infections. *Journal of the American Geriatrics Society* 61(1):62–66.

de Boer, B., H. C. Beerens, M. A. Katterbach, M. Viduka, B. M. Willemse, and H. Verbeek. 2018. The physical environment of nursing homes for people with dementia: Traditional nursing homes, small-scale living facilities, and green care farms. *Healthcare* 6(4):137.

Deandrea, S., F. Bravi, F. Turati, E. Lucenteforte, C. La Vecchia, and E. Negri. 2013. Risk factors for falls in older people in nursing homes and hospitals. A systematic review and meta-analysis. *Archives of Gerontology and Geriatrics* 56(3):407–415.

Demiris, G., D. P. Oliver, G. Dickey, M. Skubic, and M. Rantz. 2008. Findings from a participatory evaluation of a smart home application for older adults. *Technology and Health Care* 16(2):111–118.

Demiris, G., D. P. Oliver, J. Giger, M. Skubic, and M. Rantz. 2009. Older adults' privacy considerations for vision based recognition methods of eldercare applications. *Technology and Health Care* 17(1):41–48.

Denny-Brown, N., D. Stone, B. Hays, and D. Gallaghe. 2020. *COVID-19 intesifies nursing home workforce challenges.* Washington DC: Office of the Assistant Secretary for Planning and Evaluation, U.S. Department of Health and Human Services.

Desai, R., C. E. Williams, S. B. Greene, S. Pierson, and R. A. Hansen. 2011. Medication errors during patient transitions into nursing homes: Characteristics and association with patient harm. *American Journal of Geriatric Pharmacotherapy* 9(6):413–422.

Dichter, M. N., A. Berg, J. Hylla, D. Eggers, D. Wilfling, R. Möhler, B. Haastert, G. Meyer, M. Halek, and S. Köpke. 2021. Evaluation of a multi-component, non-pharmacological intervention to prevent and reduce sleep disturbances in people with dementia living in nursing homes (MoNoPol-sleep): Study protocol for a cluster-randomized exploratory trial. *BMC Geriatrics* 21(1):40.

DOJ (Department of Justice, Office of Public Affairs). 2015. *Nation's second-largest nursing home pharmacy to pay $9.25 million to settle kickback allegations.* https://www.justice.gov/opa/pr/nations-second-largest-nursing-home-pharmacy-pay-925-million-settle-kickback-allegations (accessed January 18, 2022).

Donelli, D., M. Antonelli, C. Bellinazzi, G. F. Gensini, and F. Firenzuoli. 2019. Effects of lavender on anxiety: A systematic review and meta-analysis. *Phytomedicine* 65: 153099.

Dong, X., R. Chen, and M. A. Simon. 2014. Elder abuse and dementia: A review of the research and health policy. *Health Affairs* 33(4):642–649.

Dwyer, L. L., L. D. Harris-Kojetin, R. H. Valverde, J. M. Frazier, A. E. Simon, N. D. Stone, and N. D. Thompson. 2013. Infections in long-term care populations in the United States. *Journal of the American Geriatrics Society* 61(3):341–349.

Edelman, L. S., J. Drost, R. P. Moone, K. Owens, G. L. Towsley, G. Tucker-Roghi, and J. E. Morley. 2021. Editorial: Applying the age-friendly health system framework to long term care settings. *Journal of Nutrition, Health & Aging* 25(2):141–145.

Edvardsson, D., D. Fetherstonhaugh, and R. Nay. 2010. Promoting a continuation of self and normality: Person-centred care as described by people with dementia, their family members and aged care staff. *Journal of Clinical Nursing* 19(17–18):2611–2618.

Eijkelenboom, A., H. Verbeek, E. Felix, and J. van Hoof. 2017. Architectural factors influencing the sense of home in nursing homes: An operationalization for practice. *Frontiers of Architectural Research* 6(2):111–122.

Ellis, B., and M. Hicken. 2017. *Sick, dying and raped in America's nursing homes.* https://www.cnn.com/interactive/2017/02/health/nursing-home-sex-abuse-investigation/ (accessed February 4, 2022).

Fedschun, T. 2019. *Nurse arrested in rape of woman in vegetative state who gave birth at care facility.* https://www.foxnews.com/us/nurse-arrested-in-rape-of-woman-in-vegetative-state-who-gave-birth-at-care-facility (accessed February 4, 2022).

FEMA (Federal Emergency Management Agency). 2016a. *Emergency support function #8—Public health and medical services annex.* https://www.fema.gov/sites/default/files/2020-07/fema_ESF_8_Public-Health-Medical.pdf (accessed August 12, 2021).

FEMA. 2016b. *Emergency support function #15—External affairs annex.* https://www.fema.gov/sites/default/files/2020-07/fema_ESF_15_External-Affairs.pdf (accessed September 24, 2021).

FEMA. 2020. *National Response Framework.* https://www.fema.gov/emergency-managers/national-preparedness/frameworks/response (accessed August 12, 2021).

FEMA. 2021. *About us.* https://www.fema.gov/about (accessed August 12, 2021).

Figueiro, M. G., B. A. Plitnick, A. Lok, G. E. Jones, P. Higgins, T. R. Hornick, and M. S. Rea. 2014. Tailored lighting intervention improves measures of sleep, depression, and agitation in persons with Alzheimer's disease and related dementia living in long-term care facilities. *Clinical Interventions in Aging* 9:1527–1537.

Figueroa, J. F., R. K. Wadhera, I. Papanicolas, K. Riley, J. Zheng, E. J. Orav, and A. K. Jha. 2020. Association of nursing home ratings on health inspections, quality of care, and nurse staffing with COVID-19 cases. *JAMA* 324(11):1103–1105.

Fischer, B. L., C. E. Gleason, R. E. Gangnon, J. Janczewski, T. Shea, and J. E. Mahoney. 2014. Declining cognition and falls: Role of risky performance of everyday mobility activities. *Physical Therapy* 94(3):355–362.

Forbes, D., C. M. Blake, E. J. Thiessen, S. Peacock, and P. Hawranik. 2014. Light therapy for improving cognition, activities of daily living, sleep, challenging behaviour, and psychiatric disturbances in dementia. *Cochrane Database Systematic Review* 2014(2):CD003946.

Galambos, C., M. Skubic, S. Wang, and M. Rantz. 2013. Management of dementia and depression utilizing in-home passive sensor data. *Gerontechnology* 11(3):457–468.

Galambos, C., M. Rantz, A. Craver, M. Bongiorno, M. Pelts, A. J. Holik, and J. S. Jun. 2019. Living with intelligent sensors: Older adult and family member perceptions. *Computers, Informatics, Nursing* 37(12):615–627.

GAO (U.S. Government Accountability Office). 2007. *Federal actions needed to improve targeting and evaluation of assistance by quality improvement organizations.* Washington DC: U.S. Government Accountability Office.

GAO. 2019a. *Nursing homes: Improved oversight needed to better protect residents from abuse.* Washington, DC: U.S. Government Accountability Office.

GAO. 2019b. *Elder abuse: Federal requirements for oversight in nursing homes and assisted living facilities differ.* Washington, DC: U.S. Government Accountability Office.

GAO. 2019c. *Nursing homes: Better oversight needed to protect residents from abuse, a statement for the record by John E. Dicken, director, health care.* Washington, DC: U.S. Government Accountability Office.

GAO. 2020. *Infection control deficiencies were widespread and persistent in nursing homes prior to COVID-19 pandemic.* Washington, DC: U.S. Government Accountability Office.

Gates, D., E. Fitzwater, and P. Succop. 2003. Relationships of stressors, strain, and anger to caregiver assaults. *Issues in Mental Health Nursing* 24(8):775–793.

Geng, F., D. G. Stevenson, and D. C. Grabowski. 2019. Daily nursing home staffing levels highly variable, often below CMS expectations. *Health Affairs* 38(7):1095–1100.

Gillespie, S. M., L. J. Gleason, J. Karuza, and M. N. Shah. 2010. Health care providers' opinions on communication between nursing homes and emergency departments. *Journal of the American Medical Directors Association* 11(3):204–210.

Giri, S., L. M. Chenn, and R. Romero-Ortuno. 2021. Nursing homes during the COVID-19 pandemic: A scoping review of challenges and responses. *European Geriatric Medicine* 12(6):1127–1136.

Goldstein, M., and R. Gebeloff. 2019. *Dozens of nursing homes with HUD-backed mortgages have 'serious deficiencies'.* https://www.nytimes.com/2019/06/24/business/nursing-homes-hud.html (accessed February 7, 2022).

Gozalo, P., S. Prakash, D. M. Qato, P. D. Sloane, and V. Mor. 2014. Effect of the Bathing Without a Battle training intervention on bathing-associated physical and verbal outcomes in nursing home residents with dementia: A randomized crossover diffusion study. *Journal of the American Geriatrics Society* 62(5):797–804.

Green House Project. 2012. *Pilot study finds meaningful savings in the Green House® model for eldercare*. https://thegreenhouseproject.org/wp-content/uploads/Cost_Savings_Summary_2012.pdf (accessed August 26, 2021).

Gulka, H. J., V. Patel, T. Arora, C. McArthur, and A. Iaboni. 2020. Efficacy and generalizability of falls prevention interventions in nursing homes: A systematic review and meta-analysis. *Journal of the American Medical Directors Association* 21(8):1024–1035.e1024.

Hado, E., and L. Friss Feinberg. 2020. Amid the COVID-19 pandemic, meaningful communication between family caregivers and residents of long-term care facilities is imperative. *Journal of Aging & Social Policy* 32(4–5):410–415.

Harnett, P. J., S. Kennelly, and P. Williams. 2020. A 10-step framework to implement integrated care for older persons. *Ageing International* 45(3):288–304.

Harrington, C., J. M. Wiener, L. Ross, and M. Musumeci. 2017. *Key issues in long-term services and supports quality*. https://www.kff.org/medicaid/issue-brief/key-issues-in-long-term-services-and-supports-quality (accessed August 25, 2021).

Harrington, C., L. Ross, S. Chapman, E. Halifax, B. Spurlock, and D. Bakerjian. 2020. Nurse staffing and coronavirus infections in California nursing homes. *Policy, Politics, and Nursing Practice* 21(3):174–186.

Hickman, S. E., A. L. Barrick, C. S. Williams, S. Zimmerman, B. R. Connell, J. S. Preisser, C. M. Mitchell, and P. D. Sloane. 2007. The effect of ambient bright light therapy on depressive symptoms in persons with dementia. *Journal of the American Geriatrics Society* 55(11):1817–1824.

Hodgson, N. A., L. N. Gitlin, L. Winter, and K. Czekanski. 2011. Undiagnosed illness and neuropsychiatric behaviors in community residing older adults with dementia. *Alzheimer Disease and Associated Disorders* 25(2):109–115.

Hoel, R. W., R. M. Giddings Connolly, and P. Y. Takahashi. 2021. Polypharmacy management in older patients. *Mayo Clinic Proceedings* 96(1):242–256.

HRW (Human Rights Watch). 2018. *"They want docile": How nursing homes in the United States overmedicate people with dementia*. New York: Human Rights Watch.

HRW. 2021. *U.S.: Concerns of neglect in nursing homes—Pandemic exposes need for improvements in staffing, oversight, accountability*. https://www.hrw.org/news/2021/03/25/us-concerns-neglect-nursing-homes# (accessed September 8, 2021).

Hughes, R. G. 2008. *Patient safety and quality: An evidence-based handbook for nurses*. Rockville, MD: Agency for Healthcare Research and Quality.

Hyer, K., L. M. Brown, L. Polivka-West, and A. Berman. 2010. Helping nursing homes prepare for disasters. *Health Affairs* 29(10):1961–1965.

IOM (Institute of Medicine). 1986. *Improving the quality of care in nursing homes*. Washington, DC: National Academy Press.

IOM. 2001. *Crossing the quality chasm: A new health system for the 21st century*. Washington, DC: National Academy Press.

IOM. 2012. *Crisis standards of care: A systems framework for catastrophic disaster response: Volume 1: Introduction and CSC framework*. Washington, DC: The National Academies Press.

IOM and NRC (Institute of Medicine and National Research Council). 2014. *Elder abuse and its prevention: Workshop summary*. Washington, DC: The National Academies Press.

Isaksson, U., U. H. Graneheim, and S. Åström. 2009. Female caregivers' experiences of exposure to violence in nursing homes. *Journal of Psychiatric and Mental Health Nursing* 16(1):46–53.

Iversen, M. H., A. Kilvik, and W. Malmedal. 2015. Sexual abuse of older residents in nursing homes: A focus group interview of nursing home staff. *Nursing Research and Practice* 2015:716407.

Jaffe, S. 2021. *After pandemic ravaged nursing homes, new state laws protect residents.* https://khn.org/news/article/after-pandemic-ravaged-nursing-homes-new-state-laws-protect-residents (accessed August 25, 2021).

Joosse, L. L. 2011. Sound levels in nursing homes. *Journal of Gerontological Nursing* 37(8):30–35.

Jump, R. L. P., C. J. Crnich, L. Mody, S. F. Bradley, L. E. Nicolle, and T. T. Yoshikawa. 2018. Infectious diseases in older adults of long-term care facilities: Update on approach to diagnosis and management. *Journal of the American Geriatrics Society* 66(4):789–803.

Kane, R. A., T. Y. Lum, L. J. Cutler, H. B. Degenholtz, and T.-C. Yu. 2007. Resident outcomes in small-house nursing homes: A longitudinal evaluation of the initial Green House program. *Journal of the American Geriatrics Society* 55(6):832–839.

Kennedy, C., and J. Will. 2021. Interventions for preventing abuse in the elderly. *International Journal of Nursing Practice* 27(1):e12870.

King, B. J., A. L. Gilmore-Bykovskyi, R. A. Roiland, B. E. Polnaszek, B. J. Bowers, and A. J. H. Kind. 2013. The consequences of poor communication during transitions from hospital to skilled nursing facility: A qualitative study. *Journal of the American Geriatrics Society* 61(7):1095–1102.

Kristiansen, L., O. Hellzén, and K. Asplund. 2006. Swedish assistant nurses' experiences of job satisfaction when caring for persons suffering from dementia and behavioural disturbances. An interview study. *International Journal of Qualitative Studies on Health and Well-being* 1(4):245–256.

Kua, C. H., V. S. L. Mak, and S. W. Huey Lee. 2019. Health outcomes of deprescribing interventions among older residents in nursing homes: A systematic review and meta-analysis. *Journal of the American Medical Directors Association* 20(3):362–372.e311.

Lachs, M. S., T. Rosen, J. A. Teresi, J. P. Eimicke, M. Ramirez, S. Silver, and K. Pillemer. 2013. Verbal and physical aggression directed at nursing home staff by residents. *Journal of General Internal Medicine* 28(5):660–667.

Lachs, M. S., J. A. Teresi, M. Ramirez, K. van Haitsma, S. Silver, J. P. Eimicke, G. Boratgis, G. Sukha, J. Kong, A. M. Besas, M. R. Luna, and K. A. Pillemer. 2016. The prevalence of resident-to-resident elder mistreatment in nursing homes. *Annals of Internal Medicine* 165(4):229–236.

Lachs, M., L. Mosqueda, T. Rosen, and K. Pillemer. 2021. Bringing advances in elder abuse research methodology and theory to evaluation of interventions. *Journal of Applied Gerontology* 40(11):1437–1446.

Lane, K. R., C. Galambos, L. J. Phillips, L. L. Popejoy, and M. Rantz. 2019. Aging in place: Transitional housing and supported housing models. In T. Fulmer and B. Chernof (eds.), *Handbook of geriatric assessment*. Burlington, MA: Jones & Bartlett Learning. Pp. 365–371.

Lane, S. J., and E. McGrady. 2016. Nursing home self-assessment of implementation of emergency preparedness standards. *Prehospital and Disaster Medicine* 31(4):422–431.

Lane, S. J., and E. McGrady. 2018. Measures of emergency preparedness contributing to nursing home resilience. *Journal of Gerontological Social Work* 61(7):751–774.

Laxton, C. E., D. A. Nace, and A. Nazir. 2020. Solving the COVID-19 crisis in post-acute and long-term care. *Journal of the American Medical Directors Association* 21(7):885–887.

Lee, S. W. H., V. S. L. Mak, and Y. W. Tang. 2019. Pharmacist services in nursing homes: A systematic review and meta-analysis. *British Journal of Clinical Pharmacology* 85(12):2668–2688.

Leipzig, R. M., R. G. Cumming, and M. E. Tinetti. 1999a. Drugs and falls in older people: A systematic review and meta-analysis: I. Psychotropic drugs. *Journal of the American Geriatrics Society* 47(1):30–39.

Leipzig, R. M., R. G. Cumming, and M. E. Tinetti. 1999b. Drugs and falls in older people: A systematic review and meta-analysis: II. Cardiac and analgesic drugs. *Journal of the American Geriatrics Society* 47(1):40–50.

Leland, N. E., S. J. Elliott, L. O'Malley, and S. L. Murphy. 2012. Occupational therapy in fall prevention: Current evidence and future directions. *American Journal of Occupational Therapy* 66(2):149–160.

Levy, K., L. Kilgour, and C. Berridge. 2019. Regulating privacy in public/private space: The case of nursing home monitoring laws. *Elder Law Journal* 26:323–363.

Lin, P. J., D. I. Kaufer, M. L. Maciejewski, R. Ganguly, J. E. Paul, and A. K. Biddle. 2010. An examination of Alzheimer's disease case definitions using Medicare claims and survey data. *Alzheimer's & Dementia* 6(4):334–341.

Lindbloom, E. J., J. Brandt, L. D. Hough, and S. E. Meadows. 2007. Elder mistreatment in the nursing home: A systematic review. *Journal of the American Medical Directors Association* 8(9):610–616.

Lum, T. Y., R. A. Kane, L. J. Cutler, and T.-C. Yu. 2008. Effects of Green House nursing homes on residents' families. *Health Care Financing Review* 30(2):35–51.

Lynch, R. M., and R. Goring. 2020. Practical steps to improve air flow in long-term care resident rooms to reduce COVID-19 infection risk. *Journal of the American Medical Directors Association* 21(7):893–894.

Malmedal, W., M. H. Iversen, and A. Kilvik. 2015. Sexual abuse of older nursing home residents: A literature review. *Nursing Research and Practice* 2015:902515.

Martin, J. L., and S. Ancoli-Israel. 2008. Sleep disturbances in long-term care. *Clinics in Geriatric Medicine* 24(1):39–50.

McCrystal, T., M. Burghardt, and S. Ferranti. 2010. *Buyer beware: OIG shines a spotlight on provider relationships with long term care pharmacies and scrutinizes contract pricing structures.* https://www.ropesgray.com/-/media/Files/in-the-news/2010/07/impact-of-omnicare-settlement-for-pharmacy-providers-and-long-term-care-facilities.pdf (accessed January 18, 2022).

McGarry, B. E., D. C. Grabowski, and M. L. Barnett. 2020. Severe staffing and personal protective equipment shortages faced by nursing homes during the COVID-19 pandemic. *Health Affairs* 39(10):1812–1821.

McGarry, B. E., G. K. SteelFisher, D. C. Grabowski, and M. L. Barnett. 2021. COVID-19 test result turnaround time for residents and staff in US nursing homes. *JAMA Internal Medicine* 181(4):556–559.

MedPAC (Medicare Payment Advisory Commission). 2021. *March 2021 report to the congress: Medicare payment policy.* Washington, DC: Medicare Payment Advisory Commission.

Meuleners, L. B., M. L. Fraser, M. K. Bulsara, K. Chow, and J. Q. Ng. 2016. Risk factors for recurrent injurious falls that require hospitalization for older adults with dementia: A population based study. *BMC Neurology* 16(1):188.

Meyer, D. L., B. Dorbacker, J. O'Rourke, J. Dowling, J. Jacques, and M. Nicholas. 1992. Effects of a "quiet week" intervention on behavior in an Alzheimer boarding home. *American Journal of Alzheimer's Care and Related Disorders and Research* 7(4):2–7.

Mishra, A. K., M. Skubic, M. Popescu, K. Lane, M. Rantz, L. A. Despins, C. Abbott, J. Keller, E. L. Robinson, and S. Miller. 2020. Tracking personalized functional health in older adults using geriatric assessments. *BMC Medical Informatics and Decision Making* 20(1):270.

Mitchell, S. L. 2021. *Care of patients with advanced dementia.* https://www.uptodate.com/contents/care-of-patients-with-advanced-dementia (accessed February 8, 2022).

MITRE (The MITRE Corporation). 2020. *Coronavirus Commission for Safety and Quality in Nursing Homes: Commission final report.* https://sites.mitre.org/nhCOVIDcomm/wp-content/uploads/sites/14/2020/09/FINAL-REPORT-of-NH-Commission-Public-Release-Case-20-2378.pdf (accessed August 20, 2021).

Mody, L., S. L. Krein, S. Saint, L. C. Min, A. Montoya, B. Lansing, S. E. McNamara, K. Symons, J. Fisch, E. Koo, R. A. Rye, A. Galecki, M. U. Kabeto, J. T. Fitzgerald, R. N. Olmsted, C. A. Kauffman, and S. F. Bradley. 2015. A targeted infection prevention intervention in nursing home residents with indwelling devices: A randomized clinical trial. *JAMA Internal Medicine* 175(5):714–723.

Mody, L., M. T. Greene, J. Meddings, S. L. Krein, S. E. McNamara, B. W. Trautner, D. Ratz, N. D. Stone, L. Min, S. J. Schweon, A. J. Rolle, R. N. Olmsted, D. R. Burwen, J. Battles, B. Edson, and S. Saint. 2017. A national implementation project to prevent catheter-associated urinary tract infection in nursing home residents. *JAMA Internal Medicine* 177(8):1154–1162.

Mody, L., K. J. Gontjes, M. Cassone, K. E. Gibson, B. J. Lansing, J. Mantey, M. Kabeto, A. Galecki, and L. Min. 2021. Effectiveness of a multicomponent intervention to reduce multidrug-resistant organisms in nursing homes: A cluster randomized clinical trial. *JAMA Network Open* 4(7):e2116555.

Montoya, A., and L. Mody. 2011. Common infections in nursing homes: A review of current issues and challenges. *Aging Health* 7(6):889–899.

Montoya, A., M. Cassone, and L. Mody. 2016. Infections in nursing homes: Epidemiology and prevention programs. *Clinics in Geriatric Medicine* 32(3):585–607.

Muir, S. W., K. Gopaul, and M. M. Montero Odasso. 2012. The role of cognitive impairment in fall risk among older adults: A systematic review and meta-analysis. *Age and Ageing* 41(3):299–308.

Munier-Marion, E., T. Bénet, C. Régis, B. Lina, F. Morfin, and P. Vanhems. 2016. Hospitalization in double-occupancy rooms and the risk of hospital-acquired influenza: A prospective cohort study. *Clinical Microbiology and Infection* 22(5):461.e467–461.e469.

Murray, T., and J. Friedman. 2020. *Nursing home safety during COVID: PPE shortages, seven months into pandemic, 20 percent of facilities lacked enough supplies.* https://uspirg.org/feature/usp/nursing-home-safety-during-covid-ppe-shortages (accessed November 29, 2021).

Musumeci, M., and P. Chidambaram. 2020. *Key questions about nursing home regulation and oversight in the wake of COVID-19.* https://www.kff.org/coronavirus-covid-19/issue-brief/key-questions-about-nursing-home-regulation-and-oversight-in-the-wake-of-covid-19 (accessed December 7, 2020).

Myhre, J., S. Saga, W. Malmedal, J. Ostaszkiewicz, and S. Nakrem. 2020. Elder abuse and neglect: An overlooked patient safety issue. A focus group study of nursing home leaders' perceptions of elder abuse and neglect. *BMC Health Services Research* 20(1):199.

Nakrem, S., A. G. Vinsnes, G. E. Harkless, B. Paulsen, and A. Seim. 2013. Ambiguities: Residents' experience of 'nursing home as my home'. *Internal Journal of Older People Nursing* 8(3):216–225.

Narang, P., M. El-Refai, R. Parlapalli, L. Danilov, S. Manda, G. Kaur, and S. Lippmann. 2010. Antipsychotic drugs: Sudden cardiac death among elderly patients. *Psychiatry (Edgmont)* 7(10):25–29.

National Consumer Voice (The National Consumer Voice for Quality Long-Term Care). 2021. *The devasting effect of lockdowns on residents of long-term care facilities during COVID-19.* https://theconsumervoice.org/uploads/files/issues/Devasting_Effect_of_Lockdowns_on_Residents_of_LTC_Facilities.pdf (accessed September 8, 2021).

NCEA (National Center on Elder Abuse). 2021a. *Research, statistics, and data.* https://ncea.acl.gov/What-We-Do/Research/Statistics-and-Data.aspx (accessed May 20, 2021).

NCEA. 2021b. *World Elder Abuse Awareness Day is June 15th.* https://ncea.acl.gov/WEAAD.aspx (accessed November 3, 2021).

Nguyen Thi, P. L., S. Briançon, F. Empereur, and F. Guillemin. 2002. Factors determining inpatient satisfaction with care. *Social Science and Medicine* 54(4):493–504.

NIA (National Institute on Aging). 2021. *The dangers of polypharmacy and the case for deprescribing in older adults.* https://www.nia.nih.gov/news/dangers-polypharmacy-and-case-deprescribing-older-adults#:~:text=Inappropriate%20polypharmacy%20%E2%80%94%20the%20use%20of,or%20causes%20a%20new%20one (accessed February 1, 2022).

Nursing Home Abuse Guide. 2021. *Financial abuse.* https://nursinghomeabuseguide.com/elder-abuse/financial (accessed November 8, 2021).

Nursing Home Abuse Justice. 2021. *Mandated reporting laws for elder abuse.* https://www.nursinghomeabuse.org/articles/elder-abuse-reporting-laws (accessed November 3, 2021).

Nygaard, A., L. Halvorsrud, E. K. Grov, and A. Bergland. 2020. What matters to you when the nursing is your home: A qualitative study on the views of residents with dementia living in nursing homes. *BMC Geriatrics* 20(1):227.

ODPHP (Office of Disease Prevention and Health Promotion, U.S. Department of Health and Human Services). 2021. *Adverse drug events.* https://health.gov/our-work/national-health-initiatives/health-care-quality/adverse-drug-events (accessed November 3, 2021).

Ogletree, A. M., R. Mangrum, Y. Harris, D. R. Gifford, R. Barry, L. Bergofsky, and D. Perfetto. 2020. Omissions of care in nursing home settings: A narrative review. *Journal of the American Medical Directors Association* 21(5):604-614.e606.

OIG (Office of the Inspector General). 2011. *Medicare atypical antipsychotic drug claims for elderly nursing home residents.* Washington, DC: Office of the Inspector General, U.S. Department of Health and Human Services.

OIG. 2012. *Gaps continue to exist in nursing home emergency preparedness and response during disasters: 2007–2010.* Washington, DC: Office of the Inspector General, U.S. Department of Health and Human Services.

OIG. 2014a. *Adverse events in skilled nursing facilities: National incidence among Medicare beneficiaries.* Washington DC: Office of the Inspector General, U.S. Department of Health and Human Services.

OIG. 2014b. *Hospital emergency preparedness and response during Superstorm Sandy.* Washington, DC: Office of the Inspector General, U.S. Department of Health and Human Services.

OIG. 2019. *Incidents of potential abuse and neglect at skilled nursing facilities were not always reported and investigated.* Washington DC: Office of the Inspector General, U.S. Department of Health and Human Services.

OIG. 2021. *CMS could improve the data it uses to monitor antipsychotic drugs in nursing homes.* Washington, DC: Office of the Inspector General, U.S. Department of Health and Human Services.

O'Mahony, D., D. O'Sullivan, S. Byrne, M. N. O'Connor, C. Ryan, and P. Gallagher. 2014. STOPP/START criteria for potentially inappropriate prescribing in older people: Version 2. *Age and Ageing* 44(2):213–218.

Ouslander, J. G., and D. C. Grabowski. 2020. COVID-19 in nursing homes: Calming the perfect storm. *Journal of the American Geriatrics Society* 68:2153–2162.

Passini, R., H. Pigot, C. Rainville, and M.-H. Tétreault. 2000. Wayfinding in a nursing home for advanced dementia of the Alzheimer's type. *Environment and Behavior* 32(5):684–710.

Pierce, J. R., S. K. Morley, T. A. West, P. Pentecost, L. A. Upton, and L. Banks. 2017. Improving long-term care facility disaster preparedness and response: A literature review. *Disaster Medicine and Public Health Preparedness* 11(1):140–149.

Pillemer, K., D. Burnes, C. Riffin, and M. S. Lachs. 2016. Elder abuse: Global situation, risk factors, and prevention strategies. *The Gerontologist* 56(Suppl 2):S194–S205.

Poon, E. G., C. A. Keohane, C. S. Yoon, M. Ditmore, A. Bane, O. Levtzion-Korach, T. Moniz, J. M. Rothschild, A. B. Kachalia, J. Hayes, W. W. Churchill, S. Lipsitz, A. D. Whittemore, D. W. Bates, and T. K. Gandhi. 2010. Effect of bar-code technology on the safety of medication administration. *New England Journal of Medicine* 362(18):1698–1707.

Popejoy, L. L., M. A. Khalilia, M. Popescu, C. Galambos, V. Lyons, M. Rantz, L. Hicks, and F. Stetzer. 2015. Quantifying care coordination using natural language processing and domain-specific ontology. *Journal of the American Medical Informatics Association* 22(e1):e93–e103.

Powell, T., D. Hanfling, and L. O. Gostin. 2012. Emergency preparedness and public health: The lessons of Hurricane Sandy. *JAMA* 308(24):2569–2570.

Pugh, T. 2020. *Flu shot mandates for nursing home staff urged as COVID persists.* https://news.bloomberglaw.com/health-law-and-business/flu-shot-mandates-for-nursing-home-staff-urged-as-covid-persists (accessed August 25, 2021).

Rabig, J., W. Thomas, R. A. Kane, L. J. Cutler, and S. McAlilly. 2006. Radical redesign of nursing homes: Applying the Green House concept in Tupelo, Mississippi. *The Gerontologist* 46(4):533–539.

Ramsey-Klawsnik, H. 2018. *Part 1: Understanding and working with adult protective services (APS).* https://ncea.acl.gov/NCEA/media/Publication/Understanding-and-Working-with-APS_May2018.pdf (accessed November 8, 2021).

Rantz, M. J., K. D. Marek, M. Aud, H. W. Tyrer, M. Skubic, G. Demiris, and A. Hussam. 2005. A technology and nursing collaboration to help older adults age in place. *Nursing Outlook* 53(1):40–45.

Rantz, M. J., R. T. Porter, D. Cheshier, D. Otto, C. H. Servey, 3rd, R. A. Johnson, M. Aud, M. Skubic, H. Tyrer, Z. He, G. Demiris, G. L. Alexander, and G. Taylor. 2008. Tigerplace, a state-academic-private project to revolutionize traditional long-term care. *Journal of Housing for the Elderly* 22(1–2):66–85.

Rantz, M. J., L. Phillips, M. Aud, L. Popejoy, K. D. Marek, L. L. Hicks, I. Zaniletti, and S. J. Miller. 2011. Evaluation of aging in place model with home care services and registered nurse care coordination in senior housing. *Nursing Outlook* 59(1):37–46.

Rantz, M., L. L. Popejoy, C. Galambos, L. J. Phillips, K. R. Lane, K. D. Marek, L. Hicks, K. Musterman, J. Back, S. J. Miller, and B. Ge. 2014a. The continued success of registered nurse care coordination in a state evaluation of aging in place in senior housing. *Nursing Outlook* 62(4):237–246.

Rantz, M., L. Popejoy, K. Musterman, and S. J. Miller. 2014b. Influencing public policy through care coordination research. In G. Lamb (ed.), *Care coordination: The game changer.* Silver Spring, MD: American Nurses Association. Pp. 203–220.

Rantz, M., K. Lane, L. J. Phillips, L. A. Despins, C. Galambos, G. L. Alexander, R. J. Koopman, L. Hicks, M. Skubic, and S. J. Miller. 2015. Enhanced registered nurse care coordination with sensor technology: Impact on length of stay and cost in aging in place housing. *Nursing Outlook* 63(6):650–655.

Rau, J. 2020. *Coronavirus stress test: Many 5-star nursing homes have infection-control lapses.* https://khn.org/news/coronavirus-preparedness-infection-control-lapses-at-top-rated-nursing-homes/ (accessed January 27, 2022).

Redmond, P., T. C. Grimes, R. McDonnell, F. Boland, C. Hughes, and T. Fahey. 2018. Impact of medication reconciliation for improving transitions of care. *The Cochrane Database of Systematic Reviews* 8(8):CD010791-CD010791.

Regnier, V. 2018. *Housing design for an increasingly older population: Redefining assisted living for the mentally and physically frail.* Hoboken, NJ: John Wiley & Sons.

Reid, J., K. Wilson, K. E. Anderson, and C. P. Maguire. 2015. Older inpatients' room preference: Single versus shared accommodation. *Age and Ageing* 44(2):331–333.

Reiling, J., R. Hughes, and M. Murphy. 2008. The impact of facility design on patient safety. In R. Hughes (ed.), *Patient safety and quality: An evidence-based handbook for nurses*. Rockville, MD: Agency for Healthcare Research and Quality.

Riemersma-van der Lek, R. F., D. F. Swaab, J. Twisk, E. M. Hol, W. J. Hoogendijk, and E. J. Van Someren. 2008. Effect of bright light and melatonin on cognitive and noncognitive function in elderly residents of group care facilities: A randomized controlled trial. *JAMA* 299(22):2642–2655.

Roubein, R. 2021. Will the nursing home of the future be an actual home? *Politico*, April 30. https://www.politico.com/news/agenda/2021/04/30/nursing-home-future-483460 (accessed November 29, 2021).

Sabatino, C. P., and C. Harrington. 2021. Policy change to put the home back into nursing homes. *BIFOCAL, Journal of the ABA Commission on Law and Aging* 42(6):119–125.

Sandvoll, A. M., E. K. Grov, and M. Simonsen. 2020. Nursing home residents' ADL status, institution-dwelling and association with outdoor activity: A cross-sectional study. *PeerJ* 8:e10202.

Schnelle, J. F., C. A. Alessi, N. R. Al-Samarrai, R. D. Fricker, Jr., and J. G. Ouslander. 1999. The nursing home at night: Effects of an intervention on noise, light, and sleep. *Journal of the American Geriatrics Society* 47(4):430–438.

Schwarz, B. 1997. Nursing home design: A misguided architectural model. *Journal of Architectural and Planning Research* 14(4):343–359.

Scott, A. M., J. Li, S. Oyewole-Eletu, H. Q. Nguyen, B. Gass, K. B. Hirschman, S. Mitchell, S. M. Hudson, and M. V. Williams. 2017. Understanding facilitators and barriers to care transitions: Insights from project achieve site visits. *Joint Commission Journal on Quality and Patient Safety* 43(9):433–447.

Shen, K. 2020. Relationship between nursing home COVID-19 outbreaks and staff neighborhood characteristics. *medRxiv*, December 6. https://doi.org/10.1101/2020.09.10.

Shen, Y., F. Sun, A. Zhang, and K. Wang. 2021. The effectiveness of psychosocial interventions for elder abuse in community settings: A systematic review and meta-analysis. *Frontiers in Psychology* 12:679541.

Siegel, J. D., E. Rhinehart, M. Jackson, and L. Chiarello. 2017. *Management of multidrug-resistant organisms in healthcare settings, 2006*. https://www.cdc.gov/infectioncontrol/pdf/guidelines/mdro-guidelines.pdf (accessed September 8, 2021).

Silow-Carroll, S., D. Peartree, S. Tucker, and A. Pham. 2021. *Fundamental nursing home reform: Evidence on single-resident rooms to improve personal experience and public health*. https://www.healthmanagement.com/wp-content/uploads/HMA.Single-Resident-Rooms-3.22.2021_final.pdf (accessed November 5, 2021).

Simmons, S., J. Schnelle, J. Slagle, N. A. Sathe, D. Stevenson, M. Carlo, and M. L. McPheeters. 2016. *Resident safety practices in nursing home settings, Technical briefs, no. 24*. Rockville, MD: Agency for Healthcare Research and Quality

Skubic, M., R. D. Guevara, and M. Rantz. 2015. Automated health alerts using in-home sensor data for embedded health assessment. *IEEE Journal of Translational Engineering in Health and Medicine* 3:1–11.

Sloane, P. D., V. J. Honn, S. A. R. Dwyer, J. Wieselquist, C. Cain, and S. Myers. 1995. Bathing the Alzheimer's patient in long term care: Results and recommendations from three studies. *American Journal of Alzheimer's Disease* 10(4):3–11.

Sloane, P. D., C. M. Mitchell, G. Weisman, S. Zimmerman, K. M. Foley, M. Lynn, M. Calkins, M. P. Lawton, J. Teresi, L. Grant, D. Lindeman, and R. Montgomery. 2002. The Therapeutic Environment Screening Survey for Nursing Homes (TESS-NH): An observational instrument for assessing the physical environment of institutional settings for persons with dementia. *Journals of Gerontology, Series B: Psychological Sciences* 57(2):S69–S78.

Sloane, P. D., C. S. Williams, C. M. Mitchell, J. S. Preisser, W. Wood, A. L. Barrick, S. E. Hickman, K. S. Gill, B. R. Connell, J. Edinger, and S. Zimmerman. 2007a. High-intensity environmental light in dementia: Effect on sleep and activity. *Journal of the American Geriatrics Society* 55(10):1524–1533.

Sloane, P. D., L. W. Cohen, C. S. Williams, J. Munn, J. S. Preisser, M. D. Sobsey, D. A. Wait, and S. Zimmerman. 2007b. Effect of specialized bathing systems on resident cleanliness and water quality in nursing homes: A randomized controlled trial. *Journal of Water and Health* 5(2):283–294.

Sloane, P. D., N. J. Brandt, A. Cherubini, T. S. Dharmarajan, D. Dosa, J. T. Hanlon, P. Katz, R. T. C. M. Koopmans, R. D. Laird, M. Petrovic, T. P. Semla, E. C. K. Tan, and S. Zimmerman. 2021. Medications in post-acute and long-term care: Challenges and controversies. *Journal of the American Medical Directors Association* 22(1):1–5.

Spanko, A. 2020. *New CMS push to target nursing homes in hotspots "misleading," "under-resourced."* https://skillednursingnews.com/2020/07/new-cms-push-to-target-nursing-homes-in-hotspots-misleading-under-resourced (accessed August 25, 2021).

Spinewine, A., P. Evrard, and C. Hughes. 2021. Interventions to optimize medication use in nursing homes: A narrative review. *European Geriatric Medicine* 12(3):551–567.

Stall, N. M., A. Jones, K. A. Brown, P. A. Rochon, and A. P. Costa. 2020. For-profit long-term care homes and the risk of COVID-19 outbreaks and resident deaths. *Canadian Medical Association Journal* 192(33):E946–E955.

Stiller, A., F. Salm, P. Bischoff, and P. Gastmeier. 2016. Relationship between hospital ward design and healthcare-associated infection rates: A systematic review and meta-analysis. *Antimicrobial Resistance & Infection Control* 5(1):51.

Stone, E., M. Skubic, M. Rantz, C. Abbott, and S. Miller. 2015. Average in-home gait speed: Investigation of a new metric for mobility and fall risk assessment of elders. *Gait Posture* 41(1):57–62.

Stone, P. W., C. T. A. Herzig, M. Agarwal, M. Pogorzelska-Maziarz, and A. W. Dick. 2018. Nursing home infection control program characteristics, CMS citations, and implementation of antibiotic stewardship policies: A national study. *Inquiry* 55:46958018778636.

Storey, J. E. 2020. Risk factors for elder abuse and neglect: A review of the literature. *Aggression and Violent Behavior* 50:101339.

Strausbaugh, L. J., and C. L. Joseph. 2000. The burden of infection in long-term care. *Infection Control and Hospital Epidemiology* 21(10):674–679.

Strausbaugh, L. J., S. R. Sukumar, C. L. Joseph, and K. P. High. 2003. Infectious disease outbreaks in nursing homes: An unappreciated hazard for frail elderly persons. *Clinical Infectious Diseases* 36(7):870–876.

Su, B. Y., M. Enayati, K. C. Ho, M. Skubic, L. Despins, J. Keller, M. Popescu, G. Guidoboni, and M. Rantz. 2019. Monitoring the relative blood pressure using a hydraulic bed sensor system. *IEEE Transactions on Biomedical Engineering* 66(3):740–748.

Tay, E. L., S. W. H. Lee, G. H. Yong, and C. P. Wong. 2018. A systematic review and meta-analysis of the efficacy of custom game based virtual rehabilitation in improving physical functioning of patients with acquired brain injury. *Technology and Disability* 30(1–2):1–23.

Terrell, K. M., and D. K. Miller. 2006. Challenges in transitional care between nursing homes and emergency departments. *Journal of the American Medical Directors Association* 7(8):499–505.

Thomas, K., R. Gebeloff, and J. Silver-Greenberg. 2021. *Phony diagnoses hide high rates of drugging at nursing homes.* https://www.nytimes.com/2021/09/11/health/nursing-homes-schizophrenia-antipsychotics.html (accessed November 8, 2021).

Thompson, D.-C., M.-G. Barbu, C. Beiu, L. G. Popa, M. M. Mihai, M. Berteanu, and M. N. Popescu. 2020. The impact of COVID-19 pandemic on long-term care facilities worldwide: An overview on international issues. *BioMed Research International* 2020:8870249.

TROPOS (Leibniz Institute for Tropospheric Research). 2020. *COVID-19: Indoor air in hospitals and nursing homes requires more attention: Recommendations on how to reduce SARS-CoV-2 aerosol dispersal.* www.sciencedaily.com/releases/2020/12/201214104710.htm (accessed January 27, 2022).

True, S., J. Cubanski, R. Garfield, M. Rae, G. Claxton, P. Chidambaram, and K. Orgera. 2020. *COVID-19 and workers at risk: Examining the long-term care workforce.* https://www.kff.org/coronavirus-covid-19/issue-brief/covid-19-and-workers-at-risk-examining-the-long-term-care-workforce (accessed August 25, 2021).

Truitt, E., R. Thompson, D. Blazey-Martin, D. NiSai, and D. Salem. 2016. Effect of the implementation of barcode technology and an electronic medication administration record on adverse drug events. *Hospital Pharmacy* 51(6):474–483.

University of Nebraska–Lincoln. 2021. *Ventilation in residential care environments.* Washington, DC: Office of Energy Efficiency and Renewable Energy, U.S. Department of Energy.

U.S. Congress, Senate, Committee on Finance. 2019. *Not forgotten: Protecting americans from abuse and neglect in nursing homes.* 116th Cong., March 6 (statement of Maya Fischer: Daughter of Sonja Fischer, Nursing Home Rape Victim). https://www.finance.senate.gov/imo/media/doc/Fischer%20Testimony.pdf (accessed February 4, 2022).

U.S. Senate Committee on Finance. 2018. *Sheltering in danger: How poor emergency planning and response put nursing home residents at risk during hurricanes Harvey and Irma.* https://www.finance.senate.gov/imo/media/doc/Sheltering%20in%20Danger%20Report%20(2%20Nov%202018).pdf (accessed September 14, 2021).

van den Berg, M. E. L., M. Winsall, S. M. Dyer, F. Breen, M. Gresham, and M. Crotty. 2019. Understanding the barriers and enablers to using outdoor spaces in nursing homes: A systematic review. *The Gerontologist* 60(4):e254–e269.

van Hoof, J., H. Verbeek, B. M. Janssen, A. Eijkelenboom, S. L. Molony, E. Felix, K. A. Nieboer, E. L. Zwerts-Verhelst, J. J. Sijstermans, and E. J. Wouters. 2016a. A three perspective study of the sense of home of nursing home residents: The views of residents, care professionals, and relatives. *BMC Geriatrics* 16(1):169.

van Hoof, J., M. L. Janssen, C. M. C. Heesakkers, W. van Kersbergen, L. E. J. Severijns, L. A. G. Willems, H. R. Marston, B. M. Janssen, and M. E. Nieboer. 2016b. The importance of personal possessions for the development of a sense of home of nursing home residents. *Journal of Housing for the Elderly* 30(1):35–51.

van Zadelhoff, E., H. Verbeek, G. Widdershoven, E. van Rossum, and T. Abma. 2011. Good care in group home living for people with dementia. Experiences of residents, family and nursing staff. *Journal of Clinical Nursing* 20(17–18):2490–2500.

Verbeek, H., E. Van Rossum, S. M. Zwakhalen, G. I. Kempen, and J. P. Hamers. 2009. Small, homelike care environments for older people with dementia: A literature review. *International Psychogeriatrics* 21(2):252–264.

Verrue, C. L., M. Petrovic, E. Mehuys, J. P. Remon, and R. Vander Stichele. 2009. Pharmacists' interventions for optimization of medication use in nursing homes: A systematic review. *Drugs Aging* 26(1):37–49.

Vlaeyen, E., J. Coussement, G. Leysens, E. Van der Elst, K. Delbaere, D. Cambier, K. Denhaerynck, S. Goemaere, A. Wertelaers, F. Dobbels, E. Dejaeger, and K. Milisen. 2015. Characteristics and effectiveness of fall prevention programs in nursing homes: A systematic review and meta-analysis of randomized controlled trials. *Journal of the American Geriatrics Society* 63(2):211–221.

Wang, L., I. Norman, T. Xiao, Y. Li, and M. Leamy. 2021. Psychological first aid training: A scoping review of its application, outcomes and implementation. *International Journal of Environmental Research and Public Health* 18(9).

Wang, R., L. Chen, L. Fan, D. Gao, Z. Liang, J. He, W. Gong, and L. Gao. 2015. Incidence and effects of polypharmacy on clinical outcome among patients aged 80+: A five-year follow-up study. *PLoS One* 10(11):e0142123.

Waters, R. 2021. The big idea behind a new model of small nursing homes. *Health Affairs* 40(3):378–383.

Wegerer, J. 2017. *The connection between UTIs and dementia.* https://www.alzheimers.net/2014-04-03-connection-between-utis-and-dementia (accessed February 8, 2022).

Welsh, T. J., A. McGrogan, and A. Mitchell. 2020. Deprescribing in the last years of life—It's hard to STOPP. *Age and Ageing* 49(5):723–724.

Werner, R. M., A. K. Hoffman, and N. B. Coe. 2020. Long-term care policy after COVID-19—Solving the nursing home crisis. *New England Journal of Medicine* 383(10):903–905.

Wiener, J. M., M. P. Freiman, D. Brown, and RTI International. 2007. *Nursing home care quality: Twenty years after the Omnibus Budget Reconciliation Act of 1987.* Durham, North Carolina: RTI International.

Wood, K., N. Mehri, N. Hicks, and J. M. Vivoda. 2020. Family satisfaction: Differences between nursing homes and residential care facilities. *Journal of Applied Gerontology* 40(12):1733–1742.

Woodbridge, R., M. P. Sullivan, E. Harding, S. Crutch, K. J. Gilhooly, M. Gilhooly, A. McIntyre, and L. Wilson. 2018. Use of the physical environment to support everyday activities for people with dementia: A systematic review. *Dementia* 17(5):533–572.

Woolcott, J. C., K. J. Richardson, M. O. Wiens, B. Patel, J. Marin, K. M. Khan, and C. A. Marra. 2009. Meta-analysis of the impact of 9 medication classes on falls in elderly persons. *Archives of Internal Medicine* 169(21):1952–1960.

Wrublowsky, R. 2018. *Design guide for long-term care homes.* https://www.fgiguidelines.org/wp-content/uploads/2018/03/MMP_DesignGuideLongTermCareHomes_2018.01.pdf (accessed September 8, 2021).

Wu, M. C., H. C. Sung, W. L. Lee, and G. D. Smith. 2015. The effects of light therapy on depression and sleep disruption in older adults in a long-term care facility. *International Journal of Nursing Practice* 21(5):653–659.

Yon, Y., M. Ramiro-Gonzalez, C. R. Mikton, M. Huber, and D. Sethi. 2019. The prevalence of elder abuse in institutional settings: A systematic review and meta-analysis. *European Journal of Public Health* 29(1):58–67.

Yurkofsky, M., and J. G. Ouslander. 2021. *COVID-19: Management in nursing homes.* https://www.uptodate.com/contents/covid-19-management-in-nursing-homes (accessed July 8, 2021).

Zhu, X., H. Lee, H. Sang, J. Muller, H. Yang, C. Lee, and M. Ory. 2022. Nursing home design and COVID-19: Implications for guidelines and regulation. *Journal of the American Medical Directors Association* 23(2):272–279.e271.

Zimmerman, S., B. J. Bowers, L. W. Cohen, D. C. Grabowski, S. D. Horn, P. Kemper, and the THRIVE Research Collaborative. 2016. New evidence on the Green House model of nursing home care: Synthesis of findings and implications for policy, practice, and research. *Health Services Research* 51(Suppl 1):475–496.

Zimmerman, S., C. Dumond-Stryker, M. Tandan, J. S. Preisser, C. J. Wretman, A. Howell, and S. Ryan. 2021. Nontraditional small house nursing homes have fewer COVID-19 cases and deaths. *Journal of the American Medical Directors Association* 22(3):489–493.

Payment and Financing

Ideally, payment and financing for nursing home care and services would be designed to support access to services, a high quality of care, equity, and efficiency. The current system in the United States falls short in achieving those goals, however. This chapter of the report reviews the current payment and financing and framework for nursing home care and services and identifies high-priority challenges that the nation needs to address in order to improve the quality of care in nursing homes.

PAYING FOR NURSING HOME CARE

The United States devotes a significant share of national health expenditures to nursing home care. Spending on nursing homes[1] reached $172.7 billion in 2019, representing 5 percent of total health expenditures (CMS, 2019a; Martin et al., 2020). Three payers account for the majority of funds that go to nursing home services: the federal Medicare program, the federal–state Medicaid program, and private payers. In 2020, Medicaid paid for the care of 62 percent of all nursing home residents, Medicare for 12 percent of all nursing home residents, and private payers for the remaining 26 percent (KFF, 2020).[2]

Nursing homes serve two broad groups of residents: long-stay residents and those individuals who are discharged to a nursing home to receive post-acute care after a hospital stay. Within each group, there is significant diversity among the populations. Medicaid is the dominant payer for long-stay

---

[1] Total expenditures on care provided in nursing homes and continuing care retirement communities.

[2] Of the total number of nursing homes, 97.5 percent are Medicare certified, and 95.2 percent are Medicaid certified (Harris-Kojetin et al., 2019).

residents, who typically are individuals with chronic illness and who have an average length of stay in a nursing home setting of approximately 2 years. Care for this patient population consists largely of providing assistance with activities of daily living such as bathing, dressing, eating, toileting, and walking (see Chapter 4). To qualify for Medicaid-funded nursing home care, an individual must meet state-established medical eligibility criteria and satisfy income and asset thresholds (Sollitto, 2021).

Medicare is the dominant payer for post-acute care nursing home patients, also referred to as short-stay residents, who have an average length of stay of approximately 25 days (Werner et al., 2013). Medicare-certified nursing homes also provide skilled, rehabilitative care to individuals following an acute-care hospital stay (Harris-Kojetin et al., 2019). The goal of this care is to help people achieve and maintain their highest level of functioning (see Chapter 4). To qualify for services, a Medicare beneficiary covered by the traditional fee-for-service (FFS) Medicare program[3] must require daily skilled nursing or rehabilitative therapy services, generally within 30 days of an inpatient hospital stay of at least 3 days in length as an inpatient[4] and must be admitted to the nursing home as a result of a condition related to that hospital stay (CMS, 2019b).

An individual may transition between post-acute and long-stay settings over time. Consider, for example, a community-dwelling individual who is hospitalized and then discharged to a nursing home. In some cases, the nursing home will discharge the individual back to the community, while at other times the person will remain as a long-stay resident at the same facility. Similarly, a long-stay nursing home resident who is hospitalized may then return to the nursing home as a post-acute patient before transitioning back to a long-stay setting. Many of these individuals who transition across settings are beneficiaries of both Medicare and Medicaid. For these people, known as dually eligible individuals, Medicare pays for the hospital and short-stay nursing home care, and Medicaid pays for long-stay nursing home care.

This fragmented payment system, with Medicare paying for short-term post-acute care, and Medicaid paying for long-term nursing home care, often creates perverse incentives across the settings of care with significant implications for nursing home care and financing (Grabowski, 2007). For example, the Medicaid program has less incentive to prevent Medicare-financed hospitalizations, while the Medicare program has less incentive to prevent newly admitted nursing home patients from transitioning to long-stay Medicaid status.

---

[3] This refers to individuals covered under the traditional fee-for-service Medicare program, in contrast to those enrolled in Medicare Advantage plans.

[4] This requirement was waived during the COVID-19 pandemic.

Medicare Coverage and Payment

Although Medicare pays for a relatively small percentage of those receiving nursing home care, it is an important payer of health care services for nursing home residents. On average, Medicare paid for only 12 percent of the total bed-days in nursing homes nationwide, but accounted for nearly 27 percent of overall revenues in 2019 (CRS, 2020; KFF, 2020). Medicare is considered a generous payer of post-acute care nursing home services. Medicare margins, or the amount Medicare pays relative to the cost to treat beneficiaries in skilled nursing facilities (SNFs), have averaged more than 14 percent over the past 11 years. The Medicare Payment Advisory Commission (MedPAC) has called for better alignment of Medicare payments with the cost of SNF care (MedPAC, 2020).

Under traditional FFS Medicare, Part A covers inpatient hospital care, SNF care, some home health care, and as discussed further below, hospice care. Medicare Part B covers physician visits, outpatient services, preventive services, and some home health services (KFF, 2019). Medicare covers all necessary services for post-acute care patients, including room and board, nursing care, and ancillary services such as drugs, laboratory tests, and physical therapy. Medicare covers up to 100 days of nursing home care for an episode of acute illness and recovery. For the first 20 days of a benefit period, Medicare pays 100 percent of the cost of care. From day 21 on, most patients become responsible for a substantial daily copayment. For fiscal year 2021, the copayment was $185.50 per day (MedPAC, 2021a). Medicaid, for dually eligible individuals, or Medicare Supplemental insurance (Medigap), for those individuals who have purchased that coverage, typically cover that copayment (CMS, 2021a).

The Medicare Advantage (MA) program, also known as Part C, provides an alternative to traditional Medicare. Through the MA program, discussed further below, Medicare beneficiaries can sign up for coverage through a health maintenance organization or preferred provider organization and receive coverage for Medicare Part A and Part B benefits, as well as Part D (outpatient prescription drug benefits) (KFF, 2019). More than half (51 percent) of Medicare beneficiaries had traditional Medicare along with some type of supplemental coverage including Medigap, employer-sponsored insurance, and Medicaid, while 39 percent were enrolled in a Medicare Advantage plan as of 2018 (Koma et al., 2021).

Patient-Driven Payment Model

In October 2019, Medicare implemented a new payment system for nursing home care known as the patient-driven payment model (PDPM). This new payment system replaced the case-mix model, which was based on resource utilization groups[5] that heavily weighted payments according to the volume of therapy use (e.g., number of weekly therapy minutes provided to residents). The PDPM shifts the emphasis away from volume toward value, and takes into account factors related to the patient's underlying complexity of condition and clinical needs. This change is designed to be budget neutral and to align payment incentives with quality incentives (McGarry et al., 2021).

The previous payment system had long been criticized for promoting rehabilitation therapy services to nursing home residents that were often deemed excessive and unnecessary. The share of days classified as rehabilitation increased from 78 percent in 2002 to 95 percent in 2018 (MedPAC, 2020). The Department of Justice, for its part, has investigated and brought cases against nursing homes for improper billing for medically unnecessary and excessive therapy services.[6]

The implementation of the new payment model coincided with the beginning of the COVID-19 pandemic. Thus, it will take some time to understand the overall impact of the new payment model. However, early research suggests that the shift to PDPM is associated with reduced therapy staffing (McGarry et al., 2021) and services (Rahman et al., 2022). The Medicare Payment Advisory Commission has found nursing homes have continued to make double-digit Medicare margins under the PDPM (MedPAC, 2020). The COVID-19 pandemic, for its part, led to a significant reduction in post-acute care in nursing homes. One early study showed, for example, that from 2019 to 2020, admissions to nursing homes for post-acute care declined 51 percent, resulting in a 55 percent decline in spending on post-acute care (Werner and Bressman, 2021). Further research will determine whether the reduction in post-acute care admissions is a short-term response to the pandemic or an indication of a longer-term change in post-acute care utilization.

Medicare's Hospice Benefit

As discussed in Chapter 4, Medicare provides a separate hospice benefit for beneficiaries who are expected to live 6 months or less. It is important to note Medicare will not pay for nursing home care and hospice care in a nursing home simultaneously (CMS, 2022a; Fausto, 2018; Span, 2012). Medicare pays hospice agencies a per-person daily rate to provide a range of palliative care services that reflect residents' preferences for end-of-life care as specified in their care plans. Medicare first introduced the hospice benefit in 1983, and the benefit's use and associated program spending has grown

---

[5] Resource utilization groups classify nursing home residents according to their clinical and functional statuses as identified from Minimum Data Set data supplied by the nursing home.

[6] See https://www.foley.com/en/insights/publications/2020/03/skilled-nursing-facilities-target-area-doj-fca (accessed February 14, 2022).

steadily; Medicare hospice expenditures rose from less than $3 billion in 2000 to nearly $21 billion in 2019. Moreover, the share of Medicare beneficiaries who die in hospice care has increased from 22 percent in 2000 to more than 50 percent in 2019 (MedPAC, 2021a; Sheingold et al., 2015). Medicare's hospice benefit paid for services provided to more than 1.6 million beneficiaries in 2019 (MedPAC, 2021a).

Medicare's daily per-beneficiary rate is paid to hospice agencies irrespective of the amount of services provided to the patient on a given day. Hospice agencies may find caring for patients in nursing home settings more profitable than caring for patients in home settings because of the efficiencies of treating patients in a centralized location, the overlap in responsibilities between the hospice and the nursing home, and the ability of nursing homes to serve as referral sources for new patients (MedPAC, 2020; OIG, 2018).

The Medicare Payment Advisory Commission and the Office of the Inspector General have expressed concern that hospice providers may be selectively enrolling nursing home residents with longer hospice stays and less complex care needs, thereby generating higher profit margins (MedPAC, 2008; OIG, 2011; Sheingold et al., 2015; Teno and Higginson, 2018; Wachterman et al., 2011). One study found that the growth in hospice care for nursing home residents was associated with less aggressive care near death. At the same time, the study revealed that increased hospice care was associated with an overall increase in Medicare expenditures (Gozalo et al., 2015). To address these concerns, the Center for Medicare and Medicaid Innovation launched an initiative to include the Part A Hospice benefit through the Value-Based Insurance Design model, which is discussed further below.[7]

Medicaid Coverage and Payment

Medicaid is the federal–state program for low-income individuals who meet the program's eligibility requirements; Medicaid provides coverage to 20 percent of the U.S. population (KFF, 2019). Medicaid covers a range of long-term services and supports (LTSS) including home- and community-based services (HCBS) that enable individuals to live in community settings as well as institutional care provided in nursing home settings. The overall share of funds going to HCBS as compared to nursing homes has shifted significantly over the past two decades. Although HCBS spending varies considerably across states, slightly more than 40 percent of Medicaid LTSS spending went to nursing homes in fiscal year (FY) 2016, compared to 20 years ago when nursing homes received more than 80 percent of Medicaid's LTSS spending (Rudowitz et al., 2019). Despite the increased funding for

---

[7] See https://innovation.cms.gov/innovation-models/vbid-hospice-benefit-overview (accessed February 2, 2020).

HCBS, nearly 200,000 Medicaid beneficiaries are on waiting lists for home-based care services (KFF, 2018).

Medicaid pays a fixed daily rate to cover the cost of care, room, meals, and medical supplies (ACA, 2021). States are guaranteed federal matching funds for services provided to Medicaid-eligible individuals. The federal match rate is determined by a formula and varies by state, ranging from a match of at least 50 percent, to a high of 75 percent in poorer states (Rudowitz et al., 2019).

Each state's Medicaid program uses a variety of methods to set payment rates for Medicaid nursing home residents (Grabowski et al., 2004a; MACPAC, 2019). In general, nursing homes must submit cost reports which the state Medicaid programs use to establish rates which fall into two broad categories:

- *Facility-specific or cost-based:* a nursing home's rate is based on its reported per diem costs subject to certain limitations, and
- *Facility-independent or price:* the same rate is paid to a group of homes based on costs reported by homes with similar characteristics subject to certain limitations.

As an incentive for nursing homes to control costs, states will set rates prospectively using prior year (or years) cost reports. States typically group costs from the cost reports into a series of cost centers including direct care, indirect care, administration, and capital. Each cost center has an associated cap or spending limit. The incentive to control costs increases when states do not update rates using more recent cost reports but instead adjust rates over time for inflation using an exogenous measure of price changes. Most states allow bed-hold payments when a resident takes a short leave of absence from the facility for an inpatient hospital stay or a therapeutic leave (visit with family). The majority of states adjust their Medicaid payment rates for case mix to ensure access for residents with more extensive care needs. These adjustments may be for individual residents or may be tied to the average case mix of a nursing home (CMS, 2021b). As discussed below, some states also use incentive-based Medicaid payments for high-performing facilities.

Medicaid Spend Down

To qualify for Medicaid coverage for nursing home care, individuals must meet both income and asset thresholds. The asset standard is often the key barrier to qualifying for Medicaid, because individuals can treat medical expenditures against the income standard in most states. Individuals can have no more than $2,000 in assets if single and no more than $3,000 if married (Johnson et al., 2021).[8] For married individuals, there

---

[8] Income rules for Medicaid eligibility vary by state.

are also spousal impoverishment provisions that protect a certain amount of the couple's combined resources for the spouse living in the community in determining Medicaid eligibility. Some assets are also set aside and not counted when determining Medicaid nursing home eligibility such as the value of the home (up to state-set limit), one vehicle, burial space, and life insurance policies (up to a limit). If individuals have assets above the limit, they must "spend down" their assets until they qualify for Medicaid (Johnson et al., 2021).

Long-term nursing home use has been identified as a key predictor of transition into Medicaid as many older adults face significant unplanned costs of long-term care—particularly as even a semi-private room in a nursing home can cost more than $100,000 per year, far exceeding the median income and savings of older adults (Jacobson et al., 2017; Keohane et al., 2017; Wiener et al., 2013) (see Box 7-1 below).

Private Payers

A small percentage of people pay privately for nursing home services. Private-pay residents' payments are market based and reflect rates set by the nursing home. Unlike other health services for which insurers influence payment rates, long-term care insurance plays almost no role in determining private-pay nursing home rates. Only 11 percent of people over age 65 have long-term care insurance, and the policies almost always provide a specified daily dollar benefit (Johnson, 2016; McGarry and Grabowski, 2019a). A private-pay resident in a nursing home would be responsible to pay any difference between the specified benefit and the agreed-upon nursing home charge.

BOX 7-1
Family Member Perspective

"My mother had a private room because she paid out of pocket, spending the last $200,000 of my parents' lifetime savings before depleting her bank account. One more month, and she would have gone on Medicaid."

— Daughter and caregiver of two parents
with dementia who needed nursing home care

This quote was collected from the committee's online call for resident, family, and nursing home staff perspectives.

VARIABILITY BETWEEN MEDICARE AND MEDICAID PAYMENTS

The adequacy of Medicaid payment rates has been a perennial issue. A consensus exists across a broad range of stakeholders—including providers (AHCA, 2021), financial analysts (Rutledge et al., 2019), government (MedPAC, 2020), and researchers (Troyer, 2002)—that because of higher Medicare payment rates, Medicare short-stay nursing home patients generate higher profit margins than Medicaid residents (Grabowski, 2007). For its part, the MedPAC has called attention to double-digit Medicare margins in nursing homes for many years (MedPAC, 2020).

Medicaid rates may be deemed inadequate because they are lower than a nursing home's average daily cost (HHC and AHCA, 2018; Liberman, 2018). Medicaid rates may also be deemed inadequate if the nursing home's costs are insufficient to provide a minimally acceptable quality of care (HHC and AHCA, 2018; Mor et al., 2004; Rau, 2017), a condition that is particularly difficult to assess. Consequently, the following discussion will be limited to how Medicaid payment rates compare with nursing homes' actual costs.

Using Medicare cost reports, MedPAC found that non-Medicare nursing home days, for which Medicaid is the largest payer, are associated with a negative margin (MedPAC, 2021a). Cost reports reflect either expenses that the nursing homes paid or accounting costs. However, not all of the costs that a nursing home reports may be necessary for delivering care. Further contributing to the difficulty of assessing Medicaid payment adequacy is the fact that nursing home cost reports are rarely audited (Harrington et al., 2021).

Reaching a qualitative judgment about Medicaid payment adequacy is possible through a review of how Medicaid programs set nursing home rates. Rates are based on the costs that nursing homes report with limits on how much of those costs are allowed or incorporated into rates and with how frequently more recent cost information is used to update rates (Harrington and Swan, 1984; MACPAC, 2019). The likely results of such a review would be that Medicaid rates cover the cost of care for Medicaid residents for different shares of nursing homes across states (MACPAC, 2019). For example, a state with limits that exclude few costs—excluding costs only above the 80th percentile, for example—and that are rebased annually using this year's cost reports to set next year's rates would have a substantial share of nursing homes with Medicaid rates exceeding the cost of care. Another state with stricter limits—at the 50th percentile, for example—and with less frequent rebasing using cost reports that are several years old would have fewer homes with Medicaid rates exceeding care costs.

When the Medicaid payment rate exceeds the average cost of care, rates may be seen as adequate by this test. However, when the Medicaid rate is less than average costs of Medicaid residents' care, it still may be adequate to cover the incremental or marginal costs of care (HHC and AHCA, 2018; Liberman, 2018), depending on a nursing home's overall business operations and payment arrangements. As noted above, nursing homes have three major payers for care, and the prices for each payer are determined separately. The Medicare and Medicaid programs establish the price or payment rates administratively. The market or an agreement between the resident and the facility determines the private pay rate (Fiedler, 2021). Economists refer to a business operating in this situation as a *price-discriminating firm*. A price-discriminating firm maximizes revenue or profit by serving customers who pay the incremental cost of serving them and some share of fixed costs. Such a firm may want a customer who pays less than the average cost to avoid losing profit when more of the fixed costs are paid by other customers. For example, if Medicare is covering fixed costs, Medicaid only has to cover the incremental cost of treating a nursing home resident. A nursing home would be forgoing profit to turn this resident away even if the resident did not cover the average costs of care.

For this reason, nursing homes historically have served Medicaid residents when Medicaid rates were less than their average costs. However, under this scenario a nursing home could not exist on Medicaid payments alone. This is consistent with evidence suggesting that nursing homes that close are more likely to have been financed predominantly by Medicaid and located in poorer neighborhoods with greater numbers of minority residents (Feng et al., 2011; Mor et al., 2004). A considerable number of closures among high-Medicaid-financed nursing homes in rural areas have occurred over the past few years (Healy, 2019).

Existing law requires that state Medicaid programs' payments are adequate to provide access to care of sufficient quality.[9] States are required to provide assurances that their payment rates meet this criterion.[10] For certain providers, the Centers for Medicare & Medicaid Services (CMS) requires that states also submit evidence that their payment rates are indeed adequate. However, nursing home payment rates are not subject to this requirement despite Medicaid's significant role as a payer of nursing home care. The lack of transparency or accountability in payment, flow of funds, and nursing home finances makes it extremely difficult to assess the adequacy of current Medicaid payments, and is discussed further in Chapter 8.

---

[9] Social Security Act, Title XIX §1902(a)(30)(A), 42 U.S. Code §1396a, 89th Cong., 1st sess. (July 30, 1965).

[10] CMS Requirements, Medical Assistance Program—Payments for Services, 42 CFR §447 (1978).

VALUE-BASED PAYMENT MODELS AND THE IMPACT ON QUALITY OF CARE

Traditionally, the most common approach to paying for U.S. health care services has been the FFS payment system, which pays for the quantity or intensity of services rendered, regardless of patient outcomes. Payment systems based on quantity have been called out as a key barrier to quality improvement (IOM, 2001), and various approaches to improving the quality of care in nursing homes have focused on shifting from paying for quantity to paying for quality using a strategy known as value-based payment (VBP). VBP encompasses an array of initiatives and terminology, a small sampling of which are shown in Box 7-2. VBP approaches have been used to pay for both chronic and acute care in nursing homes.

Value-Based Payment for Chronic Care

Payers began experimenting with value-based payment (VBP) in the nursing home setting four decades ago, beginning with pay-for-performance (P4P) approaches. P4P approaches are designed to provide incentives to health care providers to achieve high levels of performance or improvements in performance on specific quality measures (Briesacher et al., 2009; Werner et al., 2010). For example, as part of a test of establishing P4P in nursing homes in San Diego in 1980, financial incentives were awarded to 36 randomly selected nursing homes. These incentives were in addition to regular nursing home payments, and were linked to the improved functional or health status of the patient while a resident in the nursing home. Research revealed that residents of nursing homes in the test group had a greater likelihood of going home or going to a nursing home that provided less intensive care than the control group. Moreover, residents of nursing homes in the test group had lower rates of hospitalization or death than people in the control group of nursing homes (Norton, 1992). Despite these results, P4P was not more commonly implemented in nursing homes settings until the early 2000s.

Beginning in 2002, a number of state Medicaid agencies implemented P4P programs, with financial bonuses to nursing homes linked to the quality of chronic care delivered, typically in the form of a small per diem add-on for achieving the quality goals set out in the program (Kane et al., 2007; Werner et al., 2010). Although these programs varied by state, one evaluation of these P4P programs found a similar pattern of quality improvement in some areas and not others. For example, the evaluation revealed that states that implemented P4P had higher rates of improvement on three clinical quality measures—the percentage of residents being physically restrained, the percentage in moderate to severe pain, and the percentage who developed pressure sores—than in states that did not implement P4P. The impact of P4P on structural process measures such as total number of deficiencies and

> **BOX 7-2**
> **Terminology of Value-Based Payment**
>
> **Value-based payment (VBP)** is a payment system (fee-for-service [FFS] or otherwise) with some linkage to quality, value, or infrastructure.
>
> An **accountable care organization (ACO)** is an alternative payment model in which groups of doctors, hospitals, and other health care providers come together voluntarily to provide coordinated high-quality care to their patients to ensure that patients receive the right care at the right time while avoiding unnecessary duplication of services and preventing medical errors. ACOs assume responsibility for the total cost of care for a population. When an ACO effectively provides high-quality care and controls health care spending, the ACO shares in the savings it achieves for the insurer.
>
> **The alternative payment model (APM)**, according to the Centers for Medicare & Medicaid Services, is a "specific subcategory of value-based purchasing initiatives that require providers to make fundamental changes in the way they provide care" and that "shift financial incentives further away from volume by linking provider payments to both quality and total cost of care results" (CMS, 2015). Thus, providers take on substantial financial risk to deliver high-quality care at lower costs, typically across health care providers and settings. APMs can apply to a specific medical condition, an episode of care, or a patient population.
>
> **Bundled payments** are a form of APM in which doctors, hospitals, and other health care providers receive a fixed price for an episode of care. Also known as episode-based payments, bundled payments require providers to assume risk since they are responsible for covering costs that exceed the target price for an episode of care. On the other hand, providers share in the savings if they do not exceed the target price and maintain quality.[11]
>
> **Capitated payment arrangements** can take two forms. Under a global capitation arrangement, health care providers receive a single, fixed payment for all the health care services given to a patient, including primary care, hospitalizations, and specialist care. Under partial or blended capitation agreements, health care providers receive a monthly payment that covers a set of services provided to a patient, such as laboratory services or primary care. All other care is reimbursed using an FFS model. Some but not all VBP approaches use capitated payment arrangements.
>
> **Pay-for-performance (P4P)** is a form of VBP that provides a financial bonus to health care providers if they meet or exceed agreed-upon quality or performance measures. P4P programs can also impose financial penalties on providers that fail to achieve specified goals or cost savings. Typically, P4P models add a quality or value incentive to an FFS model. Unlike APMs, P4P programs to do not put providers at substantial risk or hold providers accountable for total costs of care across providers or settings.
>
> SOURCES: CMS, 2015, 2021b; Murphy and LaPointe, 2016; Werner et al., 2021.

---

[11] In contrast to diagnosis-related group payments, which pay for hospital stays using a prospectively determined payment rate based upon the patient's diagnosis, bundled payments typically encompass an episode of care that spans care settings (e.g., hospital and post-acute care settings).

nurse staffing, however, was not associated with improvements in quality. The evaluation found that deficiency rates worsened slightly under P4P, while there was no change in staffing levels (Werner et al., 2013).

VBP for Chronic and Post-Acute Care

In 2009, CMS launched a 3-year voluntary nursing home value-based purchasing demonstration in Arizona, New York, and Wisconsin to test nursing home P4P models that included financial incentives tied to long-stay and post-acute nursing home quality measures (White et al., 2006). Evaluators judged nursing homes' performance using hospitalization rates, a set of quality measures, staffing levels, and survey inspections and found no systematic changes in the quality measures. Arizona achieved Medicare savings in the first year of the demonstration, as did Wisconsin for the first 2 years, while there were no savings in New York. Nursing homes made limited or no changes as a result of the demonstration (Grabowski et al., 2017). Given the lack of evidence for success, this 3-year demonstration project ended in 2012.

VBP for Post-Acute Care

As part of the 2014 Protecting Access to Medicare Act,[12] CMS implemented the skilled nursing facility value-based purchasing (SNF VBP)[13] program across all Medicare-certified nursing homes in 2018 (CMS, 2019c). The program assesses facility performance using a single risk-adjusted hospital readmission measure to generate performance scores and payment incentives. To date, this program has not demonstrated an effect on readmission rates. In the program's first year, FY 2019, 26 percent of facilities earned positive incentives and 72 percent earned negative incentives, compared with 19 percent positive and 65 percent negative incentives in the second year, FY 2020 (Daras et al., 2021). Nursing homes that were not-for-profit, larger in size, and located in rural areas were more likely to receive positive incentives, as were facilities that had the highest registered nurse staffing levels (Daras et al., 2021). Nursing homes in lower-income neighborhoods, those with a majority of residents who were of a minority race or ethnicity, and those with larger populations of frail older adults were more likely to be penalized (Hefele et al., 2019; Qi et al., 2020).

---

[12] Protecting Access to Medicare Act of 2014, Public Law 113-93; 42 USC 1305, 113th Cong., 2nd Sess. (April 1, 2014).

[13] As noted in Chapter 2, the term nursing home is used throughout the report for consistency, but skilled nursing facility is used in this section on post-acute care, the largest portion of which is provided in a SNF.

MedPAC is required by law to review the progress of the SNF VBP and make recommendations. In its June 2021 report, MedPAC identified five key design flaws of the program:[14]

(1) The SNF VBP program assesses performance using a single outcome measure—all-cause readmissions—despite the fact that quality entails multiple measureable dimensions.
(2) Thresholds set in advance—referred to as "cliffs"—may not be the best approach to encouraging quality improvement.
(3) The SNF VBP puts aside a share of the incentive payments as program savings instead of paying out the entire sum as incentives to nursing homes.
(4) SNF VBP's minimum stay amounts are too low to ensure that the program rewards actual performance, instead of random variation.
(5) The program does not take into account the variation in the social risk factors of nursing home patient populations; as a result, nursing homes with high-risk populations are at a disadvantage (MedPAC, 2021b).

Based on the identification of these key weaknesses, MedPAC recommended that Congress eliminate Medicare's SNF VBP program and instead establish a new nursing home value incentive program. MedPAC's recommendations called for Medicare to design the program to evaluate a limited set of performance measures, incorporate strategies to ensure reliable measure results, develop a way to reduce the impact of the "cliffs," use a peer-grouping approach to take into account differences in patient social risk factors, and distribute all the savings to providers (MedPAC, 2021b).

Impact of VBP on Health Equity

The positive impact from implementation of P4P and related VBP in nursing homes has been limited, with gains largely confined to a narrow range of targeted measures and limited, if any, evidence for meaningful improvements in the overall quality of care (Grabowski et al., 2017; Werner et al., 2013). Importantly, prior research has suggested that VBP may have unintended consequences on nursing homes that serve a high proportion of Medicaid recipients or residents from minority populations. Nursing homes located in low-income ZIP codes are more likely to have hospital readmission rates that exceed the nursing home VBP threshold and therefore must pay financial penalties (Qi et al., 2020). Nursing homes that have populations that include more than 50 percent Black residents as well as homes

---

[14] The first three items refer to elements that are required by statute.

serving Hispanic or Latinx residents and those funded by Medicaid are also more likely to receive penalties under the nursing home SNF VBP (Hefele et al., 2019). These findings are consistent with evidence in other health care sectors, where providers' structural and patient case-mix characteristics are significant predictors of provider performance in VBP programs (Chen et al., 2017; Gilman et al., 2015a,b; Ryan, 2013). These unintended effects are often the result of disparities between providers, rather than disparities within providers (Werner et al., 2013). As a result of disparities between providers, financial penalties are levied differentially on providers that care for a disproportionate share of low-income, Black, or Medicaid-insured individuals (Abrahamson, 2020; Damberg et al., 2014; Edelman, 2015; Sandhu et al., 2020).

Alternative Payment Models for Nursing Home Care

Partially in response to the lack of effectiveness of P4P approaches, more recent Medicare and Medicaid programs have implemented alternative payment models (APMs) for nursing home care. APMs are a type of VBP that holds providers financially accountable for the quality and cost of care delivered to patients. The majority of P4P models add a quality or value incentive to an FFS model (Delbanco, 2014). In contrast, APMs place greater emphasis on shifting as much revenue as possible to risk-based or population-based payments.

More than 40 percent of Medicare beneficiaries receive post-acute care after a hospital discharge (Tian, 2016), the largest portion of which takes place in a SNF (Werner and Konetzka, 2018). Medicare FFS is the predominant payer of SNF stays (Singletary et al., 2021). In 2018, for example, Medicare paid for 2.2 million SNF stays among Traditional Medicare beneficiaries, which cost a total of $28.5 billion (MedPAC, 2020). The amount spent on SNF stays is not only large but growing: between 2004 and 2010, Medicare spending on SNF stays increased an average of almost 8 percent a year and, since then, has continued to trend upwards, though at a slower rate (MedPAC, 2020). Large geographic variation in post-acute care spending (Newhouse and Garber, 2013) has led many to question the value of post-acute care, and has fueled payment reform efforts designed to control spending on post-acute care. APMs have been introduced, in part, to limit the growing cost of post-acute SNF care.

Increases in post-acute SNF care are driven in part by Medicare's fee-for-service payment system, which pays separately for acute and post-acute care. Additionally, Medicare pays a *per diem* rate for SNF care, which may result in SNF stays that are longer than optimal—where the costs to the payer of one additional day in a SNF may outweigh the marginal benefit to the patient for that day (Werner et al., 2019a).

In an effort to reduce unnecessary SNF utilization, Medicare has had a long-standing copayment policy for FFS beneficiaries. Medicare pays in full for the first 20 days of a SNF benefit period. The 21st day however, triggers an increase in the daily copayment from $0 to more than $185 (MedPAC, 2021a; Werner et al., 2019a). The result of this policy is that a large number of patients are discharged on their 20th day of a SNF stay (Chatterjee et al., 2019a). It may also result in stays that are longer than necessary preceding the 20th day of a SNF stay, as the FFS payment may encourage SNFs to keep patients in the facility as long as possible (Werner et al., 2019a).

Until recently, few incentives existed to minimize SNF use or SNF length of stay. Recent developments, including Medicare payment reforms focused on controlling total costs of care combined with the growing number of enrollees in MA plans, have led to the availability of other options to control costs and reduce unnecessary utilization (Werner et al., 2021). Most notably, bundled payment and accountable care organizations (ACOs) are increasingly holding providers accountable for the costs of care across provider types and episodes of care. Post-acute care has become a common target as providers seek ways to reduce the costs of care.

As a result of these financial pressures, post-acute care utilization is changing, both in terms of the number of people receiving post-acute care services as well as in terms of the intensity of use of post-acute care, reflected in changes in measures of intensity (such as length of stay or number of therapy hours). Patients are being discharged to the home setting more frequently (potentially with arrangements for home health care) instead of being discharged to a SNF (Barnett et al., 2019a; Finkelstein et al., 2018; McWilliams et al., 2018). Discharge to the home may be a suitable option for only the healthiest patients (Werner et al., 2019b) and SNF use remains a common and costly option (Tian, 2016). Among those who are admitted to SNFs, the intensity of care they receive is also changing as a result of APMs, with shorter lengths of SNF stays among people who are discharged to a SNF after a hospital stay (Barnett et al., 2019a; McWilliams et al., 2018).

Research indicates that the declines in SNF utilization may be associated with documented increases in the need for care at home (Bressman et al., 2021), as Medicare beneficiaries increasingly require assistance from informal caregivers and other non-Medicare-reimbursed home care aides after hospital discharge. These trends in increasing caregiver burden may intensify with the implementation of APMs (Chatterjee et al., 2019b), which are accelerating the decline of SNF utilization. Such effects, however, could be mitigated by increasing home-based supports for older adults and by providing enhanced support to caregivers through training and financial compensation, such as the Money Follows the Person demonstration project (Musumeci et al., 2019).

Episode-Based Payment for Post-Acute Care

Under the existing FFS payment system, hospitals and nursing homes receive separate payments for care and do not coordinate the care they provide to patients across these settings. To control costs while improving quality of care, Medicare introduced the Bundled Payments for Care Improvement Initiative (BPCI) in 2013[15] and the Comprehensive Care for Joint Replacement Model (CJR) in 2016,[16] both authorized by the 2010 Affordable Care Act. BPCI pays hospitals and health care providers based on episodes of care rather than on a FFS basis (Parekh et al., 2017). BCPI is a voluntary program designed to shift overall financial responsibility to hospitals for all hospital and post-hospital services associated with a single episode of care. At its inception, BPCI included coverage for 48 clinical episodes ranging from treatment for congestive heart failure and stroke to lower joint replacement (mainly hip and knee), the latter of which is the most common clinical category of post-acute care (Rolnick et al., 2020). CJR, in contrast, is a mandatory program implemented in 67 markets at its inception that covers all hip and knee replacements. While BPCI ended in 2018, it was replaced by BPCI Advanced,[17] which extends BPCI to include more episodes, longer episode windows, and more downside risk (CMS, 2022b).

Hospitals have developed a number of strategies to strengthen their relationships with SNFs to exert influence over the quality and cost of post-acute SNF care for their referred patients. A study of 22 hospitals and health systems participating in either Medicare's Comprehensive Care for Joint Replacement model or the BCPI model found that common strategies hospitals used to strengthen their relationships with SNFs included creating networks of preferred SNFs to monitor the quality and cost of SNF post-acute care. "Common coordination strategies included sharing access to electronic medical records, embedding providers across facilities, hiring dedicated care coordination staff, and creating platforms for data sharing" (Zhu et al., 2018). (See Chapter 9 for discussion of health information technology in nursing homes.)

Research has found that cost savings achieved under alternative payment models are driven almost entirely by a decrease in the use of institutional post-acute care, with patients being discharged to home settings more frequently instead of being discharged to a nursing home (Finkelstein et al., 2018). In addition, some studies observed declines in nursing home

---

[15] See https://innovation.cms.gov/innovation-models/bundled-payments (accessed October 21, 2021).

[16] See https://innovation.cms.gov/innovation-models/cjr (accessed October 21, 2021).

[17] BPCI Advanced qualifies as an Advanced APM under the Quality Payment Program. See https://innovation.cms.gov/innovation-models/bpci-advanced (accessed February 14, 2022).

length of stay under episode-based payments which ranged from 0.1 days to 2.1 days; these reductions were not associated with an increase in readmission rates for patients (Barnett et al., 2019a; McWilliams et al., 2018).

There is concern about potential unintended consequences of any new payment approach; thus, careful monitoring for signs of such consequences is critical as bundled payments are applied to a broader array of conditions. The BPCI Advanced program will generate additional data critical to strengthening the existing evidence base on bundled payments. These data, and data specifically collected to monitor the effects of the program on health equity, should be used to monitor and address any unintended consequences of this payment model (Liao et al., 2020).

Bundled payment models are not unique to the U.S. health care system. Payers in other nations are also looking to alternative payment models that offer incentives to health care providers to increase value while containing costs of care. An eight-country study of the impact of bundled-payment models on health care value examined 23 bundled payment–model initiatives in the United States and seven other nations.[18] The study reviewed a total of 35 research studies on various aspects of the bundled-payment model. Nearly all the studies (32 out of 35) examined the impact of the model on health care quality and spending, and a majority of those studies (20 out of 32) found that bundled-payment initiatives were associated with limited savings or modest reduction in the growth of health care spending. More than half of the studies (18 out of 32) noted improvements in most of the measures of quality that were evaluated. The study concluded that bundled-payment models have the potential to result in lower health care spending with either an improvement in or no impact on quality. Importantly, the studies did not evaluate patient experiences of care under the payment model (Struijs et al., 2020).

Accountable Care Organizations

The other common APM implemented in nursing homes is an accountable care organization. An ACO typically consists of a group of clinicians, hospitals, and other health care providers who work together to provide coordinated, high-quality care to their Medicare patients. According to CMS, the goal of establishing an ACO is "to ensure that patients get the right care at the right time, while avoiding unnecessary duplication of services and preventing medical errors. When an ACO succeeds both in delivering high-quality care and spending health care dollars more wisely, the ACO will share in the savings it achieves for the Medicare program" (CMS, 2021c).

---

[18] Other countries studied included Denmark, England, Netherlands, New Zealand, Portugal, Sweden, and Taiwan.

Currently, the largest Medicare ACO is the Medicare Shared Savings Program. Medicare ACOs affect nursing home care in three main ways: (1) when a nursing home is a provider in an ACO; (2) when nursing home residents are attributed to an ACO; and (3) when a nursing home leads an ACO, focusing on managing all care for long-term care residents. Accumulating evidence suggests that the first two cases result in higher quality for post-acute care and chronic care, and in nursing homes being more appropriately used for post-acute care (Agarwal and Werner, 2018; Chang et al., 2019, 2021; Colla et al., 2016). There is little evidence to date, however, of the effect of nursing home–led ACOs, which may have the largest potential impact in terms of addressing the misalignment introduced by multiple payers for nursing home care (Chang et al., 2019, 2021).

Accountable Care Organizations for Post-Acute Care

In theory, ACOs may seek to reduce unnecessary nursing home use to reduce costs and, in cases when individuals do use nursing home care, to coordinate care across hospitals and nursing homes. In practice, however, the evidence suggests that ACOs largely generate savings by reducing nursing home use (Barnett et al., 2019b; McWilliams et al., 2017). Although an increasing number of hospitals participate in an ACO, fewer nursing homes do: half of all ACOs formally include at least one post-acute service in the ACO, and only 18 to 33 percent of ACOs include a nursing home (Colla et al., 2016; OIG, 2017). Those ACOs that reported having a formal relationship with a post-acute provider were more likely to report providing care aimed at improving transitions and coordinating care for patients (Colla et al., 2016). Those Medicare beneficiaries who were discharged from ACO-affiliated hospitals to ACO-affiliated skilled nursing facilities had better patient outcomes—lower hospital readmission rates, shorter hospital lengths of stay, and lower Medicare costs—than beneficiaries cared for by non-ACO-participating providers and also than beneficiaries treated at the ACO-affiliated hospitals before their ACO affiliation (Agarwal and Werner, 2018).

Accountable Care Organizations for Chronic Care

ACOs for long-stay nursing home residents are relatively limited; less than 25 percent are attributed to a Medicare ACO, and approximately 1.6 percent of all U.S. nursing homes are ACO providers (Chang et al., 2019). Available research indicates a potential beneficial effect of ACOs in a number of key domains, including enhancing care coordination across multiple settings, reducing unnecessary hospitalizations, and lessening the fragmentation caused by multiple payers. A study that examined outcomes among ACO-attributed nursing home residents found that compared with a matched cohort of non-attributed residents, ACO-attributed residents had fewer hospitalizations for ambulatory care–sensitive conditions and fewer outpatient visits. The study did not find any difference, however, in total expenditures between the two resident cohorts (Chang et al., 2021).

There are few examples of nursing home–led ACOs. One known example is the long-term care (LTC) ACO, the first ACO focused on Medicare beneficiaries residing in long-term care facilities. More than 200 long-term care facilities participate in the LTC ACO, which launched in 2016 and is a subsidiary of Genesis HealthCare. A formal evaluation of this ACO has not been completed.

State Medicaid programs are also beginning to offer ACO programs that, in addition to primary and acute medical care, may also be responsible for long-term care. However, the challenge for nursing home-led Medicare ACOs and Medicaid ACOs is that to effectively serve Medicare–Medicaid enrollees they must operate across both the Medicare and Medicaid programs. This has been difficult to coordinate and often creates conflicting financial incentives (Collette, 2020; Leavitt Partners, 2017; Matulis and Lloyd, 2018).

Alternative Payment Models and Health Disparities

Many experts believe that APMs are promising approaches to meaningfully improve quality of care and constrain health care spending. Although the evidence is not yet complete (Baicker and Chernew, 2017; Burns and Pauly, 2018), early research in nursing home settings suggests this may be the case. At the same time, concerns about the impact of APMs on disparities exist, much as they do for P4P programs. Because sicker patients who need more care become economically unattractive under APMs, providers may avoid caring for complex patients. Evidence to date from settings outside of nursing homes does not support this concern, with evidence of no decrease in access to care for vulnerable older adults or Black patients under BPCI (Joynt Maddox et al., 2019a; Navathe et al., 2018). Similarly, while ACOs are more likely to locate in well-resourced communities (Yasaitis et al., 2016), once they do, research suggests that they do not decrease access to care for Black or low-income patients (Lee et al., 2020).

APMs may nonetheless worsen disparities between participating providers. Hospitals that participate in the voluntary BPCI programs tended to be better resourced (Joynt Maddox et al., 2019b). For-profit and public hospitals that participated in BPCI were less likely to drop out of the program than nonprofits (Joynt Maddox et al., 2018).

Managed Care in Medicare and Medicaid

Managed care in the Medicare program takes the shape of what are known as Medicare Advantage (MA) plans. These plans cover chronic care and post-acute care services.

Medicare Advantage Plans for Chronic Care

MA does not typically pay directly for long-stay care in a nursing home. However, Medicare special needs plans (SNPs) are a subcategory of coordinated care plans limited to beneficiaries with specific diseases or characteristics. These SNPs customize benefits, provider choices, and drug formularies to align with the specific needs of their beneficiaries. Authorized by Congress in 2003, SNPs were first available in 2006. Various laws, including the Affordable Care Act in 2010, have extended authority for SNPs, and more recently the Bipartisan Budget Act of 2018, which included the CHRONIC Care Act (SNP Alliance, 2021),[19] permanently authorized SNPs. Nearly 4 million Medicare beneficiaries are currently enrolled in SNPs, and these beneficiaries accounted for approximately 15 percent of total MA enrollment in 2021 (Freed et al., 2021).

There are three types of SNPs. The first type, the chronic condition SNP (C-SNP), is limited to Medicare beneficiaries with severe or disabling chronic conditions. Currently there are 15 SNP-specific chronic conditions that allow eligibility for C-SNP benefits.[20] Approximately 10 percent of SNP enrollees are in C-SNPs (Freed et al., 2021). C-SNPs might be applicable to the long-term care setting as those individuals may receive post-acute care in a nursing home following a hospital stay (Stefanacci and Pakizegee, 2020).

The second type of SNP, the institutional SNP (I-SNP), is a specialized form of MA that is limited to Medicare beneficiaries who are long-term residents of a nursing home (CMS, 2016). These plans were designed to facilitate the alignment of financial incentives of nursing homes and Medicare with the companion goal of improving care delivery across various health care settings (MedPAC, 2013). Individuals in I-SNPs account for 2 percent of SNP enrollees (Freed et al., 2021). While Medicaid (or a private payer) is still responsible for the costs of long-term nursing home care, the I-SNP plan is financially responsible for Medicare-eligible health care costs, which provides a strong incentive for the plans to make investments to improve care provided in nursing home settings (Goldfeld et al., 2013).

---

[19] Bipartisan Budget Act of 2018, Public Law 115-123; 115th Cong., 2nd sess. 42 USC 1305 (February 9, 2018).

[20] For the complete list of conditions, see https://www.cms.gov/Medicare/Health-Plans/SpecialNeedsPlans/C-SNPs (accessed November 4, 2021).

Developed out of a demonstration of the Evercare model[21] (Kane et al., 2002), I-SNPs use advanced practice clinicians, such as nurse practitioners (NPs), to coordinate and deliver care in conjunction with I-SNP members' primary care physicians, nursing home staff, and other providers. This enhanced care is provided with no additional cost to the patient or nursing facility. The advanced practice clinicians create a comprehensive care plan for each I-SNP member, which is then shared with all members of the care team. APRNs and NPs provide primary, acute, and preventive care for I-SNP members and hold family care conferences to help identify the resident's medical, behavioral, and social needs; to establish goals of care; to specify therapeutic approaches; to coordinate care with specialists; and to manage the resident's treatment. The goal of this enhanced care model is to use onsite advanced practice clinicians to reduce residents' unnecessary hospitalizations, working together with a health plan that is responsible financially for the nursing home and medical care of the residents. Regulations require that an individual must have a 3-day stay in a hospital to qualify for Medicare Part A benefits in a SNF. An important feature of the I-SNP is that the plan waives that requirement and enables an individual to receive SNF skilled services without a qualifying hospital stay. The I-SNP's team of advanced practice clinicians is focused on effective medical management to enable them to identify and treat a patient's change in condition early and thereby reduce unnecessary and avoidable ED visits and hospitalizations (McGarry and Grabowski, 2019b).

An early CMS-sponsored evaluation of the I-SNP model showed improvement in quality for I-SNP-insured nursing home residents, with 50 percent lower rates of hospitalizations compared with other nursing home residents and resulting reductions in spending. The evaluation estimated that each NP saved an average of approximately $103,000 a year in hospital costs per NP (Kane et al., 2003).

A more recent evaluation found that compared with traditional Medicare FFS nursing home residents, I-SNP beneficiaries had lower rates of use of inpatient and emergency department services and higher use of skilled nursing facility care, which resulted in lower overall spending (McGarry and Grabowski, 2019b).

The third type of SNP is the dual SNP or D-SNP. Nearly 90 percent of SNP enrollees are in D-SNPs (Freed et al., 2021). The Affordable Care Act of 2010 authorized a type of D-SNP known as the fully integrated dual eligible (FIDE) SNP. FIDE SNPs give states expanded authority and flexibility to more closely integrate Medicare and Medicaid services. FIDE SNPs are required to provide Medicaid LTSS as well as Medicare benefits

---

[21] See https://innovation.cms.gov/Medicare-demonstrations/evercare-demonstration (accessed October 21, 2021).

and are required to have established arrangements to promote alignment between the two programs. FIDE SNPs are the most integrated delivery model outside of the Program of All Inclusive Care for the Elderly[22] and the Financial Alignment Initiative demonstrations, and they are the only D-SNP plans that are financially at risk for all Medicare and Medicaid services (Verdier et al., 2015).

Little evidence exists about the effects of FIDE SNPs on the value of nursing home care. One study reviewed the Minnesota Senior Health Option, a care model administered by FIDE SNPs, and found decreased hospitalizations and emergency department use (Anderson and Feng, 2016). Another study found that enrollment in the FIDE SNP reduced hospital readmission among dually enrolled members in a program in California (Sorbero et al., 2018).

More recently, the Bipartisan Budget Act of 2018[23] provided permanent legal authorization for D-SNPs and included requirements for a new D-SNP category, the highly integrated dual eligible (HIDE) SNP, introduced in 2021. In contrast to a FIDE SNP, a HIDE SNP is required to provide (directly or through a Medicaid managed care plan) either LTSS or behavioral health services as well as other Medicaid services to its dual eligible members (CMCS, 2019; MACPAC, 2021; Serna et al., 2022).

Medicare Advantage (MA) Plans for Post-Acute Care

MA plans cover post-acute SNF care for beneficiaries with a demonstrated need. These plans, unlike FFS plans, are able to negotiate contracts with nursing homes. MA plans pay for beneficiaries' services out of the monthly capitated payments the plans receive for each covered member. MA plans have a greater ability to manage their enrollees' use of nursing homes and can restrict the enrollees' choice of providers to those considered to be high-value providers (MedPAC, 2015). Some research has found that MA beneficiaries are more likely than FFS beneficiaries to enter low-quality nursing homes after hospital discharge (Meyers et al., 2018). Other studies, however, have found that MA beneficiaries also have better outcomes than their FFS Medicare counterparts, including lower rates of hospital readmission and higher rates of return to the community, though they also appeared to be healthier at baseline (Huckfeldt et al., 2017).

Prior research revealed lower SNF use and shorter SNF length of stay for common conditions among MA beneficiaries than among those enrolled

---

[22] For more information, see https://www.medicaid.gov/medicaid/long-term-services-supports/program-all-inclusive-care-elderly/index.html (accessed November 4, 2021).

[23] Bipartisan Budget Act of 2018, Public Law 115-123; 42 USC 1305, 115th Cong., 2nd Sess. (February 9, 2018).

in traditional Medicare (Huckfeldt et al., 2017). Some of this difference may be related to healthier beneficiaries enrolling in MA plans (Kumar et al., 2018). It may also reflect the higher level of cost sharing that MA beneficiaries might assume for SNF care (depending upon the specific MA plan they are enrolled in) compared with FFS beneficiaries, or the use of management strategies that MA plans apply to limit the use of SNF services (Gadbois et al., 2018; Keohane et al., 2015). Research also indicates that MA enrollees tend to enter lower-star-rated nursing homes than traditional Medicare beneficiaries (Meyers et al., 2018).

Including Hospice in Medicare Advantage Plans

CMS launched a 4-year demonstration of a new value-based insurance design model for hospice care in January 2021. The demonstration, known as the hospice "carve-in," addresses the fragmentation of care and fiscal responsibility for hospice care discussed earlier in this chapter. The model will evaluate the inclusion of the Medicare Part A hospice benefits in MA plans with the provision of palliative care, transitional concurrent care, and supplemental benefits. Participating MA plans will be financially responsible for Medicare Part A and Part B benefits.

Patients will have the choice of an in-network or out-of-network provider in the first 2 years of the demonstration, though palliative care, transitional concurrent care, and supplemental benefits will be available only to patients receiving care from in-network providers. MA plans participating in the demonstration program cannot implement cost sharing that would be higher than the amount allowed under original Medicare for hospice services provided in network or out of network (CMS, 2021d).

Medicaid Managed Care

In recent years, state Medicaid programs have started to turn to managed care plans to administer LTSS benefits. About half of all states have managed care contractors, though not all of those states use managed care plans to administer the nursing home benefit. Instead, they may focus only on in-home and community LTSS services. Using the Medicaid Section 1115 demonstrations, 25 states offered Medicaid managed care programs as of 2020, up from 8 states in 2004 (Libersky et al., 2018; MACPAC, 2022). States using a managed care plan for nursing homes may set payment rates for nursing homes or delegate that responsibility to the managed care plan (Nelb, 2020).

Research has yet to shed much light on the quality of nursing home care in managed care organization (MCO) networks. One study of a demonstration project in California found that the MCOs developed a wide network of nursing homes but selected nursing homes for the network without paying sufficient attention to quality criteria. Nursing homes in the network scored significantly lower on selected quality measures than non-network nursing homes (Graham et al., 2018).

Achieving Health Equity through Alternative Payment Models

Research has not yet provided evidence that VBP has improved—or even directly focused on—access to care or health outcomes for populations with social risk factors, including racial and ethnic minorities, rural populations, and individuals with disabilities (Liao et al., 2020). CMS has focused on monitoring the unintended effects of VBP among populations with social risk factors (Liao et al., 2020). For VBP to be effective, however, it must tackle head on the root causes of persistent health inequities and disparities in access and quality, namely, systemic bias and underperformance in the health care system for at-risk populations (Werner et al., 2021).

An explicit part of paying nursing homes under new models such as APMs must be a concentrated focus on reducing disparities. Toward that end, the quality measurement and quality goals that APMs use to determine payment should include measures of improving outcomes for disadvantaged populations and reducing existing disparities (Damberg and Elliot, 2021). It is also imperative that all new payment programs include explicit monitoring and evaluation of health care disparities.

The biggest challenge for achieving health equity under APMs is related to the distinct financial resources across providers. Ample evidence exists that those nursing homes caring for a disproportionate share of Medicaid-insured individuals have lower quality of care (Gandhi et al., 2021; Grabowski, 2004; Grabowski et al., 2004b; Mor et al., 2004; Sharma et al., 2020). An essential first step to avoid further exacerbating disparities will be to address payment inequities across nursing homes by increasing Medicaid payment rates to levels adequate to cover the costs of caring for residents.

FINANCING NURSING HOME CARE

As the discussion of payment mechanisms in this chapter has illustrated, the U.S. approach to financing nursing home care is not so much an intentional system as a set of circumstances that has evolved over time to fill the largest gaps. Private insurance is rare, and few people can pay out of pocket for an extended nursing home stay (Dong et al., 2021; Konetzka, 2014a). The result is that Medicaid plays a dominant role as the default payer of nursing home care, but it is constantly subject to state budget constraints.

Medicare revenues from post-acute care play a disproportionate role in financial sustainability, and services such as hospice are paid for separately and are not well integrated into standard care.

One implication of this unsystematic financing system is a lack of equity in access to high-quality nursing home care. Such heavy reliance on Medicaid to fund nursing home care, with strict financial and health-related eligibility rules, means that many individuals may go without needed care or may receive care that is inadequate in quality or quantity. High-quality nursing homes have long considered prospective residents on Medicaid to be the least attractive financially (He and Konetzka, 2015). Extensive research has shown that dependence on Medicaid is associated with admission to lower-quality facilities with lower staffing ratio, more regulatory deficiencies, and a higher proportion of residents of color (Konetzka and Werner, 2009; Mor et al., 2004). Eligibility rules also differ across sites of care and across states, even within Medicaid, which may lead to inequities across states.

The lack of equity in access to high-quality nursing home care may also reinforce broader issues of systemic racism. Individuals who need Medicaid funding for long-term care must first "spend down" all their assets, thereby impoverishing themselves. By some estimates, up to two-thirds of the population would rely on Medicaid should they end up needing nursing home care (Brown and Finkelstein, 2008); many of those would not consider themselves poor throughout their lives. Thus, unlike many other types of health care for which the risk of financial burden is diversified across insured populations, those who end up needing nursing home care experience a large financial shock from spending down their assets (Sloane et al., 2021).

A second implication of this unsystematic financing system is site-specific payment, creating often irrational payment and eligibility differentials which can lead to unintended consequences. It has long been recognized that health care in the United States, and especially long-term care, is too fragmented in its payment and delivery across types and sites of services. Nursing home care is one segment of a continuum of care that people might need for assistance with functional and cognitive impairment during their lifetimes. In particular, separate financing and payment systems for home- and community-based care and institutional care create a false dichotomy and present barriers to the rational allocation of resources across settings that takes into account costs as well as an individual's needs and preferences (Konetzka, 2014b; Ng et al., 2010). All too often, Medicaid recipients do not have a choice of long-term care settings, and despite the expansion in Medicaid home- and community-based care, the program still has an institutional bias toward nursing home care.

State and federal policy efforts have focused on identifying individuals who can be cared for in the community. These include both nursing home diversion efforts for community elders (Bardo et al., 2014) and nursing home transition efforts for residents to return to the community (Haas et al., 2019; Robison et al., 2020). Despite these efforts, research suggests that individuals who require a relatively low level of care—who conceivably could be cared for in the community—are still residing in nursing homes (Mor et al., 2007). Moreover, there are a series of risk factors that have been identified as predicting transition from home- and community-based care to long-stay nursing home care, including Alzheimer's disease, money management issues, living alone, and prior short-stay nursing home stays (Greiner et al., 2014). The supply of community alternatives has been found to be negatively associated with the prevalence of residents with low care needs in nursing homes (Cornell et al., 2020; Kane et al., 2013).

Robust financing for both home- and community-based care and nursing home care services is needed to address the broad range of long-term care needs of older adults, as has been discussed throughout this report. There will always be a portion of the older adult population who require nursing home care based on a range of factors, not least of which is the level and intensity of required health care services. This is particularly the case as increasing numbers of older adults are living with multiple complex conditions, which is likely to render a nursing home a care setting preferred by individuals and their families. Many older adults lack the resources to be able to live at home and are thus unable to receive care in a home and community setting, while many older adults living at home suffer from social isolation and loneliness (Grabowski, 2021; Guo et al., 2015; Wolff et al., 2008). On the other hand, there are also a number of residents with relatively low levels of care needs who do not require a nursing-home level of care but often have minimal or no access to community alternatives for reasons including personal financial limitations and low investment in community alternatives (Cornell et al., 2020; Hass et al., 2019; Mor et al., 2007; Segelman et al., 2017; Wang et al., 2021).

Various proposals for some type of federal long-term care insurance (LTCFC, 2016), one that covers the continuum of care, including nursing home care, have been studied over the past few decades, such as the Community Living Assistance Services and Supports (CLASS) Act that Congress passed as part of the Affordable Care Act (Favreault et al., 2015, 2016). Neither CLASS, a voluntary, federal, long-term care insurance program, nor any previous effort to expand long-term care coverage has been implemented.[24]

---

[24] For more information, see https://www.kff.org/health-costs/issue-brief/health-care-reform-and-the-class-act and https://khn.org/news/class-act-implementation-halted-by-obama-administration (accessed November 4, 2021).

In theory, relative to state-specific Medicaid programs, a federal long-term care benefit that covers everyone could be more easily integrated and aligned with Medicare, and in so doing, address the fragmentation across long-term care, post-acute care, hospice, and other health care services discussed above.

As of this writing, Congress is considering the Well-Being Insurance for Seniors to be at Home Act, a proposal based on public–private partnerships to provide catastrophic coverage for long-term care (Cohen and Butler, 2021). States, for their part, are considering enacting public long-term care insurance programs. The state of Washington created a long-term care insurance program in 2019. Other states, such as California, Illinois, Michigan, and Minnesota, are looking at alternative long-term care financing approaches (Cohen et al., 2020; Gleckman, 2019). In addition, the proposed legislation known as the Build Back Better Act, H.R. 5376 (BBB) includes provisions for increased funding for HCBS (Cox et al., 2021).

Many other high-income countries have implemented and sustained national long-term care coverage for their populations, incorporating both institutional and home-based care; the structure of some of these programs could serve as models for the United States (Chen et al., 2020; Gleckman, 2010; Grabowski, 2021; Merlis, 2004; Weiner et al., 2020). The establishment of a federal long-term care benefit to replace the existing fragmented financing arrangements certainly has both advantages and disadvantages (summarized in Table 7-1). The major advantage would be increased access to services. As discussed, Medicaid recipients often lack access to both community-based long-term care options and high-quality nursing home care. Similarly, many middle-income Americans who do not qualify for Medicaid still cannot afford high-quality long-term care. One study projects that by 2029, more than half of the nation's middle-income older adults will be unable to afford the level of care they require for their health and functional needs (Pearson et al., 2019). These middle-income individuals often also cannot purchase private long-term care insurance given medical underwriting (Cornell et al., 2016). A federal benefit would eliminate individual underwriting (no one would be excluded from the program because they have a high risk of needing long-term care). As a result, a federal benefit system would provide broader access to nursing homes and other long-term care services.

Under the existing financing arrangements, the lowest-quality nursing homes disproportionately care for Medicaid recipients and persons of color. The new federal benefit would help to address some of the inequities across facilities and individuals by payer status and race. The system also requires families to spend down their assets to qualify for Medicaid and rely heavily on unpaid caregiving from family members. A federal benefit would protect families against catastrophic long-term care costs, and also lower the reliance on unpaid caregivers because they would have more comprehensive coverage and better overall quality of care.

TABLE 7-1 Advantages and Disadvantages of a Federal Long-Term Care Benefit

ADVANTAGES
A federal long-term care benefit could serve as a sustainable funding model to broaden access to all long-term care services for all, featuring robust financing for both nursing home and home- and community-based care, with the financial costs and risk of all long-term care services spread across the population.
A new federal long-term care benefit could • Reduce the *existing fragmentation* between payers because Medicare pays only for short-stay SNF post-acute care and Medicaid pays only for long-stay nursing home care. • Eliminate the *cross-subsidies and perverse incentives* in the current system that lead nursing homes to pursue more financially attractive short-stay residents over Medicaid-financed long-term residents. • Eliminate the requirement that *individuals spend down most of their assets* to qualify for Medicaid long-term care. • Provide *options to middle-income individuals* who cannot afford to pay privately for long-term care but are too wealthy to qualify for Medicaid. • Ensure *adequate financing for comprehensive, high-quality long-term care for all* and so reduce current inequities. • Reduce burden on family caregivers through more comprehensive coverage. • Provide *uniform coverage*, in contrast to the system of Medicaid long-term care benefits, which vary across states. • Be designed *to align with/integrate with Medicare* coverage. • Facilitate the *elimination of existing disparities* created by heavy reliance on Medicaid to fund long-term care; dependence on Medicaid financing for long-term care is associated with lower-quality nursing homes. • Address the current *disparities in long-term care* wherein individuals of color covered by Medicaid typically receive care in low-quality nursing homes. • Address the *false dichotomy and barriers to the rational allocation of resources across settings* created by separate financing and payment systems for home and community-based services and institutional care. • Provide *protection against catastrophic long-term care costs* and, like most social insurance would *spread the financial risk across the population.* • Shift responsibility for regulatory oversight, financial transparency, and accountability of nursing homes from the states to the federal government, providing consistency across states.
DISADVANTAGES
• The cost of a new federal long-term care benefit will be significant, will require additional sources of revenue, and might lead to increased taxes to help finance long-term care services. • States will be less able to tailor benefits to their populations; incentives for state innovation in benefit design will be reduced. • Due to the costs, the political challenges of enacting a new federal benefit program will be significant.

Finally, a new federal long-term care benefit would help address the disconnect and fragmentation both within Medicaid and across Medicaid and Medicare for long-term care recipients (Grabowski, 2007). A federal benefit would eliminate Medicaid's current institutional bias in most states, whereby community-based care is less generously covered. Moreover, the federal benefit could be aligned and integrated with Medicare coverage. Because a federal benefit would cover all long-term care recipients, it could be more easily integrated with Medicare coverage relative to existing Medicaid benefits, which vary across states and are available only to qualifying individuals.

A key challenge related to enactment of a federal long-term care benefit is the potential cost of such a program. The program would likely be self-funded by contributions from participants along with public subsidies for lower-income individuals. On an individual level, this would likely shift the burden of paying for long-term care to a broader group of taxpayers. On a broader societal level, this new federal benefit will shift the current burden of funding care for lower-income individuals from Medicaid to this new federal program.

A federal benefit may be associated with a risk of fewer opportunities for innovation in care delivery or limited ability to customize the program to align with state-specific needs. However, such risks have been addressed in the federal Medicare program, such as through innovative options, including MA plans, that offer greater flexibility.

An important consideration is whether a federal benefit would be feasible politically given historical resistance to this type of social insurance program in this country. As with any new such program, a critical decision will be whether to cover everyone from the beginning or only those who are vested in the program (i.e., paid in long enough to be eligible). This will have major implications in terms of the role of public financing for the early years of the program. Ultimately, a federal benefit would be designed to cover the continuum of long-term care settings while paying a rate commensurate with the delivery of high-quality care.

KEY FINDINGS AND CONCLUSIONS

Through its review of the evidence on nursing home payment and financing, the committee identified several important problems with the current system. First, there has been insufficient investment in quality care in nursing homes, with nursing homes dependent to some degree on Medicaid payment rates. Medicaid plays a dominant role as the default payer of nursing home care, but it is constantly subject to state budget constraints. Second, the system is fragmented across post-acute care, long-term care, hospice, and other services. This fragmentation creates inefficiencies and unintended incentives for overuse of some services, underuse of others, and cost shifting among more lucrative and less lucrative services. The current system is not one that anyone would have designed from the outset.

The fragmentation and potential cost shifting between Medicare-funded post-acute care services and mostly Medicaid-funded long-term care services is particularly problematic. Given that Medicare profit margins are much higher than Medicaid profit margins and that the delivery of post-acute services is, in some ways, separable from the delivery of long-term care services, economists would expect increased specialization over time in a free and competitive market. However, there appear to be institutional, regulatory, and economic obstacles in the nursing home market to doing so, given the current payment rates and capital stock. Even new entrants to the nursing home sector maintain a mix of long-term care and post-acute care beds.

To move toward a more efficient system and reduce fragmentation, the committee considered the potential of moving post-acute care out of the domain of nursing homes. This shift would enable nursing homes to specialize in long-term care, reduce fragmentation among payers, and encourage higher-quality care without the need for cost shifting. The committee recognized that such a change would require (1) ensuring that payment for long-term care is sufficient to sustain nursing homes without cross-subsidization from other services, and (2) identifying which providers should be responsible for post-acute care and aligning the economic incentives such that they are willing to do so.

The committee considered whether a promising approach would be to shift the provision of post-acute care to hospitals, as has been called for by a number of nursing home experts (Fulmer et al., 2021; Grabowski and Mor, 2020). The committee initially considered this change to be feasible for several reasons. First, the average patient census in hospitals has been declining, so hospitals may have the necessary capacity. Second, hospitals have already been increasing their responsibility for post-acute care costs through payment reforms such as bundled payments. Third, many hospitals have historical experience providing post-acute care on site, though the economics of this model in the past few decades have not been favorable. Hospitals might also increase the number of people getting post-acute care at home rather than on site.

In the course of its considerations, the committee assessed the unintended consequences of implementing such a change. Medicare, for example, could evaluate and set payment rates for post-acute care without considering the spillover effects on long-stay residents or the financial viability of nursing homes. If the underlying payment rates are insufficient, there could be an exit from the nursing home market and a shortage of nursing home care providers. As a result, more people might be encouraged to receive post-acute care at home than would be optimal for their health. For those too sick to go home, hospitals might prefer to pay for post-acute care in a nursing home rather than provide such care in the hospital setting. Allowing such arrangements would change the flow of funds, but ultimately it would not address the financial fragmentation in nursing homes. Based on careful consideration of all these factors, the committee ultimately decided not to recommend the separation of short-stay from long-stay nursing home residents, given the potential for greater risk of unintended consequences for both short- and long-stay patient populations.

The committee identified a number of additional financing and payment findings and conclusions:

- Medicare and Medicaid provide conflicting incentives between short-stay and long-stay payments, resulting in fragmentation and cross-subsidization across payers.
- Current incentives encourage nursing homes to transfer residents to hospitals rather than caring for people in the nursing home and then have them return to the nursing home after a qualifying hospital stay for post-acute care, with higher Medicare reimbursement, before transitioning back to long-stay care, with lower Medicaid reimbursement.
- Although an extensive body of research supports the strong connection between spending on direct care for residents and the quality of care, nursing homes are not required by law to devote a specific portion of their payment to direct care for residents.
- Value-based payment arrangements in Medicare, which link payment directly to the quality of care rather than the volume of services, are associated with lower rates of nursing home use and shorter lengths of stay than traditional Medicare payments.
- The impact of APMs for long-stay nursing home care is unknown but warrants exploration and testing in real-world situations.
- The quality measurement and quality goals that APMs use to determine payment should include measures of improving outcomes for disadvantaged populations and reducing existing disparities.
- The COVID-19 pandemic has resulted in a decline in admissions to nursing homes for post-acute short stays which persisted even after the rates of home health use rebounded, providing the opportunity to rethink and reshape the model of providing post-acute care in nursing homes.

REFERENCES

Abrahamson, K. 2020. *Technical report: Nursing home value-based reimbursement and quality literature review—Study of the Minnesota nursing home nursing home value-based reimbursement system.* https://mn.gov/dhs/assets/Cost-care-quality-literature-review-technical-report_tcm1053-472796.pdf (accessed November 17, 2021).

ACA (American Council on Aging). 2021. *Medicaid coverage of nursing home care: When, where and how much they pay.* https://www.medicaidplanningassistance.org/medicaid-and-nursing-homes (accessed October 21, 2021).

Agarwal, D., and R. M. Werner. 2018. Effect of hospital and post-acute care provider participation in accountable care organizations on patient outcomes and Medicare spending. *Health Services Research* 53(6):5035–5056.

AHCA (American Health Care Association, National Center for Assisted Living). 2021. *Preserve and protect Medicaid funding for long term care.* https://www.ahcancal.org/Advocacy/IssueBriefs/Medicaid.pdf (accessed September 30, 2021).

Anderson, W. L., and Z. Feng. 2016. *Minnesota managed care longitudinal data analysis.* Washington, DC: Assistant Secretary for Planning and Evaluation, U.S. Department of Health and Human Services.

Baicker, K., and M. E. Chernew. 2017. Alternative alternative payment models. *JAMA Internal Medicine* 177(2):222–223.

Bardo, A. R., R. A. Applebaum, S. R. Kunkel, and E. A. Carpio. 2014. Everyone's talking about it, but does it work? Nursing home diversion and transition. *Journal of Applied Gerontology* 33(2):207–226.

Barnett, M. L., A. Wilcock, J. M. McWilliams, A. M. Epstein, K. E. Joynt Maddox, E. J. Orav, D. C. Grabowski, and A. Mehrotra. 2019a. Two-year evaluation of mandatory bundled payments for joint replacement. *New England Journal of Medicine* 380(3):252–262.

Barnett, M. L., A. Mehrotra, and D. C. Grabowski. 2019b. Postacute care—The piggy bank for savings in alternative payment models? *New England Journal of Medicine* 381(4):302–303.

Bressman, E., N. B. Coe, X. Chen, R. T. Konetzka, and R. M. Werner. 2021. Trends in receipt of help at home after hospital discharge among older adults in the us. *JAMA Network Open* 4(11):e2135346.

Briesacher, B. A., T. S. Field, J. Baril, and J. H. Gurwitz. 2009. Pay-for-performance in nursing homes. *Health Care Financing Review* 30(3):1–13.

Brown, J. R., and A. Finkelstein. 2008. The interaction of public and private insurance: Medicaid and the long-term care insurance market. *American Economic Review* 98(3):1083–1102.

Burns, L. R., and M. V. Pauly. 2018. Transformation of the health care industry: Curb your enthusiasm? *The Milbank Quarterly* 96(1):57–109.

Chang, C. H., A. Mainor, S. Raymond, K. Peck, C. Colla, and J. Bynum. 2019. Inclusion of nursing homes and long-term residents in Medicare ACOs. *Medical Care* 57(12):990–995.

Chang, C. H., A. Mainor, C. Colla, and J. Bynum. 2021. Utilization by long-term nursing home residents under accountable care organizations. *Journal of the American Medical Directors Association* 22(2):406–412.

Chatterjee, P., M. Qi, N. B. Coe, R. T. Konetzka, and R. M. Werner. 2019a. Association between high discharge rates of vulnerable patients and skilled nursing facility copayments. *JAMA Internal Medicine* 179(9):1296–1298.

Chatterjee, P., A. K. Hoffman, and R. M. Werner. 2019b. *Shifting the burden? Consequences of postacute care payment reform on informal caregivers.* https://www.healthaffairs.org/do/10.1377/forefront.20190828.894278/full/ (accessed January 31, 2022).

Chen, L. M., A. M. Epstein, E. J. Orav, C. E. Filice, L. W. Samson, and K. E. Joynt Maddox. 2017. Association of practice-level social and medical risk with performance in the Medicare physician value-based payment modifier program. *JAMA* 318(5):453–461.

Chen, L., L. Zhang, and X. Xu. 2020. Review of evolution of the public long-term care insurance (LTCI) system in different countries: Influence and challenge. *BMC Health Services Research* 20(1):1057.

CMCS (Center for Medicaid and CHIP Services). 2019. *Medicare-Medicaid integration and unified appeals and grievance requirements for state Medicaid agency contracts with Medicare Advantage dual eligible special needs plans (D-SNPs) for contract year 2021.* https://www.medicaid.gov/federal-policy-guidance/downloads/cib111419-2.pdf (accessed January 31, 2022).

CMS (Centers for Medicare & Medicaid Services). 2015. *Report to Congress: Alternative payment models & Medicare Advantage.* Washington, DC: Centers for Medicare & Medicaid Services.

CMS. 2016. *Institutional special needs plans (I-SNPs).* https://www.cms.gov/Medicare/Health-Plans/SpecialNeedsPlans/I-SNPs (accessed April 29, 2021).

CMS. 2019a. *National health expenditures 2019 highlights.* https://www.cms.gov/files/document/highlights.pdf (accessed July 13, 2021).

CMS. 2019b. *Medicare coverage of skilled nursing facility care.* https://www.medicare.gov/Pubs/pdf/10153-Medicare-Skilled-Nursing-Facility-Care.pdf (accessed April 29, 2021).

CMS. 2019c. *Skilled nursing facility value-based purchasing program: Frequently asked questions.* Washington, DC: Centers for Medicare & Medicaid Services.

CMS. 2021a. *What's Medicare supplement insurance (Medigap)?* https://www.medicare.gov/supplements-other-insurance/whats-medicare-supplement-insurance-medigap (accessed April 29, 2021).

CMS. 2021b. *Skilled nursing facility PPS.* https://www.cms.gov/Medicare/Medicare-Fee-for-Service-Payment/SNFPPS (accessed April 29, 2021).

CMS. 2021c. *Accountable care organizations (ACOs).* https://www.cms.gov/Medicare/Medicare-Fee-for-Service-Payment/ACO (accessed October 19, 2021).

CMS. 2021d. *Medicare Advantage value-based insurance design model.* https://innovation.cms.gov/innovation-models/vbid (accessed October 29, 2021).

CMS. 2022a. *Hospice care.* https://www.medicare.gov/coverage/hospice-care (accessed January 28, 2022).

CMS. 2022b. *BPCI advanced.* https://innovation.cms.gov/innovation-models/bpci-advanced (accessed February 7, 2022).

Cohen, M. A., and S. M. Butler. 2021. The middle ground for fixing long-term care costs: The WISH Act. *Health Affairs Forefront*, August 9. https://www.healthaffairs.org/do/10.1377/hblog20210729.585743/full (accessed August 25, 2021).

Cohen, M. A., E. J. Tell, E. A. Miller, A. Hwang, and M. Miller. 2020. *Learning from new state initiatives in financing long-term services and supports.* https://www.healthinnovation.org/resources/publications/body/State-LTSS-Financing-Full-Report-July-2020.pdf (accessed November 17, 2021).

Colla, C. H., V. A. Lewis, S. L. Bergquist, and S. M. Shortell. 2016. Accountability across the continuum: The participation of postacute care providers in accountable care organizations. *Health Services Research* 51(4):1595–1611.

Collette, R. M. 2020. *Integrated care models are better for dual-eligibles.* https://www.arnoldventures.org/stories/report-integrated-care-models-are-better-for-dual-eligibles (accessed November 8, 2021).

Cornell, P. Y., D. C. Grabowski, M. A. Cohen, X. Shi, and D. G. Stevenson. 2016. Medical underwriting in long-term care insurance: Market conditions limit options for higher-risk consumers. *Health Affairs* 35(8):1494–1503.

Cornell, P. Y., W. Zhang, and K. S. Thomas. 2020. Changes in long-term care markets: Assisted living supply and the prevalence of low-care residents in nursing homes. *Journal of the American Medical Directors Association* 21(8):1161–1165.e1164.

Cox, C., R. Rudowitz, J. Cubanski, K. Pollitz, M. Musumeci, U. Ranji, M. Long, M. Freed, and T. Neuman. 2021. *Potential costs and impact of health provisions in the Build Back Better Act.* https://www.kff.org/health-costs/issue-brief/potential-costs-and-impact-of-health-provisions-in-the-build-back-better-act (accessed February 16, 2022).

CRS (Congressional Research Service). 2020. *Medicare financial status: In brief.* Washington, DC: Congressional Research Service.

Damberg, C. L., and M. N. Elliott. 2021. Opportunities to address health disparities in performance-based accountability and payment programs. *JAMA Health Forum* 2(6):e211143.

Damberg, C. L., M. E. Sorbero, S. L. Lovejoy, G. Martsolf, L. Raaen, and D. Mandel. 2014. *Measuring success in health care value-based purchasing programs: Findings from an environmental scan, literature review, and expert panel discussions.* Washington, DC: RAND Corporation and Office of the Assistant Secretary for Planning and Evaluation, U.S. Department of Health and Human Services.

Daras, L. C., A. Vadnais, Y. Z. Pogue, M. DiBello, C. Karwaski, M. Ingber, F. He, M. Segelman, L. Le, and J. Poyer. 2021. Nearly one in five skilled nursing facilities awarded positive incentives under value-based purchasing. *Health Affairs* 40(1):146–155.

Delbanco, S. F. 2014. The payment reform landscape: Pay-for-performance. *Health Affairs Forefront*, March 4. https://www.healthaffairs.org/do/10.1377/hblog20140304.037471/full (accessed November 4, 2021).

Dong, J., D. He, J. A. Nyman, and R. T. Konetzka. 2021. Wealth and the utilization of long-term care services: Evidence from the United States. *International Journal of Health Economics and Management* 21(3):345–366.

Edelman, T. 2015. *Yet again, value-based purchasing did not improve quality.* https://medicareadvocacy.org/yet-again-value-based-purchasing-did-not-improve-quality (accessed November 17, 2021).

Fausto, J. 2018. *Filling the void: Making end-of-life care a medicare "skilled need" to span the spectrum of care needed for high-quality, end-of-life care in the United States.* https://www.healthaffairs.org/do/10.1377/forefront.20180313.475221/full (accessed January 28, 2022).

Favreault, M. M., H. Gleckman, and R. W. Johnson. 2015. Financing long-term services and supports: Options reflect trade-offs for older Americans and federal spending. *Health Affairs* 34(12):2181–2191.

Favreault, M. M., H. Gleckman, and R. W. Johnson. 2016. *How much might new insurance programs improve financing for long-term services and supports?* https://www.urban.org/sites/default/files/publication/77471/2000602-How-Much-Might-New-Insurance-Programs-Improve-Financing-for-Long-Term-Services-and-Supports.pdf (accessed November 17, 2021).

Feng, Z., M. Lepore, M. A. Clark, D. Tyler, D. B. Smith, V. Mor, and M. L. Fennell. 2011. Geographic concentration and correlates of nursing home closures: 1999–2008. *Archives of Internal Medicine* 171(9):806–813.

Fiedler, M. 2021. *Designing a public option that would reduce health care provider prices.* https://www.brookings.edu/essay/designing-a-public-option-that-would-reduce-health-care-provider-prices (accessed October 20, 2021).

Finkelstein, A., Y. Ji, N. Mahoney, and J. Skinner. 2018. Mandatory Medicare bundled payment program for lower extremity joint replacement and discharge to institutional postacute care: Interim analysis of the first year of a 5-year randomized trial. *JAMA* 320(9):892–900.

Freed, M., J. F. Biniek, A. Damico, and T. Neuman. 2021. *Medicare Advantage in 2021: Enrollment update and key trends.* https://www.kff.org/medicare/issue-brief/Medicare-advantage-in-2021-enrollment-update-and-key-trends (accessed October 19, 2021).

Fulmer, T., D. B. Reuben, J. Auerbach, D. M. Fick, C. Galambos, and K. S. Johnson. 2021. Actualizing better health and health care for older adults. *Health Affairs* 40(2): 219–225.
Gadbois, E. A., D. A. Tyler, R. R. Shield, J. P. McHugh, U. Winblad, A. Trivedi, and V. Mor. 2018. Medicare Advantage control of postacute costs: Perspectives from stakeholders. *American Journal of Managed Care* 24(12):e386–e392.
Gandhi, A., H. Yu, and D. C. Grabowski. 2021. High nursing staff turnover in nursing homes offers important quality information. *Health Affairs* 40(3):384–391.
Gilman, M., E. K. Adams, J. M. Hockenberry, A. S. Milstein, I. B. Wilson, and E. R. Becker. 2015a. Safety-net hospitals more likely than other hospitals to fare poorly under Medicare's value-based purchasing. *Health Affairs (Millwood)* 34(3):398–405.
Gilman, M., J. M. Hockenberry, E. K. Adams, A. S. Milstein, I. B. Wilson, and E. R. Becker. 2015b. The financial effect of value-based purchasing and the hospital readmissions reduction program on safety-net hospitals in 2014: A cohort study. *Annals of Internal Medicine* 163(6):427–436.
Gleckman, H. 2010. *Long-term care financing reform: Lessons from the U.S. and abroad.* New York: Commonwealth Fund.
Gleckman, H. 2019. *Washington state's public long-term care insurance program is on the verge of becoming law.* https://howardgleckman.com/2019/04/18/washington-states-public-long-term-care-insurance-program-is-on-the-verge-of-becoming-law (accessed November 17, 2021).
Goldfeld, K. S., D. C. Grabowski, D. J. Caudry, and S. L. Mitchell. 2013. Health insurance status and the care of nursing home residents with advanced dementia. *JAMA Internal Medicine* 173(22):2047–2053.
Gozalo, P., M. Plotzke, V. Mor, S. C. Miller, and J. M. Teno. 2015. Changes in Medicare costs with the growth of hospice care in nursing homes. *New England Journal of Medicine* 372(19):1823–1831.
Grabowski, D. C. 2004. A longitudinal study of Medicaid payment, private-pay price and nursing home quality. *International Journal of Health Care Finance and Economics* 4(1):5–26.
Grabowski, D. C. 2007. Medicare and Medicaid: Conflicting incentives for long-term care. *The Milbank Quarterly* 85(4):579–610.
Grabowski, D. C. 2021. The future of long-term care requires investment in both facility- and home-based services. *Nature Aging* 1(1):10–11.
Grabowski, D. C., and V. Mor. 2020. Nursing home care in crisis in the wake of COVID-19. *JAMA* 324(1):23–24.
Grabowski, D. C., Z. Feng, O. Intrator, and V. Mor. 2004a. Recent trends in state nursing home payment policies. *Health Affairs (Millwood)* Suppl Web Exclusives:W4-363–373.
Grabowski, D. C., J. J. Angelelli, and V. Mor. 2004b. Medicaid payment and risk-adjusted nursing home quality measures. *Health Affairs* 23(5):243–252.
Grabowski, D. C., D. G. Stevenson, D. J. Caudry, A. J. O'Malley, L. H. Green, J. A. Doherty, and R. G. Frank. 2017. The impact of nursing home pay-for-performance on quality and Medicare spending: Results from the nursing home value-based purchasing demonstration. *Health Services Research* 52(4):1387–1408.
Graham, C., L. Ross, E. B. Bueno, and C. Harrington. 2018. Assessing the quality of nursing homes in managed care organizations: Integrating LTSS for dually eligible beneficiaries. *Inquiry: A Journal of Medical Care Organization, Provision and Financing* 55:46958018800090.
Greiner, M. A., L. G. Qualls, I. Iwata, H. K. White, S. L. Molony, M. T. Sullivan, B. Burke, K. A. Schulman, and S. Setoguchi. 2014. Predicting nursing home placement among home- and community-based services program participants. *American Journal of Managed Care* 20(12):e535–e536.

Guo, J., R. T. Konetzka, E. Magett, and W. Dale. 2015. Quantifying long-term care preferences. *Medical Decision Making* 35(1):106–113.

Harrington, C., and J. H. Swan. 1984. Medicaid nursing home reimbursement policies, rates, and expenditures. *Health Care Financing Review* 6(1):39–49.

Harrington, C., A. Montgomery, T. King, D. C. Grabowski, and M. Wasserman. 2021. These administrative actions would improve nursing home ownership and financial transparency in the post COVID-19 period. *Health Affairs Forefront*, February 11. https://www.healthaffairs.org/do/10.1377/hblog20210208.597573/full (accessed February 25, 2021).

Harris-Kojetin, L., M. Sengupta, J. P. Lendon, V. Rome, R. Valverde, C. Caffrey. 2019. *Long-term care providers and services users in the United States, 2015–2016.* https://www.cdc.gov/nchs/data/series/sr_03/sr03_43-508.pdf (accessed April 2, 2021).

Hass, Z., M. Woodhouse, D. C. Grabowski, and G. Arling. 2019. Assessing the impact of Minnesota's return to community initiative for newly admitted nursing home residents. *Health Services Research* 54(3):555–563.

He, D., and R. T. Konetzka. 2015. Public reporting and demand rationing: Evidence from the nursing home industry. *Health Economics* 24(11):1437–1451.

Healy, J. 2019. Nursing homes are closing across rural America, scattering residents. *The New York Times*, March 4. https://www.nytimes.com/2019/03/04/us/rural-nursing-homes-closure.html (accessed December 16, 2020).

Hefele, J. G., X. J. Wang, and E. Lim. 2019. Fewer bonuses, more penalties at skilled nursing facilities serving vulnerable populations. *Health Affairs (Millwood)* 38(7):1127–1131.

HHC and AHCA (Hansen, Hunter, & Company, PC and the American Health Care Association). 2018. *A report on shortfalls in Medicaid funding for nursing center care.* https://www.ahcancal.org/Reimbursement/Medicaid/Documents/2017%20Shortfall%20Methodology%20Summary.pdf (accessed October 20, 2021).

Huckfeldt, P. J., J. J. Escarce, B. Rabideau, P. Karaca-Mandic, and N. Sood. 2017. Less intense postacute care, better outcomes for enrollees in Medicare Advantage than those in fee-for-service. *Health Affairs* 36(1):91–100.

IOM (Institute of Medicine). 2001. *Crossing the quality chasm: A new health system for the 21st century.* Washington, DC: National Academy Press.

Jacobson, G., S. Griffin, T. Neuman, and K. Smith. 2017. *Income and assets of Medicare beneficiaries, 2016–2035.* https://www.kff.org/medicare/issue-brief/income-and-assets-of-medicare-beneficiaries-2016-2035 (accessed February 16, 2022).

Johnson, R. W. 2016. *Who is covered by private long-term care insurance?* https://www.urban.org/research/publication/who-covered-private-long-term-care-insurance (accessed December 1, 2021).

Johnson, R. W., M. M. Favreault, J. Dey, W. Marton, and L. Anderson. 2021. *Extended LTSS utilization makes older adults more reliant on Medicaid issue brief: ASPE issue brief.* Washington, DC: Office of the Assistant Secretary for Planning and Evaluation, U.S. Department of Health and Human Services.

Joynt Maddox, K. E., E. J. Orav, J. Zheng, and A. M. Epstein. 2018. Participation and dropout in the bundled payments for care improvement initiative. *JAMA* 319(2):191–193.

Joynt Maddox, K. E., E. J. Orav, J. Zheng, and A. M. Epstein. 2019a. How do frail Medicare beneficiaries fare under bundled payments? *Journal of the American Geriatrics Society* 67(11):2245–2253.

Joynt Maddox, K. E., E. J. Orav, J. Zheng, and A. M. Epstein. 2019b. Characteristics of hospitals that did and did not join the Bundled Payments for Care Improvement—Advanced Program. *JAMA* 322(4):362–364.

Kane, R. L., S. Flood, G. Keckhafer, B. Bershadsky, and Y.-S. Lum. 2002. Nursing home residents covered by Medicare risk contracts: Early findings from the Evercare evaluation project. *Journal of the American Geriatrics Society* 50(4):719–727.

Kane, R. L., G. Keckhafer, S. Flood, B. Bershadsky, and M. S. Siadaty. 2003. The effect of Evercare on hospital use. *Journal of the American Geriatrics Society* 51(10):1427–1434.

Kane, R. L., G. Arling, C. Mueller, R. Held, and V. Cooke. 2007. A quality-based payment strategy for nursing home care in Minnesota. *The Gerontologist* 47(1):108–115.

Kane, R. L., T. Y. Lum, R. A. Kane, P. Homyak, S. Parashuram, and A. Wysocki. 2013. Does home- and community-based care affect nursing home use? *Journal of Aging and Social Policy* 25(2):146–160.

Keohane, L. M., R. C. Grebla, V. Mor, and A. N. Trivedi. 2015. Medicare Advantage members' expected out-of-pocket spending for inpatient and skilled nursing facility services. *Health Affairs (Millwood)* 34(6):1019–1027.

Keohane, L. M., A. N. Trivedi, and V. Mor. 2017. Recent health care use and Medicaid entry of Medicare beneficiaries. *The Gerontologist* 57(5):977–986.

KFF (Kaiser Family Foundation). 2018. *Waiting list enrollment for Medicaid section 1915(c) home and community-based services waivers.* https://www.kff.org/health-reform/state-indicator/waiting-lists-for-hcbs-waivers/ (accessed May 25, 2021).

KFF. 2019. *An overview of Medicare.* https://www.kff.org/medicare/issue-brief/an-overview-of-medicare/ (accessed February 7, 2022).

KFF. 2020. *Distribution of certified nursing facility residents by primary payer source.* https://www.kff.org/other/state-indicator/distribution-of-certified-nursing-facilities-by-primary-payer-source/?currentTimeframe=0&sortModel=%7B%22colId%22:%22Location%22,%22sort%22:%22asc%22%7D (accessed April 29, 2021).

Koma, W., J. Cubanski, and T. Neuman. 2021. *A snapshot of sources of coverage among Medicare beneficiaries in 2018.* https://www.kff.org/medicare/issue-brief/a-snapshot-of-sources-of-coverage-among-medicare-beneficiaries-in-2018/ (accessed February 7, 2022).

Konetzka, R. T. 2014a. Long-term care insurance. In A. J. Culyer (ed.), *Encyclopedia of health economics*, vol. 2. San Diego: Elsevier. Pp. 152–159.

Konetzka, R. T. 2014b. The hidden costs of rebalancing long-term care. *Health Services Research* 49(3):771–777.

Konetzka, R. T., and R. M. Werner. 2009. Disparities in long-term care: Building equity into market-based reforms. *Medical Care Research and Review* 66(5):491–521.

Kumar, A., M. Rahman, A. N. Trivedi, L. Resnik, P. Gozalo, and V. Mor. 2018. Comparing post-acute rehabilitation use, length of stay, and outcomes experienced by Medicare fee-for-service and Medicare Advantage beneficiaries with hip fracture in the United States: A secondary analysis of administrative data. *PLoS Medicine* 15(6):e1002592.

Leavitt Partners. 2017. The Medicare–Medicaid ACO model: *Addressing dual 30 ligible' costs.* https://leavittpartners.com/medicare-medicaid-aco-model-addressing-dual-eligibles-costs (accessed November 8, 2021).

Lee, J. T., D. Polsky, R. Fitzsimmons, and R. M. Werner. 2020. Proportion of racial minority patients and patients with low socioeconomic status cared for by physician groups after joining accountable care organizations. *JAMA Network Open* 3(5):e204439.

Liao, J. M., A. S. Navathe, and R. M. Werner. 2020. The impact of Medicare's alternative payment models on the value of care. *Annual Review of Public Health* 41(1):551–565.

Liberman, L. 2018. *Medicaid reimbursement rates draw attention.* https://www.nic.org/blog/Medicaid-reimbursement-rates-draw-attention (accessed October 20, 2021).

Libersky, J., S. Liu, L. Turoff, J. Gellar, D. Lipson, A. Collins, J. Li, and C. Irvin. 2018. *Managed long-term services and supports: Interim evaluation report.* Baltimore, MD: Centers for Medicare & Medicaid Services.

LTCFC (Long-Term Care Financing Collaborative). 2016. *A consensus framework for long-term care financing reform.* https://www.taxpolicycenter.org/publications/consensus-framework-long-term-care-financing-reform/full (accessed November 17, 2021).

MACPAC (Medicaid and CHIP Payment and Access Commission). 2019. *Nursing facility fee-for-service payment policy.* Washington, DC: Medicaid and CHIP Payment and Access Commission.

MACPAC. 2021. *Improving integration for dually eligible beneficiaries: Strategies for state contracts with dual eligible special needs plans.* Washington, DC: Medicaid and CHIP Payment and Access Commission.

MACPAC. 2022. *Medicare advantage dual eligible special needs plans.* https://www.macpac.gov/subtopic/medicare-advantage-dual-eligible-special-needs-plans-aligned-with-medicaid-managed-long-term-services-and-supports (accessed January 31, 2022).

Martin, A. B., M. Hartman, D. Lassman, and A. Catlin. 2020. National health care spending in 2019: Steady growth for the fourth consecutive year. *Health Affairs* 40(1):14–24.

Matulis, R., and J. Lloyd. 2018. *The history, evolution, and future of Medicaid accountable care organizations.* Center for Health Care Strategies brief. https://www.chcs.org/media/ACO-Policy-Paper_022718.pdf (accessed November 8, 2021).

McGarry, B. E., and D. C. Grabowski. 2019a. What do clinicians caring for aging patients need to know about private long-term care insurance? *Journal of the American Geriatrics Society* 67(10):2167–2173.

McGarry, B. E., and D. C. Grabowski. 2019b. Managed care for long-stay nursing home residents: An evaluation of institutional special needs plans. *American Journal of Managed Care* 25(9):438–443.

McGarry, B. E., E. M. White, L. J. Resnik, M. Rahman, and D. C. Grabowski. 2021. Medicare's new patient driven payment model resulted in reductions in therapy staffing in skilled nursing facilities. *Health Affairs* 40(3):392–399.

McWilliams, J. M., L. G. Gilstrap, D. G. Stevenson, M. E. Chernew, H. A. Huskamp, and D. C. Grabowski. 2017. Changes in postacute care in the Medicare shared savings program. *JAMA Internal Medicine* 177(4):518–526.

McWilliams, J. M., L. A. Hatfield, B. E. Landon, P. Hamed, and M. E. Chernew. 2018. Medicare spending after 3 years of the Medicare shared savings program. *New England Journal of Medicine* 379(12):1139–1149.

MedPAC (Medicare Payment Advisory Commission). 2008. *June 2008 report to the Congress: Reforming the delivery system.* Washington, DC: Medicare Payment Advisory Commission.

MedPAC. 2013. *March 2013 report to the Congress: Medicare payment policy.* Washington, DC: Medicare Payment Advisory Commission. Original edition, Chapter 14.

MedPAC. 2015. *March 2015 report to the Congress: Medicare payment policy.* Washington DC: Medicare Payment Advisory Commission. Original edition, Chapter 7.

MedPAC. 2020. *March 2020 report to the Congress: Medicare payment policy.* Washington, DC: Medicare Payment Advisory Commission. Original edition, Chapter 12.

MedPAC. 2021a. *March 2021 report to the Congress: Medicare payment policy.* Washington, DC: Medicare Payment Advisory Commission.

MedPAC. 2021b. *June 2021 report to the Congress: Medicare and the health care delivery system.* Washington, DC: Medicare Payment Advisory Commission.

Merlis, M. 2004. *Long-term care financing: Models and issues.* https://www.nasi.org/research/long-term-care-financing-models-and-issues (accessed November 17, 2021).

Meyers, D. J., V. Mor, and M. Rahman. 2018. Medicare advantage enrollees more likely to enter lower-quality nursing homes compared to fee-for-service enrollees. *Health Affairs* 37(1):78–85.

Mor, V., J. Zinn, J. Angelelli, J. M. Teno, and S. C. Miller. 2004. Driven to tiers: Socioeconomic and racial disparities in the quality of nursing home care. *The Milbank Quarterly* 82(2):227–256.

Mor, V., J. Zinn, P. Gozalo, Z. Feng, O. Intrator, and D. C. Grabowski. 2007. Prospects for transferring nursing home residents to the community. *Health Affairs* 26(6):1762–1771.

Murphy, K. S., and J. LaPointe. 2016. *Understanding the value-based reimbursement model landscape.* https://revcycleintelligence.com/features/understanding-the-value-based-reimbursement-model-landscape (accessed October 19, 2021).

Musumeci, M., P. Chidambaram, and M. O. M. Watts. 2019. *Medicaid's money follows the person program: State progress and uncertainty pending federal funding reauthorization.* https://www.kff.org/medicaid/issue-brief/medicaids-money-follows-the-person-program-state-progress-and-uncertainty-pending-federal-funding-reauthorization/ (accessed January 31, 2022).

Navathe, A. S., J. M. Liao, S. E. Dykstra, E. Wang, Z. M. Lyon, Y. Shah, J. Martinez, D. S. Small, R. M. Werner, C. Dinh, X. Ma, and E. J. Emanuel. 2018. Association of hospital participation in a Medicare bundled payment program with volume and case mix of lower extremity joint replacement episodes. *JAMA* 320(9):901–910.

Nelb, R. 2020. *Themes from interviews on the development of nursing facility payment methods.* Paper presented at the December 11, 2020 Medicaid and CHIP Payment and Access Commission (MACPAC) Meeting. https://www.macpac.gov/wp-content/uploads/2020/12/Themes-from-Interviews-on-the-Development-of-Nursing-Facility-Payment-Methods.pdf (accessed November 24, 2021).

Newhouse, J. P., and A. M. Garber. 2013. Geographic variation in medicare services. *New England Journal of Medicine* 368(16):1465–1468.

Ng, T., C. Harrington, and M. Kitchener. 2010. Medicare and Medicaid in long-term care. *Health Affairs (Millwood)* 29(1):22–28.

Norton, E. C. 1992. Incentive regulation of nursing homes. *Journal of Health Economics* 11(2):105–128.

OIG (Office of the Inspector General). 2011. *Medicare hospices that focus on nursing facility residents.* Washington DC: Office of the Inspector General, U.S. Department of Health and Human Services.

OIG. 2017. *Medicare program shared savings accountable care organizations have shown potential for reducing spending and improving quality.* Washington, DC: Office of the Inspector General, U.S. Department of Health and Human Services.

OIG. 2018. *Vulnerabilities in the Medicare hospice program affect quality care and program integrity: An OIG portfolio.* Washington, DC: Office of the Inspector General, U.S. Department of Health and Human Services.

Parekh, T. M., S. P. Bhatt, A. O. Westfall, J. M. Wells, D. Kirkpatrick, A. S. Iyer, M. Mugavero, J. H. Willig, and M. T. Dransfield. 2017. Implications of drg classification in a bundled payment initiative for COPD. *American Journal of Accountable Care* 5(4):12–18.

Pearson, C. F., C. C. Quinn, S. Loganathan, A. R. Datta, B. B. Mace, and D. C. Grabowski. 2019. The forgotten middle: Many middle-income seniors will have insufficient resources for housing and health care. *Health Affairs* 38(5). https://doi.org/10.1377/hlthaff.2018.05233.

Qi, A. C., A. A. Luke, C. Crecelius, and K. E. Joynt Maddox. 2020. Performance and penalties in year 1 of the skilled nursing facility value-based purchasing program. *Journal of the American Geriatrics Society* 68(4):826–834.

Rahman, M., E. M. White, B. E. McGarry, C. Santostefano, P. Shewmaker, L. Resnik, and D. C. Grabowski. 2022. Association between the patient driven payment model and therapy utilization and patient outcomes in US skilled nursing facilities. *JAMA Health Forum* 3(1):e214366.

Rau, J. 2017. *Why glaring quality gaps among nursing homes are likely to grow if Medicaid is cut.* https://khn.org/news/why-glaring-quality-gaps-among-nursing-homes-are-likely-to-grow-if-medicaid-is-cut/ (accessed October 30, 2020).

Robison, J., N. Shugrue, M. Porter, and K. Baker. 2020. Challenges to community transitions through money follows the person. *Health Services Research* 55(3):357–366.

Rolnick, J. A., J. M. Liao, E. J. Emanuel, Q. Huang, X. Ma, E. Z. Shan, C. Dinh, J. Zhu, E. Wang, D. Cousins, and A. S. Navathe. 2020. Spending and quality after three years of Medicare's bundled payments for medical conditions: Quasi-experimental difference-in-differences study. *BMJ (Clinical Research Ed.)* 369:m1780.

Rudowitz, R., R. Garfield, and E. Hinton. 2019. *10 things to know about Medicaid: Setting the facts straight.* https://files.kff.org/attachment/Issue-Brief-10-Things-to-Know-about-Medicaid-Setting-the-Facts-Straight (accessed February 16, 2022).

Rutledge, C., M. Wocken, and S. Wilson. 2019. *34th SNF cost comparison and industry trends report: National themes, local insights.* https://www.claconnect.com/resources/white-papers/2019/-/media/files/white-papers/2019-snf-cost-comparison-and-industry-trends-report-cla.pdf (accessed September 30, 2021).

Ryan, A. M. 2013. Will value-based purchasing increase disparities in care? *New England Journal of Medicine* 369(26):2472–2474.

Sandhu, S., R. S. Saunders, M. B. McClellan, and C. A. Wong. 2020. Health equity should be a key value in value-based payment and delivery reform. *Health Affairs Forefront*, November 25. https://www.healthaffairs.org/do/10.1377/hblog20201119.836369/full (accessed November 17, 2021).

Segelman, M., O. Intrator, Y. Li, D. Mukamel, P. Veazie, and H. Temkin-Greener. 2017. HCBS spending and nursing home admissions for 1915(c) waiver enrollees. *Journal of Aging & Social Policy* 29(5):395–412.

Serna, L., A. Johnson, and E. Rollins. 2022. *The Medicare Advantage program: Status report and mandated report on dual-eligible special needs plans.* https://www.medpac.gov/wp-content/uploads/2021/10/MA-status-MedPAC-Jan22.pdf (accessed January 31, 2022).

Sharma, H., M. C. Perraillon, R. M. Werner, D. C. Grabowski, and R. T. Konetzka. 2020. Medicaid and nursing home choice: Why do duals end up in low-quality facilities? *Journal of Applied Gerontology* 39(9):981–990.

Sheingold, S., S. Bogasky, and S. Stearns. 2015. *Medicare's hospice benefit: Revising the payment system to better reflect visit intensity.* Washington, DC: Office of the Assistant Secretary for Planning and Evaluation, U.S. Department of Health and Human Services.

Singletary, E., R. Roiland, M. Harker, D. H. Taylor Jr., and R. S. Saunders. 2021. *Value-based payment and skilled nursing facilities: Supporting SNFs during COVID-19 and beyond.* https://healthpolicy.duke.edu/sites/default/files/2021-05/Margolis%20SNF.pdf (accessed February 1, 2021).

Sloane, P. D., R. Yearby, R. T. Konetzka, Y. Li, R. Espinoza, and S. Zimmerman. 2021. Addressing systemic racism in nursing homes: A time for action. *Journal of the American Medical Directors Association* 22(4):886–892.

SNP Alliance. 2021. *About special needs plans (SNPs).* https://snpalliance.org/what-we-do/about-snps (accessed April 29, 2021).

Sollitto, M. 2021. *Qualifying for Medicaid long-term care.* https://www.agingcare.com/articles/Medicaid-and-long-term-care-133719.htm (accessed October 29, 2021).

Sorbero, M. E., A. M. Kranz, K. E. Bouskill, R. Ross, A. I. Palimaru, and A. Meyer. 2018. *Addressing social determinants of health needs of dually enrolled beneficiaries in Medicare Advantage plans: Findings from interviews and case studies.* Santa Monica, CA: RAND Corporation.

Span, P. 2012. *Forced to choose: Nursing home vs. hospice.* https://newoldage.blogs.nytimes.com/2012/11/30/forced-to-choose-nursing-home-vs-hospice/ (accessed January 28, 2022).

Stefanacci, R. G., and M. Pakizegee. 2020. *Special needs plans are special for long-term care.* https://www.hmpgloballearningnetwork.com/site/altc/articles/special-needs-plans-are-special-long-term-care (accessed November 4, 2021).

Struijs, J., E. F. de Vries, C. A. Baan, P. F. van Gils, and M. B. Rosenthal. 2020. *Bundled-payment models around the world: How they work and what their impact has been.* https://www.commonwealthfund.org/publications/2020/apr/bundled-payment-models-around-world-how-they-work-their-impact (accessed February 16, 2022).

Teno, J. M., and I. Higginson. 2018. Paying for value: Lessons from the Medicare hospice benefit. *Health Affairs Forefront*, May 2. https://www.healthaffairs.org/do/10.1377/hblog20180427.522132/full (accessed November 17, 2021).

Tian, W. 2016. *Statistical brief #205: An all-payer view of hospital discharge to postacute care, 2013.* https://www.hcup-us.ahrq.gov/reports/statbriefs/sb205-Hospital-Discharge-Postacute-Care.jsp (accessed January 31, 2022).

Troyer, J. L. 2002. Cross-subsidization in nursing homes: Explaining rate differentials among payer types. *Southern Economic Journal* 68(4):750–773.

Verdier, J., A. Kruse, R. S. Lester, A. M. Philip, and D. Chelminsky. 2015. *State contracting with Medicare Advantage dual eligible special needs plans: Issues and options.* http://www.chcs.org/media/ICRC-Issues-and-Options-in-Contracting-with-D-SNPs-FINAL.pdf (accessed October 7, 2021).

Wachterman, M. W., E. R. Marcantonio, R. B. Davis, and E. P. McCarthy. 2011. Association of hospice agency profit status with patient diagnosis, location of care, and length of stay. *JAMA* 305(5):472–479.

Wang, S., H. Temkin-Greener, A. Simning, R. T. Konetzka, and S. Cai. 2021. Medicaid home- and community-based services and discharge from skilled nursing facilities. *Health Services Research* 56(6):1156–1167.

Weiner, J., N. B. Coe, A. K. Hoffman, and R. M. Werner. 2020. *Policy options for financing long-term care in the U.S.* https://ldi.upenn.edu/our-work/research-updates/policy-options-for-financing-long-term-care-in-the-u-s (accessed November 17, 2021).

Werner, R. M., and E. Bressman. 2021. Trends in post-acute care utilization during the COVID-19 pandemic. *Journal of the American Medical Directors Association* 22(12):2496–2499.

Werner, R. M., and R. T. Konetzka. 2018. Trends in post–acute care use among medicare beneficiaries: 2000 to 2015. *JAMA* 319(15):1616–1617.

Werner, R. M., R. T. Konetzka, and K. Liang. 2010. State adoption of nursing home pay-for-performance. *Medical Care Research and Review* 67(3):364–377.

Werner, R. M., R. T. Konetzka, and D. Polsky. 2013. The effect of pay-for-performance in nursing homes: Evidence from state Medicaid programs. *Health Services Research* 48(4):1393–1414.

Werner, R. M., R. T. Konetzka, M. Qi, and N. B. Coe. 2019a. The impact of Medicare copayments for skilled nursing facilities on length of stay, outcomes, and costs. *Health Services Research* 54(6):1184–1192.

Werner, R. M., N. B. Coe, M. Qi, and R. T. Konetzka. 2019b. Patient outcomes after hospital discharge to home with home health care vs to a skilled nursing facility. *JAMA Internal Medicine* 179(5):617–623.

Werner, R. M., E. J. Emanuel, H. H. Pham, and A. S. Navathe. 2021. *The future of value-based payment: A road map to 2030.* https://ldi.upenn.edu/wp-content/uploads/archive/pdf/PennLDI-Future-of-Value-Based-Payment-WhitePaper.pdf (accessed October 19, 2021).

White, A., D. Hurd, T. Moore, D. Warner, N. Wu, and R. Sweetland. 2006. *Quality monitoring for Medicare global payment demonstrations: Nursing home quality-based purchasing demonstration.* Abt Associates. https://www.abtassociates.com/insights/publications/report/quality-monitoring-for-Medicare-global-payment-demonstrations-nursing (accessed February 25, 2021).

Wiener, J. M., W. L. Anderson, G. Khatutsky, Y. Kaganova, and J. O'Keeffe. 2013. *Medicaid spend down: New estimates and implications for longterm services and supports financing reform: Final report.* Washington, DC: RTI International.

Wolff, J. L., J. D. Kasper, and A. D. Shore. 2008. Long-term care preferences among older adults: A moving target? *Journal of Aging & Social Policy* 20(2):182–200.

Yasaitis, L. C., W. Pajerowski, D. Polsky, and R. M. Werner. 2016. Physicians' participation in ACOS is lower in places with vulnerable populations than in more affluent communities. *Health Affairs (Project Hope)* 35(8):1382–1390.

Zhu, J. M., V. Patel, J. A. Shea, M. D. Neuman, and R. M. Werner. 2018. Hospitals using bundled payment report reducing skilled nursing facility use and improving care integration. *Health Affairs (Project Hope)* 37(8):1282–1289.

Quality Assurance: Oversight and Regulation

Regulation is common to a wide range of products and services, such as food, construction, pharmaceuticals, transportation, and electronics. The purpose of regulation is to assure that products and services are safe and meet certain standards for minimum acceptable quality. A standard economic justification for why nursing home care needs regulation is that regulations can help address market failures, such as consumers' difficulty in accessing, monitoring, and responding to information about the quality of care (GAO, 1997; Grabowski and Stevenson, 2006; IOM, 2001; Shugarman and Brown, 2006). The typically frail health of the nursing home resident population, combined with the relatively high level of government financing for nursing home care in the United States, further bolsters the political and policy justifications for governmental oversight of the sector. In that respect, government regulations are intended to protect consumers and ensure accountability in the use of public funds by developing quality standards, evaluating whether nursing homes meet those standards, and enforcing sanctions when necessary (IOM, 2001). This chapter reviews the history and current state of quality assurance, accomplished largely through oversight and regulation, of the nursing home sector.

HISTORY OF QUALITY ASSURANCE IN NURSING HOMES

The federal government's formal involvement with the oversight of nursing homes started with the enactment of Medicare and Medicaid in 1965. Over the decades, various laws and federal regulations sought to improve the quality of care in nursing homes and also improve the oversight and regulation of nursing homes' performance (see Box 8-1).

BOX 8-1
Brief Timeline of Nursing Home Regulation

- The **1965 Social Security Act** enacted Medicare and Medicaid and gave the U.S. Department of Health, Education, and Welfare (HEW) (predecessor to the U.S. Department of Health and Human Services) the authority to set requirements of participation for nursing homes.
- The **1965 Older Americans Act** was amended in 1973 and again in 1987 to add important quality standards and create the ombudsman program.
- In **1971**, the Office of Nursing Home Affairs was created within HEW and tasked with enforcing quality improvement measures in nursing homes, reviewing federal long-term care policies, and providing guidance for agencies overseeing nursing homes.
- The **Social Security Amendments of 1972** included full federal funding of state survey and certification activities and directed HEW to develop quality standards for nursing homes that participate in Medicare and Medicaid.
- In **1974**, HEW issued federal certification criteria for nursing homes. These regulations were clarified in 1978 but remained essentially unchanged.
- The **1987 Nursing Home Reform Act**, part of the Omnibus Budget Reconciliation Act of 1987 (OBRA 87), renewed focus on residents' mental, psychosocial, and physical well-being and included provisions on education and training standards for nursing home staff, safety and sanitation practices, survey processes, and transparency.
- The subsequent Residents' Bill of Rights included the right to privacy, self-determination, freedom from abuse, and voicing grievances without reprisal
- The **2010 Patient Protection and Affordable Care Act** sought to improve the transparency and accountability of nursing home quality, improve oversight and enforcement mechanisms, improve staff training requirements, improve data collection and reporting, and prevent elder abuse through several acts. For example,
    - **The Nursing Home Transparency and Improvement Act** required public transparency of ownership, quality, and staffing information and established Nursing Home Compare (now Care Compare; see Chapter 3).
    - **The Elder Justice Act** and the **Patient Safety and Abuse Prevention Act** set forth requirements to prevent and report abuse and other crimes against older adults in long-term care settings.
- The **2015 Improving Medicare Post-Acute Care Transformation Act of 2014 (IMPACT Act)** was revised to improve the 5-Star Quality rating system.
- In **2016, the Centers for Medicare & Medicaid Services released a final rule** updating requirements of participation for long-term care facilities in Medicare and Medicaid programs.
- The **January 2019 executive order** "Reducing Regulation and Controlling Regulatory Costs" scaled back the oversight of nursing homes in several areas as part of a broader movement to reduce bureaucracy and government intervention.

SOURCES: ACL, 2021a; Brinker and Walker, 1962; CMS, 2016, 2018a; Grabowski, 2007; IOM, 1986; KFF, 2015; Klauber and Wright, 2001; Musumeci and Chidambaram, 2020; Public Law 81-734, 1950; Public Law 92-603, 1972; Public Law 109-171, 2005; Public Law 111-148, 2009; Public Law 113-185, 2014; Rau, 2017; Walshe, 2001; Watson, 2012; Wells and Harrington, 2013.

OMNIBUS BUDGET RECONCILIATION ACT OF 1987

The 1986 Institute of Medicine (IOM) report *Improving the Quality of Care in Nursing Homes* cited widespread quality-of-care problems and substantial concerns about the ineffectiveness—and unevenness—of oversight at that point in time (IOM, 1986). Specifically, the report stated

> The implicit goal of the regulatory system is to ensure that any person requiring nursing home care be able to enter any certified nursing home and receive appropriate care, be treated with courtesy, and enjoy continued civil and legal rights. This happens in many nursing homes in all parts of this country. But in many other government-certified nursing homes, individuals who are admitted receive very inadequate—sometimes shockingly deficient—care that is likely to hasten the deterioration of their physical, mental, and emotional health. (p. 2)

Soon after the release of the 1986 IOM report, Congress enacted the Nursing Home Reform Act as part of the Omnibus Budget Reconciliation Act of 1987 (OBRA 87).[1] OBRA 87 regulations raised the expectations for nursing homes considerably by establishing uniform and tougher nationwide standards. The regulations strengthened and consolidated quality standards (including standards related to quality of life and residents' rights), expanded the types of sanctions that could be imposed, and required data collection using the Minimum Data Set. Overall, the regulations in OBRA 87 established the modern survey and enforcement system, detailing the expectation that facilities be surveyed once every 9 to 15 months at times that were unannounced to the facilities and adding several intermediate sanctions that would be available to aid in enforcement. For family member perspectives on the importance of regulations to the quality of care in nursing homes, see Box 8-2.

Quality Assurance and Nursing Homes in the 21st Century

For more than 30 years, the statutory requirements of OBRA 87 and associated regulations promulgated by the Centers for Medicare & Medicaid Services (CMS) have largely defined nursing home quality assurance activities. To remain eligible for Medicare and Medicaid payments, nursing homes must meet requirements of participation[2] covering a range of dimensions such as residents' rights, quality of care, and the physical environment

---

[1] Omnibus Budget Reconciliation Act of 1987, Public Law 100-203; 100th Cong., 1st sess. (December 22, 1987).

[2] CMS Requirements for Long Term Care Facilities—Quality of Life, 42 CFR Part §483, Subpart B (2016).

> **BOX 8-2**
> **Family Member Perspectives**
>
> "How did we get this culture change in Mama's facility? Regulations! Without the power of federal regulations, change would not have occurred. Quality of care, quality of life, and fundamental resident rights to a safe and dignified existence mean very little without regulations and strong enforcement. My experience with my mother and in my 33-year 'paid' career are ample evidence that providers will not police themselves."
>
> — **Kathy Bradley, Family Member and Founder, CEO, and Board President of Our Mother's Voice**
>
> "We need actual regulation—surprise visits and regular visits from inspectors and real penalties for violations (and information made available to the public)."
>
> — **Family Member, Berkeley, California**
>
> *These quotes were collected from the Quality of Care in Nursing Homes Public Webinars and the committee's online call for resident, family and nursing home staff perspectives.*

(CMS, 2021a; Kapp, 2000). However, while substantial changes have occurred in nursing home care since the implementation of the OBRA 87 regulations, the general structure of the oversight and regulation of nursing homes has, for the most part, remained the same. A notable exception is the incorporation of new regulations as part of the Patient Protection and Affordable Care Act (ACA)[3] (see Box 8-1) (Wells and Harrington, 2013). The ACA includes provisions such as requiring facilities to disclose information concerning ownership and governance, directing CMS to collect payroll data on direct care staffing, and establishing the Civil Monetary Penalty Reinvestment Program (KFF, 2013). In 2016, CMS released a final rule updating its requirements of participation.[4] The full rule, the first significant revision of federal regulations of nursing homes in over 25 years, was designed to streamline existing nursing home regulations, remove duplication, and align with current legislation. The 2016 rule expanded regulations to facilitate person-centered care, infection control, and quality improvement activities. The 2016 rule also restricted the ability of nursing homes to require that residents enter into pre-dispute arbitration agreements, a

---

[3] Patient Protection and Affordable Care Act of 2010, Public Law 111-148; 111th Cong., 2nd sess. (March 23, 2010).
[4] CMS Requirements for Long Term Care Facilities, 42 CFR § 483 (2016).

provision the nursing home industry challenged almost immediately. As a result, the July 2019 final rule allowed nursing homes to offer residents pre-dispute binding arbitration but not require it.

In accordance with the January 2017 executive order "Reducing Regulation and Controlling Regulatory Costs," the oversight and enforcement of the requirements of participation were scaled back as part of a broader movement to reduce bureaucracy and government intervention, including the encouragement of regulators to not impose fines for "one-time" events (Musumeci and Chidambaram, 2020; Rau, 2017). The executive order proposed relaxing regulations in other areas, such as emergency preparedness, as well (CMS, 2018a).

Today, challenges are evident in the current quality assurance framework. While great progress has been made since the passage of OBRA 87, substantial quality problems have persisted. With its emphasis on minimum standards for operation, the main purpose of regulation is to identify and deter poor-quality care practices. In 1998, a report to Congress by the Health Care Financing Administration (HCFA) noted that "ongoing press reports of questionable practice reinforce a widespread negative perception of the quality of nursing home care and underscore the importance of the Federal government's responsibilities" (HCFA, 1998, p. i). However, recent investigative and government reports have documented substantial lapses in nursing home oversight processes across multiple states (see later in this chapter for more on oversight of the state survey process). The following sections will provide an overview of quality assurance roles and responsibilities today.

FEDERAL AND STATE REGULATION

The 1986 IOM report noted three components of government regulation of nursing homes that are important to quality assurance:

1. Criteria to determine quality;
2. Determining compliance with these criteria; and
3. Enforcing compliance with the criteria (IOM, 1986).

Chapter 3 of this report examines quality measurement in nursing homes as a means of determining the quality of care. This section gives a high-level overview of the role that the federal government, state governments, and the private sector play in the oversight of nursing homes by determining their compliance with regulations.

States have the primary responsibility for licensing providers, giving each state some control over nursing home market entry and retention. State licensure imposes minimum standard requirements that a home must meet in order to continue operating. Historically, however, state licensing decisions have excluded few facilities, as regulators consider the loss or denial of a license to operate to be a drastic remedy that should be reserved for only serious breaches of resident safety and quality-of-care standards (Li et al., 2010). States could potentially take a more active role in screening applications to assess the quality of performance at facilities owned by applicants for the license to operate.

Consequently, the primary locus of regulatory stringency lies in the federal requirements of participation as a Medicare- or Medicaid-certified nursing home provider (Furrow et al., 2008; IOM, 2001, p. 21; Walshe, 2001). The requirements of participation include requirements that likely parallel most states' licensure standards but that also specify the minimum quality of care that a nursing home must provide. For example, the requirements of participation state that nursing homes must provide services and activities to "attain or maintain the highest practicable physical, mental, and psychosocial well-being of each resident" according to a written plan of care.[5]

Even though requirements of participation go beyond what might be considered the absolute minimum standards of quality, the increased requirements are rather modest. On the other hand, some have argued that the sheer number of requirements of participation creates long checklists that encourage technical compliance but do not adequately allow providers to focus on their residents' quality of life (Harrar et al., 2021; Jaffe, 2020; Walshe, 2001). This tension emerged prominently between the 2016 revision of nursing home standards and the subsequent repeated efforts to scale these standards back (Justice in Aging, 2020; Musumeci and Chidambaram, 2020; National Consumer Voice, 2019). Despite the ideological nature of this particular dispute, there is still potential merit to the exercise of ensuring that the requirements of participation are both thorough in ensuring quality and maintain a focus on what matters to nursing home residents.

Medicare and Medicaid are the predominant purchasers of nursing home care, and the need to maintain beneficiary access limits the ability of Medicare and Medicaid to demand quality that exceeds the requirements of participation. More demanding requirements of participation also need to be balanced with potential increases in program payments that ensure sufficient numbers of nursing homes will continue to serve beneficiaries.

Certificate of Need and Construction Moratoria

As part of the licensing process, some states maintain certificate-of-need requirements to regulate expansions in the health care market as a strategy to constrain health care spending. Certificate-of-need policies

---

[5] CMS Requirements for Long Term Care Facilities—Administration, 42 CFR § 483.70 (2016).

employ a need-based evaluation of all applications for new construction or additions to existing facilities that would increase the number of beds. Additionally, some states have implemented construction moratoria that prohibit the building of new health care facilities. By 1979, almost all states had certificate-of-need regulations, and these policies typically included nursing homes (Feder and Scanlon, 1980). As of December 2021, 35 states and Washington, DC, have certificate-of-need policies in place, with wide variability among the states in how these policies are structured, including how "need" is defined (Cavanaugh et al., 2020; NCSL, 2021; Wiener et al., 1998).

Impact of Certificate-of-Need Policies in Health Care

The general rationale for certificate-of-need and construction moratorium regulations rests on Roemer's law, which states "a built bed is a filled bed is a billed bed" (Shain and Roemer, 1959). That is, these policies seek to compensate for a concern that the principles of supply and demand in a third-party payment system may result in overinvestment in health care facilities, misdistribution of health care resources, and delivery of more services than actually needed, given that consumers are not impacted by the cost of services (Bruneau, 2014; Feder and Scanlon, 1980; Havighurst, 2005). For health care in general, certificate-of-need regulations have been found to be largely ineffective, and "in fact, by limiting supply and monopolizing local health care, [they] seem to raise costs and undermine quality care. More than anything, though, they limit access to health care services" (Mitchell, 2021). In 2004, the Department of Justice (DOJ) and the Federal Trade Commission recommended reconsidering these regulations, stating that they believed that "on balance, [they] are not successful in containing health care costs, and that they pose serious anticompetitive risks that usually outweigh their purported economic benefits. Market incumbents can too easily use [certificate-of-need] procedures to forestall competitors from entering an incumbent's market" (DOJ and FTC, 2004, p. 22). In 2016, Mitchell and Koopman noted that "forty years of peer-reviewed academic research suggests that [certificate-of-need] laws have not only failed to achieve their goals but have in many cases led to the opposite of what those who enacted the laws intended" (Mitchell and Koopman, 2016).

Impact of Certificate-of-Need and Construction Moratoria on Nursing Homes

The general principles behind certificate-of-need regulations may not apply to the nursing home setting, in that residents and their families often do have out-of-pocket expenditures for care (see Chapter 7) (Feder and

Scanlon, 1980). The logic behind these regulations for nursing homes specifically is that limiting the number of beds will, in turn, limit the number of Medicaid beneficiaries in nursing home settings, thus keeping state Medicaid spending low. However, the evidence does not suggest that the regulations have much effect (Grabowski et al., 2003; Rahman et al., 2016). As noted by Wiener and colleagues, "most states feel that supply controls have contributed to cost containment, although none could quantify the effect" (Wiener et al., 1998, p. 10). In fact, Medicare and Medicaid spending on nursing home care has been shown to grow faster in states with certificate-of-need laws (as compared to states without those laws) (Rahman et al., 2016). Moreover, when states repeal certificate-of-need laws, they do not experience increases in nursing home spending, with the likely reason being that most families will exhaust every community option before seeking nursing home care (Grabowski and Gruber, 2007; Grabowski et al., 2003; Konetzka et al., 2019; Mattimore et al., 1997). The cost of compliance with certificate-of-need regulations may also exceed their benefits and decrease social welfare (Conover and Bailey, 2020).

While certificate-of-need regulations do not appear to have their intended effect of holding down Medicaid nursing home spending, they can have the unintended effect of harming consumers. Studies have found that these regulations limit choice and lower access to medical services and health care resources, especially for those in rural areas (Feder and Scanlon, 1980; Mitchell, 2017; Wiener et al., 1998); decrease the quality of care for some measures of quality (Fayissa et al., 2020; Grabowski et al., 2008; Stratmann and Wille, 2016; Zinn, 1994); and increase private-pay prices (Nyman, 1994). For example, Fayissa and colleagues (2020) found that nursing homes in states with such regulations (as compared to nursing homes in states without these regulations) had lower health survey scores (by 18 to 24 percent) and lower levels of employment for registered nurses and licensed practical nurses (along with increased employment of certified nurse aides) (Fayissa et al., 2020). Additionally, the presence of these policies did not result in fewer complaints.

Certificate-of-need regulations and construction moratoria can also discourage innovation by preventing the entry of more modern and desirable nursing home options and restricting facility renovation and remodeling (Grabowski, 2017; Mitchell, 2021; Reinhard and Hado, 2021; Wiener et al., 1998). As Chapter 6 notes, many of today's nursing homes were built using design features adapted from hospitals constructed in the 1960s and 1970s and therefore have an institutional environment (Eijkelenboom et al., 2017; Schwarz, 1997). Furthermore, certificate-of-need regulations may contribute to the perpetuation of larger nursing homes, rather than the smaller, more home-like settings that are more desirable. These regulations have been associated with a higher average nursing home size (Ferdows and Rahman, 2020; Kosar and Rahman, 2021; Nastasi, 2020; Rahman, 2016); the average number of beds is roughly 110 in states without such a regulation and 131 in states with one (Rahman et al., 2016). The experience of small-home models such as the Green House (see Chapter 6) have highlighted the importance of capital investments for developing higher-quality models of nursing home care.

Some have argued that certificate-of-need policies and construction moratoria are needed because of the decreasing occupancy rates in nursing homes. However, one examination of nursing home moratoria in Indiana noted that "focusing solely on occupancy rates ignores the underlying reasons why the beds are unoccupied" (Glans, 2015). The author suggests that lower occupancy rates may reflect that "they are older and are not offering the services consumers want or need" and that new facilities will naturally replace older, less desirable nursing homes (rather than "forcing" residents into older facilities) (Glans, 2015). Others have raised concerns that lifting certificate-of-need regulations will increase Medicaid spending on institutional care and so reduce investment in home- and community-based settings of long-term care (Kitchener et al., 2005; Miller et al., 2002; Williams, 2019). However, no evidence suggests that this has occurred. In fact, limited evidence demonstrates that between 1992 and 2009, "spending on home health care by both Medicare and Medicaid increased at a much faster rate in states without [certificate of need]" (Rahman et al., 2016).

At the height of the COVID-19 pandemic in spring of 2020, 24 states eased, suspended, or temporarily lifted certificate-of-need regulations to increase flexibility (Erickson, 2021). Several other states introduced legislation to repeal or reform such restrictions (Mitchell, 2021).

State Surveys

States assist with the assessment of facilities' compliance with requirements of participation and, as necessary, with the investigation of complaints and adverse incidents. States have some discretion in how they administer these responsibilities, but all states are expected to adhere to the detailed protocols outlined in the State Operations Manual (CMS, 2017a). Using the federal survey protocol and other federal guidance, states report state survey findings about the scope and severity of deficiencies as well as their recommendations for enforcement actions to CMS. However, CMS has the ultimate authority to sanction facilities and to audit all state inspection activities (CMS, 2018b; IOM, 1986). Accordingly, the federal government has the statutory power to review state decisions and overrule them, known as the "look behind" provision (Walshe and Harrington, 2002).

The overall survey process (Figure 8-1) is uniform across states. In 2017, the process was updated to use "as much structure as possible to

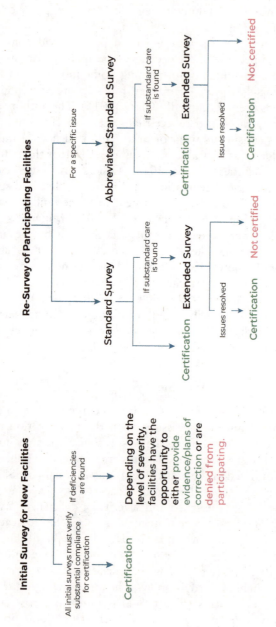

FIGURE 8-1 Nursing home Medicare/Medicaid certification survey process.
SOURCE: Adapted from CMS, 2018b.

ensure consistency while allowing surveyors the autonomy to make decisions based on their expertise and judgment" (CMS, 2017b). The process is also completely automated (instead of using paper as was previously done in some surveys). Most commonly, facilities receive a standard survey. However, if a surveyor finds evidence of substandard care, the choice can be made to then conduct an extended survey, which evaluates additional participation requirements. The survey agency then compiles its findings of deficiencies and recommends action to CMS and the state. It is up to CMS and the state to determine whether they give a facility the opportunity to correct its deficiencies before CMS imposes penalties. If CMS and the state give a facility the opportunity to correct deficiencies, it must submit an acceptable plan of correction or proof of correction for past noncompliance (CMS, 2018b).

Upon completing the entire survey process, facilities have the opportunity to dispute cited deficiencies through an informal dispute resolution process beyond the plans of correction. However, if there is evidence of "immediate jeopardy—a situation in which the facility's noncompliance with one or more requirements of participation has caused, or is likely to cause, serious injury, harm, impairment, or death to a resident"—the regional office or state Medicaid agency will immediately terminate the facility's Medicare/Medicaid participation, mandate installing temporary management, or impose other penalties (CMS, 2018b).

State Surveyors for Long-Term Care

Minimum standards to be a federal surveyor in long-term care facilities for the determination of Medicare/Medicaid compliance include

- Appropriate background in the health professions or health administration;
- Completion of an orientation program and basic surveyor training course;
- Passing the Surveyor Minimum Qualifications Test;
- Annual job-related training courses;
- Lack of conflict of interest; and
- Dedication of at least 50 percent of one's working time to survey activities or to meeting the professional qualifications for the surveyor's health profession (CMS, 2019a).

The survey team's composition and size varies, depending primarily on the following factors: the number of beds in the facility, whether the facility has a history of deficiencies, if a facility has a special care unit, and whether the team includes surveyors-in-training. CMS guidance calls for states to staff the survey teams with multidisciplinary individuals who have expertise and knowledge of best practices in working with the care population. Ultimately, "the state (or, for federal teams, the regional office) decides what the composition of the survey team will be," as long as it meets statutory and regulatory requirements (CMS, 2016). In addition, a multidisciplinary team of professionals, at least one of whom is a registered nurse, must conduct nursing home standard surveys.

The 1986 IOM report *Improving the Quality of Long-Term Care* included several recommendations regarding the training of nursing home surveyors, including

- Implementation of programs for effective training and monitoring of surveyor performance to reduce inconsistency;
- A revision of guidelines to be more specific about the qualifications of surveyors and the composition and numbers of survey team staff; and
- Increased federal training efforts and support of state-level training programs.

A 1999 report from the Office of the Inspector General (OIG) also called for evaluating surveyor staff to ensure that there is adequate staffing, additional training for state surveyors with a forum to meet and discuss common issues to ensure consistency, and standardized ongoing training requirements across states (OIG, 1999). Several reports note the challenges in hiring qualified surveyor staff. For example, a 2005 report from the Government Accountability Office (GAO) highlighted "continuing problems in hiring and retaining qualified surveyors, a factor that states indicated can contribute to variability in the citation of serious deficiencies" (GAO, 2005, p. 37). In 2008, the GAO noted two factors that contributed to significant understatement of serious care problems by surveyors: weaknesses in surveyors' investigative skills and weaknesses in surveyors' ability to properly analyze the information they had collected (GAO, 2008). A follow-up study in 2009 concluded that "workforce shortages and training inadequacies affected states' ability to complete thorough surveys, contributing to the understatement of nursing home deficiencies" (GAO, 2009a, p. 22). States often identify staffing as a key factor in their inability to meet the standard for survey timeliness, noting "the most common staffing-related description centered on the inability to attract and retain surveyors, often due to not being able to offer high enough salaries to compete in local markets" (OIG, 2022a, p. 11).

Similar to recruiting care providers to the nursing home setting, recruiting qualified surveyors can also be a challenge. In her testimony to this committee, Alice Bonner, a senior advisor with the Institute for Healthcare Improvement (IHI), noted

> How are we training surveyors? [. . . .] How [can] we get really good, dedicated people to want to become surveyors? This is one of the most important jobs in health care. And it's critical to people who live in nursing homes and who work in nursing homes. And to the care partners in the community. So how can we recruit really good people who are registered nurses and social workers, who can make a lot more money doing something else in a lot of states?

Overall, state survey agencies need more surveyors (in sheer numbers), competitive compensation, and enhanced training to ensure that surveyors have the qualifications and supports needed to effectively carry out their responsibilities.

Funding of the Survey Process

The survey process is funded by a combination of Medicare, Medicaid, and non-Medicaid state funds (GAO, 2009b). Medicare surveys are funded by a discretionary appropriation from Congress based on budget requests submitted by CMS while states receive 75 percent federal matching funds for Medicaid surveys (GAO, 2009b; OIG, 2022a). CMS' budget for these activities remained flat since fiscal year (FY) 2014, at about $397 million annually (OIG, 2022a). However, during that time period, CMS increased the allotment to states by about 4 percent. In 2020, CMS received additional funding through the Coronavirus Aid, Relief, and Economic Security Act[6] for survey and certification expenses during the COVID-19 pandemic. In addition to paying the 25 percent of Medicare-covered expenditures for surveys, states are also expected to contribute additional funds for other reasons, including the costs associated with state licensure (GAO, 2009b). In 2009, the GAO noted that "CMS oversight of states' use of survey funds is limited because it relies on state-reported data, has inadequate information about non-Medicaid state funding, and does not require states to justify supplemental funding" (GAO, 2009b, p. 15). See later in this chapter for more on CMS oversight of the state survey process.

---

[6] Coronavirus Aid, Relief, and Economic Security Act, Public Law 116-136; 116th Cong., 2nd sess. (March 27, 2020).

Complaints

In addition to standard survey inspections that nursing homes undergo, residents and other parties may file complaints with the state or federal regulatory agency related to adverse events or general dissatisfaction with the quality of care. Medicare- and Medicaid-certified nursing homes are required to have established procedures for complaints by residents and people acting on the resident's behalf. Specifically, nursing homes must

- Make survey, certification, and complaint investigation reports available;
- Investigate complaints and monitor compliance; and
- Make information about what complaint forms are, how they are used, and how to file a complaint with the state survey and certification program and the state long-term care ombudsman program available.[7,8]

States are responsible for receiving, prioritizing, and investigating complaints. The most serious complaints are categorized as either "immediate jeopardy" or "high priority" (also known as non-immediate jeopardy–high) and require immediate attention (see Box 8-3). Less serious complaints may require onsite investigation by the state, desk review, or referral, but do not have a specific timeframe for action.

While there are many ways to file a complaint at a nursing home, states must have standard complaint forms for residents to file with the state survey agency and a state long-term care ombudsman program (depending on the facility). They also must have a formal complaint resolution process. The ACA sought to make filing such complaints easier by providing standardized complaint forms and streamlining the complaint resolution process (KFF, 2013). However, substantial barriers still exist—including barriers related to the process itself as well as those related to fear of reprisal (Carlson, 2015; Lee et al., 2021). For example, according to reports by ombudsmen, racial and ethnic minority residents may avoid filing complaints out of fear of retaliation (Lee et al., 2021).

Data on consumer complaints have improved in recent years with Care Compare's addition of information on complaints and deficiencies. As shown in Table 8-1, the number of overall complaints per 1,000 nursing homes increased steadily between 2011 and 2018 (OIG, 2020a). The percentage of complaints prioritized as either immediate jeopardy or high priority remained relatively consistent. As shown in Table 8-2, between

---

[7] Social Security Act, Title XVIII §1819 (d)(1)(C), 42 U.S. Code 1395i-3, 89th Cong., 1st sess. (July 30, 1965).

[8] Social Security Act, Title XI §1128I (f), 42 U.S. Code § 1320a-7j, 89th Cong., 1st sess. (July 30, 1965).

> **BOX 8-3**
> **Definitions of Nursing Home Complaints**
>
> **Immediate jeopardy complaints** allege serious injury, harm, impairment, or death to a resident, and indicate an immediate risk unless immediate corrective action is taken. State survey agencies are required to start an onsite investigation within 2 business days.
>
> **High priority (non-Immediate Jeopardy - High) complaints** allege harm that negatively impacts the individual's mental, physical, or psychosocial status and are of such consequence to the person's well-being that a rapid response is indicated. State survey agencies are required to start an onsite survey within 10 business days.
>
> SOURCES: CMS, 2019b; OIG, 2019a, 2020a.

TABLE 8-1 Numbers and Prioritization of Complaints, 2011–2018

	2011	2015	2016	2018
Total number of complaints	47,279	62,790	66,077	71,602
Number of complaints per 1,000 nursing home residents	32.7	44.9	47.3	52.3
Percentage of complaints prioritized as immediate jeopardy	6%	8.5%	9%	7%
Percentage of complaints prioritized as high priority	49.1%	50.6%	50%	47%

SOURCE: OIG, 2020a.

TABLE 8-2 Numbers and Investigations of Immediate Jeopardy and High Priority Complaints, 2016–2018

	2016	2017	2018
Immediate Jeopardy Complaints			
Number of immediate jeopardy complaints	6,039	5,451	5,245
Percentage of immediate jeopardy complaints not investigated within 2 days	24.0%	17.7%	12.8%
High Priority Complaints			
Number of high priority complaints	32,774	32,722	33,974
Percentage of high priority complaints not investigated within 10 days	15.4%	16.2%	19.3%

SOURCE: OIG, 2019a.

2016 and 2018, the percentage of immediate jeopardy complaints that were not investigated within the required timeline decreased, but the percentage of high-priority complaints that were not investigated within the required timeline increased. Moreover, from 2016 through 2018, "twenty-one states failed to meet CMS' timeliness threshold for high priority complaints in all three years" (OIG, 2020a, p. 6); among these states, 10 did not meet performance thresholds for timeliness for 8 consecutive years (2011–2018). (See more on timeliness of survey activities later in this chapter.)

In one example, as of April 2014, long-term care facilities in California had more than 10,000 open complaints and facility-reported incidents (California State Auditor, 2014). A 2014 report from the California State Auditor recommended establishing specific timelines for the investigation of these complaints, ensuring adequate staff, and following specific procedures for review and approval; as of November 2019, these recommendations had not been implemented (California State Auditor, 2014, 2020).

For a nursing home staff perspective on the complaints process, see Box 8-4.

For more on states' performance in addressing complaints, see later in this chapter for a discussion of CMS oversight and performance of the state survey process.

Additional State-Based Roles

Although the most important role of states in nursing home oversight is assessing compliance with federal requirements, states that wish to increase the stringency of nursing home quality control have additional mechanisms available. For instance, states might impose more stringent

---

BOX 8-4
Nursing Home Staff Perspective

"There is a great need for staff to follow up on requests/complaints in a more timely and thorough manner; after six years of quarterly care plan meetings discussing the same concerns, there was still no change/improvement in the system which delegated tasks from the top down but then NEVER checked to confirm action was completed."

— **Anonymous, St. Louis, Missouri**

This quote was collected from the committee's online call for resident, family, and nursing home staff perspectives.

staffing standards than those in federal guidelines (Harrington et al., 2020). States also have primary oversight responsibility for the very small portion of nursing homes that do not participate in the Medicare or Medicaid programs and therefore are not subject to the detailed requirements of participation.

PRIVATE ACCREDITATION

Beyond the required government oversight, nursing homes can elect to undergo additional voluntary scrutiny through private accrediting entities such as The Joint Commission. Typically funded by fees from participating facilities, private accrediting agencies generally set detailed accreditation standards, assess facilities' compliance with those standards, and subsequently work with providers to address identified shortcomings and improve operations (Castle et al., 2011). Relative to government oversight, the approach of private accrediting agencies is oriented more to quality improvement, something that is outside the standard purview of regulatory agencies. There is very little evidence, however, suggesting that nursing home providers who choose to engage in voluntary accreditation efforts have subsequently improved care practices (Wagner et al., 2012).

CMS allows certain health care organizations to receive a "deemed status"—that is, the organization can participate in Medicare and Medicaid but be exempt from the Medicare survey and certification process if a qualifying private accrediting entity determines that the organization meets or exceeds federal requirements of participation (ASHE, 2021; CMS, 2008). However, a 1998 report to Congress from HCFA found that private accreditation (as compared to the traditional survey process) emphasized process and structure measures over resident-centeredness, were less transparent than the traditional nursing home survey process, and tended to miss serious deficiencies; the authors concluded that "the potential cost savings to deeming would not appear to justify the risk to the health and safety of the vulnerable nursing home population" (HCFA, 1998, p. iv). Determinations by private accrediting bodies are not sufficient for nursing homes' participation in Medicare and Medicaid, and are strictly voluntary.

ENFORCEMENT AND PENALTIES

After the determination of compliance with quality criteria through requirements of participation, the third component of regulation for nursing homes is the enforcement of compliance with these criteria, largely through various sanctions.

Sanctions by CMS and State Survey Agencies

To enforce compliance and penalize poor performers, CMS and state survey agencies can levy a range of sanctions against nursing homes. Depending on the seriousness of the deficiency, penalties can range from directed plans of correction and in-service trainings to the imposition of civil monetary (or money) penalties (CMPs), the appointment of temporary management, denial of payment, and termination from participation in the Medicare and Medicaid programs.

Prior to OBRA 87, termination from participating in Medicare and Medicaid programs was the only available sanction for noncompliant facilities, but today there are a wider variety of intermediate options for penalizing noncompliant nursing homes. As noted earlier, states report survey findings about the scope and severity of deficiencies as well as their recommendations for enforcement actions to CMS. Despite the range of enforcement options available, CMPs have by far been the most common remedy used in recent years to sanction nursing homes. Specifically, as Table 8-3 shows, CMPs accounted for nearly 72 percent of the 28,077 enforcement actions taken from FY 2016 through FY 2020. (See below for more on CMPs.)

More stringent sanctions, such as temporary management and termination from participation in Medicare and Medicaid, are rarely used (CMS, 2021b; GAO, 2009c; Li et al., 2010; OIG, 2006a). For example, in 2006, OIG found that CMS terminated the participation of only 45 percent of the facilities that warranted that sanction (OIG, 2006a).

Civil Monetary Penalties

CMPs are fines imposed by CMS for noncompliance with requirements of participation—either a total fine based on the number of days out of compliance for a single infraction (per day) or for each instance of noncompliance (CMS, 2021c). In 2019, almost $120 million was collected in CMPs (about $100 million from per day penalties and nearly $20 million from per instance penalties); the average total dollar amount was $68,126 for per day penalties and $9,950 for per instance penalties (CMS, 2022). The average days in effect for per day penalties was 57 days (CMS, 2022). In 2005, the OIG found that CMS tended to impose penalties at the lower end of the range (OIG, 2005). Additionally, some studies have found interstate variability in how CMP is enforced and how the funds are used (Harrington et al., 2008; Wang et al., 2019).

Through the CMP Reinvestment Program, a portion of these funds are returned to states to be used for activities to improve the quality of care for nursing home residents. Examples of permissible use of the funds include assistance for residents of facilities that are closed or decertified,

QUALITY ASSURANCE 417

TABLE 8-3 Enforcement Actions Report, FY 2016–2019

Enforcement Action	2016	2017	2018	2019	TOTAL
State Monitoring	67	100	95	38	300
Directed Plan of Correction	37	46	63	75	221
Temporary Management	3	5	1	7	16
Discretionary Denial of Payment for New Admits	445	551	453	577	2,026
Mandatory Denial of Payment for New Admits—3 Months	221	161	191	162	735
Denial of Payment for All Residents	5	5	7	3	20
Directed In-Service Training	337	278	275	292	1,182
Civil Monetary Penalty	2,726	4,206	3,399	3,421	13,752
CMS-Approved Alternative or Additional	5	11	8	8	32
Transfer of Residents/Closure of Facility	0	1	1	0	2
Transfer of Residents	2	0	0	0	2
Discretionary Termination	8	7	3	2	20
Mandatory Termination	15	12	7	12	46
Total Number of Enforcement Actions	3,871	5,383	4,503	4,597	18,354
Total Number of Nursing Homes with Enforcement Actions*	2,537	3,474	2,944	2,991	11,946

SOURCE: CMS, 2021b.
NOTE: While more recent data are available, the impact of the COVID-19 pandemic on enforcement actions may skew data trends, and require separate analysis.
*These data come from the Certification and Survey Provider Enhanced Reporting (CASPER) system. CASPER notes that the provider (i.e., nursing home) count is "valid for the subset of providers or suppliers for which there are survey records in CASPER." For more information, see https://qcor.cms.gov (accessed November 10, 2021).

relocation of residents, support for resident and family councils, training of nursing home staff and surveyors, and technical assistance for quality improvement in nursing homes (CMS, 2021c). CMP funds cannot be used for expenses such as research, capital improvements, nursing home employee salaries, and expenses associated with requirements of participation (CMS, 2019c).

Civil and Criminal Action

Distinct from the mechanisms described above, the government can hold nursing homes liable for damages under fraud and abuse laws, such as under the federal False Claims Act (Landsberg and Keville, 2001). This law provides sanctions against any health care provider that defrauds the government, either by billing CMS for services it did not actually render or, in some cases, for delivering services that do not meet baseline standards. Although regulators use the False Claims Act relatively infrequently to police nursing home quality, it can be an option for extreme cases of noncompliance with requirements of participation.

Additionally, government agencies are not the only entities that can impose penalties; the courts can hold nursing homes liable for certain violations (Stevenson and Studdert, 2003). As with traditional medical malpractice claims, nursing home residents and their families have a private right of action against facilities for damages and potentially even for breach of contract. While some argue that liability for harm increases the incentives for delivering high-quality care, evidence shows little difference in the susceptibility to claims of harm among lower-quality and higher-quality homes (Studdert and Stevenson, 2004; Studdert et al., 2011). Furthermore, liability claims have little impact on the subsequent care that facilities provide (Konetzka et al., 2013; Stevenson et al., 2013a).

Many states have passed tort reform legislation, most notably caps on non-economic damages, which can have a particularly negative impact on nursing home cases (Studdert and Stevenson, 2004). Furthermore, during the COVID-19 pandemic, several states passed liability protections for nursing homes against pandemic-related claims or enhanced existing laws (Associated Press, 2021; Brown, 2021; Critchfield, 2021). In July 2020, the American Bar Association noted that more than half of all states "have granted some sort of immunity from civil liability to long-term care facilities and health care providers. Three states have granted facilities and providers immunity from criminal *and* civil liability" (Brooks et al., 2021). Most of the states provide protections from accusations of negligence, requiring proof of willful or gross negligence.

In 1998, President Clinton announced a large initiative to improve the quality of care in nursing homes (White House, 1998). Part of this initiative directed HCFA (in conjunction with the Office of the Inspector General and DOJ) to "refer egregious violations of quality of care standards for criminal or civil investigation and prosecution when appropriate." In March 2020, the DOJ announced the National Nursing Home Initiative (NNHI), a program coordinated by the Elder Justice Initiative in collaboration with the U.S. Attorneys' Offices. NNHI aims to pursue civil and criminal actions against nursing homes that provide substandard care and "owners and operators who have profited at the expense of their residents" (DOJ, 2020). NNHI looks for facilities that lack proper hygiene and infection control protocols, fail to provide proper food to residents, withhold pain medication from residents, fail to provide adequate staffing, or use chemical and physical restraints. DOJ plans to scrutinize data from whistleblowers, wrongful death lawsuits, federal and state inspections and audits, and COVID-19 reporting data from federal agencies (e.g., CMS) (Hall et al.,

2020). NNHI will also work to ensure compliance with the False Claims Act (Yoder, 2020). DOJ has not released more information about NNHI since it launched the program.

Corporate Integrity Agreements

Beyond the traditional survey process, a corporate integrity agreement allows nursing homes with identified quality-of-care problems to remain in the Medicare and Medicaid programs if they contract with an independent quality monitor that has been authorized by OIG to oversee clinical improvement and compliance. Corporate integrity agreements generally last for 5 years (OIG, 2022b). The OIG sometimes negotiates a corporate integrity agreement as part of a settlement for investigations of fraud arising under the False Claims Act (DOJ, 2014, 2016; OIG, 2022b).

In 2009, the OIG studied 15 nursing home corporations that had entered into corporate integrity agreements (OIG, 2009). While all 15 corporations ultimately instituted structures and processes related to quality, the OIG was unable to determine the actual impact on the quality of care because of the "lack of agreed-upon benchmarks for quality of care outcome measures throughout the nursing home industry" (OIG, 2009, p. 17). In 2018, in response to media coverage of the use of corporate integrity agreements in the settlements of False Claims Act cases, the Center for Medicare Advocacy called for more transparency of corporate integrity agreements (Edelman, 2018). It noted

> Transparency would both enable the monitor to receive comprehensive, timely information that is relevant to determining the company's compliance with the [corporate integrity agreement] (or whether there has been a material breach) and inform the public about the ongoing status of the company's compliance. (Edelman, 2018)

The Special Focus Facility Program

The Special Focus Facility (SFF) program, created in 1998, is a program in which CMS and states identify the lowest-performing facilities as determined by numbers of deficiencies found during survey, the severity of those citations, and patterns of serious problems over time and then subject those facilities to more frequent inspections and quality improvement activities (CMS, 2021d). States use a points-based system to create a list of candidates for the program. The states then select a subset of the candidate list to participate in the SFF program. CMS regulations state,

"Once a state selects a facility as an SFF, the state survey agency, on CMS's behalf, conducts a full, onsite inspection of all Medicare health and safety requirements every six months and recommends progressive enforcement (e.g., fines, denial of Medicare payment) until the nursing home either (1) graduates from the SFF program; or (2) is terminated from the Medicare and/or Medicaid program(s)" (CMS, 2021d). According to CMS, most SFF nursing homes improve significantly within 18 to 24 months, with CMS terminating about 10 percent from participating in Medicare and Medicaid (CMS, 2021d). Improving this small program has been a recent focus of federal policy makers and is a central component of the proposed Nursing Home Reform Modernization Act. However, many graduates fail to sustain improvement (or may even regress) and the budget for the SFF program only allows for oversight of a small fraction of the nursing homes deemed to be among the most poorly performing (CMA, 2019; GAO, 2010a; Rau, 2017).

CMS OVERSIGHT AND PERFORMANCE OF THE STATE SURVEY AND CERTIFICATION PROCESSES

As noted earlier, CMS holds responsibility for overseeing the state survey process. Several reports from GAO and OIG over the past two decades have found failures in the survey process to properly identify serious care problems, fully correct and prevent recurrence of identified problems, and investigate complaints in a timely manner, as well as failures in CMS's oversight of these surveys (GAO, 1999, 2003, 2007, 2008, 2009a, 2010b, 2018, 2019; OIG, 2006b, 2019b,c, 2020a, 2022a). For example, a 2008 GAO study found that surveyors "sometimes understate the extent of serious care problems in homes because they miss deficiencies" (GAO, 2008, p. 2). In January 2022, OIG reported that "just over half of states repeatedly failed to meet requirements for conducting nursing home surveys, most commonly for failures of survey timeliness" (OIG, 2022a, p. 8); 23 percent of failures for timeliness were for failure to conduct high-priority complaints within 10 days of the allegation. In 2020, OIG raised questions about "some states' ability to address serious nursing home complaints and also about the effectiveness of CMS' oversight of states" (OIG, 2020a, p. 14). Furthermore, investigative reports have also highlighted stories of failures in the regulatory process to detect or report serious issues (e.g., abuse, neglect) (Gebeloff et al., 2021; Levinson, 2017; Rau, 2018a; Silver-Greenberg and Gebeloff, 2021).

Improving the survey and certification process requires consideration of several overarching issues, including CMS's oversight of state performance, variability in survey performance, and the limited ability of surveyors to tailor the process based on a facility's previous performance.

Evaluating State Performance of Surveys

A major part of CMS's oversight responsibility includes evaluating state performance in survey and certification activities. The State Performance Standards System allows CMS regional offices to monitor state performance and identify areas for improvement through the use of performance metrics across three domains:

1. Frequency (number and time frame of surveys),
2. Quality (surveys conducted in accordance with federal guidelines and accurately identify deficiencies), and
3. Enforcement and remedy (effectiveness of enforcement) (OIG, 2022a).

If a state is found to have performed inadequately, CMS can impose remedies (e.g., training, technical assistance, and corrective action plans) or sanctions (e.g., meeting with governor and other state officials, reducing federal financial participation, and terminating the state's agreement) (OIG, 2022a). Financial penalties can be imposed in addition to such remedies and sanctions. A 2008 GAO report found that CMS was "not using the database to oversee consistent implementation of the program by the regional offices—for example, the agency is not using the database to identify inconsistencies between comparative and observational survey results" (GAO, 2008, p. 2). In January 2022, OIG reported that many corrective action plans were missing or lacked detail, CMS often did not track training and technical assistance efforts, and CMS rarely imposed formal sanctions (OIG, 2022a). OIG's recommendations included better tracking of the outcomes of remedies, establishing guidelines for progressive enforcement actions on the state, and actively disseminating state performance metrics with other stakeholders.

Variability in Survey Performance

Whether in the implementation of routine inspection responsibilities, imposition of sanctions, or in the investigation of complaints, considerable variation in processes and outcomes exists across states (Castle et al., 2007; CMS, 2021e; GAO, 2005, 2011a; Hansen et al., 2017; Harrington et al., 2008; OIG, 2003, 2019a, 2020a, 2022a; Stevenson, 2006). For example, a 2003 OIG report found that states use different deficiency tags to cite the same problem (OIG, 2003). A 2005 GAO report identified inconsistency in how states conduct surveys (as demonstrated by "wide interstate variability in the proportion of homes found to have serious deficiencies") as a challenge to ensuring high-quality care (GAO, 2005). As mentioned earlier, the responsibility for surveying and enforcing compliance with nursing home standards falls largely to individual states. This approach may increase bureaucracy and inevitably introduces state-level variation in the regulatory process (OIG, 2003). Such variation in implementing federal oversight standards and processes may occur both within and across states. However, it can be difficult to determine what portion of this variation reflects true quality-of-care differences and what portion reflects different state approaches to regulation. For example, states may interpret regulations differently (GAO, 2011a). States can also have limited capacity to faithfully execute oversight responsibilities, and these constraints are especially acute in some states.

Responsiveness to Previous Performance

Nursing home oversight in the United States is largely a standardized enterprise, with almost all facilities inspected for compliance with the same standards on a roughly annual basis. In contrast, a more targeted approach to regulation would scrutinize low- and high-quality performers with differing intensity. The idea of targeted or responsive regulation has a broad theoretical foundation aimed at making oversight more effective. Regulatory theorists have outlined the potential strengths and limitations of the approach (Braithwaite et al., 2007; Walshe, 2001), and both the 1986 and 2001 IOM reports on long-term care quality raised the notion of targeting inspection efforts more efficiently (IOM, 1986, 2001). In 1986, the IOM noted

> the introduction into the survey cycle of flexibility that is tied to performance and key events should enable survey resources to be targeted to those facilities most in need of attention: problem or marginal facilities and facilities where new circumstances could adversely affect residents. Facilities that are performing well would be rewarded for their good behavior by less-intense monitoring. That will allow survey agency staff to be used for more urgent tasks. (IOM, 1986, p. 112)

In fact, the current approach to nursing home oversight already incorporates elements of responsive regulation, albeit primarily at the lower end of the quality spectrum, such as through the SFF program. CMS's Quality Improvement Organization program (see Chapter 3) has also targeted relatively poor performers (Stevenson and Mor, 2009). Federal regulations also allow states to vary inspection frequencies between 9 and 15 months and to tailor the inspections themselves based on the anticipated quality of care in the facility. One analysis of the most recent Community Assessment for Public Health Emergency Response survey found that this happens only to a small extent. In 2018, for example, one- and five-star nursing homes differed in survey frequency by only 11 days on average, with an average of 399 days between surveys for all facilities (Stevenson, 2019).

Still, many advocates oppose targeted survey efforts and argue that "the approach fails to recognize our current ability to identify high-performing facilities and how quickly quality of care can decline at even the best nursing homes" (Stevenson, 2019; see also Edelman, 2019). In particular, it has been challenging to conceptualize and implement a revised or scaled-back survey approach for better-performing nursing homes. Such an approach would depend on two key elements: regulators being able to reliably identify better facilities deserving of less scrutiny, and the oversight system being sufficiently responsive to detect and respond if care faltered. At a recent Senate Finance Committee hearing on nursing homes, Senator Ron Wyden (D-OR) characterized the five-star quality rating system as a "mess," in part because of the fact that four- and five-star facilities were among those that had cases of reported abuse and neglect (Wyden, 2019). In addition, a March 2021 *New York Times* article raised additional concerns about the veracity of the data underlying the five-star system, some of which are self-reported (Silver-Greenberg and Gebeloff, 2021). (See Chapter 3 for more on the five-star quality reporting system.)

Collaboration for Quality Improvement

Federal statutes currently preclude survey agencies from consulting with or guiding the nursing homes they oversee, based on the assumption that if surveyors are too collegial with nursing homes, they may be less likely to cite deficiencies or impose sanctions (Li et al., 2012; Stevenson, 2018). Examples of possible collaborations include that state survey agencies could require nursing homes to develop and implement plans of correction for areas where they are falling short, or in advance of imposing fines, survey agencies could encourage nursing homes to work with quality improvement technical-assistance programs to help them identify and address the root causes of their problems (Stevenson and Mor, 2009). In its 1998 report to Congress, HCFA found little evidence that quality improvement initiatives could supplant the normal survey process (HCFA, 1998).

LONG-TERM CARE OMBUDSMAN PROGRAMS

Long-term care ombudsman programs, administered by the Administration for Community Living, represent the only type of entity within the nursing home system whose sole mission is to be an advocate for the residents to ensure that they receive the care to which they are entitled (NORC, 2019). State ombudsmen work to (1) monitor, protect, and promote resident rights by investigating and resolving complaints from nursing home residents; (2) advocate for systems-level change; and (3) perform outreach activities and educate residents, their loved ones, staff, and collaborating agencies on the rights of residents (NORC, 2019). The program plays an important extra-regulatory role in nursing home quality assurance in that these complaints and investigations are distinct from the legally required complaint mechanisms that state regulatory agencies direct (Berish et al., 2019; Hunt, 2008). Ombudsmen can serve as liaisons between the government and facilities by communicating information about best practices to nursing homes, responding to concerns about oversight and quality of care, and alerting government agencies to problems that require their attention (Berish et al., 2019). One study noted, "Though ombudsmen have limited power in their oversight and have no binding regulatory authority, they play three major roles in the long-term care environment: mediator, informal therapist, and resident advocate" (Berish et al., 2019, p. 1326).

The Long-Term Care Ombudsman Program began as a demonstration program in 1972 and was elevated to a statutory level in 1978 through an amendment to the Older Americans Act which required each state to establish an ombudsman program (ACL, 2021b; Hunt, 2008; NASUAD, 2019). Over time, additional amendments expanded the program to other long-term care settings, provided various legal protections for the ombudsmen themselves, established the National Long-Term Care Ombudsman Resource Center,[9] and required all ombudsmen to participate in training provided by that center. In 2016, the State Long-Term Care Ombudsman Programs Final Rule provided guidance for operating state-based programs, including defining the responsibilities of key figures and entities, criteria and roles for approaches to resolving complaints, and conflicts of interest (ACL, 2021b; NASUAD, 2019). Today, the Long-Term Care Ombudsman Program has an official Office of the State Long-Term Care Ombudsman in all U.S. states, the District of Columbia, Puerto Rico, and Guam (ACL, 2021b). By statute, ombudsmen are required to

- Identify, investigate, and resolve complaints made by or on behalf of residents;
- Provide information to residents about long-term services and supports;
- Ensure that residents have regular and timely access to ombudsman services;
- Represent the interests of residents before governmental agencies and seek administrative, legal, and other remedies to protect residents; and
- Analyze, comment on, and recommend changes in laws and regulations pertaining to the health, safety, welfare, and rights of residents (ACL, 2021b).

---

[9] For more information, see https://ltcombudsman.org (accessed August 16, 2021).

Structure and Funding of Long-Term Care Ombudsman Programs

The Administration for Community Living provides grants to each State Unit on Aging to develop an annual state plan for its long-term care ombudsman program and establish an Office of the State Long-Term Care Ombudsman. The state ombudsman administers the state program and oversees designated representatives of the state office who serve as local staff as well as volunteers (NORC, 2019); long-term care ombudsman programs often have few paid staff at the state and local level, with volunteers conducting most of their activities (Berish et al., 2019). In FY 2017, the program overall had 1,319 full-time paid staff and 8,810 total volunteers (NORC, 2019). Having a lower full-time staff to facility ratio correlates with a higher percentage of facilities being visited at least quarterly. Expenditures on these programs totaled $106.7 million across all funding sources in FY 2017; the federal government provided 50 percent, states provided 43 percent, and local governments 7 percent of this funding (NORC, 2019).

While regulations require state units on aging to ensure that the ombudsman programs have sufficient resources and protections to conduct their legislatively mandated functions, there is considerable variation in the amount of resources, funding, and staffing among all programs, with limited funding affecting many programs' abilities to meet federal mandates. For example,

- Only 23 percent of state ombudsmen report having sufficient financial resources,
- Only 27 percent of state ombudsmen report having sufficient staff,
- Only 15 percent of state ombudsmen report having enough volunteers, and
- Only 56 percent of state ombudsmen report having adequate legal counsel (NORC, 2019).

At least half of state ombudsmen report that a lack of resources hinders their ability to fully conduct the following activities: recruitment and retention of volunteers, development and support of resident and family council development and support, community education, legal assistance for residents, and regular nursing home visits (NORC, 2019).

Extent of Services

In FY 2017, ombudsmen visited 68 percent of all nursing homes on at least a quarterly basis for routine visits and, when also including complaint investigations, 79 percent of nursing homes (NORC, 2019). While state ombudsmen do some onsite visits, they are primarily responsible for overseeing the program, and local and volunteer ombudsmen

TABLE 8-4 Services Provided by Long-Term Care Ombudsmen and Level of Activity, FY 2017

Services Provided by Long-Term Care Ombudsmen	Level of Activity in FY 2017
Complaints	201,460*
Provision of information to individuals and staff	529,098
Attendance at resident and family council meetings	22,999
Community education sessions	10,170

SOURCE: NORC, 2019.
NOTES: *The top three categories for complaints are discharge/eviction, failure to respond to requests for assistance, and issues related to dignity and respect. Complaints were most often received from residents (40 percent), nursing home staff (19 percent), and relatives and friends (18 percent).

typically perform the in-person visits (NORC, 2019). Among the paid state ombudsmen who reported visiting nursing homes, 45 percent did so on a routine basis, compared with 81 percent of local ombudsmen and 95 percent of volunteer ombudsmen (NORC, 2019). Table 8-4 above provides an overview of the extent of services provided by ombudsmen to nursing home residents in 2017.

Evidence of Impact

Although few rigorous studies have quantified the program's impact, researchers have noted that the "existence of a local [long-term care ombudsman program] is a significant predictor of quality of care, suggesting a positive preventative presence," (Estes et al., 2010, p. 775) especially given the modest investment of governmental resources (Hollister and Estes, 2013). The presence of an ombudsman has been associated with increased levels of complaints and deficiency citations, which suggests that ombudsmen are able to bring more issues to the attention of surveyors; additionally, ombudsman are more likely to be present at surveys of nursing homes with persistently poorer quality (Berish et al., 2019). Studies have found that the effectiveness of ombudsmen increases significantly with more autonomy and investment of resources, including funding; a larger number of paid staff; and minimum staffing requirements, smaller case-loads, and higher percentages of nursing facilities visited (Estes et al., 2004).

Seventy-eight percent of volunteer ombudsmen, but only 51 percent of state ombudsmen and 66 percent of local ombudsmen, report that the majority of their relationships in nursing homes are effective (NORC, 2019). The volunteers attributed this effectiveness to "the ongoing presence they maintain in facilities and the positive working relationships they develop with facility staff who come to view them as a resource" (NORC, 2019).

Local ombudsman also reported that "their knowledge, confidence and experience level are crucial factors in determining the effectiveness of their relationships with facility staff" (NORC, 2019).

RESIDENT AND FAMILY COUNCILS

As described in Chapter 4, resident and family councils are independent groups for residents and families to discuss and address any issues or concerns within a facility. The primary goal of such councils is to improve the quality of care and life within nursing homes (Grant, 2021). Additionally, councils meet to discuss issues and policies that affect resident care, plan activities, provide education, and serve as a bridge between residents and the facility, among other activities (Grant, 2021; LTCCC, 2017).

OBRA 87 first included regulatory requirements for family and resident councils. The act requires facilities to[10]

- Provide existing councils with private meeting spaces,
- Designate a staff person to assist with council requests, and
- Respond to concerns and recommendations of the council regarding resident care and quality of life (Legal Aid Justice Center, 2013).

The 2016 federal regulations updated and strengthened the requirements for these councils. Specifically, the new 2016 regulations updated the requirements concerning resident and family councils with the following:[11]

- Residents must invite their families/individuals to participate in the councils;
- Councils must include people beyond family members, called resident representatives, if a resident chooses;
- Residents themselves can participate in the councils;
- The facility and council must both approve the designated staff person;
- The facility must make residents, family members, and resident representatives aware of upcoming council meetings in a way that the council approves;
- The facility must act promptly upon grievances and recommendations from the council and provide a rationale for their response (Justice in Aging, National Consumer Voice, and CMA, 2021; National Consumer Voice, 2017).

For more on resident and family councils, see Box 4-7 in Chapter 4.

---

[10] Omnibus Budget Reconciliation Act of 1987, Public Law 100-203; 42 USC §1396r(c).
[11] CMS Requirements for Long Term Care Facilities—Resident Rights, 42 CFR § 483.10 (2016).

EFFECTIVENESS OF QUALITY ASSURANCE FOR IMPROVING THE QUALITY OF CARE

Despite the prominent role of nursing home oversight and regulation, there is relatively modest evidence concerning its effectiveness in ensuring a minimum standard of quality. Much of the evidence is observational and follows the national implementation of OBRA 87. Measuring how well nursing home oversight activities minimize poor-quality care is challenging, not only because all U.S. nursing homes are subject to the same minimum federal standards, but also because of the many other changes that have occurred in the nursing home sector over the decades since OBRA 87 was passed. With this caveat, many studies have documented improvements in resident outcomes and care practices in the years following the implementation of OBRA 87. Nursing home regulations seem particularly effective at improving quality in certain easily measured and discrete categories. For example, in the years following OBRA 87, there was a substantial decrease in the use of restraints and catheters; reductions in dehydration rates and pressure ulcers; more discussions between residents and care providers about care plans, end-of-life plans, and other issues; and increased overall staffing levels (Fashaw et al., 2020; Hawes, 1996; Hawes et al., 1997; HCFA, 1998; IOM, 1996; Wiener et al., 2007; Zhang and Grabowski, 2004). Although notable improvements in care practices and selected quality measures followed the implementation of OBRA 87, nursing home care still demonstrates persistent quality challenges, at least among a subset of facilities. It is unclear whether these recurring challenges reflect inadequate implementation and enforcement of existing standards (as described earlier in this chapter) or deeper limitations in what quality-directed regulation can achieve.

Regulation specifies that the role of the federal government is to ensure the requirements of participation are enforced and "are adequate to protect the health, safety, welfare, and rights of residents and to promote the effective and efficient use of public moneys."[12] (See later in this chapter for more on transparency related to the financing of nursing home care.) It is difficult to calculate the total costs to federal and state governments of regulating nursing homes, and few studies have done so. A 2001 study estimated the annual costs of the nursing home survey and certification process at $382 million, or $22,000 per home (Walshe, 2001). After accounting for inflation and other changes in the nursing home sector over the past two decades, the direct costs to the government today are likely to be considerably higher. Moreover, in addition to the costs of regulation for government,

---

[12] Nursing Home Reform Law of 1987, Public Law 100-203, 42 USC 1395i-3(f)(1), 100th Cong., 1st sess. (December 22, 1987).

the direct and indirect costs of regulatory oversight to nursing homes are important to consider against the benefits to residents' quality of care and quality of life (Mor, 2011; Mukamel et al., 2011, 2012, 2014; Stevenson, 2019). Some of the only research in this area found that greater regulatory stringency was significantly associated with better quality for four of seven quality measures studied and that the cost-effectiveness for the activities of daily living measure in particular was estimated to be around $72,000 per quality-adjusted life year in 2011 (Mukamel et al., 2012).

Most resident advocates and nursing home providers are dissatisfied with the effectiveness of the current nursing home regulatory model, yet little consensus exists on how to improve the system (Stevenson, 2018). Nursing home advocates highlight the fact that, as noted earlier, existing regulations are often not being completely and consistently enforced and suggest that additional regulations need to be put in place to fully protect residents. Alternatively, many providers believe that the existing regulations are excessive and impede innovation and good-quality care. Unlike other areas of nursing home care, little common ground exists between the two groups. The lack of empirical evidence to guide policy makers is a further barrier to progress.

TRANSPARENCY AND ACCOUNTABILITY

A key aim of nursing home oversight over the past decade has been to ensure greater transparency in ownership and financing. Most nursing homes have been for-profit entities for decades. In the early 2000s, increased private equity investment and ownership complexity spurred a renewed focus on this topic (Duhigg, 2007; Stevenson and Grabowski, 2008), culminating with the ACA including provisions to encourage the disclosure of ownership and financial relationships (KFF, 2013). Still, it is clear that such transparency has not occurred. The committee recognizes that these issues are prevalent across the entire health care system, and not limited to nursing homes. However, the following sections highlight the implications of this lack of transparency on improving the quality of nursing home care.

Nursing Home Ownership

Nursing homes can be classified as either for-profit, nonprofit, or government-owned nursing homes. As Chapter 2 notes, 69.3 percent of nursing homes are for-profit entities, and nearly 60 percent are affiliated with companies that own or operate more than one nursing home (chain ownership) (Harris-Kojetin et al., 2019).

Despite important nuances related to the case mix of certain nursing homes and nursing home chains, the literature suggests that, in general, for-profit nursing homes consistently demonstrate lower levels of quality, including satisfaction with care, than not-for-profit nursing homes (Banaszak-Holl et al., 2002; Comondore et al., 2009; GAO, 2011b; Grabowski and Hirth, 2003; Grabowski et al., 2013; Harrington et al., 2001; Hillmer et al., 2005; Stevenson and Grabowski, 2008; You et al., 2016). For example, for-profit nursing homes, compared with nonprofit or government-owned nursing homes, have been associated with fewer registered nurse and total nurse staffing hours, fewer nurses per resident, and more deficiencies (Harrington et al., 2012; O'Neill et al., 2003; Rau and Lucas, 2018). In addition, nursing homes designated as SFFs are more likely to be for-profit facilities or part of a chain (GAO, 2009d). Studies suggest a possible association between for-profit ownership and higher rates of COVID-19 cases and deaths (as compared to nonprofit or government-owned nursing homes) (Bach-Mortensen et al., 2021; Ochieng et al., 2021). The relationship between quality of care and ownership status has also been observed when for-profit nursing homes convert to not-for-profit ownership and subsequently demonstrate improvements in quality, nonprofit nursing homes convert to for-profit and show a decline in performance (Grabowski and Stevenson, 2008), or chains are purchased by private equity companies (Harrington et al., 2012).

Data from the first 5 years (2009–2013) of the five-star rating system reveal that for-profit nursing homes had lower ratings than the nonprofit and government-owned nursing homes (Abt Associates Inc., 2014). "Indeed nearly twice as many non-profit as for-profit nursing homes a five-star overall quality rating (35.6 percent vs. 19.7 percent)" (Abt Associates Inc., 2014, p. 8). Furthermore, only 5.7 percent of for-profit nursing homes received five stars in the staffing domain, compared to 21 percent of nonprofit nursing homes and 26 percent of government-owned nursing homes. (See Chapter 3 for more on the five-star quality rating.) Nursing home chains are more likely to acquire nursing homes of lower quality, and these quality problems persist after the acquisition (Grabowski et al., 2016).

One challenge associated with chain ownership is that chain owners may have pressures to prioritize corporate interests over the residents' needs (Banaszak-Holl et al., 2002; Harrington et al., 2001; You et al., 2016). Beyond chain ownership, nursing home ownership has become more complex over the past few decades. For example, private equity ownership and real estate investment trusts (REITs) have been expanding in health care, including among nursing homes (Cockburn, 2020; Finn, 2020; GAO, 2010c; Harrington et al., 2017, 2021; Stevenson and Grabowski, 2008). Private equity ownership of nursing homes has been associated with higher short-term mortality; lower measures of well-being, such as mobility; higher numbers of total deficiencies; lower total nurse staffing ratios (i.e., fewer hours per resident day); and increased costs (Braun et al., 2021; GAO, 2011b; Gupta et al., 2021). Private equity ownership of nursing homes has also been associated with a lower likelihood of having adequate supply of personal protective equipment (PPE) (Braun et al., 2020). Private equity and REIT engagement helped fuel a restructuring in how nursing home companies are organized. Harrington and colleagues (2021) found that

> Many nursing homes separated their operating companies from their asset and property companies in an effort to shield parent companies from liability and reduce regulatory oversight. Real estate investment companies (REITs) have dramatically expanded their ownership since the Housing and Economic Recovery Act of 2008 allowed REITs to buy health care facilities. These companies lease their facilities and property to nursing home operating companies at sometimes exorbitant rents.

Given the influence of ownership status on the quality of care in nursing homes, enhanced transparency regarding the details of ownership, including corporate structure and spending priorities, would provide important insights. Nursing homes are required to report certain details about their ownership structures, which is captured in CMS's Provider Enrollment Chain and Ownership System (PECOS). However, PECOS data are incomplete and somewhat difficult for consumers, payers, regulators, and others to use (GAO, 2010c). Furthermore, CMS does not audit the data for accuracy and has not enforced reporting requirements related to the nursing home's organization (e.g., parent companies, related-party entities) (Harrington et al., 2021).

As discussed earlier in this chapter, the assurance of nursing home quality centers largely on public-sector oversight through licensure and certification. The focus of these efforts is on whether an individual nursing home is performing acceptably. When problems are present, the nursing home must make corrections or, in cases of extremely deficient care, a nursing home may face a range of sanctions (or, rarely, lose its certification to serve Medicare or Medicaid residents). However, with some exceptions (e.g., fraud and abuse), regulatory policy focuses on and sanctions the facility-level provider rather than looking at performance across nursing homes with a common owner or management company. Similarly, information available on Care Compare, including the five-star rating system, is all at the level of the individual facility (see Chapter 3). Consumers, payers, regulators, and others could benefit from a readily available capacity to examine facilities and other related entities in which owners have a stake. Publicly available ownership information needs to reflect and capture the complexity of today's nursing home sector (e.g., operations, ownership structures) to enable tracking quality across nursing homes with a common owner, understand which entities are responsible for care, and determine which entities are benefiting from Medicare and Medicaid payments or favorable tax policies that might further entice them into the sector (e.g., REIT investors).

Financing

Quality assurance efforts have not focused extensively on the potential labyrinth of financial ties that shape what facilities are able to do, including how they are able to respond during a crisis. For example, while many for-profit nursing homes receive funds from the federal government (i.e., CMS), there are no specific requirements for how these funds are spent (in spite of the federal government's responsibility, noted earlier, in overseeing how public funds are spent). Improving the ability to understand where nursing homes spend their resources and gaining a more accurate sense of their overall financial well-being are essential elements of transparency. Progress has been made in simplifying nursing home cost reporting, yet substantial questions remain regarding the accuracy and completeness of these data (GAO, 2016). In fact, a significant lack of transparency characterizes the overall state of nursing home financing.

While nursing homes report low operating margins, with potential negative impacts on patient care and quality, some are using third-party transactions or unrelated business entities to hide profits (Cenziper et al., 2020; Harrington et al., 2015, 2021; Rau, 2017, 2018b). For example, a case study of a for-profit nursing home chain in California found that "the chain's complex, interlocking individual and corporate owners and property companies obscured its ownership structure and financial arrangements" (Harrington et al., 2015, p. 779). In addition, it has become more apparent over the last few decades that nursing homes' real estate assets are central to the entities that choose to invest in this sector. Furthermore, the engagement of private equity and REITs is fueled by the tax advantages of these arrangements, including their potential role in operating facilities.

Moreover, Rau (2017) reported that owners of nursing homes "outsource a wide variety of goods and services to companies in which they have a financial interest or that they control" through related-party transactions, sometimes at prices that are well over the market rates in order to accrue higher profits that nursing homes do not record in their financial accounts. In 2018, Rau reported that related party transactions accounted for $11 billion in nursing home expenditures in 2015 (one-tenth of their costs) and that "homes with related companies were fined 22 percent more often for serious health violations than independent homes" (Rau, 2018b); nursing homes that outsource to related organizations tend to have lower staffing levels, higher rates of patient injuries and unsafe practices, and almost twice as many complaints as independent homes (Rau, 2017).

Evidence suggests that this outsourcing practice may be widespread. A 2009 study from the Office of the Assistant Secretary for Planning and Evaluation, for example, found that an increasing number of nursing homes were changing hands to regionally focused private-investment-owned facilities that increasingly used limited liability corporation structures and partnership structures, such as general partnerships and limited partnerships (ASPE, 2009). Owners had also arranged for additional corporations to create layers in between themselves and their nursing homes, an arrangement that replaced previous basic for-profit and not-for-profit owner-operator structures (ASPE, 2009; Stevenson et al., 2013b). For a family member perspective on nursing home ownership and financing, see Box 8-5.

The lack of transparency or accountability in payment, funds flow, and nursing home finances makes it extremely difficult to assess the adequacy of current Medicaid payments. (See Chapter 7 for more on financing of nursing homes.) Though it is not an illegal practice, advocates have raised concerns that nursing home operators may use public Medicare and Medicaid funds to cover non-direct-care services (e.g., administrative costs) and earn significant profit while reporting low margins (LTCCC, 2021). For example, in the aforementioned case study of a California for-profit nursing home chain, the authors found that "profits were hidden in the chain's management fees, lease agreements, interest payments to owners, and purchases from related-party companies" (Harrington et al., 2015, p. 779). Furthermore, despite claims of financial challenges during the COVID-19 pandemic, one analysis of 11 publicly traded nursing home companies found that they had suffered relatively little financial impact (Kingsley and Harrington, 2021).

Consolidated annual reports that include data from operators and entities related by common ownership or management could help provide greater transparency and financial accountability needed to improve regulatory oversight (Harrington et al., 2021). For example, in 2021, California passed legislation requiring such a report, including information about the owner/operator and all related parties that have an ownership or control

---

BOX 8-5
Family Member Perspective

"My experience validated everything I know about the difference between non-profit and for-profit nursing homes. I want to emphasize the need to change how privately owned nursing homes are allowed to separate ownership into real estate and operations, allowed to create related-party businesses that siphon off profits that should go to staff and care."

— Daughter and caregiver of two parents with
dementia who needed nursing home care

This quote was collected from the committee's online call for resident, family, and nursing home staff perspectives.

interest of 5 percent or more and provide any service, facility, or supply to the nursing home (Grajeda and Yood, 2021). Sponsors of the legislation argued that large, for-profit nursing homes were "using complex ownership structures to increase profitability by shielding funds behind the corporate family so that these funds cannot be fully considered by the state when it sets rates and reimbursements for care" and that the reports would allow the state to evaluate if nursing homes were diverting revenues into related entities rather than directing the funds toward resident care (Grajeda and Yood, 2021).

NURSING HOME OVERSIGHT DURING COVID-19

The threat posed by COVID-19 resulted in a different approach to oversight. More immediate and effective regulation could have helped guide facilities to better protect nursing home residents, staff, and families. For example, CMS did not require routine COVID-19 testing until 6 months after the pandemic started, facilities did not have access to a reliable supply of PPE, and no state imposed limitations on part-time or agency staff who visited multiple facilities (Kohn, 2021). Chronic underenforcement (i.e., lack of proper identification of deficiencies and imposition of penalties) exacerbated these problems. In fact, at the start of the pandemic, per-day fines for noncompliance were replaced with per-instance fines, key requirements were waived, and nursing homes restricted access to surveyors and ombudsmen (Kohn, 2021).

To limit the spread of COVID-19 in nursing homes, outside visitation by anyone other than essential health care personnel (including family, surveyors, and ombudsmen) was restricted (except in some very limited circumstances), and group activities and communal dining were eliminated. The initial CMS regulatory guidance emphasized flexibility and prioritized protecting residents over compliance with certain regulations. For example, CMS temporarily suspended specific reporting requirements such as resident assessment and staffing data, and it also waived some requirements related to residents' rights in the name of physical safety (Stevenson and Bonner, 2020; Stevenson and Cheng, 2021). CMS also directed state survey agencies to stop regular inspection efforts and instead focus inspection efforts on infection control and investigating allegations of immediate jeopardy to residents (CMS, 2020a,b; 2021f). See Figure 8-2 for CMS guidance changes early in the pandemic.

Regulators had a difficult balance to strike during the public health emergency—"maintaining general protections and accountability while ensuring that nursing homes had sufficient flexibility and resources to meet residents' needs" (Stevenson and Bonner, 2020). Early in the pandemic, these steps were seen as essential for resident safety, but the repercussions

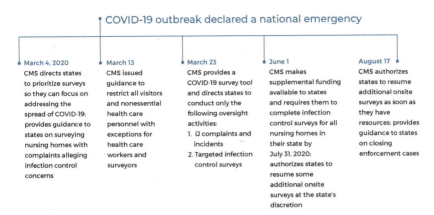

FIGURE 8-2 Timeline of key CMS guidance to states early in the COVID-19 pandemic.
SOURCE: OIG, 2020b.

of these actions were substantial and carried separate harms of their own (Dolan and Mejia, 2020a; Mo and Shi, 2020; Montgomery et al., 2020; Rodney et al., 2021). Disaster planning focused on the physical safety of residents and overlooked other aspects of psychosocial well-being. The sudden loss of connections to family, friends, and volunteers and the new barriers to health and social services staff undercut modern expectations for high-quality nursing home care. For example, findings from a national survey revealed that 76 percent of nursing home residents felt lonelier than usual and 64 percent did not even leave their rooms to socialize (Montgomery et al., 2020). Families expressed concern that their loved ones in nursing homes seemed more lethargic, had worse physical health, and stopped smiling and laughing amidst the visitation restrictions and reduced oversight (HRW, 2021; Nash et al., 2021). For family member perspectives on the impact of visitation policies during the COVID-19 pandemic, see Box 8-6. (See Chapters 2 and 4 for more on social isolation and loneliness during the pandemic.)

As a result of this guidance, surveys were less thorough, and there were fewer documented complaints from ombudsman, families, and residents (OIG, 2020b; Stevenson and Cheng, 2021). In fact, "Deficiency citations generally decreased to near zero by April 2020 with the exception of infection prevention and control deficiencies and citations for failure to report COVID-19 data to the national health safety network" (Stevenson and Cheng, 2021). Consequently, nursing homes were not being held liable or accountable for deficiencies, such as understaffing (Kohn, 2021). Backlogs for standard surveys grew exponentially during the pandemic,

> **BOX 8-6**
> **Family Member Perspectives**
>
> "The social isolation that my mother suffered during her end of life was heartbreaking, wrong, and unconscionable. She suffered an inhuman end of life, denied both family and clergy to ease her suffering."
>
> — E.
>
> "My mother was in from July until she just die in March. What I would change is the elimination of visitation for a year. The isolation worsened my mom's heart failure and dementia."
>
> — Anonymous, Brunswick, Ohio
>
> *These quotes were collected from the committee's online call for resident, family, and nursing home staff perspectives.*

ranging from 22 to 96 percent of nursing homes by state (with a national average of 71 percent) going without a standard survey for at least 16 months from February 1, 2020, through May 31, 2021 (OIG, 2021). Furthermore, investigative reports drew attention to cases of inappropriate evictions and unsafe transfers of older adults and people with disabilities from nursing homes, many to homeless shelters, ostensibly as a way to make room for more lucrative short-stay residents with COVID-19 coming from hospitals (Dolan and Mejia, 2020b; Silver-Greenberg and Harris, 2020).

With facilities in lockdown, oversight was needed to ensure not only the adequacy of infection controls but the quality of resident care more generally. Quality assurance was challenging before the pandemic, and the "significantly scaled back oversight and data reporting was concerning, even if temporary" (Stevenson and Bonner, 2020). For example, problem facilities such as SFFs still needed to be monitored for general quality, but guidance did not prioritize or distinguish the continued need for enhanced oversight of these facilities during the pandemic.

Careful emergency planning and regulatory changes can help facilities better respond to emergencies—both event-specific emergencies such as hurricanes, but also broader and longer-lasting public health emergencies, such as COVID-19—and prevent such disproportionate devastation on nursing home communities in the future. (See Chapter 6 for more on emergency planning.) Contingency plans to address the lack of PPE and in-person visitation "should be viewed as essential for bolstering care oversight, residents' mental and physical health, and delivering high quality care" (Stevenson and Cheng, 2021). This may include options such as virtual monitoring activities, equipping facilities with PPE resources and technology for safe in-person or virtual visitation, and improving data collection and communication between facilities and regulatory bodies (Stevenson and Bonner, 2020; Stevenson and Cheng, 2021). Maintaining regulatory activities, transparency, and oversight will be a critical part of protecting residents' health, well-being, and quality of life during future emergencies.

KEY FINDINGS AND CONCLUSIONS

General Oversight and Regulation

- While substantial changes have occurred in nursing home care since the implementation of OBRA 87 regulations, the general structure of the oversight and regulation of nursing homes has largely remained the same.
- The oversight and enforcement of nursing home rules were scaled back in 2017 as part of a broader movement to reduce bureaucracy and government intervention.
- Requirements of participation provide the primary focus for regulation and cover a range of dimensions, such as residents' rights, quality of care, quality of life, and the physical environment.
- States have the primary responsibility for licensure of nursing home providers as a way to control the market, but few facilities have been denied licensure.
- Certificate-of-need regulations and construction moratoria do not appear to have had their intended effect of holding down Medicaid nursing home spending; rather, these laws can discourage innovation and decrease access.
- Certificate-of-need regulations may contribute to the perpetuation of larger nursing homes.
- Despite the prominent role of nursing home oversight and regulation, the evidence base for its effectiveness in ensuring a minimum standard of quality is relatively modest.
- Many resident advocates and nursing home providers are dissatisfied with the effectiveness of the current nursing home regulatory model. Yet, little consensus exists on how to improve the system.

State Surveys and Sanctions

- States assist with the assessment of facilities' compliance with requirements of participation and, as necessary, with the investigation of complaints and adverse incidents. States have some discretion in how they administer these responsibilities, but all states are expected to adhere to the detailed protocols outlined in the State Operations Manual.
- Nursing home oversight in the United States is largely a standardized process, with almost all facilities inspected for compliance with the same standards on a roughly annual basis. However, there is considerable variation in processes and outcomes in the implementation of routine inspection responsibilities, in the imposition of sanctions, and in the investigation of complaints.
- There is some evidence that states have difficulty finding qualified surveyors, and limited evidence on the quality of training and effectiveness of state surveyors.
- CMS and state survey agencies can levy a range of sanctions against out-of-compliance nursing homes, but the imposition of CMPs is most common.
- State survey agencies may not have adequate capacity or resources to fulfill all their responsibilities.
- Decades of evidence document failures in the survey process to properly identify serious care problems, to fully correct and prevent recurrence of identified problems, to investigate complaints in a timely manner, and in CMS's oversight of these surveys.
- CMS is able to impose remedies or sanctions if a state is found to have performed inadequately, but CMS does not fully track performance and rarely imposes formal sanctions.
- While the current regulatory process needs significant improvement, particularly in relation to the uneven enforcement of regulations, there is a dearth of evidence to suggest which approaches would ultimately lead to improvement in the quality of care.
- Real-time metrics need to be used in the testing of new approaches to surveys (e.g., changed frequency) in order to monitor for signals of decreasing quality.
- The budget of the SFF program allows for oversight of only a very small fraction of low-performing nursing homes, and many facilities that graduate from the program fail to sustain improvement.

Long-Term Care Ombudsman Program

- There is considerable variation in the resources, funding, and staffing among ombudsman programs, and limited funding affects programs' abilities to meet federal and state requirements and to fully

- provide nursing home residents and their families with the best support possible.
- The impact of the Long-Term Care Ombudsman Program has been largely positive, especially given the modest investment of governmental resources.

Transparency and Accountability

- Current data sources provide little insight into the corporate structure, finances, and operations of individual nursing homes.
- In general, for-profit nursing homes consistently demonstrate lower levels of quality, including satisfaction with care, than not-for-profit nursing homes.
- Current data sources do not allow for an examination of performance across nursing homes by a common owner.
- Nursing homes may use related-party transactions or unrelated business entities to hide profits. There is a lack of transparency regarding these transactions.
- Progress has been made in simplifying nursing home cost reporting, yet there are still substantial questions about the accuracy and completeness of these data.
- Increased transparency and accountability of the finances, operations, and ownership of nursing homes is important for improving the financial investment in nursing home care as well as to improve quality assurance, all toward the common goal of improving the quality of care in nursing homes.

COVID-19

- During the pandemic, regulators had a difficult balance to strike—maintaining general protections and accountability while ensuring that nursing homes had sufficient flexibility and resources to meet residents' needs.
- Early responses to the pandemic prioritized resident safety over other aspects of psychosocial well-being.
- Limiting visitation by family, surveyors, and ombudsmen affected the quality of care.
- CMS directed state survey agencies to scale back regular inspection efforts in order to focus on infection control and investigations of immediate jeopardy.
- Surveys were less thorough, and there were fewer documented complaints from ombudsman, families, and residents.
- During the COVID-19 pandemic, many states sought liability protections for nursing homes against pandemic-related claims of negligence.

- Maintaining regulatory activities, transparency, and oversight will be a critical part of protecting residents' health, well-being, and quality of life during future emergencies.

REFERENCES

Abt Associates. 2014. *Nursing home compare five-star quality rating system: Year five report [public version]*. Baltimore, MD: Abt Associates Inc.

ACL (Administration for Community Living). 2021a. *Older Americans Act*. https://acl.gov/about-acl/authorizing-statutes/older-americans-act (accessed December 2, 2021).

ACL. 2021b. *Long-Term Care Ombudsman Program*. https://acl.gov/programs/Protecting-Rights-and-Preventing-Abuse/Long-term-Care-Ombudsman-Program (accessed August 19, 2021).

ASHE (American Society for Health Care Engineering). 2021. *Deemed status*. https://www.ashe.org/advocacy/orgs/deemedstatus (accessed September 2, 2021).

ASPE (Assistant Secretary for Planning and Evaluation). 2009. *Nursing home ownership trends and their impact on quality of care*. Washington, DC: HHS Office of the Assistant Secretary for Planning and Evaluation.

Associated Press. 2021. Critics say Indiana COVID-19 law allows nursing home neglect. *NPR*, May 8. https://www.wfyi.org/news/articles/critics-say-indiana-COVID-19-law-allows-nursing-home-neglect (accessed November 17, 2021).

Bach-Mortensen, A. M., B. Verboom, A. Movsisyan, and M. D. Esposti. 2021. A systematic review of the associations between care home ownership and COVID-19 outbreaks, infections and mortality. *Nature Aging* 1:948–961.

Banaszak-Holl, J., W. B. Berta, D. M. Bowman, J. A. Baum, and W. Mitchell. 2002. The rise of human service chains: Antecedents to acquisitions and their effects on the quality of care in U.S. nursing homes. *Managerial and Decision Economics* 23(4–5):261–282.

Berish, D. E., J. Bornstein, and J. R. Bowblis. 2019. The impact of long-term care ombudsman presence on nursing home survey deficiencies. *Journal of the American Medical Directors Association* 20(10):1325–1330.

Braithwaite, J., T. Makkai, and V. A. Braithwaite. 2007. *Regulating aged care: Ritualism and the new pyramid*. Cheltenham, UK: Edward Elgar Publishing.

Braun, R. T., H. Yun, L. P. Casalino, Z. Myslinski, F. M. Kuwonza, H. Jung, and M. A. Unruh. 2020. Comparative performance of private equity-owned U.S. nursing homes during the COVID-19 pandemic. *JAMA Network Open* 3(10). https://doi.org/10.1001/jamanetworkopen.2020.26702.

Braun, R. T., H. Jung, L. P. Casalino, Z. Myslinski, and M. A. Unruh. 2021. Association of private equity investments in U.S. nursing homes with the quality and cost of care for long-stay residents. *JAMA Health Forum* 2(11). https://doi.org/10.1001/jamahealthforum.2021.3817.

Brinker, P. A., and B. Walker. 1962. The Hill-Burton Act: 1948–1954. *Review of Economics and Statistics* 44(2):208–212.

Brooks, S., R. Grant, and M. F. Bonamarte. 2020. States move to shield LTC facilities from civil liability. *Bifocal* 41(6): July 6. https://www.americanbar.org/groups/law_aging/publications/bifocal/vol-41/vol-41--issue-no-6--july-august-2020-/states-move-to-shield-ltc-facilities-from-liability/ (accessed January 25, 2022).

Brown, D. 2021. Providers rejoice after receiving liability protections for nursing homes. *McKnights Long-Term Care News*, April 7. https://www.mcknights.com/news/providers-rejoice-after-receiving-liability-protections-for-nursing-homes (accessed November 17, 2021).

Bruneau, J. 2014. *The great healthcare CON.* https://fee.org/articles/the-great-healthcare-con (accessed February 4, 2022).

California State Auditor. 2014. *California Department of Public Health: It has not effectively managed investigations of complaints related to long-term health care facilities: Report 2014-111.* https://www.auditor.ca.gov/pdfs/reports/2014-111.pdf (accessed February 5, 2022).

California State Auditor. 2020. *State high risk: The California State Auditor's updated assessment of high-risk issues faced by the state and select state agencies.* https://www.bsa.ca.gov/pdfs/reports/2019-601.pdf (accessed February 5, 2022).

Carlson, E. 2015. *20 common nursing home problems—and how to resolve them.* https://www.waombudsman.org/files/2015/10/20CommonNurseHomeProblems.pdf (accessed November 16, 2021).

Castle, N. G., J. Engberg, and A. Men. 2007. Variation in the use of nursing home deficiency citations. *Journal of Healthcare Quality* 29(6):12–23.

Castle, N. G., L. M. Wagner, J. C. Ferguson, and S. M. Handler. 2011. Safety culture of nursing homes: Opinions of top managers. *Health Care Management Review* 36(2):175–187.

Cavanaugh, J., C. G. Brothers, A. Griffin, R. Hoover, M. LoPresti, and J. Wrench. 2020. *Conning the competition: A nationwide survey of certificate of need laws.* Arlington, VA: Institute for Justice.

Cenziper, D., J. Jacobs, A. Crites, and W. Englund. 2020. Profit and pain: How California's largest nursing home chain amassed millions as scrutiny mounted. *The Washington Post*, December 31. https://www.washingtonpost.com/business/2020/12/31/brius-nursing-home (accessed November 8, 2021).

CMA (Center for Medicare Advocacy). 2019. *Special report: "Graduates" from the Special Focus Facility Program provide poor care.* https://medicareadvocacy.org/graduates-from-the-special-focus-facility-program-provided-poor-care (accessed February 5, 2022).

CMS (Centers for Medicare & Medicaid Services). 2008. *Center for Medicaid and State Operations/Survey and Certification Group: Accreditation and its impact on various survey and certification scenarios.* https://www.cms.gov/Medicare/Provider-Enrollment-and-Certification/SurveyCertificationGenInfo/downloads/SCLetter09-08.pdf (accessed September 2, 2021).

CMS. 2016. *Chapter 7 state operations manual—Survey and enforcement process for skilled nursing facilities and nursing facilities.* Washington, DC: Centers for Medicare & Medicaid Services.

CMS. 2017a. *State operations manual: Appendix PP—Guidance to surveyors for long term care facilities.* https://www.cms.gov/Medicare/Provider-Enrollment-and-Certification/GuidanceforLawsAndRegulations/Downloads/Appendix-PP-State-Operations-Manual.pdf (accessed July 8, 2021).

CMS. 2017b. *New long-term care survey process.* https://www.cms.gov/Medicare/Provider-Enrollment-andCertification/GuidanceforLawsAndRegulations/Downloads/New-Long-term-Care-Survey-Process%E2%80%93Slide-Deck-andSpeaker-Notes.pptx (accessed February 1, 2022).

CMS. 2018a. *Medicare and Medicaid programs; proposed regulatory provisions to promote program efficiency, transparency, and burden reduction.* https://www.cms.gov/newsroom/fact-sheets/Medicare-and-Medicaid-programs-proposed-regulatory-provisions-promote-program-efficiency-0 (accessed March 4, 2019).

CMS. 2018b. *State operations manual: Chapter 7—Survey and enforcement process for skilled nursing facilities and nursing facilities.* https://www.cms.gov/regulations-and-guidance/guidance/manuals/downloads/som107c07pdf.pdf (accessed August 10, 2021).

CMS. 2019a. *State operations manual: Chapter 4—Program administration and fiscal management.* https://www.cms.gov/regulations-and-guidance/guidance/manuals/downloads/som107c04pdf.pdf (accessed November 9, 2021).

CMS. 2019b. *State operations manual: Chapter 5—complaint procedures.* https://www.cms.gov/Regulations-and-Guidance/Guidance/Manuals/Downloads/som107c05pdf.pdf (accessed February 2, 2022).

CMS. 2019c. *Examples of non-allowable uses of CMP reinvestment funds.* Washington, DC: Centers for Medicare & Medicaid Services.

CMS. 2020a. *Prioritization of survey activities.* https://www.cms.gov/files/document/qso-20-20-all.pdf (accessed January 12, 2022).

CMS. 2020b. *Guidance for infection control and prevention of coronavirus disease 2019 (COVID-19) in nursing homes (revised).* https://www.cms.gov/files/document/qso-20-14-nh-revised.pdf (accessed November 15, 2021).

CMS. 2021a. *Nursing homes.* https://www.cms.gov/Medicare/Provider-Enrollment-and-Certification/GuidanceforLawsAndRegulations/Nursing-Homes (accessed February 7, 2021).

CMS. 2021b. *S&C's Quality, Certification and Oversight Reports (QCOR).* https://qcor.cms.gov/report_select.jsp?which=0 (accessed October 25, 2021).

CMS. 2021c. *Civil Money Penalty Reinvestment Program.* https://www.cms.gov/Medicare/Provider-Enrollment-and-Certification/SurveyCertificationGenInfo/LTC-CMP-Reinvestment (accessed February 5, 2022).

CMS. 2021d. *Special Focus Facility ("SFF") program.* https://www.cms.gov/Medicare/Provider-Enrollment-and-certification/CertificationandComplianc/downloads/sfflist.pdf (accessed April 29, 2021).

CMS, 2021e. *Fiscal year (FY) 2020 state performance standards system (SPSS) findings, FY 2021 SPSS guidance, and FY 2019 results.* https://www.cms.gov/files/document/admin-info-letter-21-08-all.pdf (accessed February 1, 2022).

CMS. 2021f. *Prioritization of survey activities.* https://www.cms.gov/files/document/qso-20-20-allpdf.pdf-0 (accessed April 6, 2021).

CMS. 2022. *Civil money penalty (CMP) report.* https://qcor.cms.gov/nh_wizard.jsp?which=0&report=enf_cmp.jsp (accessed February 5, 2022).

Cockburn, A. 2020. *Elder abuse: Nursing homes, the coronavirus, and the bottom line.* https://harpers.org/archive/2020/09/elder-abuse-nursing-homes-covid-19 (accessed February 6, 2022).

Comondore, V. R., P. J. Devereaux, Q. Zhou, S. B. Stone, J. W. Busse, N. C. Ravindran, K. E. Burns, T. Haines, B. Stringer, D. J. Cook, S. D. Walter, T. Sullivan, O. Berwanger, M. Bhandari, S. Banglawala, J. N. Lavis, B. Patrisor, H. Schunemann, K. Walsh, N. Bhatnager, and G. H. Guyatt. 2009. Quality of care in for-profit and not-for-profit nursing homes: Systematic review and meta-analysis. *BMJ* 339:b2732.

Conover, C. J., and J. Bailey. 2020. Certificate of need laws: A systematic review and cost-effectiveness analysis. *BMC Health Services Research* 20:748.

Critchfield, H. 2021. Florida protected nursing homes from COVID lawsuits. Then cases began to spike. *Tampa Bay Times*, September 28. https://www.tampabay.com/news/health/2021/09/28/florida-protected-nursing-homes-from-COVID-lawsuits-then-cases-began-to-spike (accessed November 17, 2021).

DOJ (U.S. Department of Justice). 2014. *Extendicare Health Services Inc. agrees to pay $38 million to settle False Claims Act allegations relating to the provision of substandard nursing care and medically unnecessary rehabilitation therapy.* https://www.justice.gov/opa/pr/extendicare-health-services-inc-agrees-pay-38-million-settle-false-claims-act-allegations (accessed February 6, 2022).

DOJ. 2016. *Nursing home chain to pay $5.3 million to resolve False Claims Act allegations.* https://www.justice.gov/usao-ndtx/pr/nursing-home-chain-pay-53-million-resolve-false-claims-act-allegations (accessed February 6, 2022).

DOJ. 2020. *Department of Justice launches a national nursing home initiative.* https://www.justice.gov/opa/pr/department-justice-launches-national-nursing-home-initiative (accessed March 30, 2021).

DOJ and FTC (Federal Trade Commission). 2004. *Improving health care: A dose of competition.* https://www.ftc.gov/sites/default/files/documents/reports/improving-health-care-dose-competition-report-federal-trade-commission-and-department-justice/040723healthcarerpt.pdf (accessed February 4, 2022).
Dolan, J., and B. Mejia. 2020a. *As coronavirus raged through nursing homes, inspectors found nothing wrong.* https://www.latimes.com/california/story/2020-06-28/coronavirus-nursing-homes-state-inspector-covid-19 (accessed February 5, 2022).
Dolan, J., and B. Mejia. 2020b. *Coronavirus patients could be cash cows for nursing homes.* https://canhrnews.com/coronavirus-patients-could-be-cash-cows-for-nursing-homes (accessed February 5, 2022).
Duhigg, C. 2007. Nursing homes owned by private equity face U.S. inquiries. *The New York Times*, October 24. https://www.nytimes.com/2007/10/24/business/worldbusiness/24iht-nursing.4.8037461.html (accessed April 29, 2021).
Edelman, T. 2018. *Corporate integrity agreements and nursing homes.* https://medicareadvocacy.org/corporate-integrity-agreements-and-nursing-homes (accessed April 29, 2021).
Edelman, T. 2019. *Annual surveys at nursing facilities are essential to protect residents.* https://medicareadvocacy.org/annual-surveys-at-nursing-facilities-are-essential-to-protect-residents (accessed November 16, 2021).
Eijkelenboom, A., H. Verbeek, E. Felix, and J. van Hoof. 2017. Architectural factors influencing the sense of home in nursing homes: An operationalization for practice. *Frontiers of Architectural Research* 6(2):111–122.
Erickson, A. C. 2021. *States are suspending certificate-of-need laws in the wake of COVID-19 but the damage might already be done.* https://pacificlegal.org/certificate-of-need-laws-COVID-19 (accessed November 9, 2021).
Estes, C. L., D. M. Zulman, S. C. Goldberg, and D. D. Ogawa. 2004. State long term care ombudsman programs: Factors associated with perceived effectiveness. *The Gerontologist* 44(1):104–115.
Estes, C. L., S. P. Lohrer, S. Goldberg, B. R. Grossman, M. Nelson, M. J. Koren, and B. Hollister. 2010. Factors associated with perceived effectiveness of local long-term care ombudsman programs in New York and California. *Journal of Aging and Health* 22(6):772–803.
Fashaw, S. A., K. S. Thomas, E. McCreedy, and V. Mor. 2020. Thirty-year trends in nursing home composition and quality since the passage of the Omnibus Reconciliation Act. *Journal of the American Medical Directors Association* 21(2):233–239.
Fayissa, B., S. Alsaif, F. Mansour, T. E. Leonce, and F. G. Mixon, Jr. 2020. Certificate-of-need regulation and healthcare service quality: Evidence from the nursing home industry. *Healthcare* 8(4):423.
Feder, J., and W. Scanlon. 1980. Regulating the bed supply in nursing homes. *Milbank Memorial Fund Quarterly: Health and Society* 58(1):54–88.
Ferdows, N. B., and M. Rahman. 2020. Evolution of the nursing home industry in states with different certificate of need policies. *Journal of the American Medical Directors Association* 21(4):559–561.
Finn, I. 2020. *U.S. nursing homes: A goldmine for real estate and private equity firms.* https://www.wsws.org/en/articles/2020/04/27/nur2-a27.html (accessed February 6, 2022).
Furrow, B. R., T. L. Greaney, S. H. Johnson, T. S. Jost, and R. L. Schwartz. 2008. *Health law: Cases, materials and problems.* St. Paul, MN: West Publishing.
GAO (U.S. Government Accountability Office). 1997. *Long-term care: Consumer protection and quality-of-care issues in assisted living.* Washington, DC: U.S. Government Accountability Office.
GAO. 1999. *Nursing home care: Enhanced HCFA oversight of state programs would better ensure quality.* Washington, DC: U.S. Government Accountability Office.
GAO. 2003. *Nursing home quality: Prevalence of serious problems, while declining, reinforces importance of enhanced oversight.* Washington, DC: U.S. Government Accountability Office.

GAO. 2005. *Nursing homes: Despite increased oversight, challenges remain in ensuring high-quality care and resident safety.* Washington, DC: U.S. Government Accountability Office.

GAO. 2007. *Nursing homes: Efforts to strengthen federal enforcement have not deterred some homes from repeatedly harming residents.* Washington, DC: U.S. Government Accountability Office.

GAO. 2008. *Federal monitoring surveys demonstrate continued understatement of serious care problems and CMS oversight weakness.* Washington, DC: U.S. Government Accountability Office.

GAO. 2009a. *Nursing homes: Addressing the factors underlying understatement of serious care problems requires sustained CMS and state commitment.* Washington, DC: U.S. Government Accountability Office.

GAO. 2009b. *Medicare and Medicaid participating facilities: CMS needs to reexamine its approach for funding state oversight of health care facilities.* Washington, DC: U.S. Government Accountability Office.

GAO. 2009c. *Nursing homes: Opportunities exist to facilitate the use of the temporary management sanction.* Washington, DC: U.S. Government Accountability Office.

GAO. 2009d. *Nursing homes: CMS's special focus facility methodology should better target the most poorly performing homes, which tended to be chain affiliated and for-profit.* Washington, DC: U.S. Government Accountability Office.

GAO, 2010a. *Poorly performing nursing homes: Special focus facilities are often improving, but CMS's program could be strengthened.* Washington, DC: U.S. Government Accountability Office.

GAO, 2010b. *Nursing homes: Some improvement seen in understatement of serious deficiencies, but implications for the longer-term trend are unclear.* Washington, DC: U.S. Government Accountability Office.

GAO, 2010c. *Nursing homes: Complexity of private investment purchases demonstrates need for CMS to improve the usability and completeness of ownership data.* Washington, DC: U.S. Government Accountability Office.

GAO. 2011a. *Nursing homes: More reliable data and consistent guidance would improve CMS oversight of state complaint investigations.* Washington, DC: U.S. Government Accountability Office.

GAO. 2011b. *Nursing homes: Private investment homes sometimes differed from others in deficiencies, staffing, and financial performance.* Washington, DC: U.S. Government Accountability Office.

GAO. 2016. *Skilled nursing facilities: CMS should improve accessibility and reliability of expenditure data.* Washington, DC: U.S. Government Accountability Office.

GAO. 2018. *Nursing home quality: Continued improvements needed in CMS's data and oversight. (GAO-18-694T):1-17.* https://www.gao.gov/products/GAO-18-694T (accessed August 27, 2020).

GAO. 2019. *Nursing homes: Improved oversight needed to better protect residents from abuse.* Washington, DC: U.S. Government Accountability Office.

Gebeloff, R., K. Thomas, and J. Silver-Greenberg. 2021. *How nursing homes' worst offenses are hidden from the public.* https://www.nytimes.com/2021/12/09/business/nursing-home-abuse-inspection.html?smid=em-share (accessed February 2, 2022).

Glans, M. 2015. *Indiana nursing home moratorium.* https://www.jamesmadison.org/the-heartland-institute-research-commentary-indiana-nursing-home-moratorium (accessed February 4, 2022).

Grabowski, D. C. 2007. Medicare and Medicaid: Conflicting incentives for long-term care. *The Milbank Quarterly* 85(4):579–610.

Grabowski, D. C., and D. G. Stevenson. 2008. Ownership conversions and nursing home performance. *Health Services Research* 43(4):1184–1203.

Grabowski, D. C. 2017. Nursing home certificate-of-need laws should be repealed. *Health Affairs Forefront*, June 9. https://www.healthaffairs.org/do/10.1377/hblog20170609.060529/full (accessed February 10, 2021).

Grabowski, D. C., and J. Gruber. 2007. Moral hazard in nursing home use. *Journal of Health Economics* 26(3):560–577.

Grabowski, D. C., and R. A. Hirth. 2003. Competitive spillovers across non-profit and for-profit nursing homes. *Journal of Health Economics* 22(1):1–22.

Grabowski, D. C., and D. G. Stevenson. 2006. Long-term care regulation. In R. Schulz (ed.), *The encyclopedia of aging*, 4th ed. New York: Springer Publishing. Pp. 701–704.

Grabowski, D. C., R. L. Ohsfeldt, and M. A. Morrisey. 2003. The effects of CON repeal on Medicaid nursing home and long-term care expenditures. *Inquiry* 40(2):146–157.

Grabowski, D. C., J. Gruber, and J. J. Angelelli. 2008. Nursing home quality as a common good. *Review of Economics and Statistics* 90(4):754–764.

Grabowski, D. C., Z. Feng, R. Hirth, M. Rahman, and V. Mor. 2013. Effect of nursing home ownership on the quality of post-acute care: An instrumental variables approach. *Journal of Health Economics* 32(1):12–21.

Grabowski, D. C., R. A. Hirth, O. Intrator, Y. Li, J. Richardson, D. G. Stevenson, Q. Zheng, and J. Banaszak-Holl. 2016. Low-quality nursing homes were more likely than other nursing homes to be bought or sold by chains in 1993–2010. *Health Affairs* 35(5):907–914.

Grajeda, H., and K. Yood. 2021. *What price transparency? California SB 650 shines light on skilled nursing facility ownership while creating new reporting burdens for California skilled nursing facilities*. https://www.jdsupra.com/legalnews/what-price-transparency-california-sb-3985939/ (accessed February 2, 2022).

Grant, R. 2021. *Family guide to effective family councils*. National Long-Term Care Ombudsman Resource Center and National Citizens' Coalition for Nursing Home Reform. https://theconsumervoice.org/uploads/files/family-member/Guide-toEffective-Family-Councils.pdf (accessed August 5, 2021).

Gupta, A., S. T. Howell, C. Yannelis, and A. Gupta. 2021. *Does private equity investment in healthcare benefit patients? Evidence from nursing homes*. National Bureau of Economic Research working paper no. 28474. https://www.nber.org/papers/w28474 (accessed February 25, 2021).

Hall, S. M., C. R. Haper, and B. K. Steinwascher. 2020. Insight: Nursing homes face heightened criminal enforcement during COVID-19. *Bloomberg Law*, June 15. https://news.bloomberglaw.com/us-law-week/insight-nursing-homes-face-heightened-criminal-enforcement-during-COVID-19 (accessed March 30, 2021).

Hansen, K. E., K. Hyer, A. A. Holup, K. M. Smith, and B. J. Small. 2017. Analyses of complaints, investigations of allegations, and deficiency citations in United States nursing homes. *Medical Care Research and Review* 76(6): 736–757.

Harrar, S., J. Eaton, and H. Meyer. 2021. *10 steps to reform and improve nursing homes*. https://www.aarp.org/caregiving/health/info-2021/steps-to-improve-nursing-homes (accessed January 13, 2021).

Harrington, C., S. Woolhandler, J. Mullan, H. Carrillo, and D. U. Himmelstein. 2001. Does investor ownership of nursing homes compromise the quality of care? *American Journal of Public Health* 91(9):1452–1455.

Harrington, C., T. Tsoukalas, C. Rudder, R. J. Mollot, and H. Carrillo. 2008. Variation in the use of federal and state civil money penalties for nursing homes. *The Gerontologist* 48(5):679–691.

Harrington, C., B. Olney, H. Carrillo, and T. Kang. 2012. Nurse staffing and deficiencies in the largest for-profit nursing home chains and chains owned by private equity companies. *Health Services Research* 47(1 Pt 1):106–128.

Harrington, C., L. Ross, and T. Kang. 2015. Hidden owners, hidden profits, and poor nursing home care: A case study. *International Journal of Health Services* 45(4):779–800.

Harrington, C., F. F. Jacobsen, J. Panos, A. Pollock, S. Sutaria, and M. Szebehely. 2017. Marketization in long-term care: A cross-country comparison of large for-profit nursing home chains. *Health Services Insights* 10:1–23.

Harrington, C., M. E. Dellefield, E. Halifax, M. L. Fleming, and D. Bakerjian. 2020. Appropriate nurse staffing levels for U.S. nursing homes. *Health Services Insights* 13:1–14.

Harrington, C., A. Montgomery, T. King, D. C. Grabowski, and M. Wasserman. 2021. These administrative actions would improve nursing home ownership and financial transparency in the post COVID-19 period. *Health Affairs Forefront*, February 11. https://www.healthaffairs.org/do/10.1377/hblog20210208.597573/full (accessed February 25, 2021).

Harris-Kojetin, L., M. Sengupta, J. P. Lendon, V. Rome, R. Valverde, and C. Caffrey. 2019. *Long-term care providers and services users in the United States, 2015–2016*. DHHS publication no. 2019-1427. https://www.cdc.gov/nchs/data/series/sr_03/sr03_43-508.pdf (accessed November 19, 2021).

Havighurst, C. C. 2005. Monopoly is not the answer. *Health Affairs* 24(Suppl1):W5-373–W5-375.

Hawes, C. 1996. *Assuring nursing home quality: The history and impact of federal standards in OBRA-87*. https://www.commonwealthfund.org/publications/fund-reports/1996/dec/assuring-nursing-home-quality-history-and-impact-federal (accessed February 10, 2021).

Hawes, C., V. Mor, C. D. Phillips, B. E. Fries, J. N. Morris, E. Steele-Friedlob, A. M. Greene, and M. Nennstiel. 1997. The OBRA-87 nursing home regulations and implementation of the resident assessment instrument: Effects on process quality. *Journal of the American Geriatrics Society* 45(8):977–985.

HCFA (Health Care Financing Administration). 1998. *Report to Congress: Study of private accreditation (deeming) of nursing homes, regulatory incentives and non-regulatory initiatives, and effectiveness of the survey and certification system*. https://ia801605.us.archive.org/3/items/reporttocongress00unit_11/reporttocongress00unit_11.pdf (accessed February 23, 2022).

Hillmer, M. P., W. P. Wodchis, S. S. Gill, G. M. Anderson, and P. A. Rochon. 2005. Nursing home profit status and quality of care: Is there any evidence of an association? *Medical Care Research and Review* 62(2):139–166.

Hollister, B. A., and C. L. Estes. 2013. Local long-term care ombudsman program effectiveness and the measurement of program resources. *Journal of Applied Gerontology* 32(6):708–728.

HRW (Human Rights Watch). 2021. *U.S.: Concerns of neglect in nursing homes—Pandemic exposes need for improvements in staffing, oversight, accountability*. https://www.hrw.org/news/2021/03/25/us-concerns-neglect-nursing-homes# (accessed September 8, 2021).

Hunt, S. S. 2008. *History and role of the Long-Term Care Ombudsman Program*. https://ltcombudsman.org/uploads/files/support/history-and-role.pdf (accessed May 7, 2021).

IOM (Institute of Medicine). 1986. *Improving the quality of care in nursing homes*. Washington, DC: National Academy Press.

IOM. 1996. *Nursing staff in hospitals and nursing homes: Is it adequate?* Washington, DC: National Academy Press.

IOM. 2001. *Improving the quality of long-term care*. Washington, DC: National Academy Press.

Jaffe, I. 2020. Ideal nursing homes: Individual rooms, better staffing, more accountability. *NPR*, May 21. https://www.npr.org/2020/05/21/855821083/ideal-nursing-homes-individual-rooms-better-staffing-more-accountability (accessed September 2, 2021).

Justice in Aging. 2020. *Fighting the rollback of nursing home protections*. https://justiceinaging.org/fighting-rollback-nursing-home-protections (accessed April 16, 2021).

Justice in Aging, National Consumer Voice, and CMA (Justice in Aging, the National Consumer Voice for Quality Long-Term Care, and the Center for Medicare Advocacy). 2021. *A closer look at the revised nursing facility regulations: Grievances and resident/family councils*. https://www.justiceinaging.org/wp-content/uploads/2017/05/Revised-Nursing-Facility-Regulations_Grievances-and-Resident-or-Family-Councils.pdf (accessed August 5, 2021).

Kapp, M. 2000. Quality of care and quality of life in nursing facilities: What's regulation got to do with it? *McGeorge Law Review* 31:707–731.

KFF (Kaiser Family Foundation). 2013. *Implementation of Affordable Care Act provisions to improve nursing home transparency, care quality, and abuse prevention.* https://www.kff.org/medicaid/report/implementation-of-affordable-care-act-provisions-to-improve-nursing-home-transparency-care-quality-and-abuse-prevention (accessed February 10, 2021).

KFF. 2015. *Long-term care in the United States: A timeline.* https://www.kff.org/medicaid/timeline/long-term-care-in-the-united-states-a-timeline/#1978 (accessed October 23, 2020).

Kingsley, D. E., and C. Harrington. 2021. COVID-19 had little financial impact on publicly traded nursing home companies. *American Geriatrics Society* 69:2099–2102.

Kitchener, M., T. Ng, N. Miller, and C. Harrington. 2005. Medicaid and home and community-based services: National program trends. *Health Affairs* 24(1):206–212.

Klauber, M., and B. Wright. 2001. *The 1987 Nursing Home Reform Act.* https://www.aarp.org/home-garden/livable-communities/info-2001/the_1987_nursing_home_reform_act.html (accessed October 20, 2020).

Kohn, N. A. 2021. Nursing homes, COVID-19, and the consequences of regulatory failure. *Georgetown Law Journal Online* 110. https://www.law.georgetown.edu/georgetown-law-journal/wp-content/uploads/sites/26/2021/04/Kohn_Nursing-Homes-COVID-19-and-the-Consequences-of-Regulatory-Failure.pdf (accessed January 25, 2022).

Konetzka, R. T., J. Park, R. Ellis, and E. Abbo. 2013. Malpractice litigation and nursing home quality of care. *Health Services Research* 48(6 Pt 1):1920–1938.

Konetzka, R. T., H. Daifeng, J. Dong, and J. A. Nyman. 2019. Moral hazard and long-term care insurance. *The Geneva Papers on Risk and Insurance—Issues and Practice* 44:231–251.

Kosar, C. M., and M. Rahman. 2021. Early acceleration of COVID-19 in areas with larger nursing homes and certificate of need laws. *Journal of General Internal Medicine* 36(4):990–997.

Landsberg, B. S., and T. D. Keville. 2001. Nursing homes face quality-of-care scrutiny under the False Claims Act. *Healthcare Financial Management* 55(1):54–58.

Lee, K., R. L. Mauldin, W. Tang, J. Connolly, J. Harwerth, and K. Magruder. 2021. Examining racial and ethnic disparities among older adults in long-term care facilities. *The Gerontologist* 61(6):858–869.

Legal Aid Justice Center. 2013. *The rights of family councils in nursing homes.* https://www.justice4all.org/wp-content/uploads/2013/05/Rights-of-Family-Councils.pdf (accessed August 10, 2021).

Levinson, D. R. 2017. *Early alert: The Centers for Medicare & Medicaid Services has inadequate procedures to ensure that incidents of potential abuse or neglect at skilled nursing facilities are identified and reported in accordance with applicable requirements (A-01-17-00504).* https://oig.hhs.gov/oas/reports/region1/11700504.pdf (accessed November 1, 2021).

Li, Y., C. Harrington, W. D. Spector, and D. B. Mukamel. 2010. State regulatory enforcement and nursing home termination from the Medicare and Medicaid programs. *Health Services Research* 45(6 Pt 1):1796–1814.

Li, Y., W. D. Spector, L. G. Glance, and D. B. Mukamel. 2012. State "technical assistance programs" for nursing home quality improvement: Variations and potential implications. *Journal of Aging & Social Policy* 24(4):349–367.

LTCCC (Long Term Care Community Coalition). 2017. *Consumer factsheet: Resident & family councils.* https://nursinghome411.org/wp-content/uploads/2017/05/LTCCC-Factsheet-Resident-Family-Councils.pdf (accessed August 5, 1997).

LTCCC. 2021. *Nursing home Medicaid funding: Separating fact from fiction.* https://nursinghome411.org/wp-content/uploads/2021/01/LTCCC-Policy-Brief-Medicaid-Funding-Facts-vs-Fiction.pdf (accessed November 17, 2021).

Mattimore, T. J., N. S. Wenger, N. A. Desbiens, J. M. Teno, M. B. Hamel, H. Liu, R. Califf, A. F. Connors, Jr., J. Lynn, and R. K. Oye. 1997. Surrogate and physician understanding of patients' preferences for living permanently in a nursing home. *Journal of the American Geriatrics Society* 45(7):818–824.

Miller, N. A., C. Harrington, and E. Goldstein. 2002. Access to community-based long-term care: Medicaid's role. *Journal of Aging and Health* 14(1):138–159.

Mitchell, M. D. 2017. *Certificate-of-need laws: Are they achieving their goals?* https://www.mercatus.org/system/files/mitchell-con-qa-mop-mercatus-v2.pdf (accessed November 9, 2021).

Mitchell, M. 2021. It's time for states to ditch certificate-of-need laws. *U.S. News and World Report*, July 9. https://www.usnews.com/news/best-states/articles/2021-07-09/on-the-heels-of-the-pandemic-states-should-get-rid-of-certificate-of-need-laws (accessed November 9, 2021).

Mitchell, M. D., and C. Koopman. 2016. *40 years of certificate-of-need laws across America.* https://www.mercatus.org/publications/corporate-welfare/40-years-certificate-need-laws-across-america (accessed February 4, 2022).

Mo, S., and J. Shi. 2020. The psychological consequences of the COVID-19 on residents and staff in nursing homes. *Work, Aging and Retirement* 6(4):254–259.

Montgomery, A., S. Slocum, and C. Stanik. 2020. *Experiences of nursing home residents during the pandemic.* https://altarum.org/sites/default/files/uploaded-publication-files/Nursing-Home-Resident-Survey_Altarum-Special-Report_FINAL.pdf (accessed October 22, 2020).

Mor, V. 2011. Cost of nursing home regulation: Building a research agenda. *Medical Care* 49(6):535–537.

Mukamel, D. B., Y. Li, C. Harrington, W. D. Spector, D. L. Weimer, and L. Bailey. 2011. Does state regulation of quality impose costs on nursing homes? *Medical Care* 49(6):529–534.

Mukamel, D. B., D. L. Weimer, C. Harrington, W. D. Spector, H. Ladd, and Y. Li. 2012. The effect of state regulatory stringency on nursing home quality. *Health Services Research* 47(5):1791–1813.

Mukamel, D. B., S. F. Haeder, and D. L. Weimer. 2014. Top-down and bottom-up approaches to health care quality: The impacts of regulation and report cards. *Annual Review of Public Health* 35(1):477–497.

Musumeci, M., and P. Chidambaram. 2020. *Key questions about nursing home regulation and oversight in the wake of COVID-19.* https://www.kff.org/coronavirus-COVID-19/issue-brief/key-questions-about-nursing-home-regulation-and-oversight-in-the-wake-of-COVID-19 (accessed December 7, 2020).

Nash, W. A., L. M. Harris, K. E. Heller, and B. D. Mitchell. 2021. "We are saving their bodies and destroying their souls": Family caregivers' experiences of formal care setting visitation restrictions during the COVID-19 pandemic. *Journal of Aging & Social Policy* 33(4–5):398–413.

Nastasi, V. 2020. *Protecting Florida's most vulnerable: Market-based reform to improve nursing home care.* https://www.jamesmadison.org/wp-content/uploads/2021/01/Policy-Brief_Nursing_Homes_Dec2020_v02.pdf (accessed February 4, 2022).

NASUAD (National Association of States United for Aging and Disabilities, National Long-Term Care Ombudsman Resource Center, and National Consumer Voice for Quality Long-Term Care). 2019. *State Long-Term Care Ombudsman Program: 2019 revised primer for state agencies.* Washington, DC: National Association of States United for Aging and Disabilities, National Long-Term Care Ombudsman Resource Center, and National Consumer Voice for Quality Long-Term Care.

National Consumer Voice (The National Consumer Voice for Quality Long-Term Care). 2017. *Factsheet: Resident council rights in nursing homes.* https://theconsumervoice.org/uploads/files/long-term-care-recipient/Resident_Council_Rights_Fact_Sheet.pdf (accessed August 10, 2021).

National Consumer Voice. 2019. *Side-by-side comparison of current & proposed federal nursing home regulations (including arbitration agreements).* https://theconsumervoice.org/uploads/files/general/Side-by-Side_Comparison_of_Proposed_and_Current_ROP_8-2-2019.pdf (accessed August 10, 2021).

NCSL (National Conference of State Legislatures). 2021. *Certificate of need (CON) state laws.* https://www.ncsl.org/research/health/con-certificate-of-need-state-laws.aspx (accessed February 4, 2022).

NORC (NORC at the University of Chicago). 2019. *Final report: Process evaluation of the Long-Term Care Ombudsman Program (LTCOP).* https://acl.gov/sites/default/files/programs/2020-10/LTCOPProcessEvaluationFinalReport_2.pdf (accessed August 19, 2021).

Nyman, J. A. 1994. The effects of market concentration and excess demand on the price of nursing home care. *Journal of Industrial Economics* 42:193–204.

Ochieng, N., P. Chidambaram, R. Garfield, and T. Neuman. 2021. *Factors associated with COVID-19 cases and deaths in long-term care facilities: Findings from a literature review.* https://www.kff.org/coronavirus-covid-19/issue-brief/factors-associated-with-covid-19-cases-and-deaths-in-long-term-care-facilities-findings-from-a-literature-review (accessed February 1, 2022).

OIG (Office of the Inspector General). 1999. *Nursing home survey and certification overall capacity.* Washington, DC: Office of the Inspector General, U.S. Department of Health and Human Services.

OIG. 2003. *Nursing home deficiency trends and survey and certification process consistency.* Washington, DC: Office of the Inspector General, U.S. Department of Health and Human Services.

OIG. 2005. *Nursing home enforcement: The use of civil money penalties.* Washington, DC: HHS Office of the Inspector General, U.S. Department of Health and Human Services.

OIG. 2006a. *Nursing home enforcement: Application of mandatory remedies.* Washington, DC: HHS Office of the Inspector General, U.S. Department of Health and Human Services.

OIG. 2006b. *Nursing home complaint investigations.* Washington, DC: HHS Office of the Inspector General, U.S. Department of Health and Human Services.

OIG. 2009. *Nursing home corporations under quality of care corporate integrity agreements.* Washington, DC: Office of the Inspector General, U.S. Department of Health and Human Services.

OIG. 2019a. *Trends in nursing home complaints: Text-based data.* https://oig.hhs.gov/oei/maps/2019-nursing-home/text-map.asp (accessed February 1, 2022).

OIG. 2019b. *CMS guidance to state survey agencies on verifying correction of deficiencies needs to be improved to help ensure the health and safety of nursing home residents.* Washington, DC: HHS Office of the Inspector General.

OIG. 2019c. *Incidents of potential abuse and neglect at skilled nursing facilities were not always reported and investigated.* Washington, DC: HHS Office of the Inspector General.

OIG. 2020a. *States continued to fall short in meeting required timeframes for investigating nursing home complaints: 2016–2018.* Washington, DC: Office of the Inspector General, U.S. Department of Health and Human Services.

OIG. 2020b. *Onsite surveys of nursing homes during the COVID-19 pandemic: March 23–May 30, 2020* Washington, DC: Office of the Inspector General, U.S. Department of Health and Human Services.

OIG. 2021. *States' backlogs of standard surveys of nursing homes grew substantially during the COVID-19 pandemic: Addendum to oei-01-20-00430.* Washington, DC: Office of the Inspector General, U.S. Department of Health and Human Services.

OIG. 2022a. *CMS should take further action to address states with poor performance in conducting nursing home surveys.* Washington, DC: Office of the Inspector General, U.S. Department of Health and Human Services.

OIG. 2022b. *Corporate integrity agreements.* https://oig.hhs.gov/compliance/corporate-integrity-agreements (accessed February 6, 2022).

O'Neill, C., C. Harrington, M. Kitchener, and D. Saliba. 2003. Quality of care in nursing homes: An analysis of relationships among profit, quality, and ownership. *Medical Care* 41(12):1318–1330.

Rahman, M., O. Galarraga, J. S. Zinn, D. C. Grabowski, and V. Mor. 2016. The impact of certificate-of-need laws on nursing home and home health care expenditures. *Medical Care Research and Review* 73(1):85–105.

Rau, J. 2017. Trump administration eases nursing home fines in victory for industry. *The New York Times*, December 24. https://www.nytimes.com/2017/12/24/business/trump-administration-nursing-home-penalties.html (accessed April 29, 2021).

Rau, J. 2018a. "It's almost like a ghost town." Most nursing homes overstated staffing for years. *The New York Times*, August 7. https://www.nytimes.com/2018/07/07/health/nursing-homes-staffing-medicare.html (accessed April 29, 2021).

Rau, J. 2018b. Care suffers as more nursing homes feed money into corporate webs. *The New York Times*, January 2. https://www.nytimes.com/2018/01/02/business/nursing-homes-care-corporate.html (accessed February 2, 2021).

Rau, J., and E. Lucas. 2018. *1,400 nursing homes get lower Medicare ratings because of staffing concerns.* https://khn.org/news/1400-nursing-homes-get-lower-medicare-ratings-because-of-staffing-concerns (accessed February 6, 2022).

Reinhard, S. C., and E. Hado. 2021. *LTSS choices: Small-house nursing homes.* https://www.aarp.org/ppi/info-2021/ltss-choices-small-house-nursing-homes (accessed February 25, 2021).

Rodney, T., N. Josiah, and D.-L. Baptiste. 2021. Loneliness in the time of COVID-19: Impact on older adults. *Journal of Advanced Nursing* 77(9):e24–e26.

Schwarz, B. 1997. Nursing home design: A misguided architectural model. *Journal of Architectural and Planning Research* 14(4):343–359.

Shain, M., and M. I. Roemer. 1959. Hospital costs relate to the supply of beds. *Modern Hospital* 92(4):71–73.

Shugarman, L. R., and J. A. Brown. 2006. *Nursing home selection: How do consumers choose? Volume I: Findings from Focus Groups of Consumers and Information Intermediaries.* https://aspe.hhs.gov/basic-report/nursing-home-selection-how-do-consumers-choose-volume-i-findings-focus-groups-consumers-and-information-intermediaries (accessed February 25, 2021).

Silver-Greenberg, J., and R. Gebeloff. 2021. Maggots, rape and yet five stars: How U.S. ratings of nursing homes mislead the public. *The New York Times*, March 13. https://www.nytimes.com/2021/03/13/business/nursing-homes-ratings-Medicare-COVID.html?campaign_id=9&emc=edit_nn_20210313&instance_id=28051&nl=the-morning&regi_id=98348276&segment_id=53394&te=1&user_id=d3b6076e56d56335bd158430d6fd0d63 (accessed March 15, 2021).

Silver-Greenberg, J., and A. J. Harris. 2020. 'They just dumped him like trash': Nursing homes evict vulnerable residents. https://www.nytimes.com/2020/06/21/business/nursing-homes-evictions-discharges-coronavirus.html?action=click&module=Top%20Stories&pgtype=Homepage (accessed February 5, 2022).

Stevenson, D. G. 2006. Nursing home consumer complaints and quality of care: A national view. *Medical Care Research and Review* 63(3):347–368.

Stevenson, D. G. 2018. *The future of nursing home regulation: Time for a conversation?* https://www.healthaffairs.org/do/10.1377/hblog20180820.660365/full (accessed September 3, 2020).

Stevenson, D. G. 2019. *Pushing past the status quo to protect nursing home residents.* https://www.healthaffairs.org/do/10.1377/hblog20190926.292183/full (accessed November 9, 2021).

Stevenson, D. G., and A. Bonner. 2020. The importance of nursing home transparency and oversight, even in the midst of a pandemic. *Health Affairs Forefront,* May 12. https://www.healthaffairs.org/do/10.1377/hblog20200511.431267/full (accessed November 15, 2021).

Stevenson, D. G., and A. K. Cheng. 2021. Nursing home oversight during the COVID-19 pandemic. *Journal of the American Geriatrics Society* 69(4):850–860.

Stevenson, D. G., and D. C. Grabowski. 2008. Private equity investment and nursing home care: Is it a big deal? *Health Affairs* 27(5):1399–1408.

Stevenson, D. G., and V. Mor. 2009. Targeting nursing homes under the Quality Improvement Organization program's 9th statement of work. *Journal of the American Geriatrics Society* 57(9):1678–1684.

Stevenson, D. G., and D. M. Studdert. 2003. The rise of nursing home litigation: Findings from a national survey of attorneys. *Health Affairs (Millwood)* 22(2):219–229.

Stevenson, D. G., M. J. Spittal, and D. M. Studdert. 2013a. Does litigation increase or decrease health care quality? A national study of negligence claims against nursing homes. *Medical Care* 51(5):430–436.

Stevenson, D. G., J. S. Bramson, and D. C. Grabowski. 2013b. Nursing home ownership trends and their impacts on quality of care: A study using detailed ownership data from Texas. *Journal of Aging & Social Policy* 25(1):30–47.

Stratmann, T., and D. Wille. 2016. *Certificate-of-need laws and hospital quality.* https://www.mercatus.org/system/files/mercatus-stratmann-wille-con-hospital-quality-v1.pdf (accessed November 9, 2021).

Studdert, D. M., and D. G. Stevenson. 2004. Nursing home litigation and tort reform: A case for exceptionalism. *The Gerontologist* 44(5):588–595.

Studdert, D. M., M. J. Spittal, M. M. Mello, A. J. O'Malley, and D. G. Stevenson. 2011. Relationship between quality of care and negligence litigation in nursing homes. *New England Journal of Medicine* 364(13):1243–1250.

Wagner, L. M., S. M. McDonald, and N. G. Castle. 2012. Impact of voluntary accreditation on deficiency citations in U.S. nursing homes. *The Gerontologist* 52(4):561–570.

Walshe, K. 2001. Regulating U.S. nursing homes: Are we learning from experience? *Health Affairs* 20(6):128–144.

Walshe, K., and C. Harrington. 2002. Regulation of nursing facilities in the United States: An analysis of resources and performance of state survey agencies. *The Gerontologist* 42(4):475–487.

Wang, X., D. Gammonley, and F. Bender. 2019. Civil money penalty enforcement actions for quality deficiencies in nursing homes. *The Gerontologist* 60(5):868–877.

Watson, S. D. 2012. From almshouses to nursing homes and community care: Lessons from Medicaid's history. *Georgia State University Law Review* 26(3):937–969.

Wells, J., and C. Harrington. 2013. *Implementation of Affordable Care Act provisions to improve nursing home transparency, care quality, and abuse prevention.* https://www.kff.org/medicaid/report/implementation-of-affordable-care-act-provisions-to-improve-nursing-home-transparency-care-quality-and-abuse-prevention (accessed February 25, 2021).

White House. 1998. *President Clinton announces initiative to improve the quality of nursing homes.* https://clintonwhitehouse6.archives.gov/1998/07/1998-07-21-president-announces-initiative-to-improve-nursing-homes.html (accessed January 24, 2022).

Wiener, J. M., D. G. Stevenson, and S. M. Goldenson. 1998. *Controlling the supply of long-term care providers at the state level.* Washington, DC: The Urban Institute.

Wiener, J. M., M. P. Freiman, D. Brown, and RTI International. 2007. *Nursing home care quality: Twenty years after the Omnibus Budget Reconciliation Act of 1987.* https://www.kff.org/wp-content/uploads/2013/01/7717.pdf (accessed January 29, 2021).

Williams, B. 2019. *Opening the floodgates: Repealing certificate of needs laws could drown nursing home care.* https://papers.ssrn.com/sol3/papers.cfm?abstract_id=3447410 (accessed February 4, 2022).

Wyden, R. 2019. *Wyden statement at Finance Committee hearing on nursing homes and elder abuse.* https://www.finance.senate.gov/wyden-statement-at-finance-committee-hearing-on-nursing-homes-and-elder-abuse (accessed April 29, 2021).

Yoder, T. 2020. DOJ announces initiative to combat substandard care in nursing homes; emphasizes importance of whistleblowers. *National Law Review* 10(70), March 10. https://www.natlawreview.com/article/doj-announces-initiative-to-combat-substandard-care-nursing-homes-emphasizes (accessed January 25, 2022).

You, K., Y. Li, O. Intrator, D. Stevenson, R. Hirth, D. Grabowski, and J. Banaszak-Holl. 2016. Do nursing home chain size and proprietary status affect experiences with care? *Medical Care* 54(3):229–234.

Zhang, X., and D. C. Grabowski. 2004. Nursing home staffing and quality under the Nursing Home Reform Act. *The Gerontologist* 44(1):13–23.

Zinn, J. S. 1994. Market competition and the quality of nursing home care. *Journal of Health Politics, Policy and Law* 19(3):555–582.

9

Health Information Technology

Health information technology (HIT) systems designed to facilitate health care delivery, management, and payment have become pervasive throughout the U.S. health care system. One of the more common forms of HIT is the electronic health record (EHR),[1] which has a wide array of uses, ranging from clinical support functions, digital prescriptions, and automated medication dispensing, to functions related to billing, reimbursement, and administration, to patient safety and quality improvement (Alexander and Madsen, 2018; Cherry et al., 2011; Kruse et al., 2017; Rantz et al., 2010a; Scott et al., 2017; Shiells et al., 2019). The capabilities of HIT in effectively promoting patient safety, enhancing the effectiveness of patient care delivery, facilitating the management of chronic conditions, and improving the efficiency of health care professionals are particularly important in nursing home settings, given the characteristics of the patient population. Nursing home residents typically have complex conditions, take multiple medications, and frequently undergo transitions in care (e.g., visits to the emergency department and hospital admissions) (Vest et al., 2019). Moreover, a nursing home resident's stay tends to be extended rather

---

[1] Although the terms "electronic health record" (EHR) and "electronic medical record" (EMR) are often used interchangeably, they are not the same. EMRs are the traditional patient medical chart in digital rather than paper format and are typically tied to one organization. EMRs enable providers to track data over time, identify patients for preventive visits and screenings, monitor patients, and improve health care quality. EHRs go beyond EMRs in their capacity to collect and store information from all the clinicians providing care to the patient (including laboratories and specialists). Importantly, all authorized clinicians involved in a patient's care can access the information in an EHR (ONC, 2019a). For more information, see https://www.healthit.gov/faq/what-are-differences-between-electronic-medical-records-electronic-health-records-and-personal (accessed December 1, 2021).

than episodic, with care typically lasting years rather than weeks or months. This requires more extensive ongoing communication, care coordination activities, and different HIT reporting mechanisms that can support the clinical staff in identifying, monitoring, and responding to changes in a resident's condition over an extended period of time (Rantz et al., 2010a,b). Effective integration of HIT into care delivery has the potential to improve communication and data sharing for treatment referrals, allow providers to securely share data in real time, and provide better and more efficient care to beneficiaries (MACPAC, 2021).

Used appropriately, EHRs have the potential to prevent medical errors, expedite team decisions, reduce health care costs, increase administrative efficiencies, decrease paperwork, promote patient safety, and expand access to health care in nursing home settings (Bjarnadottir et al., 2017; Kruse et al., 2017; Lee, 2015; ONC, 2019b). Thus, members of the nursing home interdisciplinary care team, with appropriate training (DiAngi et al., 2019; Longhurst et al., 2019; Pantaleoni et al., 2015), can call upon the multiple functions of EHRs to improve the overall quality of care for nursing home residents (Spinelli-Moraski and Richards, 2013).

Other health technologies such as telehealth, videoconferencing, and personal monitoring devices are also effective tools in nursing home settings. The importance of these technologies became evident during the COVID-19 pandemic when measures such as locking down nursing home facilities to protect vulnerable residents from infection limited access to in-person clinical services as well as residents' contact with friends and family members (Whitelaw et al., 2020). Thus, health technologies that serve dual roles as alternatives to face-to-face clinical visits as well as tools to mitigate the negative health outcomes of social isolation and loneliness have a key role to play in improving the quality of care and quality of life of nursing home residents.

This chapter of the report explores the role of HIT systems in nursing home settings, beginning with a brief background on the introduction and use of HIT in nursing homes. The discussion then turns to an examination of how HIT aligns with and supports the components of the committee's conceptual model for high-quality nursing home care. From there, the chapter explores HIT's role in facilitating and operationalizing the components of the committee's model of high-quality care in nursing homes as it relates to quality measurement and improvement (Chapter 3), resident care planning (Chapter 4), and workforce productivity (Chapter 5). The discussion in this chapter will also include a review of HIT's impact on advancing patient safety and will touch on issues related to the nursing home physical environment (Chapter 6) as well as HIT's role in value-based payment (Chapter 7). The chapter concludes with a discussion of the use of other HIT applications, such as telehealth, during the COVID-19 pandemic.

EVOLUTION OF HEALTH INFORMATION TECHNOLOGY IN NURSING HOMES

The evidence base supporting the role of HIT systems in improving the quality of care in nursing homes has been steadily evolving over the past three decades. As discussed in Chapter 2, the Institute of Medicine[2] (IOM) 1986 report *Improving the Quality of Care in Nursing Homes* outlined many urgently needed measures to improve the quality of care in nursing homes. The committee's extensive reform plan reflected the recognition of the significance of HIT systems for monitoring and sustaining quality in nursing home care. The report recommended developing large national datasets derived from standardized resident assessments (IOM, 1986). This recommendation led to the creation of the Minimum Data Set (MDS), a standardized instrument used in every U.S. nursing home to assess the condition of residents. As discussed in Chapter 4 and explored further below, the MDS was designed for three key purposes: to collect data to describe each resident's condition and create individualized resident care plans, generate quality indicators to evaluate nursing homes and guide improvement efforts, and serve a reimbursement role. Notably, MDS data are also used to develop publicly reported quality measures (Rahman and Applebaum, 2009).

Subsequent IOM reports focused on the key role of HIT in improving health care quality, with a call for the widespread use of computerized patient records systems to replace paper-based patient health records within 10 years (IOM, 1991). The 2000 IOM report, *To Err Is Human: Building a Safer Health System,* shone a bright light on the safety issues affecting all types of health care delivery systems and promoted technology as a solution (IOM, 2000). That report recommended that all health care organizations implement computerized capabilities—such as computerized drug order entry systems—that could improve the safety of health care delivery. A subsequent IOM report also emphasized the importance of using HIT systems in long-term care facilities for clinical assessment, quality monitoring, and reimbursement (IOM, 2001a).

The steadily growing evidence base supporting the key role of HIT systems in clinical assessment, health care safety, and quality monitoring and improvement provided support for the enactment of a number of legislative actions to promote the widespread adoption of HIT throughout the health care system (see Box 9-1). The first of such legislation, the Health Information Technology for Economic and Clinical Health (HITECH) Act of 2009, authorized $35 billion to support health care providers such as hospitals, acute care, and ambulatory care providers to implement EHRs.

---

[2] As of March 2016, the Health and Medicine Division of the National Academies of Sciences, Engineering and Medicine (NASEM) continues the consensus studies and convening activities previously carried out by the Institute of Medicine (IOM). The IOM name is used to refer to reports issued prior to July 2015.

> **BOX 9-1**
> **Federal Policy Environment: Legislation to Advance HIT**
>
> Under the HITECH Act, enacted as part of the American Recovery and Reinvestment Act of 2009,[3] the Centers for Medicare & Medicaid Services launched a program to provide incentives to hospitals and acute care health care providers to adopt EHRs. This program, known as meaningful use, aimed to apply certified EHR technology for multiple uses including quality, safety, efficiency, and the coordination of care and reduction of health disparities.
>
> The Improving Medicare Post-Acute Care Transformation Act of 2014[4] required all long-term care organizations to report standardized patient assessment data, providing a new impetus for those organizations to implement HIT systems.
>
> The Medicare Access and CHIP Reauthorization Act of 2015[5] established the Quality Payment Program, which contains two tracks. One is the Merit-Based Incentive Payment System (MIPS). The second is the advanced alternative payment models (APMs). In MIPS, the Promoting Interoperability category focuses on meaningful use of certified EHR technology and represents a transition from the initial EHR Incentive Program to a new phase with a heightened focus on interoperability and advancing patient access to health information. Advanced APMs have specific requirements for participants to use certified EHR technology (CMS, 2022; ONC, 2019c).
>
> The 21st Century Cures Act of 2016[6] contains several provisions designed to accelerate the effective use of HIT to promote interoperability, or the seamless and secure access, exchange, and use of electronic health information, to support better access to health care information for all stakeholders, including nursing homes (ONC, 2021a).

Notably, nursing homes were not included among the group of health care providers eligible to participate in CMS' EHR Incentive Program,[7] which was renamed Promoting Interoperability Programs[8] (Adler-Milstein et al., 2016; Gold and McLaughlin, 2016). As a result, nursing homes have

---

[3] American Recovery and Reinvestment Act of 2009, Public Law 111-5; 111th Cong., 1st sess. (February 17, 2009).

[4] Improving Medicare Post-Acute Care Transformation (IMPACT) Act of 2014, Public Law 113-185; 113th Cong., 2nd sess. (October 6, 2014).

[5] Medicare Access and CHIP Reauthorization Act of 2015, Public Law 114-10; 114th Cong., 1st sess. (April 16, 2015).

[6] 21st Century Cures Act of 2016, Public Law 114-255; 114th Cong., 2nd sess. (December 13, 2016).

[7] American Recovery and Reinvestment Act of 2009, Public Law 111-5; 111th Cong., 1st sess. (February 17, 2009).

[8] See https://www.cms.gov/Regulations-and-Guidance/Legislation/EHRIncentivePrograms (accessed October 27, 2021).

not benefited from the significant financial support for EHR adoption that has been provided to other sectors of the health care system (Alexander et al., 2019a, 2020a; Kistler et al., 2021; MACPAC, 2021; ONC, 2021b; Walker et al., 2016).

Bolstered by federal financial incentives and other factors, EHRs have been adopted at a steadily increasing rate across all sectors of the health care system over the past decade. The level of EHR adoption among all nonfederal acute care hospitals was 96 percent in 2016 (ONC, 2017a), while nearly 90 percent of office-based physicians used an EMR or EHR as of 2019 (CDC, 2021a). In contrast, an Office of the National Coordinator for Health Information Technology survey estimated that as of 2016 less than two-thirds of all nursing homes had adopted an EHR (Alvarado et al., 2017). By 2019, a survey of nearly 600 nursing homes indicated the nationwide prevalence of EHR adoption among nursing homes to be 84 percent (Vest et al., 2019). Nursing homes that have not implemented EHRs continue to rely on inefficient paper-based, rather than electronic, exchange of health information. The urgency of the need for accurate, efficient exchange of health information has been underscored by the COVID-19 pandemic and its devastating effect on nursing home residents (Alexander et al., 2022).

Even those nursing homes that have an EHR in place are not necessarily taking advantage of the full benefits of EHR adoption. A lack of interoperability, or the inability to electronically share health information between different HITs such as hospital and nursing home EHRs, is a key barrier to the full and effective use of EHRs. Only a small share of the 600 nursing homes surveyed in the study referenced above indicated that they were able to perform the key functions associated with the benefits of interoperability, namely sending, receiving, searching, and integrating patients' electronic health information across care settings. As the study authors point out, "without engagement in interoperability, EHRs risk becoming just another data silo" (Vest et al., 2019). This finding aligns with earlier research that nursing homes have not taken full advantage of their investments in health information technology (Alexander et al., 2017a). Thus, it is important not only for nursing homes to adopt HIT but also for them to ensure that HIT is used to its full capacity to foster the seamless exchange of health information to support quality care for nursing home residents.

ROLE OF HIT IN QUALITY CARE IN NURSING HOMES

As discussed in Chapter 1, the committee's conceptual model for quality care in nursing homes (depicted in Figure 9-1) includes such key components as effective, timely, and equitable care; responsive and caring communication and collaboration; and an empowered staff that is knowledgeable, consistent, compassionate, and engages in team-based

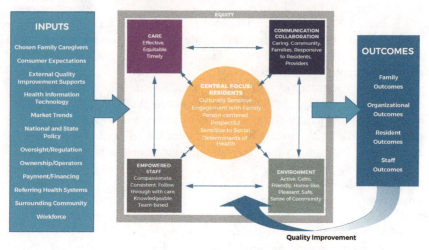

FIGURE 9-1 Conceptual model of the quality of care in nursing homes.

follow-through with care—all centered on providing person-centered, culturally sensitive, respectful care. As will be discussed below, HIT facilitates effective operationalization of the model's components and, in so doing, is key to delivering quality, person-centered care in nursing homes.

The implementation of HIT in nursing homes, if done well, holds the potential to yield benefits for nursing home residents, their families, and the people who care for them. Effective use of HIT can improve the quality of care and quality of life of nursing home residents, reduce medical errors, increase the efficiency of nursing home staff, provide the data needed to drive quality improvement and quality assurance efforts, and increase person-centered care. A number of barriers to successfully implementing EHRs and other HIT systems to their full capacity in nursing homes exist, calling for greater attention to address those challenges.

Use of HIT to Support Quality Measurement

The MDS was first fully implemented nationwide in 1991 as part of the federally required process for the clinical assessment of all residents in Medicare- and Medicaid-certified nursing homes. Described as "a powerful tool for implementing standardized assessment and for facilitating care management in nursing homes" (CMS, 2021a), the MDS enables an extensive evaluation of nursing homes, both on a facility level as well as on the level of individual resident's characteristics such as their medical, social, and functional status (Wu et al., 2009). The required MDS information also provides data for quality measurement and improvement purposes (AHRQ, 2018a). The MDS has been updated periodically since it was first introduced, with the most recent version, MDS 3.0, released in 2010.

Although concerns have been raised about the accuracy and completeness of the MDS (Rahman and Applebaum, 2009; Wu et al., 2009), it is a key resource within the broader portfolio of data sources critical to the quality of care in nursing homes. The MDS data collected during resident assessments include information about the resident's health and functioning and about changes in resident status. Importantly, this standardized data collection enables nursing homes to monitor the quality of resident care, and MDS data were critical to the development of quality indicators (Rantz and Connolly, 2004; Saliba and Buchanan, 2012) (see Chapter 3). The MDS provides the basis for the National Quality Forum–endorsed nursing home measures (AHRQ, 2018b).

EHRs can facilitate the effective, efficient, and accurate collection of data on nursing home residents required as part of the MDS process (Rantz et al., 2011). Indeed, the MDS serves as the basis for most commercially available EHRs for nursing home use. Effective EHR implementation can lead to quality improvement as reflected in lower deficiency scores, fewer medication errors and adverse drug reactions, improved compliance with practice guidelines, and improved resident outcomes regarding activities of daily living, among other quality measures (Alexander and Madsen, 2021; ONC, 2019b; Rantz et al., 2010a; Silow-Carroll et al., 2012). EHR implementation also has been found to contribute to improving other quality measures, such as increased vaccination rates, in nursing home settings (Bjarnadottir et al., 2017).

HIT and Quality Improvement

Given its capacity to facilitate communication between health care providers and advance patient safety across all health care settings, including nursing homes, HIT is viewed as an effective tool for improving the quality of care. Studies have explored the role of HIT in quality improvement related to patient safety, error reduction, improved communication, avoidable hospitalization, medication management, and health equity.

Harm reduction is particularly important in the nursing home setting, given that one in five Medicare beneficiaries experiences an adverse event within 35 days of admission to a nursing home. Moreover, nearly 60 percent of adverse events are preventable episodes associated with substandard treatment, inadequate monitoring, and delays in giving or failure to give necessary care (OIG, 2014). Adverse events are defined as harm or injury resulting from medical care (including the failure to provide needed care). Examples of adverse events include falls with injury, pressure injuries, health-care–acquired infections, and adverse drug events (Kapoor et al., 2019). Such events result, in part, from missing or inadequate information about functional, mental, and behavioral status in the communications carried out at the point of nursing home admission or discharge to a nursing home (Adler-Milstein et al., 2021). Ensuring that nursing home HIT systems are linked to the broader health care system could help address such information shortcomings (King et al., 2013; Popejoy et al., 2014; Vogelsmeier, 2014).

HIT is also associated with improved communication and the documentation of risk assessments for falls, a key area of patient safety in nursing homes (discussed in Chapter 6). For example, HIT systems have been used to facilitate the collection of longitudinal data on older adults by embedding sensors in their living spaces to detect small changes in gait speed and stride length over time. These measures are used to compare older adults who had a fall versus those who did not. Studies have shown that individuals that have cumulative changes in gait speed over time (3 weeks) have a 4.2 times greater likelihood of falling than those who have not experienced changes in their gait speed (Phillips et al., 2017). More research is needed to better understand the ways in which such data can most effectively be used by the interdisciplinary team to develop successful fall-prevention strategies for older adults (Dowding et al., 2012).

HIT has also been instrumental in another area of patient safety: that of risk assessment concerning the prevention of pressure ulcers, another prevalent condition among nursing home residents (discussed in Chapter 4). HIT has been used to improve communication about evidence-based pressure ulcer prevention strategies. One study of more than 200 nursing assistants in 16 nursing homes, for example, found that sophisticated HIT systems improved the nursing assistants' ability to pass clinical information on to other staff members, enhanced their ability to keep track of resident needs, and improved their access to clinical information overall (Alexander, 2015). Although this one study revealed a positive impact, other studies about EHR implementations and interventions using EHR data in nursing homes have demonstrated mixed impacts of technology on pressure ulcer outcomes (Dendere et al., 2021).

HIT has also shown significant promise in reducing avoidable hospitalizations and their associated costs by targeting ineffective and insufficient communication that can lead to unnecessary transfers of nursing home residents to hospitals (Ashcraft and Owen, 2017). One study of communication strategies used to reduce avoidable hospitalizations identified improvement strategies in a range of areas, including appointment scheduling, laboratory specimen drawing and results reporting, pharmacy orders and reconciliation, communication related to social work discharge planning, and tracing admission and preadmission data (Alexander et al., 2015). In each situation, nursing home staff suggested that HIT systems would improve data use efficiency and workflow and reduce the possibility of human error–associated information transfer. The study found that when nursing homes implemented these strategies, the average hospital transfer rates declined from nearly 2.5 per 1,000 resident days in 2014 to less than 2 per 1,000 resident days in 2018 (Vogelsmeier et al., 2021).

Another example of the ways in which the effective use of EHRs can advance patient safety in nursing homes is in the area of medication management. Polypharmacy, defined as the regular use of five or more medications (discussed further in Chapter 6), provides one example of how data integration is closely linked to patient safety. Structured EHR data, when integrated with computerized physician order entry and electronic prescribing, can enable decision-support functions that can promote compliance with guidelines and alert clinicians to potential medication interactions or allergies (Krüger et al., 2011). One study, for example, found that an electronic clinical decision-support system identified 57 to 73 percent of potentially inappropriate prescribing (depending on the criteria used) in seniors with multiple conditions (Rogero-Blanco et al., 2020). A review of 20 studies concluded that EHR-enabled clinical decision-support systems were effective in reducing potentially inappropriate prescribing in hospitals, though the results in nursing home settings were mixed (Scott et al., 2018).

In addition to HIT's potential role in advancing patient safety, it is also important to consider the role of HIT in advancing equity—another key domain of health care quality (IOM, 2001b; Lee, 2015; NASEM, 2021; NORC, 2010). As discussed in Chapter 2, the COVID-19 pandemic had a disproportionate impact on racial and ethnic minorities, both in the community (CDC, 2021b) and in nursing home settings (Gorges and Konetzka, 2021). HIT can support critical data collection and record demographic information such as race, ethnicity, and language preferences (Wyatt et al., 2016). The lack of data on race and ethnicity served as a barrier to developing targeted response efforts to the COVID-19 pandemic (Artiga et al., 2020).

Health information technology builds organizational capacity, which in turn enables nursing home staff to better identify resident care needs and track and manage care delivery processes; it also optimizes the nursing home staff's ability to access information important for making decisions about care delivery (Alexander, 2015). However, more evidence is needed, particularly in nursing home settings, on the specific effects of information systems components on quality measurement and quality reporting. The first step in this process would be to create sustained regular reporting mechanisms linking nursing home HIT adoption trends as a measure of quality improvement and HIT's influence on resident, family, staff, and organizational outcomes.

HIT and Care Planning

As discussed in Chapter 4, the resident care plan developed through the use of the MDS is central to the delivery of high-quality, person-centered care in nursing homes. By providing more holistic views of individual residents, including their past as well as current needs, standardized electronic documentation of resident information advances person-centered care (Zhang et al., 2012). Studies have shown that EHRs, with some customization, have the ability to increase fidelity to person-centered care plans, which is an important component of achieving person-centered care (Stanhope and Matthews, 2019).

Given the "information intensive" nature of health care (Shiells et al., 2019), documenting resident conditions is very time consuming for nursing home staff. The use of traditional, paper-based documentation is viewed as outdated, incomplete, inconsistent, and difficult to update, and it increases the opportunity for errors and may have a negative impact on the quality of care provided. EHRs, for their part, may be used for assessment and care planning with the associated benefits of effective chronic care management, improvement in quality of care, and ability to provide person-centered care (Shiells et al., 2019). Studies have shown that nursing home staff have positive views on the use of electronic documentation for care planning (Zhang et al., 2012) and that they have found templates that provide prompts to staff to identify potential problems to be particularly useful (Cherry et al., 2011). Research has provided a robust evidence base showing that EHRs can improve the accuracy and accessibility of resident documentation and contribute to a positive impact on the quality of care (Cherry et al., 2008; Kruse et al., 2017; Meehan, 2017).

Moreover, a proactive person-centered longitudinal plan of care is critical to care coordination (Dykes et al., 2014). The EHR designs most likely to advance person-centered care and care coordination would include specialized data formats whose precise form would depend on whether a person was a receiver or sender of information. This is particularly important when patient information is shared between nursing homes and hospitals during transitions of care because nursing homes often collect very specific and unique types of clinical data related to patient outcomes, while hospitals may not. Moreover, nursing home residents have very specific care needs related to chronic health conditions and care management. Without attending to specific physical as well as cognitive care needs, the individual may be at risk for rapid decline in function, and it is often very difficult or impossible for them to return to their former level of functional/mental abilities. While many common data elements in EHRs, such as code status, are represented across different health care settings, some unique fields (e.g., the activities of daily living collected by nursing homes) can create information gaps when one health care provider collects data, but another one does not. These differences could be addressed with an increased focus on standardizing HIT systems across the continuum of care so that the most useful data could be collected continuously and exchanged seamlessly between settings (ONC, 2017b; Skrocki, 2013; Suter et al., 2009).

Resident transitions between the nursing home and the hospital settings have been found to have missing, inaccurate, or conflicting information, which contributes to the risk of rehospitalization and inappropriate care for residents (King et al., 2013) as discussed in Chapter 6. Research highlights the importance of high-quality communication among health care professionals, including the effective use of EHRs to facilitate care transitions (Scott et al., 2017).

Advance Care Planning

As discussed, the care plan is instrumental in the delivery of person-centered care to nursing home residents. The pandemic amplified the importance of one element of care planning—advance care planning (ACP)—as nursing home residents are extremely vulnerable to contracting the life-threatening virus. ACP, a key component of end-of-life care, is associated with promoting person-centered care that reflects an individual's values, preferences, and beliefs, preventing unwanted care as well as reducing unnecessary hospitalizations (see Chapter 4). Individual preferences for end-of-life care are captured in written documents such as advance directives. Having a complete advance care plan in place that is accessible to clinicians is essential to the provision of care that aligns with the individual resident's preferences, values, and goals of care. The absence of an accurate advance care plan renders residents vulnerable to receiving treatment that may be aggressive and does not reflect the resident's preferences.

Studies suggest that the use of EHRs could address challenges related to documenting advance directives and thereby provide benefits for patients, families, and providers (Lemon et al., 2019). Ideally, the EHR would include electronic triggers to prompt clinicians to have goals-of-care conversations with patients and their families. In addition, EHRs would provide templates to guide the clinician through the conversation, and would generate data for quality improvement and reporting. Most importantly, given that people transition between care settings across the lifespan, using an EHR for documenting advance directives would ensure easy access to the necessary documentation to help ensure that patients receive care that is aligned with their preferences (Lamas et al., 2018).

HIT and the Workforce

HIT has the potential to improve staff efficiency with an associated positive impact on resident outcomes. One study, for example, found that 6 months after implementation of an EHR, nurses were able to spend significantly more time engaging with patients in their rooms and in purposeful interactions and less time at the nurses' station (Gomes et al., 2016). Using health information technology to capture resident health information in real time at the bedside can also reduce staff fatigue and the burden of relying on short-term memory, while also improving patient safety by enhancing the accuracy of the patient information (McAllen et al., 2018). Many nursing homes, however, only have computers located at central nursing stations and not close to residents' rooms. To take full advantage of real-time patient data collection in the EHR, mobile charting platforms are required, including tablets or point-of-care mobile workstations (Edelman et al., 2020).

Using the full capabilities of an EHR can improve the collection and documentation of patient assessment information. Ideally, the collection and recording of patient data and information should occur as close as possible to the provision of patient care, which in the nursing home setting is often at the bedside. (Rantz et al., 2011). Such real-time data entry has been shown to improve patient care, allowing for quicker results of laboratory tests and medication orders and providing more decision-making support to the clinicians (Alotaibi and Federico, 2017; Kruse et al., 2015). One study identified improvements in range of motion and reduction of high-risk pressure sores associated with the implementation of a bedside EMR with the capability of prompting staff to provide necessary care (Rantz et al., 2010a). Moreover, such improved care leads to greater patient satisfaction. Finally, real-time data entry can reduce the duplication of documentation and, in doing so, contribute to clinicians' overall efficiency (Classen et al., 2018; Gliklich et al., 2014).

Studies highlight the central role of training and education as predictors of positive workforce experience with EHRs, and emphasize that health care professionals who are not trained to use the EHR appropriately are unlikely to realize any gains in efficiency, nor will they be able to use the EHR to improve the quality of care. Research highlights not only EHR training in general, but specifically the need for initial, follow-up, and ongoing training for nursing home staff on using the EHR appropriately and to the full range of its capabilities. Additional training may have to be targeted to those nursing home staff who might lack general computer experience or who are not adept at using technology for documentation purposes (Cherry et al., 2008; Kruse et al., 2015).

Satisfaction with EHRs—on the part of clinicians as well as residents and their families—is a critically important factor in successful EHR adoption and use. If an EHR system is not easy to use or is perceived as making more work for nursing home staff rather than decreasing their workload, it will not be used to its full potential (Staggers et al., 2018). Moreover, poor EHR usability can lead to errors, which can potentially have a negative impact on patient safety (Gardner et al., 2018; Howe et al., 2018).

HIT usability needs to be assessed in terms of HIT's impact on resident, family, staff, and organizational outcomes as well as in terms of advancing equity and reducing disparities in nursing home care. Priority areas include the fit of the technology to tasks conducted by nursing home staff, user satisfaction, perceived workflows, and perceptions of system integration among processes of care. These issues are part of a growing area of research addressing the effect of clinician burden and burnout (Alexander and Ballou, 2018; Gardner et al., 2018; Zsenits et al., 2019).

HIT and Value-Based Payment

As discussed further in Chapter 7, the Centers for Medicare & Medicaid Services (CMS) continues to promote value-based programs as a way of advancing high-quality care and lowering health care costs. Launched in 2018, the Skilled Nursing Facility Value-Based Purchasing (SNF VBP) program awards or penalizes facilities for the quality of care provided to Medicare beneficiaries (see discussion in Chapter 7) (CMS, 2021b). Under this program, facilities are evaluated and receive incentives for improvements and achievements in hospital readmission measures, with additional measures expected to be introduced in the future. In a recent study, researchers reported that most U.S. skilled facilities were penalized nearly 1 percent of their Medicare payments in year 1 of the SNF VBP (Qi et al., 2020). Among the facilities more likely to be penalized were those that were small, for profit, and with low staffing levels. Additionally, homes located in low-income zip codes and with a high proportion of frail residents were likely to be penalized (Qi et al., 2020).

Research on nursing home responses to performance-based accountability measures, including the adoption of quality improvement changes, indicates that the strongest correlation between quality improvement changes was the implementation of EHRs and other HIT, such as clinical decision-support tools, to help frontline staff improve care delivery (Shetty et al., 2020). Another favorable care improvement approach includes incorporating standardized protocols into care delivery, which is often facilitated by electronic means (Hughes, 2008; Skrocki, 2013). Finally, the exchange of information with community providers was another strategy adopted by skilled nursing facilities to improve their performance levels (Adler-Milstein et al., 2021; Rahman et al., 2018).

Interoperability and Health Information Exchange

Many nursing homes lack the core competence or resources to make the most effective use of EHRs and other forms of HIT beyond using them for billing and reporting purposes. Moreover, getting information from other health care providers, such as hospitals, primary care providers, and clinical laboratories, into the EHR in a readily usable form remains a challenge. EHRs are typically facility specific, located within hospitals, physician practices, and pharmacies, but they are generally not interconnected to enable the seamless flow of health information across various health care settings. This lack of connectivity is a particular problem for the care of nursing home residents. Nursing home residents often have multiple complex medical conditions, which require effective care coordination to ensure safety and quality of care as the individual transitions among different health care settings (Brownell et al., 2014; Carroll et al., 2020; Grabowski et al., 2007; Jung et al., 2016; Lee, 2015; Mor et al., 2010; Rantz et al., 2010a,b; Unruh et al., 2013a,b; Wang et al., 2011).

Interoperability and health information exchange (HIE) are often used interchangeably but are two distinct components involved in advancing the HIT ecosystem to the point where there is efficient and effective collaboration and coordination of care among health care providers and across settings of care. HIE allows patients as well as health care providers to access and share medical information electronically in a secure manner (ONC, 2019d). Interoperability is defined as the ability of two or more HIT systems to not only exchange information, but to be able to *use* the information that has been exchanged. While HIE is necessary, it is, in and of itself, not sufficient for interoperability.[9]

Among the approximately two-thirds of nursing homes that had EHRs in 2017, less than 20 percent were capable of integrating patient health information from other health care organizations (Henry et al., 2018). The absence of this capability is a significant barrier to the real-time exchange of patient information (Powell and Alexander, 2021). Some nursing homes, however, have adopted HIT systems with the capability of supporting HIE (Adler-Milstein et al, 2021; Alexander et al., 2019b). These tend to be larger urban nursing homes with 100 beds or more and with higher staffing levels as well as those affiliated with a chain of nursing homes (Zhang et al., 2016).

Research has identified enhanced communication, increased effectiveness of care, and patient safety as being among the benefits of HIE implementation, and workflow integration has been shown to be a key facilitator of HIE (Kruse et al., 2018). A key barrier is that laboratory results and

---

[9] See https://www.healthit.gov/buzz-blog/meaningful-use/interoperability-health-information-exchange-setting-record-straight (accessed January 26, 2022).

hospital discharge records are often transferred, if at all, as PDF files that are difficult for clinical staff to use and impossible to track (Alper et al., 2021; Kruse et al., 2018). Reaching the full potential of an interoperable data exchange could improve both the quality of care and the safety of residents (Kruse et al., 2018).

The use of HIE to improve and support communication and care delivery, together with full-time embedded advanced practice registered nurses and a focus on early-illness detection and end-of-life care, were the three key elements of the Missouri Quality Initiative, a CMMI demonstration project whose goal was to reduce avoidable hospitalizations among nursing home residents (discussed in Chapter 3). The 8-year effort resulted in a 40 percent decrease in hospitalizations (for any reason) and a nearly 60 percent decrease in potentially avoidable hospitalizations. HIE facilitated staff access to detailed resident health information, enabling staff members to monitor patient progress more effectively and to identify signs of possible problems, which helped to reduce avoidable hospitalizations (Ingber et al., 2017; Rantz et al., 2017a).

Policy Measures to Advance the Use of HIT

Recognizing that significant shortcomings exist related to HIT infrastructure, data flow, security, and interoperability among health systems, CMS has sought to use policy measures to encourage the use of EHRs for the exchange of clinical information between health care settings. For example, the Interoperability and Patient Access final rule went into effect in July 2021; it requires hospitals with certain EHR capabilities to send admission, discharge, and transfer data to other providers (CMS, 2021c). This rule aims to advance interoperability through application programming interfaces (APIs)[10] to facilitate and expand access to health information.

CMS is collaborating with the Office of the National Coordinator for Health Information to establish a Trusted Exchange Framework and Common Agreement[11] to develop a nationwide network that supports the use of technology to streamline processes of care and payment (HHS, 2022). Additionally, CMS is working with standards-based organizations

---

[10] "The CMS regulations include policies which require or encourage payers to implement Application Programming Interfaces (APIs) to improve the electronic exchange of health care data—sharing information with patients or exchanging information between a payer and provider or between two payers. APIs can connect to mobile apps or to a provider electronic health record (EHR) or practice management system to enable a more seamless method of exchanging information" (CMS, 2021c).

[11] See https://www.healthit.gov/topic/interoperability/trusted-exchange-framework-and-common-agreement-tefca (accessed January 26, 2022).

(i.e., HL7) using Fast Healthcare Interoperability Resources,[12] to promote transparency and exchange among providers, payers, and patients, which could enable important discussions about cost and the value of care among these stakeholders.

The inclusion of EHR-based clinical quality measures for nursing homes in Medicare's Meaningful Measures Initiative[13] serves as an impetus for nursing homes to use the EHR to its full capability, while the 21st Century Cures Act focuses on advancing HIE capabilities[14] provided additional policy support (Vest et al., 2019). As nursing homes increasingly use new measures to assess HIT adoption and interoperability, such information can be made publicly available in Care Compare (Adler-Milstein et al., 2020a; Bjarnadottir et al., 2017; Enyioha et al., 2021; Kistler et al., 2021; Kruse et al., 2017; Powell et al., 2021; Vest et al., 2019).

CHALLENGES OF HIT ADOPTION AND USE IN NURSING HOMES

The adoption, implementation, and effective use of EHRs in nursing home settings face significant challenges. Key barriers include cost, adequate staff training, clinician burden and workload, the interoperability of information systems, and disparities in uptake and infrastructure (Alexander et al., 2017b,c; Zhang et al., 2016).

Financial Barriers

Studies have demonstrated that there are significant costs associated with the adoption of HIT such as EHRs (Kruse et al., 2015; Rantz et al., 2010a). Moreover, it is important to consider that it is not only the initial cost of adopting an EHR—regular maintenance and required technology infrastructure upgrades also represent a considerable expense for nursing homes (Filipova, 2013; Holup et al., 2013; Kruse et al., 2015; Phillips et al., 2010; Resnick et al., 2009). As noted above, nursing homes were not eligible for the federally funded incentives to help cover the costs of EHR adoption. This ineligibility for financial support is critical, as costs represent a key barrier to EHR adoption in nursing homes (Abramson et

---

[12] See https://www.healthit.gov/topic/standards-technology/standards/fhir-fact-sheets (accessed January 26, 2022).

[13] For more information see https://www.cms.gov/Medicare/Quality-Initiatives-Patient-Assessment-Instruments/QualityInitiativesGenInfo/MMF/General-info-Sub-Page (accessed December 1, 2021).

[14] For more information, see https://www.federalregister.gov/documents/2020/05/01/2020-07419/21st-century-cures-act-interoperability-information-blocking-and-the-onc-health-it-certification (accessed December 1, 2021).

al., 2014; Cherry et al., 2008; Vest et al., 2019; Wang and Biedermann, 2012).

If incentives are offered to high-performing nursing homes to encourage the adoption of quality improvement strategies involving EHRs, these funds might potentially serve to offset the costs of EHR implementation. However, lower-performing nursing homes that do not receive any incentives may experience wider disparities in resident outcomes due to the inability to fund similar quality improvement strategies (Bjarnadottir et al., 2017; Kruse et al., 2015).

Clinician Burden

Another challenge to broader adoption of HIT in nursing homes is the impact of EHR use on the workforce. Issues that shape the impact of EHRs on nursing home staff and their ability to develop, implement, and monitor resident care plans include the management of documentation, the time consumed using the EHR, and effect of EHR use on productivity (e.g., time spent with patients). These elements have been identified as important factors in clinician burden and burnout related to the use of EHRs (Adler-Milstein et al., 2020b; Alexander and Ballou, 2018).

One example of clinician burden is the phenomenon known as EHR alert fatigue. The structured format of an EHR enables developers and administrators who oversee EHR implementation to add various clinical decision-support tools that can recommend specific actions or warn the EHR user of a potential issue using an electronic alert. Alerts can be very beneficial, helping busy clinicians to identify potential changes in a patient's condition (e.g., a laboratory value that is out of bounds) that need to be addressed. This is particularly important given the prevalence of polypharmacy among nursing home residents.

However, while alerts can improve care processes, alerts can be burdensome and lead to clinicians ignoring them—for example, nearly one in four medication orders generate an alert (Saiyed et al., 2017). In fact, alert override can become a habitual behavior, rendering clinical decision-support systems significantly less useful (Ancker et al., 2017; Baysari et al., 2017). Given the scope of this problem, researchers have developed processes for better managing alerts to increase their effectiveness and reduce alert burden. One approach uses targeted deactivation of low-quality or low-effectiveness alerts (Simpao et al., 2015), while another approach is to make alerts silent to start, compile data on alert performance, and use that information to inform alert implementation decisions (Saiyed et al., 2017). Some investigators have suggested developing adaptive clinical decision-support tools that learn from a clinician's behavior and filter alerts accordingly (Lee et al., 2014). Ethical frameworks have been proposed to guide the development and implementation of these and other types of EHR capabilities to articulate the appropriate use of these systems, and incorporate processes for monitoring data quality and ensuring the security of patient data (Evans and Whicher, 2018).

Although HIT has the potential to improve staff productivity and workflow, such improvements can be offset by duplicative efforts such as staff using paper documentation in addition to use of the EHR. Other factors that impede HIT use by nursing home staff include the lack of embedded decision support and the lack of standardized language. A number of studies have identified workarounds used by staff, which are associated with errors in documentation as well as in clinical care (Hudak and Sharkey, 2007; Vogelsmeier et al., 2008). Other barriers include the lack of appropriate HIT expertise within the nursing home staff as well as the designation of HIT management to staff members who have other roles and training outside the scope and experience of managing a HIT system (Alexander et al., 2020b).

HIT that is designed well and takes into account the human factor is thought to build upon organizational capacity by enabling nursing home staff to better identify resident care needs, to track and manage care delivery processes, and to access needed information for making decisions about care delivery (Alexander, 2015; Alexander and Staggers, 2009). Research is increasingly focused on the importance of human-centered designs to address the low rates of clinician satisfaction with HIT and the perception on the part of clinicians that technology should help to manage their workload, not add to it (Carayon and Hoonakker, 2019).

Lack of Standardized Language

An additional challenge is the variation in the language used to document care practices between health care organizations. Variations in content and formatting affect the utility of resident's medical records, and various studies have concluded that medical records do not accurately reflect the patient's condition or care provided, which makes it more difficult to evaluate health care services (Skrocki, 2013). One way to improve the ability of EHRs to improve care is to design systems that reap the benefits of standardization in terms of more accurate, precise, and up-to-date information transfer among all members of the interdisciplinary team. A standardized language across the continuum of care will enable the continuous retrieval and analysis of documentation over time and across care settings to improve quality, support evidence-based practice, and achieve desired outcomes (Keenan et al., 2008; Lundberg et al., 2008).

Training

Research has identified insufficient staff training as one key HIT implementation challenge. Nursing homes have not made sufficient investments in staff training in all aspects of EHR adoption and use, nor has training been ongoing after the initial adoption of the EHR (Cherry et al., 2008; Ko et al., 2018; Kruse et al., 2015, 2017; Longhurst et al., 2019; Vest et al., 2019). Studies have found staff dissatisfaction related to the limited amount of time devoted to HIT training (Fossum et al., 2011; Meehan, 2017). Staff describe situations in which they received one single training session, the duration of which ranged from 30 minutes to an all-day session, with single training sessions of a half hour or less for certified nursing assistants or personal care aides (Ko et al., 2018). One study did show staff satisfaction with training in which the staff in the study received multiple days of training (Yu et al., 2008). Researchers have emphasized the need for policy makers and health systems to make incentives and other funds available to support HIT training and technology infrastructure in nursing homes (Ko et al., 2018).

Interoperability

The ability of nursing homes to share patient data about residents as they transition from the hospital to post-acute care settings is critical to the health care professionals who are responsible for care coordination and post-acute care. Estimates indicate that, overall, only half of all EHR systems are capable of transferring medical records to other EHR systems (Kistler et al., 2021; Powell et al., 2021; Vest et al., 2019). One study of nearly 800 acute-care hospitals, for example, found that fewer than half of the hospitals had an EHR portal through which long-term care facilities could access hospital information. Moreover, less than half of all hospitals had a portal through which hospitals could send information electronically to long-term care facilities (Adler-Milstein et al., 2020a). Other studies have pointed to shortcomings related to the information-sharing capabilities of EHRs. One study, for example, examined information sharing among nearly 500 nursing homes paired with hospitals. The study found that key information on residents' functional, mental, and behavioral status as well as on the identification of the specific individual to contact at the hospital with follow-up questions was often missing, delayed (often arriving after the patient), and difficult to use (Adler-Milstein et al., 2021).

Interoperability is a challenge for the entire health care system, one that the HITECH Act and the 21st Century Cures Act of 2020[15] have attempted to address. These two initiatives have had limited success, however, because

---

[15] 21st Century Cures Act of 2020, Public Law 114-255 (December 13, 2016).

of technical, policy, governance, and funding issues; the proprietary policies of EHR vendors; and security and privacy concerns (Adler-Milstein and Pfeifer, 2017; Powell et al., 2021; Ratwani et al., 2018). Incomplete and inconsistent information in EHRs from multiple sources, inconsistent language use in EHRs, organizational resistance to sharing data, the high cost of hiring specialists to manage interoperability, information that is not shared in a timely manner, and inadequate investment in preparation, infrastructure, and training are significant barriers to achieving meaningful interoperability (Adler-Milstein et al., 2021).

Disparities in HIT Adoption

Another challenge is related to the uneven levels of HIT adoption across nursing homes. Studies exploring the use of HIT in rural and urban nursing homes, for example, have found that nursing homes in larger, more populated areas are more likely to have more extensive HIT capabilities, use, and integration than nursing homes in less populated regions of the country (Alexander et al., 2017b, 2020c). In addition to geographic location, other nursing home characteristics that have an impact on HIT development, implementation, and use include size, staffing ratios, payer mix, and financial model (Kistler et al., 2021).

HIT adoption by nursing homes in urban areas has enabled the improved integration of clinical data into laboratory and pharmacy systems. Lower rates of HIT adoption in nursing homes in rural areas, in contrast, might lead to greater disparities in care delivery, leaving rural nursing home residents increasingly vulnerable to poor outcomes. One analysis, for example, found that 60 percent of resident care systems in rural nursing homes are not at all able to interface with external entities' computerized systems, including those found in clinics, clinical laboratories, hospitals, and other nursing homes, reducing those nursing homes' capacity for health data sharing (Powell et al., 2021). Qualitative interviews conducted with administrators from these nursing home facilities identified privacy and security concerns, transparency and control, fear of lawsuits, and organizational factors as key barriers slowing the uptake of technology (Powell et al., 2021). Identifying HIT adoption standards across nursing homes may help reduce HIT inequities and disparities both within and across facilities (Kistler et al., 2021).

Infrastructure

HIT, including EHRs and virtual telehealth applications, is a resource that can enhance access to health care services and improve equity, but only if adequate infrastructure (e.g., high-speed broadband access) and resources (e.g., knowledgeable staff) are available to support the use of the technology. However, nursing homes in rural areas of the country face numerous inequities in access to these HIT resources compared with their urban counterparts. These differences can lead to negative health outcomes. For example, older adults who live in nursing homes in urban areas have better access to specialized health care providers than those in rural areas. Recent studies have shown that HIT can support health systems in advancing health equity (Brewer et al., 2020), with at least one research team developing a digital health equity framework (Crawford and Serhal, 2020).

Limited Internet access, lack of wireless connectivity, and poor integration of HIT systems are major issues reported in studies. Poor Internet connectivity and wireless "dead zones" throughout a nursing home are identified as major barriers to the successful use of HIT (Alexander et al., 2007; Meehan, 2017). A study of nearly 900 nursing home clinicians found that while nearly 90 percent of those surveyed reported having used EHRs, only 72 percent indicated that their facilities had a wireless network (Enyioha et al., 2021). In the absence of wireless networks, nursing home staff may develop temporary approaches known as workarounds[16] to bypass inefficiencies. Such workarounds can involve a range of actions that might present temporary "fixes" to workflow obstacles, but they may result in negative consequences in terms of resident safety and quality of care, which in turn can lead to poor outcomes for residents (Kandaswamy et al., 2021).

HIT AND THE COVID-19 PANDEMIC

Nursing homes used health information technology during the COVID-19 pandemic in a number of ways, including to enhance the surveillance of outbreaks and the responses to those outbreaks.[17] The Centers for Disease Control and Prevention (CDC), for example, implemented the National Healthcare Safety Network to support the nation's COVID-19 response. This mandatory electronic reporting and surveillance system enabled long-term care facilities to assess and report COVID-19 impacts, including statistics related to rates of positivity and mortality (CDC et al., 2021; ODPHP, 2022). Results are made available in an electronic dashboard.

---

[16] EHR workarounds are defined as "behaviors that may differ from organizationally prescribed or intended procedures. They circumvent or temporarily 'fix' an evident or perceived workflow hindrance in order to meet a goal or to achieve it more readily" (Debono and Braithwaite, 2015, p. 27; see also Boonstra et al., 2021; Debono et al., 2013). Workarounds in the EHR context "can involve skipping prescribed steps, entering data that should be entered by others, or registering activities later in the EHR system rather than letting the system guide these activities" (Boonstra et al., 2021, p. 2; see also Azad and King, 2008; Blijleven et al., 2017).

[17] See https://www.cdc.gov/nhsn/index.html (accessed January 26, 2022).

EHRs contain many important data elements that can support an effective response to a viral outbreak (Atreja et al., 2008; Kukafka et al., 2007). Nursing home staff with EHR capabilities used their EHRs to monitor resident symptoms and vital signs and developed electronic dashboards to track and report resident and staff COVID infections (Andersen et al., 2021). Staff also used telehealth and other technologies, as discussed below.

Telehealth

Telehealth (defined in Box 9-2 below) has been used across all sectors of the health care system, including nursing homes, for decades (Grabowski and O'Malley, 2014; Hui et al., 2001; IOM, 1996). In many ways, nursing homes represent ideal settings for the use of telehealth services. Although the medical needs of residents have grown increasingly complex over time,

---

BOX 9-2
Telehealth Defined

The Health Resources and Services Administration of the U.S. Department of Health and Human Services defines telehealth as the use of electronic information and telecommunications technologies to support and promote long-distance clinical health care, patient and professional health-related education, public health, and health administration.

Telehealth applications include

- **Live (synchronous) videoconferencing:** a two-way audiovisual link between a patient and a care provider
- **Store-and-forward (asynchronous) videoconferencing:** transmission of a recorded health history to a health practitioner, usually a specialist.
- **Remote patient monitoring:** the use of connected electronic tools to record personal health and medical data in one location for review by a provider in another location, usually at a different time.
- **Mobile health:** health care and public health information provided through mobile devices. The information may include general educational information, targeted texts, and notifications about disease outbreaks.

Telehealth differs from telemedicine as it encompasses a wider range of services. Telemedicine focuses on remote provision of clinical services; telehealth in contrast includes nonclinical services, such as provider training, administrative meetings, and continuing medical education, in addition to clinical services.

SOURCES: ONC, 2019e, 2020.

nursing home clinicians may be on site at the nursing home on an intermittent basis, creating challenges that can contribute to misdiagnoses, delayed diagnoses, overuse of emergency department visits, and avoidable hospitalizations (Driessen et al., 2016, 2018a).

Research has shown telehealth in nursing home settings to have a variety of potential benefits, such as expanding access to care, addressing gaps in coverage, reducing the burden on staff, improving resident outcomes, and achieving cost savings. Studies have also found clinicians, residents, and family members agree about the benefits of telehealth for patient care (Edelman et al., 2020; Groom et al., 2021). These results build on earlier studies that found benefits of telehealth—in terms of both clinical efficacy as well as cost savings—for the delivery of certain specialty services, such as dermatology, geriatrics, and psychiatry, to nursing home residents (Wade et al., 2010). The potential benefits and challenges of telehealth use for nursing home residents, families, and clinicians are summarized in Table 9-1.

The use of telehealth as a viable modality for health care delivery accelerated dramatically after March 2020, when CMS, under a public health emergency waiver, removed existing barriers to telehealth services.[18] This policy change, which enabled nursing homes and other health care providers to be reimbursed for telehealth visits at the same rate as a

TABLE 9-1 Potential Benefits and Challenges Associated with Telehealth Use in Nursing Homes

Potential benefits of adopting telehealth	Potential challenges to adopting telehealth
Enable residents to avoid exposure to infectious disease, and to avoid the stress associated with transportation to and from appointments outside of a facility	Greater difficulty building the resident–provider relationship
Improve access to care/providers	Variability in implementation, use, and integration of different software/platforms/devices used for telehealth visits
Improve efficiency for clinicians (e.g., less time spent traveling to nursing homes)	Lack of available, integrated, and interoperable data
Improve communication between nursing home staff and providers	Delays in follow-up care of nursing home residents
Provide opportunities for early intervention	Increased burden for nursing home staff
Provide opportunities to include family in care of the resident	
Reduce hospital readmissions	

SOURCE: Powell and Alexander, 2021.

---

[18] For more information, see https://www.cms.gov/About-CMS/Agency-Information/Emergency/EPRO/Current-Emergencies/Current-Emergencies-page (accessed November 23, 2021).

face-to-face visit (CMS, 2020), was implemented to facilitate the provision of care remotely while simultaneously keeping nursing home residents, staff, and clinicians safe through social distancing. Regulations had previously limited the reimbursement for telehealth services to rural nursing homes as originating sites of care. In addition, CMS developed a telehealth toolkit to provide guidance to health care facilities in the use of telehealth[19] (CMS, 2020; Gillespie et al., 2020). Telehealth was found to be a critical tool to assist nursing homes to provide high-quality care in the context of an underresourced workforce spread thin by the heightened challenges of caring for vulnerable older adults during the pandemic (Jen et al., 2021), though there were challenges arising from limited workforce and resident training.

Research has found that virtual care reduced stress for residents and increased access to services, but that it also worsened social isolation and caused confusion among some patients (Powell and Alexander, 2021; Seifert et al., 2020).

However, telehealth allowed the provision of remote clinical care by both primary care physicians and specialists (Jen et al., 2021; Powell and Alexander, 2021), which enabled nursing home staff to preserve limited supplies such as personal protective equipment (PPE) (Edelman et al., 2020) (as discussed further in Chapter 6).

Significant variation exists in the use of telehealth services by nursing homes. A study based on survey results of a random sample of over 700 nursing homes found that 79 percent of nursing homes reported partial implementation of telehealth, 16 percent reported no telehealth use, and only 5 percent reported the maximum use of telehealth.[20] Though telehealth use did not vary by ownership type, the use was lower for nursing homes in rural areas. Overall, the majority of nursing home administrators reported low use of telehealth relative to other health care settings, despite the supportive policy environment (Alexander et al., 2020c). One study found that geriatric, psychiatric, and palliative care telemedicine consults were the most common in nursing homes during the COVID-19 pandemic (Groom et al., 2021). A 2018 survey found that the providers showing the highest level of interest in telemedicine consults for nursing home residents were in the areas of dermatology, geriatric psychiatry, and infectious disease (Driessen et al., 2018b).

Despite the relatively limited overall use of telehealth, the study found

---

[19] For the toolkit, see https://www.cms.gov/files/document/general-telemedicine-toolkit.pdf (accessed November 8, 2021).

[20] Nursing home respondents completed surveys between January 2019 and August 2020, which, according to the study authors, provides a comparison of pre- and post-telehealth expansion use (Alexander et al., 2020c).

that compared with the pre-expansion period (prior to March 6, 2020), nursing homes were more likely to use telehealth for a number of discrete tasks. For example, nursing homes were more than 11 times more likely to use telehealth for evaluating residents and making pre-transfer arrangements and more than four times more likely to use telehealth for second opinions and consultations in the post-expansion period, compared with the pre-expansion period. The study also found that nursing homes were nearly three times more likely to use telehealth to access radiology results and for reporting activities (Alexander et al., 2020c).

Given the potential of telehealth to reduce social isolation and preserve limited PPE in the early phases of the pandemic as well as to enhance clinical decision making and medication order entry, the low rates of telehealth use are viewed as a missed opportunity to improve the quality and safety of care in nursing homes (Alexander et al., 2020c). The limited use of telehealth in nursing home settings may be due to factors such as inadequate infrastructure, limited scientific evidence on the effectiveness of telehealth interventions to improve outcomes, concerns about the discontinuation of policies supporting telehealth billing, insufficient training and support, and the competence of workforce (Alexander et al., 2020c; Ko et al., 2018).

HIT to Counter Social Isolation

The restrictions imposed by nursing homes in response to the COVID-19 pandemic intensified feelings of social isolation and loneliness among nursing home residents who were unable to see friends and family members for long periods of time. Research has documented the negative impact of social isolation and loneliness on residents' health, well-being, and quality of life (Kemp, 2020; Ruopp, 2020; Simard and Volicer, 2020). The known health impacts include cognitive decline, depression, and anxiety (NASEM, 2020). The longer-term impacts of social isolation for nursing home residents can also include rapid functional decline, pressure injuries due to limited mobility, dehydration and malnutrition, and a sense of hopelessness. Measures taken during the pandemic to protect residents and staff by limiting outside visitors were particularly severe for residents with dementia, as their cognitive impairments made it extremely difficult to understand significant changes in their routines, including not having regular visitors (Edelman et al., 2020).

Given the serious health risks associated with social isolation and loneliness, it is critical to understand the potential of various health technology applications and ways to facilitate their use in nursing home settings to ensure residents remain connected with family and friends. While some research suggests that socially assistive robots may be helpful to address social isolation in nursing homes (Bemelmans et al., 2012), the applications do not necessarily have to involve complicated technologies. One program developed during the pandemic, for example, arranged weekly phone conversations between medical school student volunteers and older adults in nursing homes. Initial reports highlight the program's potential as an effective intervention to increase social connection among nursing home residents during the pandemic (van Dyck et al., 2020). For a resident's perspective on the impact of visitation restrictions in nursing homes as a result of the COVID-19 pandemic, see Box 9-3.

Other interventions involve applications that are more complex. The use of video technology, for example, is particularly helpful to nursing home residents with hearing impairments who compensate for their limited or lack of hearing by lip reading and using visual cues. Relying on such movements is not possible when the individual speaking to them is wearing a mask, but video connection renders a mask unnecessary. Other options include video-enabled rounding of nursing home residents who may require reminders to eat or drink or who are in need of company while eating their meal (Edelman et al., 2020).

OTHER HIT CONSIDERATIONS FOR QUALITY IMPROVEMENT

As discussed in Chapter 4, the committee based its approach to exploring needs-based care in the nursing home setting on a combination of models, including Maslow's hierarchy of needs. Interestingly, HIT can support an individual nursing home resident's progression through each level of Maslow's hierarchy from basic needs to self-actualization. For example, warmth and comfort in an older person's residence are basic needs at the physical and physiological level that innovative HIT devices can address.

BOX 9-3
Resident and Family Member Perspective

"One of the great tragedies of the present era is the proliferation of this option [nursing homes] as more people live longer and are separated from their families. As well, COVID fears have caused many facilities to restrict or eliminate visitations and activities for residents. They are operating more like prisons than homes. Isolation kills too. I want to see visitations fully resumed, with mandatory vaccinations for all staff, residents and visitors."

— Anonymous, Oviedo, Florida

This quote was collected from the committee's online call for resident, family, and nursing home staff perspectives.

Smart wearable sensors, for instance, can detect body temperature fluctuations and send an electronic message to a caregiver in situations when a nursing home resident has an abnormal temperature (Chan et al., 2012).

In the higher levels of Maslow's model, networking innovations such as social robots, which respond to touch sensations, may help address issues of isolation and loneliness in older adults living alone (Alonso-Martín et al., 2017). Devices that support greater freedom of choice and mobility within the community may help older adults remain independent and maintain a greater sense of self-esteem. For example, global positioning systems can support autonomy, independence, and safety for older adults with dementia by providing information about their location to caregivers (Øderud et al., 2015). These technological innovations, many of which are newly available or still in development, represent important opportunities to enhance the quality of care and improve the quality of life of nursing home residents.

Assistive Health Technologies

Various assistive technologies, such as remote monitoring systems and interactive therapeutic robots, are increasingly being used in nursing home settings to improve quality of care and quality of life (Birks et al., 2016; McGlynn et al., 2014; Moyle et al., 2017a,b).

Use of Remote Monitoring and Robotic Technology

Applications that support remote monitoring technology have begun to change the landscape of long-term care delivery and improve nursing home resident outcomes. Remote monitoring systems use devices that can connect to the Internet (e.g., using wireless connectivity), allow objects to move around independently, and monitor and capture medical and other health data from patients and electronically transmit this information to health care providers for assessment (Adler-Milstein et al., 2021). Such information sharing is leading to new relationships and the strengthening of existing ones among multiple stakeholders, with the ultimate goals being to enhance and sustain quality improvement initiatives, align financial incentives to reduce costs, and improve care coordination activities (Carroll et al., 2020).

Other sophisticated remote monitoring innovations can improve nursing home resident safety and alert staff to medically significant physiologic changes. For example, radar and other sensing devices are able to

- Assist in detecting falls by nursing home residents,
- Provide automatic alerting mechanisms with early notifications sent to nursing home staff when a resident is alone in a room (Su et al., 2018),

- Detect change in activities of daily living and mobility resulting from worsening heart conditions, detected by wearable or non-wearable sensors (Despins et al., 2020), and
- Detect early changes in health status triggered by data from sensors, such as those that detect blood pressure change, heart rate, and respiratory rate, embedded in the residents' living environment (Rantz et al., 2012, 2017b; Su et al., 2019).

Robotic therapy provides an additional option for the use of technology in nursing home settings and may potentially represent an innovative approach to providing care to the large and growing share of nursing home residents diagnosed with dementia. A systematic review and meta-analysis of robotic therapy research on adults with dementia found that such therapy significantly decreased agitation and increased social interaction, though it did not have a significant effect on depression, anxiety, cognitive status, or quality of life (Ong et al., 2021).

Robots can also be used to help older adults maintain independence by assisting with health monitoring tasks (e.g., taking blood pressure and providing medication reminders), instrumental tasks (e.g., housekeeping) (Louie et al., 2014), and the manipulation of objects (e.g., retrieving belongings) (Gerling et al., 2016; Grönvall and Verdezoto, 2013; Lee and Dey, 2011). Other types of robots can assist staff with tasks such as lifting patients and delivering necessary care equipment and can also alert the staff of emergencies (Purtill, 2019). There is also recent interest in the potential for robots to provide social connection and support to the decreasing workforce (Girling, 2021; Philipson, 2021; Purtill, 2019).

Regardless of how promising these and other future innovations might be for the nursing home setting, developers and implementers of assistive technologies need to consider the impact of these innovations on clinician workflow, burden, and satisfaction. Moreover, it is critically important to evaluate on a systematic basis the effect of these tools on nursing home residents' quality of life, comfort, and satisfaction, including concerns for privacy and the loss of human connection (Gerling et al., 2016; Girling, 2021).

Implementing HIT in nursing homes, if done well, has the potential to yield extensive benefits for nursing home residents, their families, and the people who care for them. Effective use of HIT can improve the quality of care and quality of life of nursing home residents, reduce medical errors, increase the efficiency of nursing home staff, and provide the data needed to drive quality improvement and quality assurance efforts, and increase person-centered care. While there are a number of barriers to successfully implementing EHRs and other HIT systems in nursing homes, research has identified potential approaches to addressing those barriers. As the demand for long-term care services increases with the aging of the population, it becomes ever more critical to identify the most appropriate uses of HIT and provide the training and support to use HIT to address the needs of older adults and other individuals who receive care in nursing homes.

KEY FINDINGS AND CONCLUSIONS

- Health information technology (HIT) in the nursing home setting plays a key role in enabling the components of the committee's conceptual model by

    - promoting person-centered care,
    - improving documentation for the resident's care plan,
    - facilitating communication between health care providers across settings of care,
    - improving the safety of health care delivery (e.g., by reducing harmful errors),
    - supporting the delivery of personal health care services and managing chronic conditions, and
    - monitoring and sustaining quality.

- The long-term care sector has a different model of care delivery than acute care. A nursing home resident's length of stay is typically much longer than that of a patient in acute care, which requires extensive ongoing communication, care coordination activities, and different HIT reporting mechanisms to support, maintain and improve the resident's physical and mental functioning over time.
- HIT implementation in nursing homes, if done well, has the potential to yield far-reaching benefits for nursing home residents, their families, and the people who care for them.
- Nursing homes have not had the financial support granted to other health care providers, given their ineligibility to participate in the federal EHR incentive program.
- The adoption, implementation, and effective use of EHRs in nursing home settings face significant challenges, including cost, adequate staff training, clinician burden and workload, the interoperability of information systems, and existing nursing home infrastructure.
- Health technologies such as telehealth, videoconferencing, and personal monitoring devices are also effective tools in nursing home settings.
- Other health technology innovations to improve care in nursing homes include wireless remote monitoring devices that can collect data about residents (e.g., humanoid robots), as well as radar and other sensing devices.

REFERENCES

Abramson, E. L., S. McGinnis, J. Moore, R. Kaushal, and HITEC Investigators. 2014. A statewide assessment of electronic health record adoption and health information exchange among nursing homes. *Health Services Research* 49(1 Pt 2):361–372.

Adler-Milstein, J., and E. Pfeifer. 2017. Information blocking: Is it occurring and what policy strategies can address it? *Milbank Quarterly* 95(1):117–135.

Adler-Milstein, J., S. C. Lin, and A. K. Jha. 2016. The number of health information exchange efforts is declining, leaving the viability of broad clinical data exchange uncertain. *Health Affairs* 35(7):1278–1285.

Adler-Milstein, J., K. Raphael, A. Bonner, L. Pelton, and T. Fulmer. 2020a. Hospital adoption of electronic health record functions to support age-friendly care: Results from a national survey. *Journal of the American Medical Informatics Association* 27(8):1206–1213.

Adler-Milstein, J., W. Zhao, R. Willard-Grace, M. Knox, and K. Grumbach. 2020b. Electronic health records and burnout: Time spent on the electronic health record after hours and message volume associated with exhaustion but not with cynicism among primary care clinicians. *Journal of the American Medical Informatics Association* 27(4):531–538.

Adler-Milstein, J., K. Raphael, T. A. O'Malley, and D. A. Cross. 2021. Information sharing practices between U.S. hospitals and skilled nursing facilities to support care transitions. *JAMA Network Open* 4(1):e2033980.

AHRQ (Agency for Healthcare Research and Quality). 2018a. *Data sources for health care quality measures*. https://www.ahrq.gov/talkingquality/measures/understand/index.html (accessed January 26, 2022).

AHRQ. 2018b. *Major nursing home quality measurement sets*. https://www.ahrq.gov/talkingquality/measures/setting/long-term-care/nursing-home/measurement-sets.html (accessed January 26, 2022).

Alexander, A. G., and K. A. Ballou. 2018. Work–life balance, burnout, and the electronic health record. *American Journal of Medicine* 131(8):857–858.

Alexander, G. L. 2015. Nurse assistant communication strategies about pressure ulcers in nursing homes. *Western Journal of Nursing Research* 37(7):984–1004.

Alexander, G. L., and R. Madsen. 2018. A national report of nursing home quality and information technology: Two-year trends. *Journal of Nursing Care Quality* 33(3):200–207.

Alexander, G. L., and R. W. Madsen. 2021. A report of information technology and health deficiencies in U.S. nursing homes. *Journal of Patient Safety* 17(6):e483–e489.

Alexander, G., and N. Staggers. 2009. A systematic review of the designs of clinical technology: Findings and recommendations for future research. *Advances in Nursing Science* 32(3):252–279.

Alexander, G. L., M. Rantz, M. Flesner, M. Diekemper, and C. Siem. 2007. Clinical information systems in nursing homes: An evaluation of initial implementation strategies. *Computers Informatics Nursing* 25(4):189–197.

Alexander, G. L., M. Rantz, C. Galambos, A. Vogelsmeier, M. Flesner, L. Popejoy, J. Mueller, S. Shumate, and M. Elvin. 2015. Preparing nursing homes for the future of health information exchange. *Applied Clinical Informatics* 6(2):248–266.

Alexander, G. L., R. W. Madsen, E. L. Miller, M. K. Schaumberg, A. E. Holm, R. L. Alexander, K. K. Wise, M. L. Dougherty, and B. Gugerty. 2017a. A national report of nursing home information technology: Year 1 results. *Journal of the American Medical Informatics Association* 24(1):67–73.

Alexander, G. L., R. Madsen, and M. Newton. 2017b. Analyzing change in nursing home information technology sophistication: A 2-year survey. *Journal of Gerontological Nursing* 43(1):17–21.

Alexander, G. L., D. Madsen, E. L. Miller, D. S. Wakefield, K. Wise, and R. L. Alexander. 2017c. The state of nursing home information technology sophistication in rural and nonrural U.S. markets. *Journal of Rural Health* 33(3):266–274.

Alexander, G. L., K. Powell, C. B. Deroche, L. Popejoy, A. S. M. Mosa, R. Koopman, L. Pettit, and M. Dougherty. 2019a. Building consensus toward a national nursing home information technology maturity model. *Journal of the American Medical Informatics Association* 26(6):495–505.

Alexander, G. L., R. Madsen, C. B. Deroche, R. Alexander, and E. Miller. 2019b. Ternary trends in nursing home information technology and quality measures in the United States. *Journal of Applied Gerontology* 39(10):1134–1143.

Alexander, G. L., C. Deroche, K. Powell, A. S. M. Mosa, L. Popejoy, and R. Koopman. 2020a. Forecasting content and stage in a nursing home information technology maturity instrument using a Delphi method. *Journal of Medical Systems* 44(3):60.

Alexander, G. L., A. Georgiou, J. Siette, R. Madsen, A. Livingstone, J. Westbrook, and C. Deroche. 2020b. Exploring information technology (IT) sophistication in New South Wales residential aged care facilities. *Australian Health Review* 44(2):288–296.

Alexander, G. L., K. R. Powell, and C. B. Deroche. 2020c. An evaluation of telehealth expansion in U.S. nursing homes. *Journal of the American Medical Informatics Association* 28(2):342–348.

Alexander, G. L., C. Galambos, M. Rantz, S. Shumate, A. Vogelsmeier, L. Popejoy, and C. Crecelius. 2022. Value propositions for health information exchange toward improving nursing home hospital readmission rates. *Journal of Gerontological Nursing* 48(1):15–20.

Alonso-Martín, F., J. J. Gamboa-Montero, J. C. Castillo, Á. Castro-González, and M. Á. Salichs. 2017. Detecting and classifying human touches in a social robot through acoustic sensing and machine learning. *Sensors* 17(5):1138.

Alotaibi, Y. K., and F. Federico. 2017. The impact of health information technology on patient safety. *Saudi Medical Journal* 38(12):1173–1180.

Alper, E., T. A. O'Malley, and J. Greenwald. 2021. *Hospital discharge and readmission.* https://www.uptodate.com/contents/hospital-discharge-and-readmission (accessed January 26, 2022).

Alvarado, C. S., K. Zook, and H. JaWanna. 2017. *Electronic health record adoption and interoperability among U.S. skilled nursing facilities in 2016.* Washington DC: Office of National Coordinator.

Ancker, J. S., A. Edwards, S. Nosal, D. Hauser, E. Mauer, R. Kaushal, and the HITEC Investigators. 2017. Effects of workload, work complexity, and repeated alerts on alert fatigue in a clinical decision support system. *BMC Medical Informatics and Decision Making* 17(1):36.

Andersen, L. E., L. Tripp, J. F. Perz, N. D. Stone, A. H. Viall, S. M. Ling, and L. A. Fleisher. 2021. Protecting nursing home residents from COVID-19: Federal strike team findings and lessons learned. *NEJM Catalyst: Innovations in Care Delivery* 2(3), June 28. https://catalyst.nejm.org/doi/full/10.1056/CAT.21.0144 (accessed January 28, 2022).

Artiga, S., B. Corallo, and O. Pham. 2020. *Racial disparities in COVID-19: Key findings from available data and analysis.* https://www.kff.org/report-section/racial-disparities-in-covid-19-key-findings-from-available-data-and-analysis-issue-brief (accessed November 10, 2021).

Ashcraft, A. S., and D. C. Owen. 2017. Comparison of standardized and customized SBAR communication tools to prevent nursing home resident transfer. *Applied Nursing Research* 38:64–69.

Atreja, A., S. M. Gordon, D. A. Pollock, R. N. Olmsted, and P. J. Brennan. 2008. Opportunities and challenges in utilizing electronic health records for infection surveillance, prevention, and control. *American Journal of Infection Control* 36(3 Suppl):S37–S46.

Azad, B., and N. King. 2008. Enacting computer workaround practices within a medication dispensing system. *European Journal of Information Systems* 17(3):264–278.

Baysari, M. T., A. Tariq, R. O. Day, and J. I. Westbrook. 2017. Alert override as a habitual behavior—A new perspective on a persistent problem. *Journal of the American Medical Informatics Association* 24(2):409–412.

Bemelmans, R., G. J. Gelderblom, P. Jonker, and L. de Witte. 2012. Socially assistive robots in elderly care: A systematic review into effects and effectiveness. *Journal of the American Medical Directors Association* 13(2):114–120.e111.

Birks, M., M. Bodak, J. Barlas, J. Harwood, and M. Pether. 2016. Robotic seals as therapeutic tools in an aged care facility: A qualitative study. *Journal of Aging Research* 2016:8569602.

Bjarnadottir, R. I., C. T. A. Herzig, J. L. Travers, N. G. Castle, and P. W. Stone. 2017. Implementation of electronic health records in U.S. nursing homes. *Computers, Informatics, Nursing* 35(8):417–424.

Blijleven, V., K. Koelemeijer, M. Wetzels, and M. Jaspers. 2017. Workarounds emerging from electronic health record system usage: Consequences for patient safety, effectiveness of care, and efficiency of care. *JMIR Human Factors* 4(4):e27.

Boonstra, A., T. L. Jonker, M. A. G. van Offenbeek, and J. F. J. Vos. 2021. Persisting workarounds in electronic health record system use: Types, risks and benefits. *BMC Medical Informatics and Decision Making* 21(1):183.

Brewer, L. C., K. L. Fortuna, C. Jones, R. Walker, S. N. Hayes, C. A. Patten, and L. A. Cooper. 2020. Back to the future: Achieving health equity through health informatics and digital health. *JMIR mHealth and uHealth* 8(1):e14512.

Brownell, J., J. Wang, A. Smith, C. Stephens, and R. Y. Hsia. 2014. Trends in emergency department visits for ambulatory care sensitive conditions by elderly nursing home residents, 2001 to 2010. *JAMA Internal Medicine* 174(1):156–158.

Carayon, P., and P. Hoonakker. 2019. Human factors and usability for health information technology: Old and new challenges. *Yearbook of Medical Informatics* 28(1):71–77.

Carroll, N. W., L. R. Hearld, and R. Joseph. 2020. Hospital ownership of postacute care providers and the cost of care. *Health Care Management Review* 45(4):E35–E44.

CDC (Centers for Disease Control and Prevention). 2021a. *Electronic medical records/electronic health records (EMRs/EHRs)*. https://www.cdc.gov/nchs/fastats/electronic-medical-records.htm (accessed November 30, 2021).

CDC. 2021b. *Health equity considerations and racial and ethnic minority groups*. https://www.cdc.gov/coronavirus/2019-ncov/community/health-equity/race-ethnicity.html (accessed November 10, 2021).

CDC, National Center for Emerging and Zoonotic Infectious Diseases (NCEZID), and Division of Healthcare Quality Promotion (DHQP). 2021. *National Healthcare Safety Network (NHSN): Nursing home COVID-19 data dashboard*. https://www.cdc.gov/nhsn/covid19/ltc-report-overview.html (accessed January 26, 2022).

Chan, M., D. Estève, J. Y. Fourniols, C. Escriba, and E. Campo. 2012. Smart wearable systems: Current status and future challenges. *Artificial Intelligence in Medicine* 56(3):137–156.

Cherry, B., M. Carter, D. Owen, and C. Lockhart. 2008. Factors affecting electronic health record adoption in long-term care facilities. *Journal for Healthcare Quality* 30(2):37–47.

Cherry, B. J., E. W. Ford, and L. T. Peterson. 2011. Experiences with electronic health records: Early adopters in long-term care facilities. *Health Care Management Review* 36(3):265–274.

Classen, D., M. Li, S. Miller, and D. Ladner. 2018. An electronic health record–based real-time analytics program for patient safety surveillance and improvement. *Health Affairs* 37(11):1805–1812.

CMS (Centers for Medicare & Medicaid Services). 2020. *Long-term care nursing homes telehealth and telemedicine tool kit.* https://www.cms.gov/files/document/covid-19-nursing-home-telehealth-toolkit.pdf (accessed November 22, 2021).

CMS. 2021a. *Minimum data set (MDS) 3.0 for nursing homes and swing bed providers.* https://www.cms.gov/Medicare/Quality-Initiatives-Patient-Assessment-Instruments/NursingHomeQualityInits/NHQIMDS30 (accessed January 26, 2022).

CMS. 2021b. *The Skilled Nursing Facility Value-Based Purchasing (SNF VBP) program.* https://www.cms.gov/Medicare/Quality-Initiatives-Patient-Assessment-Instruments/Value-Based-Programs/SNF-VBP/SNF-VBP-Page (accessed January 26, 2022).

CMS. 2021c. *Policies and technology for interoperability and burden reduction.* https://www.cms.gov/Regulations-and-Guidance/Guidance/Interoperability/index (accessed January 26, 2022).

CMS. 2022. *Quality payment program overview.* https://qpp.cms.gov/about/qpp-overview (accessed February 17, 2022).

Crawford, A., and E. Serhal. 2020. Digital health equity and COVID-19: The innovation curve cannot reinforce the social gradient of health. *Journal of Medical Internet Research* 22(6):e19361.

Debono, D., and J. Braithwaite. 2015. Workarounds in nursing practice in acute care: A case of a health care arms race? In R. L. Wears, E. Hollnagel, and J. Braithwaite (eds.), *Resilient health care, vol. 2.* New York: Routledge. Pp. 23–38.

Debono, D. S., D. Greenfield, J. F. Travaglia, J. C. Long, D. Black, J. Johnson, and J. Braithwaite. 2013. Nurses' workarounds in acute healthcare settings: A scoping review. *BMC Health Services Research* 13(1):175.

Dendere, R., M. Samadbeik, and M. Janda. 2021. The impact on health outcomes of implementing electronic health records to support the care of older people in residential aged care: A scoping review. *International Journal of Medical Informatics* 151:104471.

Despins, L. A., G. Guidoboni, M. Skubic, L. Sala, M. Enayati, M. Popescu, and C. B. Deroche. 2020. Using sensor signals in the early detection of heart failure: A case study. *Journal of Gerontological Nursing* 46(7):41–46.

DiAngi, Y. T., L. A. Stevens, B. Halpern-Felsher, N. M. Pageler, and T. C. Lee. 2019. Electronic health record (EHR) training program identifies a new tool to quantify the EHR time burden and improves providers' perceived control over their workload in the EHR. *JAMIA Open* 2(2):222–230.

Dowding, D. W., M. Turley, and T. Garrido. 2012. The impact of an electronic health record on nurse sensitive patient outcomes: An interrupted time series analysis. *Journal of the American Medical Informatics Association* 19(4):615–620.

Driessen, J., A. Bonhomme, W. Chang, D. A. Nace, D. Kavalieratos, S. Perera, and S. M. Handler. 2016. Nursing home provider perceptions of telemedicine for reducing potentially avoidable hospitalizations. *Journal of the American Medical Directors Association* 17(6):519–524.

Driessen, J., N. G. Castle, and S. M. Handler. 2018a. Perceived benefits, barriers, and drivers of telemedicine from the perspective of skilled nursing facility administrative staff stakeholders. *Journal of Applied Gerontology* 37(1):110–120.

Driessen, J., W. Chang, P. Patel, R. M. Wright, K. Ernst, and S. M. Handler. 2018b. Nursing home provider perceptions of telemedicine for providing specialty consults. *Telemedicine Journal and e-Health* 24(7):510–516.

Dykes, P. C., L. Samal, M. Donahue, J. O. Greenberg, A. C. Hurley, O. Hasan, T. A. O'Malley, A. K. Venkatesh, L. A. Volk, and D. W. Bates. 2014. A patient-centered longitudinal care plan: Vision versus reality. *Journal of the American Medical Informatics Association* 21(6):1082–1090.

Edelman, L. S., E. S. McConnell, S. M. Kennerly, J. Alderden, S. D. Horn, and T. L. Yap. 2020. Mitigating the effects of a pandemic: Facilitating improved nursing home care delivery through technology. *JMIR Aging* 3(1):e20110.

Enyioha, C., S. Khairat, and C. E. Kistler. 2021. Adoption of electronic health records by practices of nursing home providers and wi-fi availability in nursing homes. *Journal of the American Medical Directors Association* 22(2):475–476.

Evans, E. L., and D. Whicher. 2018. What should oversight of clinical decision support systems look like? *AMA Journal of Ethics* 20(9):E857–E863.

Filipova, A. A. 2013. Electronic health records use and barriers and benefits to use in skilled nursing facilities. *Computers, Informatics, Nursing* 31(7):305–318.

Fossum, M., M. Ehnfors, A. Fruhling, and A. Ehrenberg. 2011. An evaluation of the usability of a computerized decision support system for nursing homes. *Applied Clinical Informatics* 2(04):420–436.

Gardner, R. L., E. Cooper, J. Haskell, D. A. Harris, S. Poplau, P. J. Kroth, and M. Linzer. 2018. Physician stress and burnout: The impact of health information technology. *Journal of the American Medical Informatics Association* 26(2):106–114.

Gerling, K., D. Hebesberger, C. Dondrup, T. Körtner, and M. Hanheide. 2016. Robot deployment in long-term care: Case study on using a mobile robot to support physiotherapy. *Zeitschrift fur Gerontologie und Geriatrie* 49(4):288–297.

Gillespie, S. M., S. M. Handler, and A. Bardakh. 2020. Innovation through regulation: COVID-19 and the evolving utility of telemedicine. *Journal of the American Medical Directors Association* 21(8):1007–1009.

Girling, R. 2021. Can care robots improve quality of life as we age? *Forbes*, January 18. https://www.forbes.com/sites/robgirling/2021/01/18/can-care-robots-improve-quality-of-life-as-we-age/ (accessed October 20, 2021).

Gliklich, R. E., N. A. Dreyer, and M. B. Leavy. 2014. AHRQ methods for effective health care. In *Registries for evaluating patient outcomes: A user's guide*. Rockville, MD: Effective Health Care Program, Agency for Healthcare Research and Quality.

Gold, M., and C. McLaughlin. 2016. Assessing HITECH implementation and lessons: 5 years later. *Milbank Quarterly* 94(3):654–687.

Gomes, M., P. Hash, L. Orsolini, A. Watkins, and A. Mazzoccoli. 2016. Connecting professional practice and technology at the bedside: Nurses' beliefs about using an electronic health record and their ability to incorporate professional and patient-centered nursing activities in patient care. *Computers, Informatics, Nursing* 34(12):578–586.

Gorges, R. J., and R. T. Konetzka. 2021. Factors associated with racial differences in deaths among nursing home residents with COVID-19 infection in the US. *JAMA Network Open* 4(2):1–10.

Grabowski, D., J. O'Malley, and N. Barhydt. 2007. The costs and potential savings associated with nursing home hospitalizations. *Health Affairs (Project Hope)* 26:1753–1761.

Grabowski, D. C., and A. J. O'Malley. 2014. Use of telemedicine can reduce hospitalizations of nursing home residents and generate savings for Medicare. *Health Affairs* 33(2):244–250.

Grönvall, E., and N. Verdezoto. 2013. Understanding challenges and opportunities of preventive blood pressure self-monitoring at home. Paper read at Proceedings of the 31st European Conference on Cognitive Ergonomics. https://dl.acm.org/doi/10.1145/2501907.2501962 (accessed November 22, 2021).

Groom, L. L., M. M. McCarthy, A. W. Stimpfel, and A. A. Brody. 2021. Telemedicine and telehealth in nursing homes: An integrative review. *Journal of the American Medical Directors Association* 22(9):1784–1801.

Henry, J., Y. Pylypchuk, and V. Patel. 2018. Electronic health record adoption and interoperability among U.S. skilled nursing facilities and home health agencies in 2017. *The Office of the National Coordinator for Health Information Technology U.S. Department of Health and Human Services*, https://www.healthit.gov/sites/default/files/page/2018-11/Electronic-Health-Record-Adoption-and-Interoperability-among-U.S.-Skilled-Nursing-Facilities-and-Home-Health-Agencies-in-2017.pdf (accessed November 10, 2021).

HHS (U.S. Department of Health and Human Services). 2022. ONC completes critical 21st Century Cures Act requirement, publishes the Trusted Exchange Framework and the Common Agreement for health information networks. https://www.hhs.gov/about/news/2022/01/18/onc-completes-critical-21st-century-cures-act-requirement-publishes-trusted-exchange-framework-common-agreement-health-information-networks.html (accessed January 26, 2022).

Holup, A. A., D. Dobbs, H. Meng, and K. Hyer. 2013. Facility characteristics associated with the use of electronic health records in residential care facilities. *Journal of the American Medical Informatics Association* 20(4):787–791.

Howe, J. L., K. T. Adams, A. Z. Hettinger, and R. M. Ratwani. 2018. Electronic health record usability issues and potential contribution to patient harm. *JAMA* 319(12):1276–1278.

Hudak, S., and S. Sharkey. 2007. *Health information technology: Are long term care providers ready?* Oakland, CA: California HealthCare Foundation.

Hughes, R. G. 2008. Chapter 44. Tools and strategies for quality improvement and patient safety. In R. Hughes (ed.), *Patient safety and quality: An evidence-based handbook for nurses*. Rockville, MD: Agency for Healthcare Research and Quality. Pp. 3-1–3-39.

Hui, E., J. Woo, M. Hjelm, Y. T. Zhang, and H. T. Tsui. 2001. Telemedicine: A pilot study in nursing home residents. *Gerontology* 47(2):82–87.

Ingber, M. J., Z. Feng, G. Khatutsky, J. M. Wang, L. E. Bercaw, N. T. Zheng, A. Vadnais, N. M. Coomer, and M. Segelman. 2017. Initiative to reduce avoidable hospitalizations among nursing facility residents shows promising results. *Health Affairs (Millwood)* 36(3):441–450.

IOM (Institute of Medicine). 1986. *Improving the quality of care in nursing homes*. Washington, DC: National Academy Press.

IOM. 1991. *Computer-based patient record: An essential technology for health care*. Washington, DC: National Academy Press.

IOM. 1996. *Telemedicine: A guide to assessing telecommunications for health care*. Washington, DC: National Academy Press.

IOM. 2000. *To err is human: Building a safer health system*. Washington, DC: National Academy Press.

IOM. 2001a. *Improving the quality of long-term care*. Washington, DC: National Academy Press.

IOM. 2001b. *Crossing the quality chasm: A new health system for the 21st century*. Washington, DC: National Academy Press.

Jen, S. P., A. Bui, and S. D. Leonard. 2021. Maximizing efficiency of telemedicine in the skilled nursing facility during the coronavirus disease 2019 pandemic. *Journal of the American Medical Directors Association* 22(6):1146–1148.e1142.

Jung, H.-Y., A. N. Trivedi, D. C. Grabowski, and V. Mor. 2016. Does more therapy in skilled nursing facilities lead to better outcomes in patients with hip fracture? *Physical Therapy* 96(1):81–89.

Kandaswamy, S., Z. Pruitt, S. Kazi, J. Marquard, S. Owens, D. J. Hoffman, R. M. Ratwani, and A. Z. Hettinger. 2021. Clinician perceptions on the use of free-text communication orders. *Applied Clinical Informatics* 12(03):484–494.

Kapoor, A., T. Field, S. Handler, K. Fisher, C. Saphirak, S. Crawford, H. Fouayzi, F. Johnson, A. Spenard, N. Zhang, and J. H. Gurwitz. 2019. Adverse events in long-term care residents transitioning from hospital back to nursing home. *JAMA Internal Medicine* 179(9):1254–1261.

Keenan, G. M., E. Yakel, D. Tschannen, and M. Mandeville. 2008. Chapter 49. Documentation and the nurse care planning process. In R. Hughes (ed.), *Patient safety and quality: An evidence-based handbook for nurses*. Rockville, MD: Agency for Healthcare Research and Quality. Pp. 3-175–3-206.

Kemp, C. L. 2020. #Morethanavisitor: Families as "essential" care partners during COVID-19. *The Gerontologist* 61(2):145–151.

King, B. J., A. L. Gilmore-Bykovskyi, R. A. Roiland, B. E. Polnaszek, B. J. Bowers, and A. J. H. Kind. 2013. The consequences of poor communication during transitions from hospital to skilled nursing facility: A qualitative study. *Journal of the American Geriatrics Society* 61(7):1095–1102.

Kistler, C. E., S. Zimmerman, and S. Khairat. 2021. Health information technology challenges and innovations in long-term care. *Journal of the American Medical Directors Association* 22(5):981–983.

Ko, M., L. Wagner, and J. Spetz. 2018. Nursing home implementation of health information technology: Review of the literature finds inadequate investment in preparation, infrastructure, and training. *Inquiry* 55:46958018778902.

Krüger, K., L. Strand, J. T. Geitung, G. E. Eide, and A. Grimsmo. 2011. Can electronic tools help improve nursing home quality? *ISRN Nursing* 2011:208142.

Kruse, C. S., M. Mileski, V. Alaytsev, E. Carol, and A. Williams. 2015. Adoption factors associated with electronic health record among long-term care facilities: A systematic review. *BMJ Open* 5(1):e006615.

Kruse, C. S., M. Mileski, A. G. Vijaykumar, S. V. Viswanathan, U. Suskandla, and Y. Chidambaram. 2017. Impact of electronic health records on long-term care facilities: Systematic review. *JMIR Medical Informatics* 5(3):e35.

Kruse, C. S., G. Marquez, D. Nelson, and O. Palomares. 2018. The use of health information exchange to augment patient handoff in long-term care: A systematic review. *Applied Clinical Informatics* 9(4):752–771.

Kukafka, R., J. S. Ancker, C. Chan, J. Chelico, S. Khan, S. Mortoti, K. Natarajan, K. Presley, and K. Stephens. 2007. Redesigning electronic health record systems to support public health. *Journal of Biomedical Informatics* 40(4):398–409.

Lamas, D., N. Panariello, N. Henrich, B. Hammes, L. C. Hanson, D. E. Meier, N. Guinn, J. Corrigan, S. Hubber, H. Luetke-Stahlman, and S. Block. 2018. Advance care planning documentation in electronic health records: Current challenges and recommendations for change. *Journal of Palliative Medicine* 21(4):522–528.

Lee, E. K., T.-L. Wu, T. Senior, and J. Jose. 2014. Medical alert management: A real-time adaptive decision support tool to reduce alert fatigue. *AMIA Symposium* 2014:845–854.

Lee, J. 2015. The impact of health information technology on disparity of process of care. *International Journal for Equity in Health* 14:34. https://doi.org/10.1186/s12939-015-0161-3.

Lee, M. L., and A. K. Dey. 2011. *Reflecting on pills and phone use: Supporting awareness of functional abilities for older adults*. Paper read at Proceedings of the SIGCHI Conference on Human Factors in Computing Systems. http://www.cs.cmu.edu/~mllee/docs/Lee2011-Reflecting_on_Pills_and_Phone_Use-CHI2011.pdf (accessed November 22, 2021).

Lemon, C., M. De Ridder, and M. Khadra. 2019. Do electronic medical records improve advance directive documentation? A systematic review. *American Journal of Hospice and Palliative Care* 36(3):255–263.

Longhurst, C. A., T. Davis, A. Maneker, H. C. Eschenroeder, Jr., R. Dunscombe, G. Reynolds, B. Clay, T. Moran, D. B. Graham, S. M. Dean, J. Adler-Milstein, and C. Arch. 2019. Local investment in training drives electronic health record user satisfaction. *Applied Clinical Informatics* 10(2):331–335.

Louie, W. G., J. Li, T. Vaquero, and G. Nejat. 2014. A focus group study on the design considerations and impressions of a socially assistive robot for long-term care. Paper read at the 23rd IEEE International Symposium on Robot and Human Interactive Communication, August 25–29, 2014.

Lundberg, C. B., J. J. Warren, J. Brokel, G. M. Bulechek, H. K. Butcher, J. M. Dochterman, M. Johnson, M. Maas, K. S. Martin, S. Moorhead, C. Spisla, E. Swanson, and S. Giarrizzo-Wilson. 2008. Selecting a standardized terminology for the electronic health record that reveals the impact of nursing on patient care. *Online Journal of Nursing Informatics* 12(2).

MACPAC (Medicaid and Children's Health Insurance Program Payment and Access Commission). 2021. Integrating clinical care through greater use of electronic health records for behavioral health. In *June 2021 report to Congress on Medicaid and CHIP*. Washington, DC: Medicaid and CHIP Payment and Access Commission.

McAllen, E. R., Jr., K. Stephens, B. Swanson-Biearman, K. Kerr, and K. Whiteman. 2018. Moving shift report to the bedside: An evidence-based quality improvement project. *Online Journal of Issues in Nursing* 23(2). https://doi.org/10.3912/OJIN.Vol23No02PPT22.

McGlynn, S., B. Snook, S. Kemple, T. L. Mitzner, and W. A. Rogers. 2014. *Therapeutic robots for older adults: Investigating the potential of paro*. Paper presented at Proceedings of the 2014 ACM/IEEE International Conference on Human-Robot Interaction, Bielefeld, Germany. https://doi.org/10.1145/2559636.2559846 (accessed November 22, 2021).

Meehan, R. 2017. Electronic health records in long-term care: Staff perspectives. *Journal of Applied Gerontology* 36(10):1175–1196.

Mor, V., O. Intrator, Z. Feng, and D. C. Grabowski. 2010. The revolving door of rehospitalization from skilled nursing facilities. *Health Affairs (Project Hope)* 29(1):57–64.

Moyle, W., C. J. Jones, J. E. Murfield, L. Thalib, E. R. A. Beattie, D. K. H. Shum, S. T. O'Dwyer, M. C. Mervin, and B. M. Draper. 2017a. Use of a robotic seal as a therapeutic tool to improve dementia symptoms: A cluster-randomized controlled trial. *Journal of the American Medical Directors Association* 18(9):766–773.

Moyle, W., U. Arnautovska, T. Ownsworth, and C. Jones. 2017b. Potential of telepresence robots to enhance social connectedness in older adults with dementia: An integrative review of feasibility. *International Psychogeriatrics* 29(12):1951–1964.

NASEM (National Academies of Sciences, Engineering, and Medicine). 2020. *Social isolation and loneliness in older adults: Opportunities for the health care system*. Washington, DC: The National Academies Press.

NASEM. 2021. *The future of nursing 2020–2030: Charting a path to achieve health equity*. Washington, DC: The National Academies Press.

NORC (NORC at the University of Chicago). 2010. *Briefing paper: Understanding the impact of health IT in underserved communities and those with health disparities*. Bethesda, MD: NORC at the University of Chicago.

Øderud, T., B. Landmark, S. Eriksen, A. B. Fossberg, S. Aketun, M. Omland, K. G. Hem, E. Østensen, and D. Ausen. 2015. Persons with dementia and their caregivers using GPS. *Studies in Health Technology and Informatics* 217:212–221.

ODPHP (Office of Disease Prevention and Health Promotion, U.S. Department of Health and Human Services). 2022. *National healthcare safety network (NHSN)*. https://health.gov/healthypeople/objectives-and-data/data-sources-and-methods/data-sources/national-healthcare-safety-network-nhsn (accessed February 17, 2022).

OIG (Office of the Inspector General). 2014. *Adverse events in skilled nursing facilities: National incidence among Medicare beneficiaries.* Washington DC: Office of the Inspector General, U.S. Department of Health and Human Services.

ONC (Office of the National Coordinator for Health Information Technology). 2017a. *Non-federal acute care hospital electronic health record adoption.* Health IT Quick-Stat #47. https://www.healthit.gov/data/quickstats/non-federal-acute-care-hospital-electronic-health-record-adoption (accessed November 30, 2021).

ONC. 2017b. *Improve care coordination.* https://www.healthit.gov/topic/health-it-and-health-information-exchange-basics/improve-care-coordination (accessed January 26, 2022).

ONC. 2019a. *What are the differences between electronic medical records, electronic health records, and personal health records?* https://www.healthit.gov/faq/what-are-differences-between-electronic-medical-records-electronic-health-records-and-personal (accessed December 1, 2021).

ONC. 2019b. *Improved diagnostics & patient outcomes.* https://www.healthit.gov/topic/health-it-and-health-information-exchange-basics/improved-diagnostics-patient-outcomes (accessed November 10, 2021).

ONC. 2019c. *Meaningful use and the shift to the merit-based incentive payment system.* https://www.healthit.gov/topic/meaningful-use-and-macra/meaningful-use (accessed October 29, 2021).

ONC. 2019d. *Health information exchange.* https://www.healthit.gov/topic/health-it-and-health-information-exchange-basics/health-information-exchange#:~:text=Read%20the%20Roadmap-,What%20is%20HIE%3F,a%20patient's%20medical%20information%20electronically (accessed February 17, 2022).

ONC. 2019e. *What is telehealth? How is telehealth different from telemedicine?* https://www.healthit.gov/faq/what-telehealth-how-telehealth-different-telemedicine (accessed November 22, 2021).

ONC. 2020. *Telemedicine and telehealth.* https://www.healthit.gov/topic/health-it-health-care-settings/telemedicine-and-telehealth (accessed November 10, 2021).

ONC. 2021a. *ONC's Cures Act final rule.* https://www.healthit.gov/curesrule (accessed October 29, 2021).

ONC. 2021b. *Health IT legislation.* https://www.healthit.gov/topic/laws-regulation-and-policy/health-it-legislation (accessed June 4, 2021).

Ong, Y. C., A. Tang, and W. Tam. 2021. Effectiveness of robot therapy in the management of behavioural and psychological symptoms for individuals with dementia: A systematic review and meta-analysis. *Journal of Psychiatric Research* 140:381–394.

Pantaleoni, J. L., L. A. Stevens, E. S. Mailes, B. A. Goad, and C. A. Longhurst. 2015. Successful physician training program for large scale EMR implementation. *Applied Clinical Informatics* 6(1):80–95.

Phillips, K., C. Wheeler, J. Campbell, and A. Coustasse. 2010. Electronic medical records in long-term care. *Journal of Hospital Marketing & Public Relations* 20(2):131–142.

Phillips, L. J., C. B. DeRoche, M. Rantz, G. L. Alexander, M. Skubic, L. Despins, C. Abbott, B. H. Harris, C. Galambos, and R. J. Koopman. 2017. Using embedded sensors in independent living to predict gait changes and falls. *Western Journal of Nursing Research* 39(1):78–94.

Philipson, A. 2021. *Robots could one day work alongside human caregivers.* https://medcitynews.com/2021/06/robots-could-one-day-work-alongside-human-caregivers (accessed October 20, 2021).

Popejoy, L., C. Galambos, and A. Vogelsmeier. 2014. Hospital to nursing home transition challenges: Perceptions of nursing home staff. *Journal of Nursing Care Quality* 29(2):103–109.

Powell, K. R., and G. L. Alexander. 2021. Consequences of rapid telehealth expansion in nursing homes: Promise and pitfalls. *Applied Clinical Informatics* 12(4):933–943.
Powell, K. R., C. B. Deroche, and G. L. Alexander. 2021. Health data sharing in U.S. nursing homes: A mixed methods study. *Journal of the American Medical Directors Association* 22(5):1052–1059.
Purtill, C. 2019. *Stop me if you've heard this one: A robot and a team of Irish scientists walk into a senior living home.* https://time.com/longform/senior-care-robot (accessed October 20, 2021).
Qi, A. C., A. A. Luke, C. Crecelius, and K. E. Joynt Maddox. 2020. Performance and penalties in year 1 of the skilled nursing facility value-based purchasing program. *Journal of the American Geriatrics Society* 68(4):826–834.
Rahman, A. N., and R. A. Applebaum. 2009. The nursing home Minimum Data Set assessment instrument: Manifest functions and unintended consequences—past, present, and future. *The Gerontologist* 49(6):727–735.
Rahman, M., E. A. Gadbois, D. A. Tyler, and V. Mor. 2018. Hospital-skilled nursing facility collaboration: A mixed-methods approach to understanding the effect of linkage strategies. *Health Services Research* 53(6):4808–4828.
Rantz, M. J., and R. P. Connolly. 2004. Measuring nursing care quality and using large data sets in non-acute care settings: State of the science. *Nursing Outlook* 52(1):23–37.
Rantz, M. J., L. Hicks, G. F. Petroski, R. W. Madsen, G. Alexander, C. Galambos, V. Conn, J. Scott-Cawiezell, M. Zwygart-Stauffacher, and L. Greenwald. 2010a. Cost, staffing and quality impact of bedside electronic medical record (EMR) in nursing homes. *Journal of the American Medical Directors Association* 11(7):485–493.
Rantz, M. J., M. Skubic, G. Alexander, M. A. Aud, B. J. Wakefield, C. Galambos, R. J. Koopman, and S. J. Miller. 2010b. Improving nurse care coordination with technology. *Computers, Informatics, Nursing* 28(6):325–332.
Rantz, M. J., G. Alexander, C. Galambos, M. K. Flesner, A. Vogelsmeier, L. Hicks, J. Scott-Cawiezell, M. Zwygart-Stauffacher, and L. Greenwald. 2011. The use of bedside electronic medical record to improve quality of care in nursing facilities: A qualitative analysis. *Computers, Informatics, Nursing* 29(3):149–156.
Rantz, M. J., M. Skubic, R. J. Koopman, G. L. Alexander, L. Phillips, K. Musterman, J. Back, M. A. Aud, C. Galambos, R. D. Guevara, and S. J. Miller. 2012. Automated technology to speed recognition of signs of illness in older adults. *Journal of Gerontological Nursing* 38(4):18–23.
Rantz, M. J., L. Popejoy, A. Vogelsmeier, C. Galambos, G. Alexander, M. Flesner, C. Crecelius, B. Ge, and G. Petroski. 2017a. Successfully reducing hospitalizations of nursing home residents: Results of the Missouri quality initiative. *Journal of the American Medical Directors Association* 18(11):960–966.
Rantz, M., L. J. Phillips, C. Galambos, K. Lane, G. L. Alexander, L. Despins, R. J. Koopman, M. Skubic, L. Hicks, S. Miller, A. Craver, B. H. Harris, and C. B. Deroche. 2017b. Randomized trial of intelligent sensor system for early illness alerts in senior housing. *Journal of the American Medical Directors Association* 18(10):860–870.
Ratwani, R. M., E. Savage, A. Will, A. Fong, D. Karavite, N. Muthu, A. J. Rivera, C. Gibson, D. Asmonga, B. Moscovitch, R. Grundmeier, and J. Rising. 2018. Identifying electronic health record usability and safety challenges in pediatric settings. *Health Affairs* 37(11):1752–1759.
Resnick, H. E., B. B. Manard, R. I. Stone, and M. Alwan. 2009. Use of electronic information systems in nursing homes: United States, 2004. *Journal of the American Medical Informatics Association* 16(2):179–186.

Rogero-Blanco, E., J. A. Lopez-Rodriguez, T. Sanz-Cuesta, M. Aza-Pascual-Salcedo, M. J. Bujalance-Zafra, I. Cura-Gonzalez, and P. A. P. G. Multi. 2020. Use of an electronic clinical decision support system in primary care to assess inappropriate polypharmacy in young seniors with multimorbidity: Observational, descriptive, cross-sectional study. *JMIR Medical Informatics* 8(3):e14130.

Ruopp, M. D. 2020. Overcoming the challenge of family separation from nursing home residents during COVID-19. *Journal of the American Medical Directors Association* 21(7):984–985.

Saiyed, S. M., P. J. Greco, G. Fernandes, and D. C. Kaelber. 2017. Optimizing drug-dose alerts using commercial software throughout an integrated health care system. *Journal of the American Medical Informatics Association* 24(6):1149–1154.

Saliba, D., and J. L. Buchanan. 2012. Making the investment count: Revision of the Minimum Data Set for nursing homes, MDS 3.0. *Journal of the American Medical Directors Association* 13(7):602–610.

Scott, A. M., J. Li, S. Oyewole-Eletu, H. Q. Nguyen, B. Gass, K. B. Hirschman, S. Mitchell, S. M. Hudson, and M. V. Williams. 2017. Understanding facilitators and barriers to care transitions: Insights from Project ACHIEVE site visits. *Joint Commission Journal on Quality and Patient Safety* 43(9):433–447.

Scott, I. A., P. I. Pillans, M. Barras, and C. Morris. 2018. Using EMR-enabled computerized decision support systems to reduce prescribing of potentially inappropriate medications: A narrative review. *Therapeutic Advances in Drug Safety* 9(9):559–573.

Seifert, A., J. A. Batsis, and A. C. Smith. 2020. Telemedicine in long-term care facilities during and beyond COVID-19: Challenges caused by the digital divide. *Frontiers in Public Health* 8:601595.

Shetty, K. D., A. A. Tolpadi, M. W. Robbins, E. A. Taylor, K. N. Campbell, and C. L. Damberg. 2020. Nursing home responses to performance-based accountability: Results of a national survey. *Journal of the American Geriatrics Society* 68(9):1979–1987.

Shiells, K., I. Holmerova, M. Steffl, and O. Stepankova. 2019. Electronic patient records as a tool to facilitate care provision in nursing homes: An integrative review. *Informatics for Health and Social Care* 44(3):262–277.

Silow-Carroll, S., J. N. Edwards, and D. Rodin. 2012. Using electronic health records to improve quality and efficiency: The experiences of leading hospitals. *Issue Brief (Commonwealth Fund)* 17:1–40.

Simard, J., and L. Volicer. 2020. Loneliness and isolation in long-term care and the COVID-19 pandemic. *Journal of the American Medical Directors Association* 21(7):966–967.

Simpao, A. F., L. M. Ahumada, B. R. Desai, C. P. Bonafide, J. A. Gálvez, M. A. Rehman, A. F. Jawad, K. L. Palma, and E. D. Shelov. 2015. Optimization of drug–drug interaction alert rules in a pediatric hospital's electronic health record system using a visual analytics dashboard. *Journal of American Medical Informatics Association* 22(2):361–369.

Skrocki, M. 2013. *Standardization needs for effective interoperability,* https://scholarworks.wmich.edu/ichita_transactions/32/ (accessed January 26, 2022).

Spinelli-Moraski, C., and K. Richards. 2013. Health information technology in nursing homes: Why and how? *Research in Gerontological Nursing* 6(3):150–151.

Staggers, N., B. L. Elias, E. Makar, and G. L. Alexander. 2018. The imperative of solving nurses' usability problems with health information technology. *Journal of Nursing Administration* 48(4):191–196.

Stanhope, V., and E. B. Matthews. 2019. Delivering person-centered care with an electronic health record. *BMC Medical Informatics and Decision Making* 19(1):168.

Su, B. Y., K. C. Ho, M. Rantz, and M. Skubic. 2018. Radar placement for fall detection: Signature and performance. *Journal of Ambient Intelligence and Smart Environments* 10:21–34.

Su, B. Y., M. Enayati, K. C. Ho, M. Skubic, L. Despins, J. Keller, M. Popescu, G. Guidoboni, and M. Rantz. 2019. Monitoring the relative blood pressure using a hydraulic bed sensor system. *IEEE Transactions on Biomedical Engineering* 66(3):740–748.

Suter, E., N. D. Oelke, C. E. Adair, and G. D. Armitage. 2009. Ten key principles for successful health systems integration. *Healthcare Quarterly (Toronto, Ont.)* 13(Spec No):16–23.

Unruh, M. A., D. C. Grabowski, A. N. Trivedi, and V. Mor. 2013a. Medicaid bed-hold policies and hospitalization of long-stay nursing home residents. *Health Services Research* 48(5):1617–1633.

Unruh, M. A., A. N. Trivedi, D. C. Grabowski, and V. Mor. 2013b. Does reducing length of stay increase rehospitalization of Medicare fee-for-service beneficiaries discharged to skilled nursing facilities? *Journal of the American Geriatrics Society* 61(9):1443–1448.

van Dyck, L. I., K. M. Wilkins, J. Ouellet, G. M. Ouellet, and M. L. Conroy. 2020. Combating heightened social isolation of nursing home elders: The Telephone Outreach in the COVID-19 Outbreak Program. *American Journal of Geriatric Psychiatry* 28(9):989–992.

Vest, J. R., H. Y. Jung, K. Wiley, Jr., H. Kooreman, L. Pettit, and M. A. Unruh. 2019. Adoption of health information technology among U.S. nursing facilities. *Journal of the American Medical Directors Association* 20(8):995–1000.e1004.

Vogelsmeier, A. 2014. Identifying medication order discrepancies during medication reconciliation: Perceptions of nursing home leaders and staff. *Journal of Nursing Management* 22(3):362–372.

Vogelsmeier, A. A., J. R. B. Halbesleben, and J. R. Scott-Cawiezell. 2008. Technology implementation and workarounds in the nursing home. *Journal of the American Medical Informatics Association* 15(1):114–119.

Vogelsmeier, A., L. Popejoy, K. Canada, C. Galambos, G. Petroski, C. Crecelius, G. L. Alexander, and M. Rantz. 2021. Results of the Missouri Quality Initiative in sustaining changes in nursing home care: Six-year trends of reducing hospitalizations of nursing home residents. *Journal of Nutrition, Health and Aging* 25(1):5–12.

Wade, V. A., J. Karnon, A. G. Elshaug, and J. E. Hiller. 2010. A systematic review of economic analyses of telehealth services using real time video communication. *BMC Health Services Research* 10(1):233.

Walker, D., A. Mora, M. M. Demosthenidy, N. Menachemi, and M. L. Diana. 2016. Meaningful use of EHRs among hospitals ineligible for incentives lags behind that of other hospitals, 2009–13. *Health Affairs* 35(3):495–501.

Wang, H. E., M. N. Shah, R. M. Allman, and M. Kilgore. 2011. Emergency department visits by nursing home residents in the United States. *Journal of the American Geriatrics Society* 59(10):1864–1872.

Wang, T., and S. Biedermann. 2012. Adoption and utilization of electronic health record systems by long-term care facilities in Texas. *Perspectives in Health Information Management* 9(Spring). https://www.ncbi.nlm.nih.gov/pmc/articles/PMC3329211 (accessed November 23, 2021)..

Whitelaw, S., M. A. Mamas, E. Topol, and H. G. C. Van Spall. 2020. Applications of digital technology in COVID-19 pandemic planning and response. *The Lancet Digital Health* 2(8):e435–e440.

Wu, N., V. Mor, and J. Roy. 2009. Resident, nursing home, and state factors affecting the reliability of minimum data set quality measures. *American Journal of Medical Quality* 24(3):229-240.

Wyatt, R., M. Laderman, L. Botwinick, K. Mate, and J. Whittington. 2016. *Achieving health equity: A guide for health care organizations*. Cambridge, MA: Institute for Healthcare Improvement.

Yu, P., D. Hailey, and H. Li. 2008. Caregivers' acceptance of electronic documentation in nursing homes. *Journal of Telemedicine and Telecare* 14(5):261-265.

Zhang, N., S. F. Lu, B. Xu, B. Wu, R. Rodriguez-Monguio, and J. Gurwitz. 2016. Health information technologies: Which nursing homes adopted them? *Journal of the American Medical Directors Association* 17(5):441–447.

Zhang, Y., P. Yu, and J. Shen. 2012. The benefits of introducing electronic health records in residential aged care facilities: A multiple case study. *International Journal of Medical Informatics* 81(10):690–704.

Zsenits, B., J. Alcantara, and R. Mayo. 2019. Impact of HIT on burnout remains unknown—for now. *Journal of the American Medical Informatics Association* 26(10):1156–1157.

10

Recommendations

The Committee on the Quality of Care in Nursing Homes was charged with examining the ways in which the United States currently delivers, finances, measures, and regulates the quality of nursing home care. After a thorough review of the evidence, the committee arrived at seven overarching conclusions.

First, **the way in which the United States finances, delivers, and regulates care in nursing home settings is ineffective, inefficient, fragmented, and unsustainable.** Despite significant measures to improve the quality of care in nursing homes in the Omnibus Budget Reconciliation Act of 1987 (OBRA 87), too few nursing home residents today receive high-quality care. Moreover, too many nursing home workers, surveyors, and others do not receive adequate and appropriate support to fulfill their critical responsibilities. Furthermore, since 1987, the acuity level, comorbidity burden, and the sophistication and complexity of care needs of nursing home residents have increased markedly, but staffing requirements and regulations have not kept pace.

Second, the committee concluded that **immediate action to initiate fundamental change is necessary.** The situation in nursing homes was dire prior to the arrival of a new and extremely contagious viral infection. The COVID-19 pandemic amplified the significant long-standing weaknesses in nursing home care. Even prior to the pandemic, the quality of care in nursing homes was neither consistently comprehensive nor of high quality. Regulations in place for 35 years have not been fully enforced, further amplifying residents' risk of harm. Those same shortcomings rendered nursing homes, their residents, and staff extremely vulnerable and unprepared to respond to the public health emergency. Heightened media attention on the disproportionate impact of the pandemic intensified demands for reform to improve the quality of care in nursing homes. Significant actions to improve nursing home care can be implemented immediately; other needed changes will take longer to be fully operational, but need to be initiated now.

Third, the committee concluded that federal and state governments, nursing homes, health care and social care providers, payers, regulators, researchers, and others need to make **clear a shared commitment to the care of nursing home residents.** Indeed, the committee recognizes that no single actor or interested party will be able to ensure high-quality nursing home care on their own. Rather, fully realizing the committee's vision will depend upon collaboration on the part of multiple public and private partners to honor this commitment to nursing home residents, their chosen families, and the staff who strive to provide the high-quality care every resident deserves.

Fourth, the committee emphasizes that extreme care needs to be taken to ensure that quality improvement initiatives are implemented using strategies that **do not exacerbate disparities in resource allocation, quality of care, or resident outcomes** (including racial and ethnic disparities), which are all too common in nursing home settings. Indeed, while the recommendations are intended to improve health equity, the committee cannot emphasize strongly enough the critical importance of close and systematic monitoring for potential unintended consequences.

Fifth, **high-quality research is needed to advance the quality of care in nursing homes.** Much of the available research relies on retrospective cohort designs and is constrained by limited available data on nursing home care. This lack of evidence presents challenges to determining the best approaches that will lead to improved quality of care in several areas.[1]

Sixth, the committee concluded that **the nursing home sector has suffered for many decades from both underinvestment in ensuring the quality of care and a lack of accountability for how resources are allocated.** Examples of inadequate investment include the following:

- Low staff salaries and benefits combined with inadequate training has made the nursing home a highly undesirable place of employment, made even worse in the pandemic.
- Inadequate support for oversight and regulatory activities has contributed to the failure of state survey agencies to meet their requirements in a timely manner.
- Quality measurement and improvement efforts have largely ignored the voice of residents and their chosen families.

---

[1] Appendix C includes tables for priority areas of measurement and research and data collection among the committee's recommendations.

- Lack of transparency regarding nursing home finances, operations, and ownership impedes the ability to fully understand how current resources are allocated.

While some reinvestment can come from increased efficiencies and improved payment policies, the committee acknowledges that the measures called for in the following recommendations will likely require significant investment of additional financial resources at the federal and state levels as well as from nursing homes themselves. However, the committee emphasizes that this investment should not be viewed as simply adding more resources to the nursing home sector as it currently operates, which would not likely result in significant improvements. Rather, the committee calls for targeted investments which, along with current funding, would be inextricably tied to requirements for transparency that are monitored through stronger and more effective oversight to ensure resources are properly allocated to improving the quality of care.

The committee recognizes that there is inherent tension when policy makers are faced with prioritizing areas of investment that require public funding. However, in order to achieve the committee's vision of comprehensive high-quality care for all nursing home residents, the investment of new federal and state resources, as well as investment of resources from nursing homes themselves, will likely be needed. The committee also recognizes that key partners, such as the Centers for Medicare & Medicaid Services (CMS) and other federal agencies, may not currently have the full authority or resources to carry out the actions recommended. Therefore, as a final overarching conclusion, the committee notes that **all relevant federal agencies need to be granted the authority and resources from the United States Congress to implement the recommendations of this report.** Furthermore, as also noted earlier, the committee realizes that many of its recommendations will require key partners to work together among federal agencies and states as well as across sectors to implement these recommendations. This coordination of efforts will require regular communication to avoid duplication of efforts and to identify gaps in responses to pressing shortcomings in nursing home care.

COMMITTEE VISION AND GUIDING PRINCIPLES

As a framework for this study, the committee created an original conceptual model of high-quality care in nursing homes (see Chapter 1). The model depicts a vision of nursing home quality in which *residents of nursing homes receive care in a safe environment that honors their values and preferences, addresses the goals of care, promotes equity, and assesses the benefits and risks of care and treatments.*

In addition to this vision, the committee developed guiding principles for high-quality nursing home care that served to form the foundation for their recommendations (see Box 10-1).

While the committee's vision identifies what high-quality nursing home care should look like, the guiding principles serve as a reminder of the very salient fact that existing regulations *require* nursing homes to provide comprehensive, person-centered care that is holistic and responds to a resident's (and their chosen family's) care needs, goals, and preferences. However, calling attention to the reality that person-centered care is not the standard of care in nursing homes today is critically important. CMS

BOX 10-1
Committee Vision and Guiding Principles for High-Quality Nursing Home Care

COMMITTEE VISION:

Nursing home residents receive care in a safe environment that honors their values and preferences, addresses the goals of care, promotes equity, and assesses the benefits and risks of care and treatments.

GUIDING PRINCIPLES:

To achieve this vision, nursing homes should deliver comprehensive, person-centered, interdisciplinary team-based care that meets or exceeds established quality standards and supports strong connections to health care and social service systems and resources, family, friends, and the community more broadly.

High-quality nursing home care provides an environment that promotes quality of life; aligns with residents' medical, behavioral, and social care needs; reflects residents' values and preferences; promotes autonomy; and manages risks to ensure residents' safety. Such comprehensive, high-quality care includes the following, as appropriate:

- Physical health care
- Behavioral health care
- Psychosocial care
- Oral health care
- Hearing and vision care
- Rehabilitative care
- Dementia care
- Palliative care
- End-of-life care

Furthermore, it is the right of every nursing home resident to have equitable access to high-quality, comprehensive, person-centered, and culturally sensitive nursing home care.

emphasized the importance of this care in its 2016 revision of nursing home regulations, specifying that person-centered care means *to focus on the resident as the locus of control and support the resident in making their own choices and having control over their daily lives.*[2] The regulations also require nursing homes to include resident preferences in the care plan. Existing regulatory requirements have not been fully or consistently met, however, with the result that high-quality, comprehensive, person-centered care is not being provided to all nursing home residents in the United States.

OVERARCHING GOALS AND RECOMMENDATIONS

The committee's goals (with associated recommendations)[3] that follow represent an integrated approach for achieving its vision of high-quality nursing home care. The committee's recommendations fall under seven critical goals:

1. Deliver **comprehensive, person-centered, equitable care** that ensures residents' health, quality of life, and safety; promotes autonomy; and manages risks.
2. Ensure a well-prepared, empowered, and appropriately compensated **workforce**.
3. Increase the **transparency and accountability** of finances, operations, and ownership.
4. Create a more rational and robust **financing system**.
5. Design a more effective and responsive system of **quality assurance**.
6. Expand and enhance **quality measurement and continuous quality improvement**.
7. Adopt **health information technology** in all nursing homes.

Consistent with the broad charge of the committee, the committee's approach to improving the quality of care in nursing homes identifies opportunities for change in a broad range of areas encompassing care delivery—from changes to the physical environment and strengthening emergency preparedness to enhancing the workforce; strengthening the payment, financing, and regulatory policy environments; improving quality measurement; and ensuring the adoption of an effective health information technology (HIT) infrastructure to support all the committee's recommendations.

---

[2] CMS Requirements for Long-Term Care Facilities—Definitions, 42 CFR § 483.5 (2022).
[3] Appendix D includes a table of recommendations organized by the key partners responsible for implementation.

Improving the quality of care in nursing homes is not only possible but also represents a critical societal and public health imperative. Achieving each of the committee's goals will entail significant revisions to how care is delivered, financed, and regulated and how its quality is measured and improved, which requires a broad-based commitment to change from owners and administrators, staff, health care providers and organizations, researchers, and policy makers. Leveraging the expertise, leadership, and influence of this broader community will advance necessary changes.

Though the recommendations focus on diverse areas for improvement, they are interlinked by an underlying premise: the challenges facing nursing homes are complex and multifaceted and require urgent attention on multiple fronts by many participants in the system. Some recommendations are intentionally broad, allowing flexibility in how they are implemented, while others are more targeted, with more specific details on how to achieve the objectives. Some can be implemented in the near term, while others will require a longer time line; some should be relatively straightforward to achieve, while others are more aspirational and will require coordinated efforts to create significant long-term changes. The committee's recommendations should be viewed and implemented as an interrelated package of reform measures. (See Appendix E for the committee's estimated implementation time line.)

Overview of Recommendations

Nursing home residents and their families are at the heart of the committee's conceptual model, and all recommended actions are designed to improve the quality of care and quality of life for those who live in nursing homes. The committee's first goal (and first recommendation) affirms person-centered care by focusing on the identification of resident preferences and the use of the care plan. Person-centered care is enabled through the development and implementation of an accurate and effective care plan that reflects the individualized needs, preferences, and goals of care of each nursing home resident.

The committee recognizes that this first recommendation, which underscores the vital role of the care plan, may not be innovative; it is already required by federal law. However, the committee intentionally and strategically placed the goal of delivering comprehensive person-centered care first to serve as the foundation that subsequent recommendations build upon. This primary focus on person-centered care is critical to the provision of high-quality care in nursing homes and bears emphasis and reinforcement because, all too often, such care is not being provided to nursing home residents. The committee's foundational goal also calls for improvements to the physical environment of nursing homes and supports the goal of establishing smaller, less institutionalized nursing homes. Given the impact of the pandemic, the committee also calls for strengthening the preparation of nursing homes for public health emergencies.

The recommendations gradually build upon the solid foundation of Goal 1. The next set of recommendations focuses on the workforce that supports and cares for residents and the myriad staffing-related factors in urgent need of attention, such as compensation, education and training, and staffing patterns (Goal 2). This is followed by a focus on increasing the transparency and accountability of finances, operations, and ownership (Goal 3). From there, the recommendations' focus continues to broaden, moving to the development of a more rational and robust system of financing nursing home care, including the committee's call for the study of a federal long-term care benefit and targeted measures to strengthen the link between payment and the quality of care (Goal 4). Underscoring the importance of linking funding to transparency and accountability, the committee calls for enhanced measures to ensure an effective and responsive system of quality assurance through strengthened oversight and regulation of nursing homes (Goal 5). Expanding and enhancing quality measurement and quality improvement across all aspects of care provision (Goal 6), and including the voices of nursing home residents and their chosen families in these efforts, will be a critical component of strengthening quality assurance. HIT plays a key role in implementing all the committee's recommended actions, from improving care planning and quality measurement and assessment, to supporting the delivery of high-quality care and enabling the secure sharing of resident information between nursing homes and hospitals and other health care settings (Goal 7). Finally, the committee emphasizes the vital importance of attention to health equity and measures to reduce inequities in nursing home care, which is woven throughout its recommendations.

GOAL 1: DELIVER COMPREHENSIVE, PERSON-CENTERED, EQUITABLE CARE THAT ENSURES RESIDENTS' HEALTH, QUALITY OF LIFE, AND SAFETY; PROMOTES AUTONOMY; AND MANAGES RISKS

While person-centered care is foundational to the basic requirements of federal law and regulations of nursing home care, such care is not yet a reality for many nursing home residents. Significant gaps and shortcomings exist in the quality of services such as behavioral health and psychosocial care as well as in vision, hearing, and oral health care and end-of-life care. Moreover, significant disparities in the quality of care exist across nursing homes.

Care Planning

In considering the most effective approaches to fully realizing person-centered, comprehensive, high-quality and equitable care in practice in the nursing home setting, the committee recognized the central role of the resident care planning process. The resident care planning process provides a very firm foundation for operationalizing person-centered, high-quality, equitable care in nursing homes. The care plan process encompasses four critical components: creating the plan, reviewing the plan, implementing and subsequently evaluating the effectiveness of the plan, and revisiting and reviewing the care plan on a regular basis. Ideally, all of the components of the process will be implemented effectively in every nursing home. The committee recognizes that despite the critical role of the care planning process, this ideal has yet to become a reality in all nursing homes.

The first step in the process is the development of the care plan through the use of the Minimum Data Set Resident Assessment Instrument (RAI) and a shared decision-making process with residents and their chosen families to explore and identify resident care needs and preferences. These needs and preferences are then documented in the written care plan, which serves as a critical road map for care targeted to the specific goals of the individual resident: the essence of person-centered care.

Second, the care plan needs to incorporate the broad range of each resident's care needs, from physical and behavioral health to activities of daily living and preferences (e.g., attending a religious service, favorite television shows, trips to the hairdresser). To ensure that the care plan is accurate and comprehensive, members of the interdisciplinary care team need to be directly involved in reviewing and evaluating all aspects of the care plan, working together with residents and their family members. Nursing home requirements updated by CMS in 2016 specify the members of the interdisciplinary care team (detailed in Box 4-2, Chapter 4). Given the critical importance of the review and evaluation of the care plan, the committee emphasizes that this step should be overseen by nursing staff at least at the level of the registered nurse (RN).

Third, once the plan is reviewed by the interdisciplinary care team and deemed to be accurate and complete, the plan needs to be implemented. Each element of the care plan needs to include specific measures for assessing the progress of implementation and whether desired results are being achieved (degree and timing).

Fourth, in recognition of the changing nature of resident needs and preferences and of physical and mental health conditions, the care plan is to be reviewed on a regular basis. This review should take place quarterly or at the request of a resident or family member, or when there is a significant change in resident's status (as specified in the RAI manual) to ensure that the plan continues to align with resident and family preferences over time.

Recognizing the central role of the care plan as a means to achieve person-centered comprehensive, high-quality, equitable care, and fully cognizant of the fact that many of the actions recommended below are already required by federal law, the committee recommends the following:

RECOMMENDATION 1A: As a critical foundation to operationalizing person-centered care that reflects resident goals and preferences, the committee recommends compliance with regulations for person-centered care. Nursing homes,[4] with oversight by CMS, should

- Identify the care preferences of residents and their chosen families using structured, shared decision-making approaches that balance resident preferences for safety and autonomy.
- Ensure that resident care preferences are accurately documented in the care plan.
  - Interdisciplinary care team members should make certain that every resident's care plan addresses psychosocial and behavioral health as well as nursing and medical needs.
  - To certify that all aspects of the resident's care needs are fully addressed in the care plan, the interdisciplinary care team should review and evaluate the care plan to ensure it is complete, with oversight of the review and evaluation process provided by nursing staff at least at the level of the RN.
  - A complete plan should include evaluation steps (i.e., specific measures and timing of measurement) to assess the degree of implementation and success of each element.
- Implement and monitor each element of every resident's care plan and evidence of effective implementation to ensure that the care delivered continues to align with the resident's preferences.
  - Nursing home staff should revisit the care plan on a regular basis for all residents—at a minimum on a quarterly basis, when requested by the family/resident, or when there has been a significant change in condition as specified in the Long-Term Care Facility Resident Assessment Instrument 3.0 Users' Manual.

---

[4] While the committee calls on nursing homes to implement many of its recommendations, it recognizes that it is the individual nursing home owners, administrators, and clinical leaders who need to be held accountable for the quality of care provided within their specific organizations. The active role of these individuals is necessary to ensure the committee's recommendations are put into place.

Models of Care

Nursing homes are required by law to provide an array of services to both short-stay and long-stay residents of all ages with a wide range of medical and behavioral health conditions. Yet despite the complexity of the care challenges faced by nursing homes, research on best practices related to clinical, behavioral, and psychosocial care delivery in nursing homes is scarce. As a result, a robust evidence base has not yet been developed for specific models of care delivery that could serve as the most effective approach to providing high-quality person-centered care to all nursing home residents while ensuring equitable care. Given these critical knowledge gaps, the committee calls out federal agencies as well as private foundations, academic institutions, and others to prioritize and fund research on effective care delivery models.

Moreover, nursing homes are often not well connected to the communities in which they are located, nor to the broader health care system. Research that examines models of care that strengthen ties to the broader community, including universities and all sectors of the health care system, is needed to improve these connections. Finally, research on care delivery needs to focus on the specific factors that affect care directly, such as optimal staffing, physical environment, financing and payment, the use of technology, leadership models, and organizational policy. Once research has successfully identified the most effective care models, this research should be translated into practice by launching demonstration projects to test specific models in nursing home settings. The projects should be designed with an eye toward sustainability. Therefore, the committee recommends the following

RECOMMENDATION 1B: The federal government (e.g., the Agency for Healthcare Research and Quality [AHRQ], CMS, the Center for Medicare and Medicaid Innovation, the Centers for Disease Control and Prevention, and the National Institutes of Health [NIH]), private foundations, academic institutions, and long-term care provider organizations should prioritize and fund rigorous, translational research and demonstration projects to identify the most effective care delivery models to provide high-quality comprehensive, person-centered care for short-stay and long-stay nursing home residents.

- This research should focus on identifying care delivery models that reduce care disparities and strengthen connections among the nursing homes, the communities in which they are located, and the broader health care and social services sectors.
- Research on care delivery models should evaluate innovations in all aspects of care, including optimal staffing, physical environment, financing and payment, the use of technology, leadership models, and organizational policy.

Emergency Preparedness and Response

The COVID-19 pandemic shone a light on the extremely harsh lack of preparedness on the part of nursing homes for a large-scale public health emergency. Prior to the COVID-19 pandemic, there were numerous examples of nursing homes being unprepared to respond to a range of emergencies and natural disasters, such as hurricanes, tornadoes, earthquakes, floods, and wildfires. In order for nursing homes to have the capability to plan and prepare for and respond to all types of emergencies, they need to be included as integral partners in emergency management planning, preparedness, and response on the national, state, and local levels. Moreover, nursing homes need not only to be prepared to provide for the physical safety of residents but also to address their behavioral and psychosocial needs during emergencies. As demonstrated by the prohibition against friend and family member visitation during the COVID-19 pandemic and the resultant harm of social isolation, it is imperative to strike a careful balance between residents' safety and their mental and behavioral health needs. Therefore, the committee recommends the following:

RECOMMENDATION 1C: In order to safeguard nursing home residents and staff against a broad range of potential emergencies, the Department of Homeland Security should direct the Federal Emergency Management Agency to reinforce and clarify the emergency support functions (ESFs) of the National Response Framework. Specifically,

- ESF 8 (Public Health and Medical Services) should be revised to give greater prominence to nursing homes with the goal of clarifying that nursing homes specifically, and long-term care facilities more broadly, are included within ESF 8 (Public Health and Medical Services) to ensure that state and local emergency management documents and plans contain specific guidance for nursing homes during an emergency.
- ESF 15 (External Affairs Annex) should be revised to specifically include residents of nursing homes as part of the target group of "individuals with disabilities and others with access and functional needs."

Local, county, and state-level public health agencies need to ensure that nursing homes "have a seat at the table." This can be accomplished through the development of formal relationships and by ensuring reliable lines of communication. In addition, nursing homes are not always included in all phases of emergency management, such as drills and exercises. Finally, while nursing homes are currently required to have written emergency plans created in partnership with local emergency management, to review and update the plan on a regular basis, and to provide staff training in critical aspects of emergency planning, these requirements are not always in place or enforced. Therefore, the committee recommends the following:

RECOMMENDATION 1D: To ensure the physical safety as well as address behavioral health/psychosocial needs of nursing home residents and staff in public health emergencies and natural disasters,

- State regulatory agencies (with federal oversight from the Federal Emergency Management Agency and CMS) should ensure the development and ongoing maintenance of formal relationships, including strong interface, coordination, and reliable lines of communication, between nursing homes and local, county, and state-level public health and emergency management departments.
- State emergency management agencies should make certain that nursing homes are represented in
  - state, county, and local emergency planning sessions and drills;
  - local government community disaster response plans; and
  - every phase of the local emergency management planning including mitigation, preparedness, response and recovery.
- State emergency management agencies should ensure that every nursing home has ready access to personal protective equipment (PPE).
- CMS (through state regulatory agencies) is to ensure that *existing* regulations are enforced, including the following:
  - Nursing home leadership ensures that there is a written emergency plan (including evacuation plans) for common public health emergencies and natural disasters in the facility's location, which is created in partnership with local emergency management and resident and family councils.
  - Nursing home leadership reviews and updates the plan at least once every year.
    - Nursing home staff are to be routinely trained in emergency response procedures and periodically review procedures.
    - Nursing home staff are to be routinely trained in the appropriate use of PPE and infection control practices.
  - Nursing home leadership ensures that there is an emergency preparedness communication plan that includes formal procedures for contacting residents' families and staff to provide information about the general condition and location of residents in the case of an emergency or disaster.

- Documentation concerning emergency plans as well as of the conduct of emergency drills and staff awareness of emergency management plans should be added to Care Compare.

The committee emphasizes that CMS needs to ensure that staff receive training in critical aspects of emergency planning upon being hired (e.g., during staff orientation) and need to receive periodic training to refresh and update their skills and knowledge.

Physical Environment

It is critical to recognize that nursing homes serve dual roles: care settings as well as places in which people reside. All aspects of the nursing home's physical environment are critical to a resident's quality of life, yet most nursing homes resemble institutions more than homes. The nursing home infrastructure is aging, with the majority of nursing homes at least 30 years old and many of them 50 years or older, and therefore, the homes may not reflect the needs and preferences of today's older adults for smaller, home-like units. Smaller, home-like environments (including single-occupancy bedrooms and private bathrooms) provide important benefits for residents and staff and play key roles in infection control as well as an enhanced quality of life for residents. The committee recognizes that these changes will require significant investment, and concluded that design changes can be operationalized through federal incentives and state licensure decisions. Therefore, the committee recommends the following

RECOMMENDATION 1E: Nursing home owners, with the support of federal and state governmental agencies, should construct and reconfigure (renovate) nursing homes to provide smaller, more home-like environments and/or smaller units within larger nursing homes that promote infection control and person-centered care and activities.

- The design of these nursing homes should include consideration for the following characteristics: unit size, activity and dining space by unit, a readily accessible therapeutic outdoor area, an open kitchen, a staff work area, and entrances and exits.
  - Smaller units should be designed to have the flexibility to address a range of resident care and rehabilitation needs.
  - New designs should prioritize private bedrooms and bathrooms.
  - This shift to more home-like settings should be implemented as part of a broader effort to integrate the principles of culture change, such as staff empowerment, consistent staff assignment, and person-centered care practices, into the management and care provided within these settings.

- CMS, the U.S. Department of Housing and Urban Development, and other governmental agencies should develop incentives to support designs for nursing home environments (both new construction and renovations).
- State licensure decisions should ensure that all new nursing homes are constructed with single-occupancy bedrooms and private bathrooms for most or all residents.

GOAL 2: ENSURE A WELL-PREPARED, EMPOWERED, AND APPROPRIATELY COMPENSATED WORKFORCE

In 2008, the Institute of Medicine (IOM) report *Retooling for an Aging America* noted that while the need for health care professionals trained in geriatric principles was escalating, few providers choose this career path due to a variety of factors, including inadequate education and training, negative stereotypes of older adults, and significant financial disincentives to working in geriatrics. The report further noted that these issues may be especially significant for long-term care settings. The culture within nursing homes, as well as how the public views both aging in general and nursing homes specifically, will need to change because high-quality care cannot be delivered without a complete transformation of worker training and social stature. These changes to the culture of nursing homes need to be driven by nursing home leaders to ensure a robust, high-quality workforce. The following recommendations provide a variety of ways to ensure that the nursing home workforce is respected, well prepared, empowered, and appropriately compensated.

The committee recommends increasing both the numbers and the qualifications of virtually all types of nursing home workers, along with providing the necessary incentives and supports to achieve these changes. The committee recognizes that increasing requirements can exacerbate the challenges of recruiting nursing home workers. This is particularly concerning given the current dire staffing situations for many nursing homes, largely due to the impact of the COVID-19 pandemic. The committee concluded, however, that robust evidence demonstrates the positive impact of enhanced requirements on the quality of care. Moreover, enhanced requirements will further professionalize the nursing home workforce, which, when accompanied by improvements in the working environment, will contribute to the desirability of working in a nursing home.

Compensation

Nursing home workers earn significantly less in nursing homes than if they chose to work in other care settings. For example, according to

2020 data from the Bureau of Labor Statistics, the annual mean wage for RNs in nursing homes is approximately $10,000 less (more than 10 percent less) than RNs in acute-care hospitals and $17,000 less (nearly 20 percent less) than RNs employed in outpatient care settings. In particular, certified nursing assistants (CNAs) typically earn low wages and have few benefits; as a result, many live in poverty or require public assistance. The 2020 mean hourly wage for CNAs in nursing homes was $15.41 and the mean annual wage was $32,050. CNAs may earn little more than workers in other comparable entry-level jobs (such as cashier, food service worker, warehouse worker, and retail sales worker), who may have lower levels of risks for injury and may even receive full benefits.

The committee concluded that the successful recruitment and retention of a high-quality nursing home workforce depends on providing more than "adequate" compensation for their work. Rather, competitive compensation is needed (comparable to other health care settings and job opportunities) for their current and expanding roles in conjunction with the many different types of efforts that will be needed to improve the desirability of these jobs. A variety of mechanisms have been tried to increase workers' compensation and benefits, and different mechanisms may be needed to achieve competitive compensation. Therefore, the committee recommends the following:

RECOMMENDATION 2A: Federal and state governments, together with nursing homes, should ensure competitive wages and benefits (including health insurance, child care, and sick pay) to recruit and retain all types of full- and part-time nursing home staff. Mechanisms that should be considered include wage floors, requirements for having a minimum percentage of service rates directed to labor costs for the provision of clinical care, wage pass-through requirements, and student loan forgiveness.

The committee recognizes that the provision of benefits may encourage some nursing homes to reduce staffing levels or hire part-time rather than full-time staff. The committee emphasizes that nursing homes need to offer full-time, consistently assigned work whenever it is possible and desired by the worker in order to ensure high-quality care.

Staffing Standards and Expertise

Minimum staffing standards in nursing homes, particularly for licensed nursing staff, have been evaluated for decades. In 2001, CMS studied the minimum appropriate staffing levels, using modeling to identify a staffing threshold below which residents are at risk for serious quality-of-care issues. However, to date the proposed CMS minimum staffing standards have not been addressed in any subsequent regulatory rules, leaving stand a vague nurse staffing requirement that nursing homes must provide ". . . sufficient nursing staff to attain or maintain the highest practicable . . . well-being of each resident." Substantial evidence demonstrates the relationship between nurse staffing and quality of care in nursing homes, particularly for RNs. The 1996 IOM report *Nursing Staff in Hospitals and Nursing Homes* recommended a requirement for 24-hour RN coverage in nursing homes by the year 2000. The recommendation was endorsed by a subsequent IOM study in 2001, and then recommended again in the 2004 IOM report *Keeping Patients Safe*. Yet today the federal requirement is a 24-hour daily presence of licensed nurse coverage with an RN fulfilling only 8 of those hours.

Furthermore, CMS has not established minimum staffing requirements for certain key members of the interdisciplinary nursing home care team. Social workers, for example, contribute to resident care and take on various complex and clinically challenging responsibilities. Social work interventions in nursing homes have been associated with significant improvements in residents' quality of life, yet current federal regulations require only those nursing homes with 120 or more beds to hire a "qualified social worker on a full-time basis." Moreover, the "qualified social worker" is not required to hold a degree in social work, despite research showing that having social service staff members in nursing homes with higher qualifications is associated with better psychosocial care, improved behavioral symptoms, and reduced use of antipsychotic medications.

Additionally, as part of CMS's 2016 final rule, nursing homes are required to designate at least one part-time or full-time staff member as the infection prevention and control specialist. The final rule suggested that an RN would assume the role of the infection prevention and control specialist in most facilities and that the individual would need to devote approximately 15 percent of his or her time to this role. The CMS Coronavirus Commission on Safety and Quality in Nursing Homes noted, however, that the current regulations yielded an "insufficient response to the demands" of COVID-19.

The committee concluded that current minimum staffing requirements are insufficient as they relate to RN coverage, social worker presence, and infection and prevention control. Therefore, the committee recommends immediate implementation of the following minimum staffing requirements:

RECOMMENDATION 2B: CMS should enhance the current minimum staffing requirements for every nursing home to include

- Onsite direct-care RN coverage (in addition to the director of nursing) at a minimum of a 24-hour, 7-days-per-week basis with additional RN coverage that reflects resident census, acuity, case mix, and the professional nursing needs for residents as determined by the residents' assessments and care plans;

- A full-time social worker with a minimum of bachelor's degree in social work from a program accredited by the Council on Social Work Education and 1 year of supervised social work experience in a health care setting (including field placements and internships) working directly with individuals to address behavioral and psychosocial care; and
- An infection prevention and control specialist who is an RN, advanced practice RN, or a physician at a level of dedicated time sufficient to meet the needs of the size and case mix of the nursing home.

Increasing RN staffing and overall nurse staffing in nursing homes has been a consistent recommendation for improving the quality of care in nursing homes. However, the same federal staffing regulations have been in place for over 30 years, even though the types of residents and the complexity of their needs have changed dramatically. Federal staffing requirements do not specify adjustments based on the size of the nursing home or resident acuity. The committee concluded that the current minimum staffing standards likely do not reflect the needs of the current population of nursing home residents and that more research is needed on both the minimum and optimal staffing standards to meet the needs of today's nursing home population. Such information is needed for all types of nurses, including advanced practice RNs (APRNs), RNs, licensed practical/vocational nurses (LPNs/LVNs), and CNAs as well as other staff who support the health and well-being of nursing home residents. Therefore, the committee recommends the following:

RECOMMENDATION 2C: The U.S. Department of Health and Human Services (HHS) (e.g., CMS, AHRQ, and NIH) should fund research to identify and rigorously test specific minimum and optimum staffing standards for direct-care staff (e.g., APRNs, RNs, LPN/LVNs, CNAs, therapists, recreational staff, social workers, and other direct-care providers), including weekend and holiday staffing, based on resident case mix and the type of staff needed to address the care needs of specific populations. Based on the results of this research, CMS and state governments should update the regulatory requirements for staffing standards in nursing homes to reflect new minimum requirements and account for case mix.

While nursing homes may meet minimum staffing standards, additional expertise is often needed to provide comprehensive, person-centered care. Such additional expertise is especially needed for the development of complex clinical care plans, staff training, and overall planning for care systems and quality improvement. Not every facility will have the ability or need to keep such expertise on staff. The committee concluded that nursing homes need to develop ongoing relationships with a variety of professionals who can provide consultation on an as-needed basis. Access to this level of expertise is also limited by barriers to direct billing and reimbursement for these professional services. Therefore, the committee recommends the following:

RECOMMENDATION 2D: To enhance the available expertise within a nursing home,

- Nursing home administrators, in consultation with their clinical staff, should establish consulting or employment relationships with qualified licensed clinical social workers at the M.S.W. or Ph.D. level, APRNs, clinical psychologists, psychiatrists, pharmacists, and others for clinical consultation, staff training, and the improvement of care systems, as needed.
- CMS should create incentives for nursing homes to hire qualified licensed clinical social workers at the M.S.W. or Ph.D. level as well as APRNs for clinical care, including allowing Medicare billing and reimbursement for these services.

The committee notes that many other types of experts may be needed, depending upon the acuity and case mix of the nursing home residents and the availability of such expertise among the nursing home's own staff, including professionals such as dentists, audiologists, physical and occupational therapists, and many others. Furthermore, the committee recognizes that allowing direct billing for certain services would require an expansion of the Medicare program, as was called for in the 2011 IOM report *The Future of Nursing*.

CNA Empowerment

Direct-care workers (primarily CNAs) provide the majority of hands-on care to nursing home residents. Such care includes everyday tasks such as assistance with eating, bathing, toileting, and dressing as well as more advanced tasks such as infection control and care of cognitively impaired residents. Tailoring these tasks to residents' preferred schedules and needs is critical to meeting residents' goals and maintaining their function, well-being, and quality of life. The demand for CNAs is increasing, yet nursing homes have persistent challenges in recruiting and retaining workers. The top reasons for direct-care workers leaving their jobs include a lack of respect and appreciation by leadership, inadequate salary and benefits, a lack of teamwork and communication among the staff, and poor relationships with supervisors, residents, and families. CNAs may be undervalued or not respected by other nursing home staff or leadership, and their responsibilities put them at high risk for injury. Furthermore, CNAs often have little opportunity for advancement. Because of the crucial role of this position in nursing homes, the committee concluded that significantly improving the quality of care for nursing home residents requires investing in quality jobs for direct-care workers and enabling more workers to enter the CNA pipeline. Therefore, in addition to the recommendation for ensuring competitive wages and benefits (Recommendation 2A), the committee recommends the following:

RECOMMENDATION 2E: To advance the role of and empower the CNA,

- Nursing homes should provide career advancement opportunities and peer mentoring;
- Federal and state governments, together with nursing homes, should enable free entry-level training and continuing education (e.g., in community colleges);
- Nursing homes should cover CNAs' time for completing education and training programs; and
- The Health Resources and Services Administration should fund training grants to advance and expand the role of the CNA and develop new models of care delivery that take advantage of the role of the CNA as a member of the interdisciplinary care team.

Education and Training

In addition to improving wages and strengthening staffing standards, the education and training of the entire nursing home workforce is key to improving the quality of care in nursing homes. Education and training requirements for a variety of nursing home staff are inadequate or nonexistent. For example, the requirements for licensure as a nursing home administrator vary by state, and about one-third of states do not even require a bachelor's degree to be a nursing home administrator. Medical directors need to have a license to practice medicine in the state, but there are no additional specific education and training or certification requirements at the national level. The director of nursing is required to be an RN (although there are waivers to this requirement), and the competencies needed by directors of nursing often exceed the preparation provided in either associate degree or baccalaureate degree nursing programs. Both the medical director and the director of nursing have key roles in infection prevention and control, yet they may not receive specific training in these skills. The director of social services oversees all social service programs and supervises social workers and social service designees within the facility, yet there typically are no formal requirements for the role. Finally, CNAs are often inadequately prepared and trained for their expanding role. The 2008

IOM report *Retooling for an Aging America* recommended increasing the federal training requirement for direct care workers (including CNAs) to 120 hours, based on the significant number of states that require training beyond the federal minimum. While some states have increased their requirements since then, the federal minimum has remained unchanged. The training standards and curricula for direct-care workers are dated and focus on basic tasks rather than on competencies to meet the needs of today's nursing home residents.

The committee concluded that the minimum education and competency requirements need to be enhanced (or established) for a variety of nursing home workers and to be made standard at the national level. The committee recognizes that many current nursing home workers may not meet these new requirements and may need assistance in achieving these standards. Additionally, the committee recognizes that increasing the education and training requirements of these personnel can exacerbate the challenges of recruiting nursing home workers. However, as noted earlier, the committee concluded that robust evidence supports these enhanced requirements because of their impact on the quality of care. Finally, the committee recognizes that a key issue underlying the preparation of all types of workers for nursing home care is the inadequate foundation for a variety of geriatrics-related topics in their education and training programs. Therefore, the committee recommends the following:

RECOMMENDATION 2F: CMS should establish minimum education and national competency requirements for nursing home staff, to include

- Nursing home administrator: minimum of a bachelor's degree and training in topics relevant to their role (e.g., culture change, leadership and team-building, administration, and financial management);
- Medical director: completion of education or certification program specific to the care of older adults and certification in infection control and prevention;
- Director of nursing: minimum of a bachelor's degree in nursing, with a preference for master's level training; training in geriatrics and long-term care; and certification in infection control and prevention;
- Director of social services: minimum of a bachelor's degree in social work from a program accredited by the Council on Social Work Education (CSWE), with a preference for master's level training from a program accredited by CSWE; and
- Certified nursing assistants: an increase in the federal minimum of training hours to become a certified nursing assistant from 75 hours to 120 hours and training content that includes competency-based training requirements.

RECOMMENDATIONS

CMS and nursing homes should give special consideration for current staff members who do not meet these enhanced requirements and provide flexible, low-cost, and high-quality pathways to achieve these baseline education and competency levels.

Furthermore, to prepare future workers for their roles, all education programs preparing health care professionals should include content related to gerontology, geriatric assessment, long-term care, and palliative care, with an additional preference for clinical experience in a nursing home.

Regarding the recommendation for competency-based training for certified nursing assistants, the committee notes that specific instruction is needed for conditions and topics relevant to nursing home populations (beyond basic care) such as dementia; infection prevention and control; behavioral health; chronic diseases such as diabetes, heart failure, and chronic obstructive pulmonary disease; the use of assistive and medical devices; and cultural sensitivity and humility.

In addition to these enhanced requirements, the committee concluded that efforts are needed to augment the education, training, and competency of the nursing home workforce on an ongoing basis. Many nursing home workers have no requirements for continuing education related to national competencies (and when such requirements exist, they generally vary by state). Furthermore, there are substantial differences in the types of jobs that racial and ethnic minority workers are sorted into within the nursing home workforce, which can affect power hierarchies within the workforce as well as compensation and benefits. In addition, nursing home residents are becoming increasingly diverse in terms of racial and ethnic groups, LGBTQ+ populations, and younger populations, yet little is known about their specific care needs in the nursing home setting or their preferences for who cares for them. As a result, the committee concluded that all nursing home workers would benefit from specific workforce-related education and training in principles of diversity, equity, and inclusion as well as cultural sensitivity and humility with respect to institutional factors such as biases (e.g., hiring, pay, and promotion practices), cultural factors (e.g., discrimination, micro-aggressions), and interpersonal factors (e.g., racial biases). Training is also needed for the needs of younger populations in nursing homes as well as training in principles of diversity, equity, and inclusion related to the unique, culturally sensitive care needs of specific populations (e.g., LGBTQ+, specific racial and ethnic groups). For example, as noted in Chapter 2, the LGBTQ+ community may face harassment and abuse in nursing homes, and efforts to improve the quality of care for this population of nursing home residents include enhanced staff training in LGBTQ+-affirming care. Finally, the committee recognizes that family caregivers are an essential and valued part of the nursing home workforce and often do not receive the support and training they need to be effective members of the care team. Therefore, the committee recommends the following:

RECOMMENDATION 2G: To enhance the education and training of the entire nursing home workforce,

- CMS should require all levels of nursing home staff to complete annual continuing education training to ensure that staff members are meeting national competency standards.
- Nursing homes should provide ongoing diversity and inclusion training (e.g., self-awareness of and approaches to addressing racism) for all workers and leadership and ensure that the training is designed to meet the unique demographic, cultural, linguistic, and transportation needs of the community in which the nursing home is situated and the community of workers within the nursing home.
- Nursing homes should provide family caregivers with resources, training, and opportunities to participate as part of the caregiving team in the manner and to the extent that residents desire their chosen family members to be involved.

Regarding opportunities to provide improved and expanded education and training experiences for nursing home staff, the committee recognizes that programs may not exist that are specific to the nursing home setting. Therefore, this is a prime opportunity for foundations, researchers, and others to develop training programs for staff and families specific to the nursing home setting.

Data Collection and Research

In addition to enhanced requirements for key leaders and workers in nursing homes, there is a need to increase the overall numbers of more highly trained professionals (e.g., physicians, APRNs, physician assistants) involved in the delivery of care in nursing homes. However, the committee found that little is known about the prevalence of these types of workers in nursing homes and the extent of their training and expertise. The committee particularly noted a dearth of information about the role, staffing patterns, and training of medical directors, social workers, physicians, APRNs, and physician assistants. Additionally, few data exist for the numbers and staffing patterns for contract and agency staff providing care in nursing homes. This is largely due to the fact that many of these care providers are not currently captured in data reported to CMS, most notably because many of them are not directly employed by the nursing home. Finally, the committee found that very little is known about the baseline demographic information for several key members of the nursing home leadership, including medical directors, administrators, and directors of nursing. The committee concluded that much more detailed information is needed about a variety of professionals working in nursing homes in order to better understand their expertise, numbers, and staffing patterns across facilities. Furthermore, while evidence exists on the association between APRNs and the quality of care in nursing homes, baseline data are needed for a variety of professionals to more fully assess their impact on the quality of care for nursing home residents and, ultimately, to determine their minimum and optimum staffing levels (as well as innovative staffing models) to provide high-quality care for nursing home residents. Therefore, the committee recommends the following:

RECOMMENDATION 2H: As a part of routine (e.g., at least annual) data collection, nursing homes should collect and report data to CMS regarding

- Baseline demographic information on medical directors, administrators, and directors of nursing, including name, licensure, contact information, and tenure in their position;
- The geriatrics or long-term care training, expertise, and staffing patterns (including time providing direct care) of medical directors, APRNs, social workers, physicians, and physician assistants providing services in nursing homes; and
- The numbers and staffing patterns (including time providing direct care) for all contract and agency staff providing services in nursing homes.

The committee notes that some of these data may be able to be captured through the Payroll Based Journal reporting system, while other information will need to be captured in other ways.

As noted earlier, the recruitment and retention of all types of nursing home workers has significant challenges. While many of the barriers to recruitment and retention are known, the committee concluded that more research is needed on persistent systemic barriers, including the influence of systemic and structural racism that has created and sustained racial and ethnic disparities among long-term care workers. Therefore, the committee recommends the following:

RECOMMENDATION 2I: HHS (e.g., CMS, AHRQ, and NIH) should fund research on systemic barriers and opportunities to improve the recruitment, training, and advancement of all nursing home workers, with a particular focus on CNAs. This research should include the collection of gender-, ethnicity-, and race-related outcomes of job quality indicators (e.g., hiring, turnover, job satisfaction).

GOAL 3: INCREASE TRANSPARENCY AND ACCOUNTABILITY OF FINANCES, OPERATIONS, AND OWNERSHIP

A key aim of nursing home oversight over the past decade has been to ensure greater transparency into finances, operations, and ownership. CMS makes some ownership information available for active nursing homes, but these data are incomplete, difficult to verify, and often difficult to use. Current data sources do not allow for the determination of corporate structure, finances, and operations of individual facilities. Furthermore, the increased complexity of nursing home ownership structures complicates the ability to understand where nursing homes spend their resources and the ability to gain a more accurate sense of their financial well-being and spending priorities. Moreover, there is currently little transparency regarding the practice of some nursing homes to contract with related-party organizations (those also owned by the nursing home owners) for services such as management, nursing, or therapy.

Progress has been made in simplifying nursing home cost reporting in recent years, yet there are still substantial questions about the accuracy and completeness of these data. For example, there is no current mechanism to audit the accuracy and completeness of reported data, and requirements related to the full disclosure of ownership have not been enforced. In 2016, the U.S. Government Accountability Office (GAO) found that while CMS collects and reports expenditure data, it "has not taken key steps to make the data readily accessible to public partners or to ensure their reliability." The committee concluded that increased transparency and accountability of the data on the finances, operations, and ownership of all nursing homes are needed for a variety of purposes. In particular, this is important for improving the financial investment in nursing home care as well as for improving regulatory oversight, all toward a common goal of improving the quality of care in nursing homes. Therefore, the committee recommends that, at the level of the individual facility,

RECOMMENDATION 3A: HHS should collect, audit, and make publicly available detailed facility-level data on the finances, operations, and ownership of all nursing homes (e.g., through Medicare and Medicaid cost reports and data from Medicare's Provider Enrollment, Chain, and Ownership System).

- HHS should ensure that the data allow the assessment of staffing patterns, deficiencies, financial arrangements and payments, related party entities, corporate structures, and objective quality indicators by common owner (i.e., chain and multifacility owners) and management company.

Once such data are available in a manner that allows for the assessment of quality by common owner or management company, the committee recommends the following:

RECOMMENDATION 3B: HHS should ensure that accurate and comprehensive data on the finances, operations, and ownership of all nursing homes are available in a real-time, readily usable, and searchable database so that consumers, payers, researchers, and federal and state regulators are able to use the data to

- Evaluate and track the quality of care for facilities with common ownership or management company, and
- Assess the impact of nursing home real estate ownership models and related-party transactions on the quality of care.

GOAL 4: CREATE A MORE RATIONAL AND ROBUST FINANCING SYSTEM

The committee's recommendations are designed to target the well-known shortcomings related to financing nursing home care in the United States. Characterized by a high degree of fragmentation, the current approach to financing nursing home care is not an intentional system, but rather a set of circumstances that has evolved over time to fill the largest gaps. Medicaid plays a dominant role as the default payer of nursing home care, but the federal–state program is constantly subject to state budget constraints. Medicare revenues from post-acute care play a disproportionate role in financial sustainability of nursing home care, and services such as hospice care are paid separately and are not well integrated into standard nursing home care. Private insurance is rare, and few people can pay out of pocket for an extended nursing home stay.

One implication of this unsystematic financing arrangement is a lack of equity in access to high-quality nursing home care. Heavy reliance on Medicaid to fund nursing home care, with strict financial and health-related eligibility rules, results in situations in which individuals may go without needed care or receive care that is inadequate in quality or quantity. A large body of literature shows that dependence on Medicaid is associated with admission to lower-quality facilities and to facilities with lower staffing ratios, more regulatory deficiencies, and a higher proportion of residents of color. Eligibility rules also differ across sites of care and across states, even within Medicaid, which may lead to inequities across states.

A second implication of this unsystematic financing approach is the occurrence of site-specific payment, which often creates irrational payment and eligibility differentials which can lead to unintended consequences.

Separate financing and payment systems for home- and community-based care and institutional care create a false dichotomy and present barriers to the rational allocation of resources across settings that considers costs as well as individuals' needs and preferences.

Previous attempts to develop more cohesive approaches to long-term care coverage have not been successful. As of the writing of this report, the U.S. Congress is considering The Well-Being Insurance for Seniors to be at Home Act, a proposal to use public–private partnerships to provide catastrophic coverage for long-term care. Many other high-income countries have implemented and sustained national long-term care coverage for their populations, incorporating both institutional and home-based care, and the structure of some of these programs could serve as models for the United States.

Improvements in the quality of nursing home care in conjunction with improving access, efficiency, and equity will require a more rational system of financing over the long term. A more rational financing system for nursing home care specifically will likely require a new federal benefit. While the committee acknowledges that enacting a new long-term care benefit will be politically challenging, there is an urgent need for a new, more comprehensive approach to long-term care financing. A federal benefit has the most potential to

- Increase access to long-term care services and reduce unmet need;
- Reduce arbitrary barriers between sites of care;
- Reduce inequities in access to high-quality care;
- Reduce differences in resources across nursing homes; and
- Guarantee that payment rates are adequate to cover the expected level of quality.

Building on lessons learned from experience of the establishment of Medicare Part D as well as the repeal of the Community Living Assistance Services and Support Act, the new benefit would likely require taxpayer subsidies in conjunction with beneficiary premiums and cost sharing. Therefore, the committee recommends the following:

RECOMMENDATION 4A:[5] **To move toward the establishment of a federal long-term care benefit that would expand access and advance equity for all adults who need long-term care, including nursing home care,**

- **The Secretary of HHS should study ways in which this federal benefit would be designed to avoid challenges faced by previous efforts to expand long-term care coverage.**
- **CMS should implement state demonstration programs to test this federal benefit model prior to national implementation.**

---

[5] One committee member declined to endorse this recommendation.

Ensuring Adequacy of Medicaid Payments

Medicaid, the federal–state program, is the dominant payer of long-stay nursing home services. Nursing homes depend on higher payments from Medicare to cross-subsidize lower Medicaid payments. This financial arrangement is inefficient for several reasons. First, many nursing homes care for a higher number of Medicaid than Medicare recipients and receive relatively little benefit from higher payments for Medicare services. Research generally finds that nursing homes with a large share of Medicaid residents provide lower-quality care. Increasing Medicaid payment rates to ensure that they are adequate to cover the cost of providing comprehensive, high-quality care to all nursing home residents will be a critical step to addressing existing disparities. Second, the subsidization from Medicare might serve as a disincentive to states to increase their Medicaid reimbursement rates. Finally, lower Medicaid rates encourage nursing homes to prefer short-stay patients covered by Medicare to long-stay nursing home residents covered by Medicaid, resulting in selective admission practices. Lower Medicaid rates relative to Medicare rates encourage the unnecessary hospitalization of long-stay residents in order to have their post-acute care paid for by Medicare upon their return to the nursing home. For these reasons, Medicaid reimbursement rates need to be commensurate with the costs of providing comprehensive, high-quality care for nursing home residents.

Existing law requires state Medicaid programs' payments to be adequate to provide access to quality care. States are required to provide assurances that their payment rates meet this criterion. For certain providers, CMS requires that states also submit evidence that their payment rates are indeed adequate. Nursing home payment rates are not subject to this requirement, despite Medicaid's significant role as a payer of nursing home care. CMS needs to fulfill its responsibility as enshrined in existing statute to ensure the adequacy of Medicaid payment rates by requiring nursing homes to provide detailed and accurate financial information (e.g., data on costs, payment levels, resident characteristics, ownership, and corporate structure) upon which the adequacy of rates may be determined. Therefore, the committee recommends the following:

RECOMMENDATION 4B: To ensure that adequate funds are invested in providing comprehensive care for long-stay nursing home residents,

- CMS should ensure compliance with existing statute by using detailed and accurate nursing home financial information to ensure that Medicaid (or eventually, federal) payments are at a level that is adequate to cover the delivery of comprehensive, high-quality, and equitable care by all providers to nursing home residents across all domains of care (as specified in Box 10-1).

Paying for Direct Care Services

An extensive body of research indicates that there is a strong connection between spending on direct care for residents and the quality of that care. The Patient Protection and Affordable Care Act required CMS to develop new Medicare cost reports to capture specific information on nursing home costs in four categories: direct and indirect care, housekeeping and dietary services, capital expenses, and administrative services. However, beyond the reporting requirements, nursing homes are not required by law to devote a specific portion of their payment to direct care for residents. This results in great variability among nursing homes in terms of the actual dollar amount devoted to direct care as opposed to non-care costs. For example, recent evidence has shown a systematic shift in nursing home operating costs toward items such as monitoring fees, interest payments, and lease payments that are associated with the acquisition of nursing homes by private equity owners. Implementing policies that require nursing homes to spend a minimum amount of their revenue on direct resident care and staffing will guard against these types of behaviors. Therefore, the committee recommends the following:

RECOMMENDATION 4C: HHS should require a specific percentage of nursing home Medicare and Medicaid payments to be designated to pay for direct-care services for nursing home residents, including staffing (including both the number of staff and their wages and benefits), behavioral health, and clinical care.

Value-Based Payment for Nursing Homes

Nursing homes are among the most common sites of post-acute care; according to the Medicare Payment Advisory Commission, for example, 20 percent of hospitalized Medicare beneficiaries were discharged to a nursing home for post-acute care in 2018. To control rising post-acute care costs, Medicare joined the prevailing trend toward creating a stronger linkage of payment to the value and quality of care rather than to the quantity of services. Medicare's entry into the world of value-based payment included the implementation of alternative payment models (APMs) such as accountable care organizations and bundled payments that hold care providers accountable for total costs of care.

Medicare bundled payment demonstrations have found evidence of declining use of nursing home–based acute care without adverse consequences on patient outcomes. Medicare Advantage plans, for their part, have demonstrated a lower use of nursing homes for post-acute care and shorter lengths of stay for common conditions among Medicare Advantage beneficiaries compared with those covered by traditional Medicare.

Given the importance of controlling costs for post-acute care provided in nursing homes, while maintaining or improving quality of care for patients, Medicare needs to build on the experience of existing value-based payment demonstrations. In contrast to the current bundled payments made to nursing homes for a limited number of conditions, however, such arrangements need to be extended to cover the costs of care for all conditions, including acute care in the hospital and post-acute care in the nursing home setting. Bundled payments will shift financial accountability, and thus risk, for nursing home post-acute care to hospitals. In addition, hospitals and other clinicians providing care during an episode of care need to work collaboratively to provide high-quality, equitable, person-centered care and be held financially accountable to this standard by linking payment to quality metrics, including patient-reported outcomes. Indeed, the committee recognizes that there is always a risk of unintended consequences with any new payment model. As bundled payments are expanded to all conditions, close monitoring and rigorous study of the impact on patient outcomes will be required to mitigate any potential unintended consequences. Therefore, the committee recommends the following:

RECOMMENDATION 4D: To improve the value of, and accountability for, Medicare payments for short-stay post-acute care in nursing homes, HHS, CMS, and the Center for Medicare and Medicaid Innovation should extend bundled payment initiatives to all conditions and, in so doing, hold hospitals financially accountable (i.e., put hospitals "at risk") for Medicare post-acute care spending and outcomes.

The committee also recognizes the importance of the use of value-based payment for long-stay nursing home care. Medicare Advantage institutional special needs plan demonstrations for long-term care in nursing homes have indicated that such arrangements have an impact on critical outcomes such as lower rates of hospitalizations. As with short-stay residents, CMS needs to build on this experience by continuing to test out the use of APMs for long-term nursing home care.

The recommended APMs for long-term care would be separate and distinct from the recommended bundled payment initiatives for short-stay post-acute care. APMs for long-stay nursing home care would rely on global capitated budgets from a single payer and would hold health care provider organizations and health plans financially accountable for the total costs of long-term care in nursing homes. The global capitated rate would cover post-acute care, long-term care, and hospice care. Grouping the entire range of services into one global rate enhances care coordination and improves the management of the overall cost of care. In recommending these APMs as demonstration projects, the committee recognizes that the impact of APMs for long-stay nursing home care is unknown, but it concludes that the evidence to date warrants further exploration and testing of APMs in real-world situations.

Moreover, the committee is aware that there is not yet strong evidence that the use of value-based payments can improve access to care or health outcomes for vulnerable populations (e.g., racial and ethnic minorities, rural populations, and individuals with disabilities). While CMS has devoted attention to monitoring the unintended impact of value-based payment on at-risk populations, it is important to consider that the tenacious inequities and disparities within the health care system are indicative of a more extensive systemic bias—both societal and at the level of the broader health care system. If value-based payment is to serve as an alternative payment model designed to increase value and enhance equity, it must be capable of influencing the issues that directly affect access to and the quality of health care services.

Equally important is that a targeted focus on reducing health disparities needs to be an explicit part of using APMs to pay for nursing home care. The quality measurement and quality goals that APMs use to determine payment need to include measures of improving outcomes for disadvantaged populations and reducing existing disparities. All new programs also need to include explicit monitoring and evaluation of health care disparities.

The biggest challenge for achieving health equity under APMs is related to the disparate financial resources across different providers of care. It is important to note that addressing payment inequities across nursing homes by increasing Medicaid payment rates to levels adequate to cover the costs of providing comprehensive care for such residents, as discussed above, will be an essential step to avoid further exacerbating disparities. Therefore, the committee recommends the following:

RECOMMENDATION 4E: To eliminate the current financial misalignment for long-stay residents introduced by Medicaid's coverage of their nursing home services and Medicare's coverage of health care services, HHS and CMS should conduct demonstration projects to explore the use of APMs for long-term nursing home care, separate from bundled payment initiatives for post-acute care. These APMs would use global capitated budgets, making care provider organizations or health plans accountable for the total costs of care.

- APM's capitated rate should include post-acute care and hospice care for long-term nursing home residents to address financial misalignment between Medicare and Medicaid payments, while supporting care coordination.

- Designs and payments of the demonstration projects should be tied to broad-based quality metrics, including staffing metrics, residents' experience of care, functional status, and end-of-life care to ensure that APMs maintain quality of care, particularly in areas such as post-acute care, end-of-life care, and hospice care.

GOAL 5: DESIGN A MORE EFFECTIVE AND RESPONSIVE SYSTEM OF QUALITY ASSURANCE

The federal government's formal involvement with the oversight of nursing homes essentially started with the enactment of Medicare and Medicaid in 1965 and the related requirements of participation for nursing homes. Over the decades, various laws and federal regulations sought to improve the quality of care in nursing homes and also improve the oversight and regulation of nursing homes' performance (see Chapter 8, Box 8-1). Nursing home quality assurance activities are largely defined by the statutory requirements of OBRA 87 and associated regulations put forward by CMS. However, substantial changes have occurred in nursing home care since the implementation of OBRA 87, but the general structure of the oversight and regulation of nursing homes has largely remained the same.

State Surveys and CMS Oversight

States assist with the assessment of facilities' compliance with requirements of participation through regular inspections (roughly once a year) and, as necessary, the investigation of complaints and adverse incidents. Although federal oversight standards and processes are uniform across states, considerable variation in processes and outcomes exists in the implementation of routine inspection responsibilities, in the imposition of sanctions, and in the investigation of complaints. Multiple organizations have called for the strengthening of surveyor qualifications, and several reports note the challenges in hiring qualified surveyor staff, but there is very little literature evaluating surveyors' qualifications or the effectiveness of their training. Moreover, several reports from the GAO and U.S. Office of the Inspector General (OIG) over the past two decades have found failures in the survey process to properly identify serious care problems, fully correct and prevent recurrence of identified problems, and investigate complaints in a timely manner. For example, ten states did not meet performance thresholds for timeliness in addressing high-priority complaints for eight consecutive years (2011–2018). And while CMS is able to impose remedies or sanctions if a state is found to have performed inadequately, in January 2022, the OIG found that CMS often did not fully track these remedies and they rarely imposed formal sanctions.

The committee concluded that state survey agencies may not have adequate capacity (including the number of trained surveyors) or resources to fulfill all their responsibilities. The committee additionally concluded that CMS does not provide sufficient oversight of or transparency in the state survey process, and they do not adequately enforce existing sanctions for failures in performance of the states' duties. Therefore, the committee recommends the following:

RECOMMENDATION 5A: CMS should ensure that state survey agencies have adequate capacity, organizational structure, and resources to fulfill their current nursing home oversight responsibilities for monitoring, investigation, and enforcement.

- In particular, CMS should ensure that state survey agencies have adequate capacity and resources to deliver a strong, consistent, responsive, and transparent process for complaints.
- Along with providing the necessary resources, CMS should refine and expand oversight performance metrics of survey agencies for annual public reporting which would facilitate greater accountability related to whether existing federal regulations are being consistently and completely enforced and would highlight shortcomings that need to be addressed.
- CMS should use existing strategies of enforcement where states have consistently fallen short of expected standards.

The committee notes that these resources need to be available for a variety of purposes, including increasing the number of survey staff, improvements in surveyor training, and enhanced compensation.

The current quality assurance process is largely a standardized enterprise, with almost all facilities inspected at the same frequency for compliance with the same standards on a roughly annual basis. Additionally, even with a range of enforcement options available, civil monetary penalties have been by far the most common remedy used in recent years to sanction nursing homes. However, the level and extent of use of these penalties may not be sufficient to effect desired changes. Furthermore, the budget of the Special Focus Facility program, a program that targets more frequent inspections and quality improvement activities to the lowest-performing facilities, only allows for oversight of a very small fraction of such nursing homes, and many participants who complete the program fail to sustain improvement.

Despite the prominent role of nursing home oversight and regulation, the evidence base for its effectiveness in ensuring a minimum standard of quality is relatively modest. Most resident advocates and nursing home providers have expressed dissatisfaction with the effectiveness of the current nursing home regulatory model, and a variety of new approaches have been suggested, yet little consensus (or evidence) exists on how exactly to improve quality assurance efforts, including the survey process. Nursing home advocates highlight the fact that, as noted earlier, existing regulations are often not being completely and consistently enforced and suggest that additional regulations need to be put in place to fully protect residents. Alternatively, many providers believe that the existing regulations are excessive and impede innovation and good-quality care. The committee concluded that while the current regulatory process needs significant improvement, particularly in relation to the uneven enforcement of regulations, there is a dearth of evidence to suggest which approaches would ultimately lead to improvement in the quality of care for nursing home residents. In order to determine the optimal use of existing and expanded resources and make the quality assurance processes more efficient and effective, the committee recommends the following:

RECOMMENDATION 5B: CMS should develop and evaluate strategies (including the evaluation of potential unintended consequences) that make nursing home quality assurance efforts more effective, efficient, and responsive, including potential longer-term reforms such as

- Enhanced data monitoring (using prior survey performance in combination with real-time quality metrics) to track performance and triage onsite inspections of facilities;
- Increased oversight across a broader segment of poorly performing facilities (e.g., through substantially improving the Special Focus Facilities program);
- Modified formal oversight activities for high-performing facilities, including the consideration of more targeted inspections, provided adequate safeguards are in place, including
  - Surveyors present on site at least annually,
  - States meeting expected standards for responding to complaints, and
  - Nursing homes continuing to meet specified, real-time quality metrics (e.g., a robust threshold of staffing hours per resident day, stable ownership); and
- Greater use of enforcement remedies beyond civil monetary penalties, including chain-wide corporate integrity agreements, denial of admissions, directed plans of correction, temporary management, and termination from Medicare and Medicaid.

The committee notes that concerns have been raised as to whether oversight can be reduced in some manner (e.g., less frequent surveys, less intense surveys) for high performers. In particular, the concern is that significant safety risks or markers of decreases in quality (e.g., significant changes in staffing patterns) might occur in the interim between surveys. Therefore, the committee emphasizes the importance of using real-time quality metrics as an "early warning system" in conjunction with testing these approaches to ensure that safety and overall quality can be monitored and that intervention can occur quickly if problems arise.

The Long-Term Care Ombudsman Program

The Long-Term Care Ombudsman Program is the only entity within the nursing home system whose sole mission is to be an advocate for the residents to ensure that they receive the care to which they are entitled. The impact of the program has been largely positive, especially given the modest investment of governmental resources. However, there is considerable variation in the amount of resources, funding, and staffing among the various state programs. The committee concluded that limited funding affects many programs' abilities to meet federal and state requirements and fully provide nursing home residents and their families with the best support possible. Therefore, the committee recommends the following:

RECOMMENDATION 5C: The Administration for Community Living should advocate for increased funding for the Long-Term Care Ombudsman Program. Additional resources should be allocated toward

- Hiring additional paid staff and training staff and volunteers,
- Bolstering programmatic infrastructure (e.g., electronic data monitoring systems to track staff and volunteer activities and track resident and family complaints),
- Making data on state long-term care ombudsman programs and activities publicly available, and
- Developing summary metrics designed to document the effectiveness of the Long-Term Care Ombudsman Program in advocating for nursing home residents.

Additionally, states should contribute funds to their long-term care ombudsman programs to address cross-state variation in the extent to which these programs have the capacity to advocate for nursing home residents. Along with additional resources, all State Units on Aging should develop plans for their long-term care ombudsman programs to interface effectively with collaborating entities such as adult protective services, state survey agencies, and state and local law enforcement agencies.

Quality Assurance, Transparency, and Accountability

As noted earlier, the committee concluded that increased transparency and accountability will help improve the quality of care in nursing homes. The committee recommended that HHS should collect, audit, and make publicly available detailed facility-level data on the finances, operations, and ownership of all nursing homes (Recommendation 3A), and that these data are made available in a real-time, readily usable, and searchable database that allows for evaluation and track the quality of care for facilities with common ownership or management company (Recommendation 3B). Accurate and complete data will enable regulators to identify poor quality of care by owner or management company and levy sanctions as appropriate. Therefore, the committee recommends the following:

RECOMMENDATION 5D: When data on the finances and ownership of nursing homes reveal a pattern of poor-quality care across facilities with a common owner (including across states), federal and state oversight agencies (e.g., CMS, state licensure and survey agencies, the Department of Justice) should impose oversight and enforcement actions on the owner. These actions may include

- Denial of new or renewed licensure,
- The imposition of sanctions, including the exclusion of individuals and entities from participation in Medicare and Medicaid, and
- The implementation of strengthened oversight (e.g., through an improved and expanded special focus facilities program).

Certificate-of-Need Regulations and Construction Moratoria

As part of quality assurance, some states maintain certificate-of-need requirements to regulate expansions in the health care market, purportedly as a strategy to constrain health care spending. Certificate-of-need policies employ a need-based evaluation of all applications for new construction or additions to existing facilities that would increase the number of beds. Additionally, some states have implemented construction moratoria that prohibit the building of new health care facilities. For health care markets in general, certificate-of-need regulations have been found to be largely ineffective.

The logic behind certificate-of-need regulations for nursing homes specifically is that limiting the number of beds will, in turn, limit the number of Medicaid beneficiaries in nursing home settings, thus keeping state Medicaid spending to a lower level. However, the evidence does not suggest that these policies have much impact on overall Medicaid nursing home spending. On the other hand, nursing home certificate-of-need regulations have been found to limit choice and lower access to medical services and health care resources, especially for those in rural areas; decrease the quality of care for some measures of quality; and increase private-pay prices. Certificate-of-need regulations and construction moratoria can also discourage innovation by preventing the entry of more modern nursing home options (such as those that embrace principles of culture change) and restricting facility renovation and remodeling. As a result, these policies may contribute to the perpetuation of larger nursing homes, rather than the smaller, more home-like settings that are more desirable. There is no evidence that lifting certificate-of-need regulations will increase Medicaid spending on institutional care or reduce investment in home- and community-based settings of long-term care.

The committee concludes that while certificate-of-need regulations do not appear to have their intended effect of holding down Medicaid nursing home spending, they can have the unintended effect of harming consumers by limiting choice and access. Therefore, the committee recommends the following:

RECOMMENDATION 5E: States should eliminate certificate-of-need requirements and construction moratoria for nursing homes to encourage the entry of innovative care models and foster robust competition in order to expand consumer choice and improve quality.

The committee emphasizes that the elimination of such restrictive policies is not intended as a mechanism to increase the use of nursing homes or to invest in nursing homes in lieu of other long-term settings of care. Rather, the committee seeks to expand consumer choice for those who need and choose nursing home care by encouraging competition on the basis of quality.

GOAL 6: EXPAND AND ENHANCE QUALITY MEASUREMENT AND CONTINUOUS QUALITY IMPROVEMENT

The primary purpose of quality measurement is to improve the quality of care and outcomes. Effective quality measures can be used for continuous quality improvement activities.

Quality Measurement

The CMS website Care Compare provides public reporting of quality measures for nursing homes. However, it does not directly report on a key domain of high-quality care—resident and family satisfaction and experience. Technical measures of care processes and outcomes are only moderately correlated with resident and family reports of the quality of the experience of care. Furthermore, obtaining residents' and families' assessment of their care experience becomes even more important in the nursing home setting, where residents have high levels of support needs and rely on the nursing home staff and environment to meet their needs on a continuing basis for weeks, months, or even years.

While many nursing home administrators report using resident and family satisfaction surveys, and satisfaction information is reported as being useful, the surveys being used vary widely and may not be adequately validated. CMS mandates the collection of Consumer Assessment of Healthcare Providers and Systems (CAHPS) surveys in several settings or populations (e.g., hospitals, Medicare Advantage, home health care, hospice care) by independent, credentialed survey vendors, and AHRQ supports the ongoing evaluation of item performance and the association of ratings with patient characteristics. Nursing home CAHPS measures had extensive item development and testing for reliability and validity. However, the collection of the nursing home CAHPS survey is not required.

The committee concluded that the lack of inclusion of measures of resident and family satisfaction and experience in Care Compare impedes the ability of individuals and their families to make fully informed choices about providers and facilities. It also disadvantages nursing homes, which cannot benefit from using consumer reports of their experiences to improve services and care delivery. Therefore, the committee recommends the following:

RECOMMENDATION 6A: CMS should add the CAHPS measures of resident and family experience (i.e., the nursing home CAHPS surveys) to Care Compare.

- Data for this measure should be collected annually by independent reviewers (i.e., not nursing home staff) in all nursing homes.
- As data are collected nationally, ongoing psychometric testing should occur to refine the measures in order to support submission for endorsement by the National Quality Forum.

The committee supports the use of the nursing home CAHPS measures given that they are by far the most well-validated measures of resident and family experience. The committee recognizes that the cost, administration, and analysis of the CAHPS nursing home survey will be expensive and present logistical challenges. However, as noted above, the committee concluded that failure to capture the voices of residents and their families in quality measurement neglects a crucial aspect of quality. The committee emphasizes that the use of these measures is not intended to replace the crucial roles of the formal complaints process or hearing from resident and family councils, as measures of resident and family satisfaction capture a different and very important aspect of the resident and family experience. Rather, all of these mechanisms provide important insights. Finally, the committee supports consideration for eventually integrating the CAHPS measure into the five-star rating, and recognizes that continued research on what matters to residents and their families is needed to refine quality measurement efforts.

In addition to adding measures that reflect the resident and family experience, the committee concluded that Care Compare needs to be enhanced and expanded through the inclusion of more measures that can help to more fully reflect the quality of care in nursing homes. Many of these measures can be readily reported from data already collected by CMS. As noted earlier, increasing the transparency of nursing home ownership should include the ability to track quality of care by common owner or management company. Finally, the current five-star rating system is unable to distinguish modest increments in the quality of care among nursing homes with average ratings, and more work is needed to improve the validity of existing measures, such as by auditing reported data for accuracy. Therefore, the committee recommends the following:

RECOMMENDATION 6B: HHS, CMS, NIH, and AHRQ should expand and enhance existing publicly reported quality measures in Care Compare by

- Increasing the weight of staffing measures within the five-star composite rating;
- Facilitating the ability to see quality performance of facilities that share common ownership (i.e., chain and other multifacility owners) or management company;
- Improving the validity of Minimum Data Set–based measures of clinical quality (e.g., better risk adjustment, auditing for accuracy, inclusion of resident preferences); and
- Conducting additional testing to improve the differentiation of the five-star composite rating so that it better distinguishes among the middle ranges of rating, not just at the extremes.

Finally, the committee found that several other key domains of high-quality care are not reflected among the measures in Care Compare and concluded that more work is needed to develop and test valid measures for these domains of care. Therefore, the committee recommends the following:

RECOMMENDATION 6C: HHS should fund the development and adoption of new nursing home measures to Care Compare related to

- Palliative care and end-of-life care;
- Implementation of the resident's care plan;

- Receipt of care that aligns with resident's goals and the attainment of those goals;
- Staff well-being and satisfaction;
- Psychosocial and behavioral health; and
- Structural measures (e.g., health information technology adoption and interoperability; the percentage of single occupancy rooms; emergency preparedness, routine training in infection prevention; emergency response management; financial performance; staff employment arrangements [e.g., full-time, part-time, contract, and agency staff]).

The areas recommended are important for consumers to consider when seeking nursing home care that best meets their needs and for nursing homes to use in improving their care and services.

Health Equity

The quality of nursing home care is particularly concerning for several high-risk populations who experience significant disparities in care, including racial and ethnic minorities and LGBTQ+ populations. For example, nursing homes in low-income neighborhoods with high numbers of minority residents have lower quality-of-care ratings. Additionally, the COVID-19 pandemic initially had a greater impact on nursing homes that serve disproportionately more non-White residents. However, the lack of robust data specific to race and ethnicity in nursing homes makes it difficult to document the true extent and impact of disparities in care. The committee concluded that while developing measures of disparities in nursing home care is needed, doing so needs to be based on an overall health equity strategy for nursing homes. Therefore, the committee recommends the following:

RECOMMENDATION 6D: HHS should develop an overall health equity strategy for nursing homes that includes defining, measuring, evaluating, and intervening on disparities in nursing home care. The strategy should include

- Definitions of health equity and disparities in nursing homes, including disparities related to race, ethnicity, LGBTQ+ populations, and sources of payment;
- The development of new measures of disparities in nursing home care, both within and across facilities, at the national, state, and ownership levels, to be included in a national report card.

As a first step, a minimum data set of information to identify and describe disparities should be established, with data collected at least annually and made publicly available. The information should include characteristics of the communities in which nursing homes are embedded as well as the ability of community members to access nursing home care.

- Research regarding disparities and the development of policies and culturally tailored interventions should be a priority for funding by HHS, NIH, and other sources.
- HHS, in partnership with state and local governments, should use data to identify the types and degree of disparity to prioritize when action is needed and to identify the promising pathways to reduce or eliminate those disparities.

Quality Improvement

Standardized, required CMS quality measures have guided quality improvement efforts. In 2016, the ACA required that all skilled nursing facilities implement quality assurance and performance-improvement programs as a requirement of participation for reimbursement by Medicare and Medicaid. The extent to which individual facilities engage in quality improvement and the effectiveness of such activities is unknown. Furthermore, many facilities lack adequate expertise and resources for effective quality improvement. Technical assistance is one of the primary mechanisms of quality improvement. The role of technical assistance depends in part upon the nursing home recognizing its need for additional knowledge and expertise. Without a motive to improve quality, little change may occur.

The committee recognizes the role of CMS's quality improvement organization (QIO) program in providing technical assistance on a variety of topics to improve the quality of health care in general. However, the focus of the QIO program varies by scope of work, and attention to nursing homes specifically has been inconsistent. Furthermore, the evidence base about the effectiveness and relative contribution of QIOs to quality improvement in health care, and particularly for nursing homes, is lacking. On the other hand, evidence suggests that state-based programs that focus on helping nursing home staff with quality improvement activities within nursing homes using onsite assistance by expert clinical staff and collaborating groups are effective in improving quality of care and that their help is widely accepted by nursing homes. State and local programs may be particularly well suited to provide technical assistance due to familiarity with the circumstances of the local community, the ability to be seen as a trusted peer, and the development of specific expertise due to a continued solitary focus on nursing home quality. For example, state and local technical assistance programs have been effective at building trusting relationships, modifying technical assistance approaches to meet local needs and skills, and keeping up to date with scientific content. Such programs may also help integrate nursing homes into their local communities as well as the broader health care system.

The committee concluded that nursing homes would benefit from the availability of technical assistance from individuals at the state (or even local) level who are most familiar with their specific communities and challenges, have specific expertise in nursing home quality, and have a consistent and ongoing focus on nursing homes. Therefore, the committee recommends the following:

RECOMMENDATION 6E: CMS should allocate funds to state governments for grants to develop and operate state-based, nonprofit, confidential technical assistance programs that have an ongoing and consistent focus on nursing homes. These programs should provide up-to-date, evidence-based education and guidance in best clinical and operational practices to help nursing homes implement effective continuous quality-improvement activities to improve care and nursing home operations.

- CMS should create explicit standards for these programs to promote comparable programs across states.
- The program should conduct ongoing analysis and reporting of effectiveness of the services provided.
- The program should provide services to all nursing homes in the state, with a focus on those identified as being at risk for poor performance, but also available to those with moderate and high performance.
- The program should coordinate with state surveyors and ombudsmen and receive referrals regarding facilities needing assistance, but maintain the confidentiality of the details of the services provided to each facility (notwithstanding the mandated reporting requirements in each state regarding resident abuse and neglect).
- The programs should consider partnering with relevant academic institutions of higher education, such as colleges of nursing, medicine, social work, rehabilitation services, and others.

GOAL 7: ADOPT HEALTH INFORMATION TECHNOLOGY IN ALL NURSING HOMES

Research increasingly demonstrates the key role of HIT in health care settings, given its potential contribution to a range of outcomes, including increasing efficiency in care delivery, enhancing care coordination, improving staff productivity, promoting patient safety, and improving quality of care. The COVID-19 pandemic underscored the critical importance of HIT applications, such as videoconferencing and telehealth, providing vitally important means of connectivity and communication when nursing home lockdowns instituted to protect vulnerable residents from infection led to limited access to in-person clinical visits as well as residents' isolation from friends and family members.

HIT includes technologies such as electronic health records (EHRs), which have a wide range of uses, including real-time data sharing capabilities, digital prescriptions, automated medication dispensing, clinical decision-support services, and support functions related to billing, reimbursement, and administrative tasks. Members of the interdisciplinary care team would benefit from application of EHRs' multiple functions to improve the quality of care for nursing home residents.

In contrast to hospitals and acute-care settings, however, the long-term care sector—and nursing homes in particular—has been slower to adopt EHRs. Nursing home residents often have complex medical conditions that require care coordination among hospitals and other care settings, further underscoring the need for nursing homes to have EHRs that communicate with other systems in order to ensure smooth and safe care transitions as patients move from one health care setting to another.

Eligible hospitals and health care providers have long benefited from financial incentives to support EHR adoption, which were initially contained in the EHR Incentive Program created by the Health Information Technology for Economic and Clinical Health (HITECH) Act of 2009, recently revised and renamed the CMS Promoting Interoperability Program. Nursing homes were not included among those hospitals and health care professionals eligible to participate in the incentive program, and thus they have not benefited from the program's financial incentives, which sunset in 2021.

Cost is a significant barrier to EHR adoption by nursing homes, and absent the federal incentives provided to other health care providers, the prevalence, quality, and comprehensiveness of EHR adoption in nursing homes is well below that in other health care settings. Given the benefits of EHRs for both residents and staff, the committee recommends the following:

RECOMMENDATION 7A: The Office of the National Coordinator (ONC) and CMS should identify a pathway to provide financial incentives to nursing homes for certified EHR adoption that supports health information exchanges to enhance person-centered longitudinal care. These incentives should be modeled on the HITECH incentives provided to eligible hospitals and professionals.

- ONC should ensure that the nursing home program complements the Promoting Interoperability Program; and

- ONC should develop appropriate nursing home EHR certification criteria that promote adoption of health information exchange of important clinical data (e.g., admission, discharge, and transfer data).

Ideally, the collection and recording of patient data and information would occur as close to the provision of patient care (i.e., at the bedside) as possible. Such real-time data entry has been shown to improve patient care, allowing for quicker results of laboratory tests and medication orders and providing more decision-making support to the clinicians. Moreover, capturing patient data in real time benefits patients who receive improved care, which leads to greater patient satisfaction. Finally, real-time data entry can reduce duplication of documentation and, in so doing, contribute to the overall efficiency of nursing home staff.

As more and more nursing homes adopt HIT, it is critical to monitor and track HIT adoption and interoperability (i.e., the ability to communicate with other EHRs). In order to comply with Merit-Based Incentive Payment System requirements, nursing homes should be expected to use HIT in resident care delivery. However, HIT adoption varies from nursing home to nursing home, with some nursing homes using complete EHRs, while others may have partial EHR capabilities. Given this variability, a baseline measure of HIT adoption needs to be developed. One option would be to measure nursing home use of real-time HIT approaches for resident care delivery. As nursing homes use new measures to assess HIT adoption and interoperability, the results need to be publicly reported in Care Compare.

In addition, the usability of HIT, which encompasses effectiveness, efficiency, and satisfaction, needs to be assessed. This is critically important because if a HIT system is not easy to use or is perceived as making more work for nursing home staff rather than decreasing their workload, then it will not be used to its full potential. It is vital to understand the various barriers and facilitators to HIT use in nursing homes and to use the results of the assessments to improve the efficiency, effectiveness of, and satisfaction with HIT—on the part of nursing home staff as well as residents and families. Therefore, the committee recommends the following:

RECOMMENDATION 7B: In order to measure and report on HIT adoption and interoperability in nursing homes, HHS should

- Develop measures for HIT adoption and interoperability, consistent with other health care organizations;
- Measure levels of HIT adoption and interoperability on an annual basis and report results in Care Compare; and
- Measure and report nursing home staff, resident, and family perceptions of HIT usability.

The ability of HIT to realize its potential to improve safety and quality of care and to increase staff productivity is contingent upon several key factors, including the training of nursing home leadership and staff. Despite research that demonstrates that training is a key contributor to staff satisfaction with HIT, most nursing homes do not provide adequate training for staff in the optimal use of HIT. Given the key role of training, the federal government should provide incentives for the training of nursing home leadership and staff members in agreed-upon HIT core competency areas. Therefore, the committee recommends the following:

RECOMMENDATION 7C: CMS and HRSA should provide financial support for the development and ongoing implementation of workforce training, emphasizing core HIT competencies for nursing home leadership and staff, such as clinical decision support, telehealth, integration of clinical processes, interoperability, and knowledge management in patient care.

In order to create an environment of continuous learning and quality improvement, evaluation studies need to be conducted to assess the impact of HIT on resident outcome, and to examine innovative ways to use HIT to improve resident care. Studies will help nursing homes understand the key challenges of HIT adoption and use by exploring the perceptions of clinicians as well as residents of HIT usability. Moreover, studies also need to explore the disparities in HIT adoption and use across nursing homes, paying particular attention to differences in geographic location (rural versus urban), ownership status, the size of the nursing home, and specific patient populations served by individual nursing homes. Therefore, the committee recommends the following:

RECOMMENDATION 7D: ONC and AHRQ should fund rigorous evaluation studies to explore

- The use of HIT to improve nursing home resident outcomes;
- Disparities in HIT adoption and use across nursing homes;
- Innovative HIT applications for resident care; and
- The assessment of clinician, resident, and family perceptions of HIT usability

WHAT WOULD QUALITY NURSING HOME CARE LOOK LIKE?

As discussed at the beginning of this report, the committee's conceptual model presents a vision for high-quality care in nursing homes, and the committee's goals and recommendations identify specific steps to achieve this vision of improving nursing home care. It is important to consider the impact of the committee's recommendations from the perspective of nursing home residents, families, and staff.

First and foremost, the resident and his or her chosen family would take center stage, according to the tenets of person-centered care to maintain the resident's dignity, maximize independence, balance autonomy and safety, and enable meaningful relationships. Quality nursing home care would be provided to all residents, both short-stay and long-stay, and respond to the substantial differences in their care needs, goals, and preferences.

Overall, the goals, values, and preferences of the individual would be known and met, and nursing home residents would experience the best possible quality of life—thriving rather than merely surviving. Residents would have independence (as appropriate), and they would have the ability to participate in meaningful and person-centered activities that meet their potential and result in a sense of self-worth. Younger residents would have access to age-appropriate activities and environments, freedom and expression, and opportunities to interact with peers. Residents and their families would experience high satisfaction with the care they are receiving, and their voices would be heard and fully integrated into processes of quality measurement, quality improvement, and quality assurance.

Every nursing home resident would receive appropriate and effective care in a timely manner. This care would be both individualized and comprehensive, including care to support basic daily needs (e.g., hydration, nutrition, and elimination), assessment, acute care needs, chronic disease management, behavioral and social care, spiritual care, the preservation of function (e.g., cognitive and physical) and comfort, palliative care, and end-of-life care. Care coordination would include seamless transitions to other settings of care (as needed), and all nursing homes would have state-of-the-art health information systems to facilitate the sharing of information across care settings.

Individuals working in nursing homes would be highly trained and appropriately compensated, and a stable nursing home leadership would help create a supportive work environment. There would be adequate numbers of staff with high job satisfaction and low turnover rates, which would enable residents to receive consistent care from an interdisciplinary team that knows them well as a person and is able to help meet their individual goals. Staff would be compassionate and have adequate time to spend with residents for iterative care planning and decision making related to their personalized goals of care as well as time to engage socially with the resident. Staff members would have the knowledge, skills, and tools to competently and confidently carry out their work, including the ability to recognize and respond to subtle changes in residents' needs, and the entire range of nursing home workers would be respected and supported by their supervisors and engaged in team-based decision making. They would be well trained in the effective use of health information technology such as electronic health records to enhance their productivity as well as improve the quality of care provided to residents. In short, nursing homes will be places where people want to work and advance their professional careers.

In addition to being places where people want to work, nursing homes will be places where people want to live. To do so, nursing homes will be redesigned and reconfigured to actually resemble home-like settings rather than medical institutions. Single-occupancy bedrooms with private bathrooms will be the standard, and nursing homes will provide a variety of activities to engage residents while ensuring residents have the opportunity to the visit with friends and family when they want. The social environment would include connections to the local community. The physical environment of the nursing home would be clean and odor free, have good lighting, and be characterized as a calm, safe, and secure environment (e.g., free of injury, abuse, theft, and acquired infections). Such features as single-occupancy rooms and private bathrooms as well as the provision of a clean, safe, and secure environment is provided for short-stay nursing home residents as well.

The financing of nursing home care would ensure adequate funding for high-quality care, including assistance with activities of daily living, behavioral health and psychosocial care, oral health, hearing and vision, and end-of-life care. Payment models for care would more closely link payment to value rather than to the volume of services provided and, in so doing, would discourage wasteful spending. No resident or family would be faced with the prospect of spending down all their assets in order to receive nursing home care. Information on the operations of the nursing home, including the ownership structure, involvement of third parties, and spending patterns would be completely transparent to residents, families, researchers, and those responsible for nursing home regulatory oversight and quality assurance.

Nursing home oversight would be carried out by surveyors who are well trained and dedicated to their work. Deficiencies in nursing homes would be identified and resolved quickly and consistently. Nursing home residents and their families would be unafraid to voice their grievances and concerns, which would be acknowledged and swiftly addressed through an efficient and transparent grievances process and a robust Long-Term Care Ombudsman Program. Nursing home owners and management companies with severe citations within and across facilities would be sanctioned appropriately; if severe violations are noted repeatedly or go unresolved, nursing homes would be terminated from participation in Medicare and Medicaid. Nursing homes would be able to receive technical assistance as desired to address quality concerns. In short, nursing home owners will be held accountable for the care provided in their facilities.

Finally, nursing home residents and their families would have access to critical information to help them choose a high-quality nursing home that is best able to meet their goals, values, and preferences. Additionally, residents, families, and other stakeholders (e.g., states, researchers) would have access to information about the finances, operation, and ownership of nursing homes and be able to understand the quality of care provided across common ownership or management.

CONCLUSION

The urgency to reform how care is financed, delivered, and regulated in nursing home settings is undeniable. Failure to act will guarantee the continuation of many shortcomings that prevent the delivery of high-quality care in all nursing homes. The COVID-19 pandemic provided powerful evidence of the deleterious impact of inaction and inattention to long-standing quality problems on residents, families, and staff. The disruption of the pandemic, however, also serves as a stark reminder that nursing homes need to be better prepared to respond effectively to the next public health emergency, and serves as an impetus to drive critically important and urgently needed innovations to improve the quality of nursing home care. Implementing the committee's integrated set of recommendations will move the nation closer to making high-quality, person-centered, and equitable care a reality.

It has been 35 years since the passage of OBRA 87 and landmark nursing home reform measures. It is of the utmost importance that all nursing home partners work together to ensure that residents, their chosen families, and staff will no longer have to wait for needed improvements to the quality of care in nursing homes. The time to act is now.

Appendix A

Biographic Sketches

COMMITTEE MEMBERS

Betty Ferrell, R.N., Ph.D., M.A., CHPN, FAAN, FPCN (NAM 2019) (*chair*), is the director of nursing research and education and a professor at the City of Hope Medical Center in Duarte, California. She has been in nursing for more than 43 years and has focused her clinical expertise and research in pain management, quality of life (QOL), and palliative care. Dr. Ferrell is a fellow of the American Academy of Nursing, and she has more than 450 publications in peer-reviewed journals and texts. She is the principal investigator of the End-of-Life Nursing Education Consortium (ELNEC) project. She directs several other funded projects related to palliative care in cancer centers and QOL issues, including ELNEC–Geriatrics for Long-Term settings. Dr. Ferrell was a co-chairperson of the National Consensus Project for Quality Palliative Care. Dr. Ferrell completed a master's degree in theology, ethics, and culture from Claremont Graduate University in 2007. She is recognized for her career as an oncology researcher addressing issues such as quality of life, family caregiving, and palliative care, to name a few. She has authored 12 books including the *Oxford Textbook of Palliative Nursing*. She is co-author of the text *The Nature of Suffering and the Goals of Nursing* (2008) and of *Making Health Care Whole: Integrating Spirituality into Patient Care* (2010). In 2013, she was named one of the 30 visionaries in the field by the American Academy of Hospice and Palliative Medicine. Dr. Ferrell was elected to the National Academy of Medicine in 2019.

Gregory L. Alexander, Ph.D., R.N., FAAN, FACMI, FIAHSI, a professor at the Columbia University School of Nursing, is an internationally recognized nursing informaticist and clinical expert with more than 25 years of research and clinical leadership. His program of research is focused on technologies used to support patient care delivery, improve patient outcomes, and to identify and address disparities with an emphasis on aging populations. He leads national research studies benchmarking trends in information technology adoption and use. In these studies, he is evaluating the impact of health information systems on quality measures, resident outcomes, and disparities in nursing homes. As a Fulbright U.S. Scholar in 2017, he has led international research teams from Australia, New Zealand, Norway, United Kingdom, Canada, and the United States who are interested in investigating information technology use as it relates to resident care, clinical support, and quality measures. Dr. Alexander is editor of the Technology Innovations section of the *Journal of Gerontological Nursing.* Dr. Alexander's book, *An Introduction to Clinical Health Information Technology for Long Term/Post-Acute Care Settings,* shows how research identifies and promotes evidence informing new models of care, including technology implementation trends and safety and quality impacts for long-term and post-acute settings.

Mary Ersek, Ph.D., R.N., FPCN, is senior scientist at the Department of Veterans Affairs and professor of palliative care at the University of Pennsylvania School of Nursing, with a secondary appointment at the Perelman School of Medicine, University of Pennsylvania. For more than 20 years, Dr. Ersek has led and collaborated with other investigators on many research projects aimed at improving care in nursing homes and for persons with dementia. These studies involved recruiting and working with facilities, staff and providers, and residents and their families from over 70 nursing homes across the United States from Seattle, Washington, to Philadelphia, Pennsylvania, to Tuscaloosa, Alabama. In addition to these studies, Dr. Ersek developed the End-of-Life Nursing Education Consortium geriatric curriculum which has been disseminated to nursing home staff and other professionals across the United States. From 2005 to 2008, Dr. Ersek served on the Washington State Board of Nursing Home Administrators.

Colleen Galambos, Ph.D., LCSW, LCSW-C, ACSW, FGSA, is professor and the Helen Bader Endowed Chair in Applied Gerontology at the University of Wisconsin–Milwaukee. She is an adjunct professor with the Medical College of Wisconsin. Dr. Galambos is a fellow of the Gerontological Society of America and the American Academy of Social Work and Social Welfare. In 2016, she was named a National Association of Social Workers Pioneer, and in 2020 she was named a Woman of Influence by the *Milwaukee*

Business Journal. Her practice experience includes clinical, administrative, policy, and research positions in a variety of health and long-term care organizations. She served on the State of Missouri Board of Nursing Home Administrators from 2004 to 2011 and was Vice President of the Board from 2010 to 2011. She was a member of the Consensus Study Committee, Health and Medical Dimensions of Social Isolation and Loneliness in Older Adults, National Academies of Sciences, Engineering, and Medicine from 2018 to 2020. Dr. Galambos' active research areas include care transitions, advance care planning/end-of-life decision making, aging in place, health and long-term care systems quality improvement, gerontechnology, older adults and behavioral health, practice approaches in work with older adults, family caregiving, and competency-based gerontological education. Most recently, she worked as an investigator on several research projects aimed at improving long-term care, funded by the Centers for Medicare & Medicaid Services, the National Institutes of Health, and the Agency for Healthcare Research and Quality, totaling over $37 million in grant support.

David C. Grabowski, Ph.D., is a professor of health care policy in the Department of Health Care Policy at Harvard Medical School. His research examines the economics of aging with a particular interest in the areas of long-term care and post-acute care. He has published more than 200 peer-reviewed research articles, and his work has been funded by the National Institute on Aging, the Agency for Healthcare Research and Quality, and a number of private foundations. He has testified in front of Congress four times on issues related to the care of older adults. Dr. Grabowski is a member of the Medicare Payment Advisory Commission. He has also served on several Centers for Medicare & Medicaid Services (CMS) technical expert panels, including the recent CMS Coronavirus Commission on Safety and Quality in Nursing Homes. He is an associate editor of the journal *Forum for Health Economics and Policy*, and he is a member of the editorial boards of the *American Journal of Health Economics, B.E. Journal of Economic Analysis & Policy*, and *Journal of the American Medical Directors Association*. Dr. Grabowski also serves on the technical expert panel that advises CMS on the Nursing Home Compare five-star rating system that publicly reports nursing home quality.

Kathy Greenlee, J.D., is the president and chief executive officer of Greenlee Global LLC. She provides independent consulting services and public speaking. She works with states on improving government programs that address aging, disability, and abuse. From 2009 to 2016, Ms. Greenlee served as the assistant secretary for aging at the U.S. Department of Health and Human Services in Washington, DC. She was appointed to the position by President Obama and confirmed by the U.S. Senate. In 2012, Assistant Secretary Greenlee became the administrator of the Administration for Community Living (ACL), an agency she created by combining the Administration on Aging, the Office on Disability, and the Administration for Developmental Disabilities. When the Workforce Investment and Opportunities Act was signed into law, the National Institute for Disabilities, Independent Living, and Rehabilitation Research was moved to ACL, as were the programs that support centers for independent living. She previously served 18 years in the Kansas state government as an assistant attorney general, general counsel for the Kansas Insurance Department, chief of staff for the Governor, State Long-Term Care Ombudsman, and Kansas Secretary of Aging. Greenlee is the board chair for the National Council on Aging. She joined the WellSky Human and Social Services Advisory Board in late 2020; board members provide general advice on key issues in aging, disability, and homelessness.

Lisa G. Kaplowitz, M.D., M.H.S.A., works for the Virginia Department of Health as a physician expert consultant for the department's COVID-19 Vaccine Unit. Up until recently, Dr. Kaplowitz was a public health physician and deputy health officer for Arlington County, Virginia. From 2010 to 2019, she worked within the U.S. Department of Health and Human Services (HHS). She was senior medical advisor within the Office of the Assistant Secretary for Preparedness and Response (ASPR) (October 2015–March 2019) and in the Substance Abuse and Mental Health Services Administration (October 2015–February 2018). From March 2010 to October 2015 she was the deputy assistant secretary for policy in the Office of the ASPR, responsible for directing and coordinating policy and strategic planning for the Office of the ASPR. Prior to joining HHS, Dr. Kaplowitz was the director of the health department for the City of Alexandria. From 2002 to 2008, she was the deputy commissioner for emergency preparedness and response in the Virginia Department of Health, responsible for the development and implementation of Virginia's public health and medical response to all natural and manmade emergencies. She was a health policy fellow with the Institute of Medicine (now the National Academy of Medicine) in Washington, DC, in 1996–1997, working in Senator Jay Rockefeller's office on health financing and end-of-life care.

R. Tamara Konetzka, Ph.D., is the Louis Block Professor of Public Health Sciences at The University of Chicago, with a secondary appointment in the Department of Medicine, Section of Geriatrics and Palliative Medicine. Konetzka is an internationally recognized expert in the health policy and economics of long-term and post-acute care. Her research focuses on the incentives created by health care policy, including payment policy, and their effects on quality of care. She has been the principal investigator on numerous major federal research grants employing state-of-the-art econometric designs and mixed methods. This body of work has led to significant advances in knowledge of the drivers of nursing home quality, how public reporting of quality changes the behavior of providers and consumers, and the unintended consequences of home-based long-term and post-acute care. She testified twice to the U.S. Senate on issues related to nursing homes during the COVID-19 pandemic. Dr. Konetzka serves on the editorial boards of *Health Services Research* and the *Journal of the American Medical Directors Association* and is editor-in-chief of *Medical Care Research and Review*. She also serves on the technical expert panel that advises the Centers for Medicare & Medicaid Services on the Nursing Home Compare five-star rating system which publicly reports nursing home quality.

Christine A. Mueller, Ph.D., R.N., FGSA, FAAN, is a professor, the senior executive associate dean for academic programs, and a long-term care professor in nursing at the School of Nursing at the University of Minnesota. Dr. Mueller's 46-year career has focused on improving the care of elders living in nursing homes, specifically on factors that can influence the quality of nursing home care, such as nurse staffing, care delivery systems, and the role of the nurse and nursing home culture change. In the 1990s she worked on the project team for the Health Care Financing Administration Multistate Nursing Home Case-Mix and Quality demonstration project that developed the Minimum Data Set (MDS) Plus (now the MDS 3.0), quality indicators, and the Resource Utilization Group case-mix classification system for nursing homes. She was a team lead for the state of Minnesota in designing a case-mix classification system for Minnesota nursing homes and a set of quality indicators which have been used for quality payment incentives and a public report card. Dr. Mueller previously served on the board of directors for the Pioneer Network, the national organization promoting person-directed care in nursing homes.

Marilyn J. Rantz, Ph.D., R.N., FAAN (NAM 2012), has been affiliated with the University of Missouri Sinclair School of Nursing since 1992. She held the named position of University Hospital Professor of Nursing, has a joint appointment in the Department of Family and Community Medicine, was the Helen E. Nahm Chair from 2008 to 2015, and was awarded the University of Missouri Curators' Professor title in 2010. In 2012, she was elected into the Institute of Medicine (now the National Academy of Medicine) and is the only individual to be twice named as an Edge Runner by the American Academy of Nursing for two different innovations: 2008 for Aging in Place and TigerPlace and 2012 for the Quality Improvement Program for Missouri. She was inducted as a Living Legend by the American Academy of Nursing in 2020. Dr. Rantz has sustained a research program to improve the quality of care for the elderly. Her innovative work in nursing home quality spans 40 years, both in practice and as a leading researcher. She is an international expert in quality measurement in nursing homes. In 2012 and 2016, she secured $14.8 million and $19.8 million in grants from the Centers for Medicare & Medicaid Services for their Initiative to Reduce Avoidable Hospitalizations among Nursing Facility Residents—Phase 1 and Phase 2. In total, Dr. Rantz and her multidisciplinary research teams have garnered over $92 million in funds to support work measuring the effectiveness of nurse care coordination, cutting-edge research in long-term care, new delivery models of care for older adults, and technology development to enhance aging in place of community-dwelling elders. Dr. Rantz has small minority shares in Foresite Healthcare, which was developed in the business incubator at the University of Missouri to commercialize the patented sensor technology to enhance aging in place—used primarily in assisted living and independent living—developed by the UM Eldertech Research team. Dr. Rantz is not on the board of directors and not involved in business operations, nor does she receive any financial support or technology from Foresite.

Debra Saliba, M.D., M.P.H., AGSF, is a professor of medicine at the University of California, Los Angeles, where she holds the Anna & Harry Borun Endowed Chair in Geriatrics. At the Los Angeles Department of Veterans Affairs (VA), she is in the Geriatric Research, Education, and Clinical Center and is the associate director for education in the Health Services Research and Development Service's Center for the Study of Healthcare Innovation, Implementation & Policy. She also is a senior natural scientist at the RAND Corporation. As a practicing geriatrician and health services researcher, Dr. Saliba's research focuses on creating tools and knowledge that can be applied to improving the quality of care and quality of life of vulnerable older adults across care settings, including clinics, hospitals, homes, post-acute care, and nursing homes. She was the principal investigator for Center for Medicare & Medicaid Services (CMS) Minimum Data Set (MDS) 3.0 revision and evaluation project and collaborative VA MDS validation project. The revised MDS included, for the first time, resident self-reports of symptoms and preferences. National testing showed significant gains in item validity, staff satisfaction, and assessment efficiency. Her current research includes developing measures of physician performance in post-acute and long-term care; the inclusion of patient and family priorities in weighting quality measures; an evaluation of the implementation of the balancing incentives program; and the relationship between nursing home quality and staffing structures. Dr. Saliba is past president and board chair of the American Geriatrics Society. She serves on the editorial boards of *The Gerontologist* and the *Journal of Post-Acute and Long-Term Care Medicine* and is an executive editor for the *Journal of the American Geriatrics Society*. She serves on several national expert panels, including the CMS five-star technical expert panel.

William Scanlon, Ph.D., is an independent consultant to West Health. He is also a member of the Medicaid and Children's Health Insurance Program Payment and Access Commission and the Academy Health Oral Health Interest Group Advisory Committee. He began conducting health services research on the Medicaid and Medicare programs in 1975, with a focus on such issues as the provision and financing of long-term care services and supports and provider payment policies. He previously held positions at Georgetown University and the Urban Institute, was the managing director of health care issues at the U.S. Government Accountability Office, and served on the Medicare Payment Advisory Commission. Dr. Scanlon received his doctorate in economics from the University of Wisconsin, Madison.

Philip D. Sloane, M.D., M.P.H., is a distinguished professor and the director of academic advancement at the University of North Carolina at Chapel Hill (UNC-CH) School of Medicine. He co-directs the Program on Aging, Disability, and Long-Term Care of the Cecil G. Sheps Center for Health Services Research at UNC-CH. He is particularly noted for his work concerning the management of behavioral symptoms in Alzheimer's disease, for which he received the prestigious Pioneer Award from the U.S. Alzheimer's Association. Dr. Sloane is also committed to the education of professionals, paraprofessionals, and consumers. He has co-edited multiple editions of *Essentials of Family Medicine and Primary Care Geriatrics*, and he co-founded the Carolina Alzheimer's Network, a program dedicated to training primary care providers in evidence-based dementia care. Recent research foci include antibiotic stewardship in long-term care, understanding sources of stress and coping among nursing assistants, assisting family caregivers of persons with dementia in assessing and managing medical symptoms, and training nursing assistants to provide better oral hygiene care. Dr. Sloane is also the co-editor-in-chief of the *Journal of the American Medical Directors Association: The Journal of Post-Acute and Long-Term Care Medicine*.

David G. Stevenson, Ph.D., is currently a professor of health policy in the Department of Health Policy at Vanderbilt University School of Medicine. Dr. Stevenson's primary research interests are long-term care and end-of-life care. His previous work has focused on a broad range of topics in these areas, including the evolution of Medicare's hospice benefit, the role of ownership in the provision of resident and patient care, and quality assurance in the nursing home and hospice sectors. Dr. Stevenson received a B.A. from Oberlin College, a S.M. in health policy and management from the Harvard T.H. Chan School of Public Health, and a Ph.D. in health policy from Harvard University. His previous faculty appointment was in the Department of Health Care Policy at Harvard Medical School. Dr. Stevenson serves on the editorial boards of *Health Services Research,* the *Journal of Pain and Symptom Management,* and the *Journal of the American Medical Director's Association.* Dr. Stevenson also serves on the technical expert panel that advises the Centers for Medicare & Medicaid Services on the Nursing Home Compare five-star rating system that publicly reports nursing home quality.

Jasmine L. Travers, Ph.D., AGPCNP-BC, CCRN, R.N., is an assistant professor of nursing at NYU Rory Meyers College of Nursing. Her career is dedicated to designing and conducting research to improve health outcomes and reduce health disparities in vulnerable older adult groups using both quantitative and qualitative approaches. Currently, Dr. Travers is the principle investigator of a Robert Wood Johnson Foundation 4-year Career Development Award through the Harold Amos Medical Faculty Development Program in which she is examining the association of neighborhood disadvantage with nursing home outcomes and a Paul B. Beeson Emerging Leader 5-year K76 Award through the National Institute on Aging which in this mixed-method study she will develop a survey instrument aimed to identify unmet needs that are disproportionately driving avoidable nursing home placements. Dr. Travers has published widely on the topics of aging, long-term care, health disparities, workforce diversity, vaccinations, and infections and sits on the National Academies of Sciences, Engineering, and Medicine Committee on the Quality of Care in Nursing Homes as well as the AARP Public Policy Institute Advisory Panel.

Reginald Tucker-Seeley, M.A., Sc.M., Sc.D., is the vice president, health equity, at ZERO—The End of Prostate Cancer. He is currently taking a leave of absence from his position as the inaugural holder of the Edward L. Schneider chair in gerontology and an assistant professor in the Leonard Davis School of Gerontology at the University of Southern California. His research has focused primarily on the social determinants of health across the life course, such as the association between the neighborhood environment and health behavior, and on individual-level socioeconomic determinants of multi-morbidity; mortality; self-rated physical, mental, and oral health; and adult height. Mr. Tucker-Seeley has a long-standing interest in the impact of health and social policy on racial/ethnic minorities and across socioeconomic groups. He has experience working on local and state-level health disparities policy and in the measuring and reporting of health disparities at the state level.

Rachel M. Werner, M.D., Ph.D., is the executive director of the Leonard Davis Institute of Health Economics. She is a professor of medicine at the University of Pennsylvania Perelman School of Medicine as well as the Robert D. Eilers Professor of Health Care Management and Economics at the Wharton School and a practicing physician at the Philadelphia Department of Veterans Affairs (VA). Over the last two decades, Dr. Werner has built a foundational research program examining the effects of health care policies on the organization and delivery of health care, with a focus on provider payment and quality-improvement incentives. This research has revealed the many intended and unintended effects of quality measurement and incentives and was among the first to recognize that public reporting of quality information may worsen racial disparities. She is a core investigator with the VA Health Services Research and Development Service's Center for Health Equity Research and Promotion. She has received numerous awards for her work, including the Alice Hersh New Investigator Award from AcademyHealth, the Presidential Early Career Award for Scientists and Engineers, and the American Federation of Medical Research Outstanding Investigator Award. Dr. Werner was elected to the National Academy of Medicine in 2018.

STAFF

Kaitlyn Friedman, M.Sc, is an associate program officer in the Health and Medicine Division of the National Academies of Sciences, Engineering, and Medicine. In this capacity she supports the Forum on Mental Health and Substance Use Disorders, the Roundtable on Quality Care for People with Serious Illness, and the Consensus Study on the Quality of Care in Nursing Homes. Outside of the Academies, Ms. Friedman volunteers on the Research Centers and Labs Committee of the Duke Global Health Institute Equity Task Force and on the Data Management Team of the COVID-19 Task Force on Domestic Violence. Prior to joining the Academies in 2019, Ms. Friedman served as a research coordinator for Duke University, exploring the associations between violence-related injuries and alcohol use as well as managing the implementation of a feasibility trial of a brief intervention for harmful and hazardous alcohol use in Moshi, Tanzania. She also interned with the World Health Organization in 2018, contributing to technical reports on drug-impaired driving and road traffic injuries. Ms. Friedman received her master of science in global health from Duke University in 2019 and her bachelor of arts in medicine, health, and society from Vanderbilt University in 2017.

Laurie Graig, M.A., is a senior program officer in the Health and Medicine Division of the National Academies of Sciences, Engineering, and

Medicine (NASEM). In this capacity, she serves as the director of the Roundtable on Quality Care for People with Serious Illness, a convening activity that brings together leaders from government, industry, academia, health professional groups and associations, and philanthropic and patient advocacy organizations to discuss key challenges related to improving care for people with serious illness. Ms. Graig also directed another convening activity, the Forum on Mental Health and Substance Use Disorders. Previously, she served as study director of the consensus committee on Policy Issues in the Clinical Development and Use of Biomarkers for Molecularly Targeted Therapies. Prior to joining NASEM in 2014, Ms. Graig worked on a broad range of health care systems research and policy issues within for-profit and not-for-profit consulting organizations. Her previous experience includes participating in an evaluation of state-level health care improvement partnerships as a consultant to AcademyHealth. She also served as a project manager with Altarum Institute, where she managed a large, multifaceted project designed to improve the operational efficiency of community health centers using the Lean process improvement methodology, and she worked on a project funded by the U.S. Department of Health and Human Services (HHS) focused on the emergency system for advance registration of volunteer health professionals. In addition, she contributed to studies and reports for HHS in the area of public health planning and emergency preparedness, such as mass casualty events and pandemic influenza. Ms. Graig previously worked for the research and information center of Watson Wyatt, a worldwide management consulting firm. During her tenure, she authored three editions of *Health of Nations: An International Perspective on U.S. Health Care Reform* published by CQ Books (1991, 3rd edition). Ms. Graig is a former Peace Corps Volunteer, having served in Burkina Faso, West Africa. Ms. Graig received her M.A. from the University of Virginia and her B.S. from Georgetown University.

Rukshana Gupta is a senior program assistant on the Board of Health Care Services at the National Academies of Sciences, Engineering, and Medicine. Ms. Gupta recently graduated from McGill University in Montreal where she earned her bachelor of arts and sciences with a double major in biology and sociology. In university, Ms. Gupta was involved with the McGill Students' Friends of Medecins sans Frontieres and the McGill Children's Health Alliance of Montreal. During her senior year, she directed the annual Global Health Case Competition, which brings together students from around Montreal to come up with solutions to a complex, current issue in global health. At the National Academies, Ms. Gupta has been supporting several projects including the Forum on Aging, Disability, and Independence.

Tracy Lustig, D.P.M., M.P.H., is a senior program officer with the Health and Medicine Division of the National Academies of Sciences, Engineering, and Medicine. Dr. Lustig was trained in podiatric medicine and surgery and spent several years in private practice. In 1999, she was awarded a congressional fellowship with the American Association for the Advancement of Science and spent 1 year working in the office of Ron Wyden of the U.S. Senate. Dr. Lustig joined the National Academies in 2004. She was the study director for consensus studies on the geriatrics workforce, oral health, ovarian cancer research, and the 2020 report *Social Isolation and Loneliness in Older Adults: Opportunities for the Health Care System*. She has also directed workshops on the allied health workforce, the use of telehealth to serve rural populations, assistive technologies, hearing loss, and biomarkers of disability. In 2009, she staffed an Academies-wide initiative on the "Grand Challenges of an Aging Society" and subsequently helped to launch the Forum on Aging, Disability, and Independence, which she currently directs. Dr. Lustig has a doctor of podiatric medicine degree from Temple University and a master of public health degree with a concentration in health policy from The George Washington University.

Sharyl J. Nass, Ph.D., serves as the director of the Board on Health Care Services and the director of the National Cancer Policy Forum at the National Academies of Sciences, Engineering, and Medicine. The National Academies provide independent, objective analysis and advice to the nation to solve complex problems and inform public policy decisions related to science, technology, and medicine. To enable the best possible care for all patients, the board undertakes scholarly analysis of the organization, financing, effectiveness, workforce, and delivery of health care, with an emphasis on quality, cost, and accessibility. The forum examines policy issues pertaining to the entire continuum of cancer research and care. For more than two decades, Dr. Nass has worked on a broad range of health and science policy topics which includes the quality and safety of health care and clinical trials, developing technologies for precision medicine, and strategies to support clinician well-being. She has a Ph.D. from Georgetown University and undertook postdoctoral training at the Johns Hopkins University School of Medicine as well as a research fellowship at the Max Planck Institute in Germany. She also holds a B.S. and an M.S. from the University of Wisconsin–Madison. She has been the recipient of the Cecil Medal for Excellence in Health Policy Research, a Distinguished Service Award from the National Academies, and the Institute of Medicine staff team achievement award (as team leader).

Nikita Varman, M.P.H., is a research associate with the Health and Medicine Division of the National Academies of Sciences, Engineering, and

Medicine. Prior to joining the National Academies, Ms. Varman interned at Boston Children's Hospital's Office of Government Relations, where she advocated for children's health care issues at the state and federal levels, and at Medecins sans Frontieres, where she researched accessibility of hepatitis C diagnostics. She is a 2020 graduate from Boston University with a master's degree in public health and concentrations in health policy and law as well as community assessment, program design, implementation, and evaluation. Ms. Varman also holds a bachelor of science in health sciences and a bachelor of arts in political science, cum laude, as a Posse Foundation Scholar and Scarlet Key recipient from Boston University in 2019.

Appendix B

Examples from the Initiative to Reduce Avoidable Hospitalizations Among Nursing Facility Residents

This appendix provides examples of successful demonstration projects in the Initiative to Reduce Avoidable Hospitalizations among Nursing Facility Residents. (Details of the initiative and the related phases are in Chapter 3.) These examples all had a strong clinical focus. Table B-1 provides an overview of each program, including program details and specific components of the intervention. Table B-2 shows the impact of the interventions on clinical outcomes and cost savings in phase one. The assessment focused on the following measures: all-cause hospitalizations, potentially avoidable hospitalizations, all-cause emergency department (ED) visits, and potentially avoidable ED visits. Table B-3 shows the impacts demonstrated in phase two of the initiative on the two different groups. In phase two, the Centers for Medicare & Medicaid Services offered payment incentives that were added to the facilities that participated in phase one (leaving registered nurse and advanced practice registered nurse support in place) and added an additional "payment only" intervention group (without the phase one supports).

TABLE B-1 Program Details and Components for Demonstration Projects

PROGRAM	PROGRAM DETAILS	COMPONENTS
Missouri Quality Initiative (MOQI) SOURCES: Nursing Home Help, 2021a,b.	- Targeted nursing homes with high hospital transfer rates - Phase one: 16 nursing homes - Phase two: 40 nursing homes - Currently continuing through New Path Health Solutions, LLC **GOALS:** - Reduce hospitalizations - Reduce Medicare expenditures - Increase use of advance directives and end-of-life planning - Improve early illness recognition - Improve management of health conditions - Increase the use of health information technology (HIT) - Reduce medication use (including antipsychotic medications among people with dementia)	Multilevel intervention included: - Hiring a full-time advanced practice registered nurse (APRN) and MOQI team member to implement the program and share best practices for each nursing home - Employing processes and tools from the Interventions to Reduce Acute Transfers (INTERACT) program - Using feedback forms of the clinical outcome measures to facilities monthly - Encouraging physician engagement - Using advance directives - Supporting homes to implement and sustain HIT - Engaging a multidisciplinary support team
New York – Reducing Avoidable Hospitalizations (NY-RAH) SOURCE: NY-RAH, 2013.	- Phase one: 29 nursing homes - Phase two: 40 nursing homes This was the only program in the initiative where the registered nurse (RN) was employed to act more in an advisory role focused on knowledge sharing rather than in a clinical role. This resulted in a much slower buy-in, implementation, and knowledge dissemination.	NY-RAH disseminated a toolkit from programs such as INTERACT and Medical Orders for Life Sustaining Treatment to onsite providers with tools and interventions to improve care, reduce hospitalizations, and improve hospital transition processes. These evidence-based interventions were complemented with initiatives to use electronic methods to share information and resources, collect data, and create and analyze metrics.

Optimizing Patient Transfers, Impacting Medical Quality, and Improving Symptoms: Transforming Institutional Care (OPTIMISTIC) SOURCES: OPTIMISTIC, 2021, 2022.	The OPTIMISTIC program ran through Indiana University and other collaborative partners in the state from September 2012 through October 2020. 19 facilities were a part of the OPTIMISTIC program in phase one and 25 additional facilities in phase two (OPTIMISTIC, 2021). **OVERALL GOALS:** - Reduce unnecessary hospitalization - Improve medical care - Enhance transitional care - Support palliative care Leaders of OPTIMISTIC subsequently helped establish the startup company Probari to implement a program modeled after OPTIMISTIC.	Train-the-trainer model to - Build nursing staff capacity - Implement evidence-based practices for care and communication - Invest in advanced care planning Two pillars of the program: - An electronic data tracking system for patient records and employing RNs - Using APRNs to facilitate standardized education on quality improvement
Reduce Avoidable Hospitalizations Using Evidence-Based Interventions for Nursing Facilities (RAVEN) SOURCE: RAVEN, 2021.	In 2012, the University of Pittsburgh Medical Center began RAVEN by implementing five interventions across 18 diverse long-term care facilities to reduce hospitalizations, improve resident health outcomes, decrease spending, and foster culture change.	The five interventions were - Facility-based enhanced care staff - Evidenced-based assessment and clinical documentation tools - Innovative education - Enhanced medication management - Telemedicine. The primary pillar of the program involved having full-time APRNs deliver clinical care and education.

TABLE B-2 Phase One: Improvements in Outcomes and Cost Savings for Demonstration Projects

	All Medicare Services	Reductions in All-Cause Hospitalization		Reductions in Potentially Avoidable Hospitalizations		Reductions in All-Cause Emergency Department (ED) Visits		Reductions in Potentially Avoidable ED Visits	
	Phase one cost savings	Phase one outcomes	Phase one cost savings	Phase one outcomes	Phase one cost savings	Phase one outcomes	Phase one cost savings	Phase one outcomes	Phase one cost savings
MOQI	6.3%	32.0%	28.6%	49.9%	40.2%	41.7%	36.3%	56.0%	42.8%
NY-RAH	1.9%	11.4%	7.3%	19.4%	13.3%	12.4%	8.7%	14.4%	9.8%
OPTIMISTIC	6.9%	24.9%	21.6%	38.1%	24.9%	7.1%	8.7%	17.6%	24.1%
RAVEN	12.3%	17.3%	27.6%	29.6%	35.3%	2.5%	20.5%	25.5%	39.9%

SOURCE: RTI International, 2017.

TABLE B-3 Phase Two: Outcomes for Different Intervention Groups

	Phase Two: Payment plus Clinical Supports Group	Phase Two: Payment Only Group
MOQI	Potentially avoidable emergency department visits and potentially avoidable all-cause transfers significantly increased for the six qualifying diagnoses	Mixed results, no significant changes across all measures
NY-RAH	Mixed direction results for use and expenditure measures, none statistically significant	No significant changes in use and expenditure measures
OPTIMISTIC	Increases in most measures for hospitalization use and expenditures, a few were statistically significant	Mixed direction for significant changes in expenditures but no significant changes in use measures
RAVEN	Significant increases in hospital use and expenditure measures	No significant changes across all

SOURCE: RTI International, 2021.

REFERENCES

Nursing Home Help. 2021a. *MOQI initiative.* https://nursinghomehelp.org/moqi-initiative (accessed March 3, 2021).

Nursing Home Help. 2021b. *The Missouri Quality Initiative for nursing homes (MOQI) (2012-2020).* https://nursinghomehelp.org/wp-content/uploads/2021/05/Missouri-Quality-Initiative-Brief-Phases-12-10-page-052521.pdf (accessed June 11, 2021).

NY-RAH. 2013. *About NY.* https://www.nyrah.org/About.aspx (accessed March 3, 2021).

OPTIMISTIC. 2021. *OPTIMISTIC.* https://www.optimistic-care.org/ (accessed March 3, 2021).

OPTIMISTIC. 2022. *Introducing Probari!* https://www.optimistic-care.org/probari (accessed February 8, 2022).

RAVEN. 2021. *About RAVEN.* https://raven.upmc.com/aboutus.htm (accessed March 3, 2021).

RTI International. 2017. *Evaluation of the Initiative to Reduce Avoidable Hospitalizations among Nursing Facility Residents: Final report.* Waltham, MA: RTI International.

RTI International. 2021. *Evaluation of the Initiative to Reduce Avoidable Hospitalizations among Nursing Facility Residents—Payment reform: Fourth annual report.* Waltham, MA: RTI International.

Appendix C

Recommendations by Area of Measurement and by Area of Research

Table C-1 provides an overview of the areas of measurement included among the committee's recommendations. For some topics, measures exist and can be added to Care Compare immediately, while other areas are in need of development and testing of measures. Table C-2 provides an overview of the priority areas for research (including demonstration projects) and data collection identified by the committee as part of their recommendations. See the committee's full recommendations in Chapter 10.

TABLE C-1 Recommended Quality Measures for Reporting or Development and Testing

DOMAIN	Measure	Recommendation
Staffing	• Staff satisfaction and well-being	6C
	• Structural measures (e.g., routine training in infection prevention, staff employment arrangements [e.g., full-time, part-time, contract and agency staff])	
Financing and Ownership	• Structural measures (e.g., financial performance)	6C
	• Performance of facilities with common ownership	6B
Care Delivery	• Degree of implementation and success of care plan	1A
	• Consumer Assessment of Healthcare Providers and Systems (CAHPS®) survey of resident/family experience	6A
	• Resident preferences	6B
	• Palliative and end-of-life care	6C
	• Receipt of care that aligns with resident's goals, and the attainment of those goals	
	• Implementation of the resident's care plan	
	• Psychosocial and behavioral health	
Quality Assurance	• Oversight performance metrics of survey agencies	5A
	• Effectiveness of long-term care ombudsman programs	5C
Equity	• Risk adjustment	6B
	• Disparities in nursing home care	6D
Health Information Technology (HIT)	• HIT adoption and interoperability	6C, 7B
	• Staff and resident/family perceptions of HIT usability	7B
Emergency Preparedness and Infection Control	• Documentation of emergency plans	1D
	• Conduct of emergency drills	
	• Staff awareness of emergency management plans	
	• Structural measures (e.g., emergency preparedness, training in infection prevention, emergency response management, percentage of single occupancy rooms)	6C

TABLE C-2 Recommended Priority Areas for Research and Data Collection

DOMAIN	Area of Research and Data Collection	Recommendation
Quality Measurement	• Development and testing of various quality measures	See Table C-1
Staffing	• Minimum and optimum staffing standards for direct care providers	2C
	• Baseline demographic information of medical directors, administrators, and directors of nursing	2H
	• Expertise and staffing patterns of medical directors, advanced practice registered nurses, social workers, physicians, and physician assistants	2H
	• Numbers and staffing patterns for all contract and agency staff	2H
	• Systemic barriers and opportunities to improve recruitment, retention, training and advancement of all nursing home workers (particularly certified nursing assistants [CNAs])	2I
Financing and Ownership	• Facility-level data on the finances, operations, and ownership of all nursing homes	3A
	• Quality of care across facilities with common ownership or management company	3B
	• Impact of real estate ownership models and related-party transactions on quality of care	3B
	• Design of a federal long-term care benefit and subsequent state demonstration programs	4A
	• Alternative payment models for long-stay residents	4E

Care Delivery	• Models of care delivery for
	  ○ short-stay and long-stay residents,
	  ○ reduction of care disparities,
	  ○ strengthening connections to community, and
	  ○ innovations in all aspects of care.
		1B

	• Models of care delivery that take advantage of the role of the CNA as a member of the interdisciplinary team	2E

continued

TABLE C-2 Continued

DOMAIN	Area of Research and Data Collection	Recommendation
Quality Assurance	• Oversight performance metrics	5A
	• Long-term reforms such as enhanced data monitoring to triage inspections, increased oversight of poorly performing facilities, modified oversight of high-performing facilities, and greater use of a variety of enforcement remedies	5B
	• Effectiveness of long-term care ombudsman programs	5C
Equity	• Gender, ethnicity, and race-related outcomes of job quality indicators (e.g., hiring, turnover, job satisfaction)	2I
	• Nursing home disparities and the development of policies and culturally tailored interventions	6D
Health Information Technology (HIT)	• Levels of HIT adoption and interoperability	7B
	• Nursing home staff, resident, and family perceptions of HIT usability	7B, 7D
	• Use of HIT to improve resident outcomes	7D
	• Disparities in HIT adoption and use	7D
	• Innovative HIT applications for resident care	1B, 7D

Appendix D

Recommendations by Responsible Partners

TABLE D-1 Implementation of the Committee's Recommendations Organized by Responsible Partners

Responsible Partner	Rec
U.S. Congress	
All relevant federal agencies need to be granted the authority and resources from the U.S. Congress to implement the recommendations of this report.	
Secretary of HHS	
Study ways to establish a new federal long-term care benefit that would expand access and advance equity for all adults who need long-term care, including nursing home care.	4A
HHS as the lead agency (includes individual agencies within HHS)	
Fund research to identify and rigorously test specific minimum and optimum staffing standards for direct-care staff based on resident case mix, and type of staff needed to address the care needs of specific populations. (HHS, e.g., CMS, AHRQ, NIH)	2C
Fund training grants to advance and expand the role of the CNA and develop new models of care delivery that take advantage of the role of the CNA as a member of the interdisciplinary care team. (HRSA)	2E
Fund research on systemic barriers and opportunities to improve the recruitment, training, and advancement of all nursing home workers, with a particular focus on CNAs. This research should include the collection of gender, ethnicity, and race-related outcomes of job quality indicators (e.g., hiring, turnover, job satisfaction). (HHS, e.g., CMS, AHRQ, NIH)	2I

continued

TABLE D-1 Continued

Responsible Partner	Rec
HHS as the lead agency (continued)	
Collect, audit, and make available detailed facility-level data on the finances, operations, and ownership of all nursing homes, ensuring that data allow assessment of staffing patterns, deficiencies, financial arrangements, and payments, related party entities, corporate structures, and objective quality indicators by common owner and management company are available in a real-time, readily usable, and searchable database.	3A, 3B
Require designation of a specific percentage of nursing home Medicare and Medicaid payments to pay for direct care, including staffing (including both the number of staff and their wages and benefits), behavioral health, and clinical care.	4C
Extend bundled payment initiatives for short-stay nursing home acute care to include all conditions, and hold hospitals financially accountable (i.e., put hospitals "at risk") for Medicare post-acute care spending and outcomes as part of effort to improve the value of and accountability for Medicare short-stay post-acute nursing home payments. (HHS/CMS/CMMI)	4D
Conduct demonstration projects to explore the use of APMs that will eliminate current misalignment for long-stay residents by fragmented payment system. APMs to use global capitated budgets from a single payer, making provider organizations or plans accountable for total costs of care. APM's capitated rate to include post-acute care and hospice care for long-term nursing home residents to address financial misalignment between Medicare and Medicaid payments while supporting care coordination. Designs and payments of the demonstration projects should be tied to broad-based quality metrics, including staffing metrics, resident experience of care, functional status, and end-of-life care to ensure that APMs maintain quality of care, particularly in areas such as post-acute care, end-of-life care, and hospice care. (HHS/CMS)	4E
Advocate for increased funding for LTC ombudsman programs with additional resources allocated toward hiring additional paid staff and training staff and volunteers, bolstering programmatic infrastructure, making data on state LTC ombudsman programs and activities publicly available, and developing summary metrics designed to document the effectiveness of these programs in advocating for nursing home residents. (ACL)	5C
Expand and enhance existing publicly reported quality measures in Care Compare: • Increase the weight of staffing measures within the five-star composite rating • Facilitate the ability to see quality performance of facilities that share common ownership • Improve validity of MDS-based clinical quality • Conduct additional testing to improve differentiation of the five-star composite rating (HHS/CMS/NIH/AHRQ)	6B
Fund the development and adoption of new nursing home measures to Care Compare related to palliative and end-of-life care, receipt of care that aligns with resident's goals and the attainment of those goals, implementation of the resident's care plan, staff satisfaction, and psychosocial and behavioral health. Also develop and adopt new structural measures (e.g., HIT adoption and interoperability; single-occupancy rooms; emergency preparedness; infection prevention training; financial performance; staff employment arrangements).	6C

TABLE D-1 Continued

Responsible Partner	Rec
HHS as the lead agency (continued)	
Develop an overall health equity strategy for nursing homes that includes defining, measuring, evaluating, and intervening on disparities in nursing home care. Specifically, strategy to include definitions of health equity and disparities in nursing homes, including race, ethnicity, LGBTQ+ populations, and sources of payment; new measures of disparities in nursing home care to be included in a national report card. Prioritize funding research regarding disparities and the development of policies and culturally tailored interventions. (HHS, NIH, and other agencies)	6D
Use data to identify the types and degree of disparity to prioritize when action is needed and to identify the promising pathways to reduce or eliminate those disparities. (HHS, in partnership with state and local governments)	
Identify a pathway to provide financial incentives to nursing homes for certified EHR adoption and develop EHR certification criteria that promote adoption of health information exchange. (CMS, ONC)	7A
Develop measures for HIT adoption and interoperability, consistent with other health care organizations; measure levels of HIT adoption and interoperability on an annual basis and report results in Care Compare; measure and report nursing home staff, resident, and family perceptions of HIT usability. (HHS)	7B
Provide financial support for the development and ongoing implementation of workforce training emphasizing core HIT competencies for nursing home leadership and staff. (CMS, HRSA)	7C
Fund rigorous evaluation studies to explore use of HIT to improve nursing home resident outcomes; disparities in HIT adoption and use across nursing homes; innovative HIT applications for resident care; and assessment of clinician, resident, and family perceptions of HIT usability. (ONC, AHRQ)	7D
CMS as lead agency	
Enhance the current minimum staffing requirements for every nursing home to include 1. Minimum on-site RN 24/7 coverage (in addition to the director of nursing) with additional RN coverage that reflects resident census, acuity, and case mix as well as needs as determined by the residents' assessments and care plans 2. Full-time social worker with a minimum of bachelor's degree in social work from a program accredited by CSWE and 1 year of supervised social work experience working directly with individuals to address behavioral and psychosocial care 3. An infection prevention and control specialist who is an RN, APRN, or a physician at a level of dedicated time sufficient to meet the needs of the size and case mix of the nursing home	2B
Create incentives for nursing homes to hire qualified licensed clinical social workers at the M.S.W. or Ph.D. level and APRNs for clinical care, including allowing Medicare billing and reimbursement for these services.	2D

continued

TABLE D-1 Continued

Responsible Partner	Rec
CMS as lead agency (continued)	
Establish minimum education and national competency requirements for nursing home staff, including nursing home administrator, medical director, director of nursing, director of social services, and CNAs.	2F
Require all levels of nursing home staff to complete annual continuing education training to meet national competency standards.	2G
Implement state demonstration programs (prior to national implementation) to test a model for a federal long-term care benefit that would expand access and advance equity for all adults who need long-term care, including nursing home care.	4A
Ensure Medicaid payments are at a level adequate to cover the delivery of comprehensive, high-quality, and equitable care to nursing home residents across all domains of care as required by existing statute.	4B
Ensure that state survey agencies have adequate capacity, organizational structure, and resources to fulfill their current nursing home oversight responsibilities for monitoring, investigation, and enforcement, particularly for complaints. Refine and expand oversight performance metrics for annual public reporting to facilitate greater accountability that existing federal regulations are being consistently and completely enforced. Use existing strategies of enforcement where states have consistently fallen short of expected standards.	5A
Develop and evaluate strategies that make nursing home quality-assurance efforts more efficient, effective, and responsive, including potential longer-term reforms such as • Enhanced data monitoring; • Increased oversight across a broader segment of poorly performing facilities; • Modified formal oversight activities for high-performing facilities, provided adequate safeguards are in place and specified, real-time quality metrics of nursing homes continue to be met; • Greater use of enforcement remedies beyond civil monetary penalties, including directed plans of correction, temporary management, and chain-wide corporate integrity agreements, denial of admissions and termination from Medicare and Medicaid.	5B
Add the CAHPS measures of resident and family experience (i.e., the nursing home CAHPS survey) to Care Compare.	6A
Allocate funds to state governments for grants to develop and operate state-based, nonprofit, confidential technical assistance programs that have an ongoing and consistent focus on nursing homes to provide up-to-date, evidence-based education and guidance in best clinical and operational practices. Create explicit standards for these programs to promote comparable programs across states.	6E

TABLE D-1 Continued

Responsible Partner	Rec
Combination of federal agencies, state governments, and nursing homes	
Fund rigorous, pragmatic, translational research and demonstration projects to identify the most effective care delivery models to provide high-quality comprehensive, person-centered care for short-stay and long-stay nursing home residents. Research to focus on identifying models that reduce care disparities and strengthen connections between nursing homes, the communities in which they are located, and the broader health care and social services sectors. (Federal agencies [e.g., AHRQ, CMS, CMMI, CDC, NIH], private foundations, academic institutions, and long-term care provider organizations)	1B
To ensure the safety of nursing home residents, enforce existing regulations, including • Every nursing home has a written emergency plan (including evacuation plans) for common public health emergencies and natural disasters in the facility's location, created in partnership with local emergency management and resident and family councils; plan reviewed and updated at least once every year. • Nursing home staff are to be routinely trained in emergency response procedures as well as in the appropriate use of PPE and infection control practices. • Every nursing home has an emergency preparedness communication plan that includes formal procedures for contacting residents' families and staff to provide information about the general condition and location of residents in the case of an emergency/disaster. Documentation of emergency plans as well as the conduct of emergency drills and staff awareness of emergency management plans to be added to Care Compare. (CMS, through state regulatory agencies)	1D
Develop incentives to support innovative, smaller, home-like designs for nursing home environments (both new construction and renovations) that support infection control and person-centered care and improve quality of life for residents. (CMS, and other governmental agencies)	1E
Ensure competitive wages and benefits (including health insurance, child care, and sick pay) to recruit and retain all types of full- and part-time nursing home staff. Consider the following mechanisms: wage floors, requirements for minimum percentage of service rates directed to labor costs for the provision of clinical care, wage pass-through requirements, and student loan forgiveness. (Federal and state governments, together with nursing homes)	2A
Update the regulatory requirements for staffing standards in nursing homes to reflect new minimum requirements and account for case mix based on research on minimum and optimum staffing standards for direct care staff. (CMS and state governments)	2C
Make available free entry-level training and continuing education for CNAs. (Federal, state governments, nursing homes)	2E
Provide flexible, low-cost, and high-quality pathways for nursing home staff to achieve baseline education and competency levels. (CMS and nursing homes)	2F

continued

TABLE D-1 Continued

Responsible Partner	Rec
Combination of federal agencies, state governments, and nursing homes	
Impose oversight and enforcement actions on the owner when data on the finances and ownership of nursing homes reveal a pattern of poor-quality care across facilities with a common owner (including across states). Actions may include: denial of new or renewed licensure, imposition of sanctions, and implementation of strengthened oversight (e.g., through a broadened special focus facilities program). (Federal and state oversight agencies [e.g., CMS, state licensure and survey agencies, DOJ])	5D
Federal Emergency Management Agency	
Reinforce and clarify the emergency support functions (ESFs) of the National Response Framework: • Revise ESF 8 to give greater prominence to nursing homes with the goal of clarifying that nursing homes, specifically, and long-term care facilities more broadly are included within ESF 8 to ensure that state and local emergency management documents and plans contain specific guidance for nursing homes during an emergency. • Revise ESF 15 to include nursing home residents as part of the target group of "individuals with disabilities and others with access and functional needs."	1C
States	
Ensure the development and ongoing maintenance of formal relationships, including strong interface, coordination, and reliable lines of communication, among nursing homes and local, county, and state-level public health and emergency management departments. (State regulatory agencies with federal oversight from FEMA and CMS)	1D
Ensure that nursing homes are represented in • State, county, and local emergency planning sessions and drills • Local government community disaster-response plans • Every phase of local emergency management planning, including mitigation, preparedness, response and recovery • Every nursing home has ready access to personal protective equipment (State emergency management agencies)	1D
Ensure that all new nursing homes are constructed with single-occupancy bedrooms and private bathrooms for most or all residents. (State licensure agencies)	1E
Advocate for funds to LTC ombudsman programs to address cross-state variations in advocacy capability. Develop plans for LTC ombudsman programs to interface effectively with collaborating entities such as adult protective services, state survey agencies, and state and local law enforcement agencies. (State units on aging)	5C
Eliminate certificate-of-need requirements and construction moratoria for nursing homes to encourage the entry of innovative care models and foster robust competition in order to expand consumer choice and improve quality.	5E

TABLE D-1 Continued

Responsible Partner	Rec
Nursing Home Owners/Administrators	
Ensure that each element of the resident care planning process is conducted in an accurate, comprehensive, and appropriate manner for each resident to promote person-centered high-quality care that reflects resident and family preferences. Interdisciplinary care team members make certain that every resident's care plan addresses psychosocial and behavioral health as well as nursing and medical needs. Care plan to be reviewed and evaluated on a regular basis. (Nursing homes, with oversight by CMS)	1A
Construct and reconfigure (renovate) nursing homes to provide smaller, more home-like environments or smaller units within larger nursing homes with single-occupancy bedrooms and private bathrooms. This shift to more home-like settings should be implemented as part of a broader effort to integrate the principles of culture change, such as staff empowerment, consistent staff assignment, and person-centered care practices, into the management and care provided within these settings. (Nursing home owners with the support of federal and state governmental agencies)	1E
Establish consulting or employment relationships with qualified licensed clinical social workers at the M.S.W. or Ph.D. level, APRNs, clinical psychologists, psychiatrists, pharmacists, and others for clinical consultation, staff training, and improvement of care systems as needed to enhance available expertise.	2D
Provide career advancement opportunities and peer mentors for CNAs; cover CNAs' time for completing education and training programs.	2E
Provide ongoing diversity and inclusion training (e.g., self-awareness of and approaches to addressing racism) for all workers and leadership, and ensure training is designed to meet the unique demographic, cultural, linguistic, and transportation needs of the community in which the nursing home is situated and the community of workers within the nursing home.	2G
Provide family caregivers with resources, training, and opportunities to participate as part of the caregiving team in the manner and to the extent that residents desire their chosen family members to be involved.	2G
Collect and report data to CMS regarding • Baseline demographic information of medical directors, administrators, and directors of nursing, including name, licensure, contact information, and tenure; • The geriatrics or long-term care training and expertise of medical directors, APRNs, social workers, physicians, and physician assistants; • The numbers and staffing patterns for these professionals; and • The numbers and staffing patterns for all contract and agency staff providing services in nursing homes.	2H

continued

TABLE D-1 Continued

Responsible Partner	Rec
Other partners (Private foundations, academic institutions, and long-term care provider organizations)	
Prioritize and fund rigorous, pragmatic, translational research and demonstration projects to identify the most effective care-delivery models to provide high-quality comprehensive, person-centered care for short-stay and long-stay nursing home residents.	1B
Include content related to gerontology, geriatric assessment, long-term care, and palliative care, with an additional preference for clinical experience in a nursing home in all education programs to prepare future health care professionals for their roles. (All education programs preparing health care professionals)	2F

NOTES: ACL = Administration for Community Living; AHRQ = Agency for Healthcare Research and Quality; APM = alternative payment model; APRN = advanced practice registered nurse; CAHPS = Consumer Assessment of Healthcare Providers and Systems; CDC = Centers for Disease Control and Protection; CE = continuing education; CMMI = Center for Medicare and Medicaid Innovation; CMS = Centers for Medicare & Medicaid Studies; CNA = certified nursing assistant; CSWE = Council on Social Work Education; DOJ = U.S. Department of Justice; EHR = electronic health record; ESF = emergency support function; FEMA = Federal Emergency Management Agency; HHS = U.S. Department of Health and Human Services; HIT = health information technology; HRSA = Health Resources and Services Administration; LGBTQ+ = lesbian, gay, bisexual, transsexual, queer, and others; LTC = long-term care; MDS = Minimum Data Set; MIPS = Merit-Based Incentive Payment System; NIH = National Institutes of Health; ONC = Office of the National Coordinator for Health Information Technology; PPE = personal protective equipment; RN = registered nurse.

Appendix E

Recommendations Timeline

While all of the recommendations in this report target areas that require immediate attention, the committee recognizes that some recommendations can be fully implemented immediately while others will require planning, coordination, and larger scale effort. Given this recognition of an incremental approach to the integrated set of recommendations, the committee has categorized each of the components of their recommendations according to an estimated implementation timeline. Recommendations that are

- marked for *immediate implementation* are urgent, and largely can move ahead using existing structures.
- identified for *short- and intermediate-term implementation* require action in the short-term to get started, but will require some amount of planning or coordination (such as the planning or coordination needed to initiate new studies or demonstration projects).
- characterized as *long-term implementation* also require initiation in the shorter term, but the committee recognizes that full implementation may take several years (e.g., action dependent upon new research to be conducted or collaboration by multiple agencies across state and federal authorities).

The committee emphasizes that even those recommendations requiring intermediate or longer-term timeframes for complete implementation still need to be initiated now.

Recommendation	Rec
Immediate Implementation	
Documentation of resident's preferences in care plan and review and evaluation of its implementation	1A
Inclusion of explicit references to nursing homes in Emergency Support Functions	1C
Representation of nursing homes in all emergency and disaster planning and management sessions and drills	1D
Enforcement of existing regulations, including • Written emergency plan and emergency preparedness communication plan • Routine training of staff (emergency response procedures, use of personal protective equipment (PPE), infection control)	1D
Pathways for ready access to PPE	1D
Development of formal relationships between nursing homes and local, county, and state-level public health and emergency management departments	1D
Competitive wages and benefits for all nursing home staff	2A
Enhancement of the current minimum staffing requirements for every nursing home to include • Onsite direct-care registered nurse (RN) coverage at a minimum of 24/7 coverage • Additional RN coverage based on resident census, acuity, and case mix • Full-time social worker (with degree in social work and relevant experience) • Infection prevention and control specialist with sufficient dedicated time	2B
Coverage of certified nursing assistant (CNA) time for completing education and training programs	2E
Compliance with existing statute to determine adequacy of Medicaid payments to cover comprehensive care	4B
Adequate capacity and resources for state survey agencies to fulfill current oversight responsibilities	5A
Strong, consistent, responsive, and transparent process for grievances and complaints	5A
Greater use of variety of existing enforcement remedies	5B
Short-Term Implementation	
Addition of documentation of emergency plans and staff training to Care Compare	1D
Enactment of state licensure decisions to ensure that all new nursing homes are constructed with single-occupancy bedrooms and private bathrooms for most or all residents	1E
Incentives for nursing homes to hire qualified licensed clinical social workers at the M.S.W. or Ph.D. level and advanced practice registered nurses (APRNs) for clinical care, including allowing Medicare billing and reimbursement for these services	2D
Free entry-level training and continuing education for CNAs (paid for by state and federal governments together with nursing homes)	2E
Minimum education and national competency requirements for all staff	2F
Annual continuing education for all nursing home staff	2G
Resources and training to support inclusion of chosen family members as part of caregiving team	2G

Recommendation	Rec
Ongoing diversity and inclusion training for all nursing home staff (including leadership)	2G
Data collection on baseline demographics, training and expertise, and staffing patterns for staff providing direct care	2H
Detailed facility-level data on the finances, operations, and ownership of all individual nursing homes	3A
Study of federal benefit design	4A
Specific percentage of payments designated for direct-care services (including staffing, behavioral health, and clinical care)	4C
Extension of bundled payment initiatives to all conditions	4D
Elimination of certificate-of-need requirements and construction moratoria	5E
Increased weight of staffing measures within five-star composite rating on Care Compare	6B
Identification of pathway to provide financial incentives for certified EHR adoption	7A
Short-Term Implementation (Initiation of Research and Grants)	
Translational research and demonstration projects to identify the most effective nursing home care delivery models • Prioritize models that reduce disparities and strengthen connections to the community • Evaluate innovation in all aspects of care	1B
Research to identify and rigorously test specific minimum and optimum staffing standards for all direct-care staff	2C
Training grants to advance and expand the role of the CNA and develop new models of care delivery that leverage the role of the CNA as a member of the interdisciplinary care team	2E
Research on recruitment, training, and retention of all nursing home workers (particularly CNAs), including gender, ethnicity, and race-related outcomes of job quality indicators	2I
Demonstration projects to explore use of alternative payment models for long-term nursing home care tied to quality metrics	4E
Development and evaluation of strategies to improve quality assurance process	5B
Measures of disparities in nursing home care within and across facilities at national, state, and ownership levels	6D
Development of policies and culturally tailored interventions for disparities	6D
Development of new measures, including • Palliative care and end-of-life care; • Implementation of care plan; • Receipt of care that aligns with resident's goals (and attainment of those goals); • Staff well-being and satisfaction; • Psychosocial and behavioral health; • HIT adoption and interoperability; and • Various structural measures	6C

continued

Recommendation	Rec
Development of new structural measures, including • Health information technology adoption and interoperability; • Percentage of single occupancy rooms; • Emergency preparedness, routine training in infection prevention; • Emergency response management; and • Financial performance; staff employment arrangements (e.g., full-time, part-time, contract and agency staff)	6C, 7B
Development and ongoing implementation of workforce training emphasizing core HIT competencies	7C
Research on use of HIT, existing structural disparities in HIT adoption, and their impact on resident outcomes	7D
Research on innovative HIT applications for resident care and assessment of clinician, resident, and family perceptions of HIT usability	7D
Intermediate-Term Implementation	
Incentives to support innovative, smaller, home-like designs	1E
Consulting or employment relationships with qualified licensed clinical social workers at the M.S.W. or Ph.D. level, APRNs, clinical psychologists, psychiatrists, pharmacists, and others	2D
Career advancement opportunities and peer mentors for CNAs	2E
Pathways for current workers to achieve minimum education and competency requirements	2F
Inclusion of geriatrics content in education programs for all health care professionals	2F
Real-time, readily usable, and searchable database that can evaluate and track quality of care for facilities with common ownership or management company	3B
Assessment of the impact of nursing home real estate ownership models and related-party transactions on quality of care	3B
Refine, expand, and report oversight performance metrics of state survey agencies	5A
Use of existing strategies of enforcement by CMS when states fall short of expected standards (based on performance metrics)	5A
Increased funding for long-term care ombudsman programs	5C
Imposition of oversight and enforcement actions on common owner (based on ability to track quality by owner [Recommendation 3B])	5D
Collection of data for CAHPS measures and reporting on Care Compare	6A
Reporting of quality performance by common owner on Care Compare	6B
Improved validity of Minimum Data Set–based clinical quality measures on Care Compare	6B
Improved differentiation in five-star composite rating	6B
Development of overall health equity strategy for nursing homes	6D
Establishment of state-based technical assistance programs	6E
Minimum Data Set to identify and describe disparities in nursing homes (collected and reported annually)	6D
Measurement of levels of HIT adoption and interoperability and reporting of results in Care Compare	7B

Recommendation	Rec
Long-Term Implementation	
Construction and reconfiguration (renovation) of nursing homes to provide smaller, more home-like environments, and/or smaller units within larger nursing homes	1E
Updated regulatory requirements for staffing standards in nursing homes to reflect completed research on minimum and optimum staffing standards for all direct-care staff	2C
Implementation of state demonstration projects based on study of federal benefit design	4A
Ongoing psychometric testing of CAHPS in nursing homes	6A
Adoption of new measures for reporting on Care Compare (as described under short-term implementation (initiation of research)	6C, 7B
Reporting of new measures of disparities in nursing home care	6D
Identification of thresholds for action on disparities, and promising pathways to reduce or eliminate disparities	6D
Evaluation of state-based technical assistance programs	6E
Measurement and reporting of clinician, resident, and family perceptions of HIT usability	7B